HANDBOOK
FOR
ITINERANT AND RESOURCE TEACHERS
OF
BLIND AND VISUALLY IMPAIRED STUDENTS

BY

Doris M. Willoughby
and
Sharon L. M. Duffy

Developed under the sponsorship of the
National Federation of the Blind
1800 Johnson Street
Baltimore, MD 21230

HANDBOOK FOR ITINERANT AND RESOURCE TEACHERS
OF BLIND AND VISUALLY IMPAIRED STUDENTS
By Doris M. Willoughby
and Sharon L. M. Duffy

1800 Johnson Street
Baltimore, MD 21230

Printed in USA

Library of Congress Cataloging-in-Publication Data

Willoughby, Doris.
Handbook for itinerant and resource teachers of blind and visually impaired students.

Includes bibliographical references.
1. Children, Blind – Education – United States. 2. Visually handicapped children – Education – United States. 3. Children, Blind – United States – Life skills guides – Study and teaching. 4. Visually handicapped children – United States – Life skills guides – Study and teaching. 5. Teachers of the blind – Training of – United States. I. Duffy, Sharon L. M. II. National Federation of the Blind. III. Title.
HV1631.W54 1989 371.91'1 89-12973
ISBN 0-9624122-0-1

TABLE OF CONTENTS

CHAPTER 1

INTRODUCTION: A PERSONAL VIEWPOINT

By

Doris M. Willoughby

When her student needed a fourth-grade English book, Grace Starry devoted 20 hours of her own time to Brailling part of it, and recruited two volunteers to finish. She had no idea that a blind fourth-grade teacher 100 miles away had already had the same text Brailled for her own use, and would have been glad to arrange for a copy.

****

Bob Bruhn, the itinerant teacher, asked the classroom teacher to integrate Kari into the regular reading program. The classroom teacher replied that it would be difficult because Kari was not at the same place as any of the three reading groups. "Surely," countered Mr. Bruhn, "you can work out a way to have another reading group." .... All that year he wondered why the primary teachers were so cool toward him.

****

"We don't know what to do," said the Lincoln County school superintendent. "We have a new first grader who is blind. His parents don't want him to go away to the special school. Might your Braille teacher be able to help us out?"

"We have all the students we can possibly handle," replied the Jefferson County special-education supervisor. "I'm really sorry, but there seems to be a shortage of teachers of blind children. Last spring we had a request from a couple of districts south of us, and we had to turn them down."

****

Loren, a blind tenth-grader, was an excellent student, especially strong in math. When he told the itinerant teacher about his interest in electrical engineering, she said, "I hope you'll also consider computer programming. That's an especially good field for blind students."

****

These three incidents illustrate problems which I hope this book can help prevent.

The Need for This Handbook

Although P.L. 94-142 has brought many new opportunities, it is not working nearly as well as it should. Some aspects of the education of blind children are actually worse than they were 25 years ago.

This *Handbook* analyzes the real causes of problems, and gives appropriate solutions in practical terms. It is intended to be helpful to both new and experienced teachers.

A Personal History

Eleven years of teaching a regular second grade in Cedar Rapids, Iowa, provided valuable experience in general education and in understanding child development. I learned how children act, and what children generally can and cannot do. I found out what it's like to be a busy classroom teacher striving to meet the individual needs of 25 or 30 children all at once. In more than 400 conferences, parents and I talked about children's strengths and weaknesses, and planned for the future.

During most of this time, I had virtually no personal contact with blindness or blind people. I knew that blind children went to schools for the blind, and that some blind adults tuned pianos. That was about all.

Then Curtis Willoughby appeared and began to attend a young adult church group to which I belonged. I noticed his white cane and thought, "Hmm, he must be blind." As he joined us in boating, hiking, and playing checkers, I thought, "Hmm, he's a nice guy." Then he began asking me out on dates, and.......we were married the following June.

As the wife of a blind electrical engineer who is successfully employed, I constantly learn methods for doing things without sight, and ways for handling the misunderstandings of others. I learned long ago that Curt will take responsibility for his own solutions. As he gets out of the car, it is helpful for me to say, "The barber shop is three doors up the hill;" but if I had not said that, he would have found the shop quickly anyway by using various clues and perhaps asking directions. As a wife who is not totally "liberated," I usually sort his shirts for him; but on a business trip he keeps track of them just fine. When a waitress asks me, "Does he want coffee?" I ignore the question and Curt answers for himself.

Curt soon introduced me to the National Federation of the Blind, and I met large numbers of blind people from various walks of life. I was very much impressed with this group, as they worked to solve their own problems.

As a teacher interested in blindness, I gradually became aware of deficiencies in the educational opportunities for blind children. Options which should have been available, easily possible with modern technology and educational principles, too often were not really available at all. Programs that did exist were often staffed too thinly. Even specialized teachers often lacked important skills and knowledge, and the confidence that blind youngsters can get along in life as well as any others. After considerable reflection, I earned the necessary Endorsement on my teaching certificate, and became qualified to teach blind and visually-impaired children.

The National Federation of the Blind works on the real problems of blindness at their roots. My association with the National Federation of the Blind has helped me to take the knowledge and experience I have gained from general education, special courses, and elsewhere, and to work to prevent or overcome the artificial barriers that tend to keep blind children and adults isolated and dependent.

I have had experience as a resource teacher in a regular public school for three years, and as an itinerant teacher for fourteen years, in addition to the eleven years' experience teaching regular classes. In this book I have tried to bring together the philosophy and the practical methods which can help you provide the very best education for blind students today, from infancy through high school.

All anecdotes and examples are drawn from real life. Some depict my own students; others are drawn from the experiences of blind children and adults whom I have met. To preserve the privacy of individuals, fictitious names have been used and circumstances disguised.

Scope and Style

This *Handbook* provides practical, comprehensive, and creative advice about the education of blind students who have varying interests, backgrounds, and abilities. Besides pulling smaller topics together into one place, this book includes many things that other publications tend to leave out.

This *Handbook* emphasizes:

- Consistently high expectations.
- Interrelationships with general education, and with the role of the classroom teacher.
- Analyzing and troubleshooting common problems in the education of the blind.
- Deciding which methods are really best for a particular student, including mode(s) of reading.
- Relationships with all the adults in contact with the blind child.
- Helping the young student become truly ready for the adult world.

This *Handbook* is directed primarily toward teachers specializing in the education of blind and visually impaired children–experienced teachers as well as those in teacher preparation courses. Administrators, paraprofessionals, and others working with blind students will also find this book helpful. Parents will find that reading this book gives them perspective on the educational process, both for themselves and (if necessary) for help in insisting that their child's school behave appropriately.

Although the wording of the text assumes that students are children, most suggestions in this *Handbook* apply to adult students as well.

Often the terms "resource teacher" and "itinerant teacher" are used rather interchangeably, since the basic approach is similar in both settings. Furthermore, most of this book applies to special schools as well as to regular public-school settings.

This book most often discusses techniques which do not require any vision, because these techniques tend to be less well known and understood. However, it is *not* only for use with students who are totally blind or nearly so. If a student is at a disadvantage in using the typical methods and materials for the fully sighted, then this book can be helpful.

Actually, the terms "visually impaired" and "blind" are used more or less interchangeably throughout most of this book. This helps to avoid artificial categorization according to visual acuity, and furthers the goal of choosing the most efficient techniques for each individual.

Books on education are notorious for being "dry," hard to read, and unduly technical. They are also notorious for saying nothing in a great many words, and for rehashing what others have already said. Sharon Duffy and I have made strenuous efforts to avoid these traps. Every sentence in this book is there for a reason.

Almost all of this *Handbook* has been composed directly out of our own personal experience or that of others with whom we are personally acquainted. Almost all is being published here for the first time. Chapters without a specific byline were written mainly by me. Other chapters were written mainly by Sharon Duffy and have her byline. We have reviewed each other's chapters in detail, and often some passages in a given chapter were written by the other author. Each of us has brought her own perspective and strengths. It has been a great pleasure to work with Sharon Duffy in this endeavor; she has very capably provided a perspective which I, as a sighted person, cannot provide.

A few chapters, as noted, were written by other authors who have in-depth knowledge of blindness and blind techniques.

All aspects of the education and life of a visually-impaired student are interrelated, and the chapters of this book are correspondingly interrelated. Headings provide convenience and organization, but they do *not* rigidly categorize and cross-reference specific topics. In other words, this book is designed to be read as a whole, rather than as a series of self-contained topics.

Although this *Handbook* discusses Braille at length, with detailed explanation of teaching methods, it does not actually contain the Braille code itself. Also, as the chapter on "Postsecondary Education and Career Development" explains, the scope of this book only extends to the end of high school.

Companion Publications

I have also written two companion volumes, available from the National Federation of the Blind (NFB). *Your School Includes a Blind Student* is directed toward classroom teachers who do not have special training in the education of the blind. *A Resource Guide for Parents and Educators of Blind Children* is written in a style directed toward parents. However, all three books actually are designed to be helpful to all three groups. Many things have not been repeated here because they have been expressed in the others. I hope you will use all three.

Also, *Future Reflections,* the periodical for parents and educators of blind children, provides continued discussion of current topics. Many other publications are mentioned in the text and listed at the end of this book.

A Matter of Perspective

Usually a parent or teacher sees the child or children clearly, but the image of the future adult remains a distant dream. Most parents and teachers have met very few blind adults. In this book, through my own experience and that of others, I have approached the education of blind children from the other direction, bringing in the clear image of blind adults from all walks of life. What encourages success in adult life? What *is* success? What causes problems, dependency, and failure? I hope to encourage *patterns* of success, and to break vicious circles which encourage failure.

Solving Problems

Let us return to those incidents mentioned at the beginning of this Introduction.

Mrs. Starry had conscientiously arranged ways to obtain materials. But she had not made many contacts outside her community, and was not acquainted with blind adults. As a result she used up tremendous time and effort producing a book which could have been obtained ready-made.

Bob Bruhn was committed to integration of blind children. However, he had little understanding of the problems of managing a large classroom. Consequently he blithely urged (in a rather high-handed tone) "creating another reading group," as though it were a simple matter.

Lincoln and Jefferson counties felt a shortage of teachers. This shortage exists largely because of inappropriate preparation of teachers and poor use of teacher time (as discussed in the chapter "Qualifications for Itinerant and Resource Teachers" in this *Handbook*).

Loren's teacher was acquainted with some blind adults, including two computer programmers. But she failed to realize that her comment encouraged unnecessary stereotyping. The phrase, "a good field for blind students" encourages the incorrect idea of a very restricted list of occupational choices. Also, this teacher was urging a strong student *away* from an appropriate choice and toward something less technical and less challenging.

This *Handbook* discusses the patterns behind problems such as these, and others which are more subtle. Sharon Duffy and I hope that this book will be helpful as you guide your young students toward independent adulthood.

Acknowledgments and Appreciation

I deeply appreciate the help of the many without whom this book could not have been written:

- Sharon Duffy, co-author.
- The other authors and co-authors of portions of this book.
- Jeannette Eyerly, author of *The Seeing Summer* novel. In addition to her gracious permission for the printing of the playlet in the Appendix, Mrs. Eyerly has given valuable advice about this *Handbook* as a whole.
- The many other members and friends of the National Federation of the Blind who contributed important information and examples.

- Educators who contributed technical information and suggestions.
- Our students and their parents (names have been changed and circumstances disguised, of course). As Anna said in *The King and I,* "If you become a teacher, by your pupils you'll be taught."
- My family, who provided perspective and enthusiastic support. Special thanks to my husband Curtis, who programmed the computer and the typesetting, including the illustrations of the abacus.
- Dr. Ralph Bartley and Dr. Jo Thomason, whose complimentary comments appear on the cover of this book.
- The National Federation of the Blind as an organization, with its positive philosophy about blindness, and practical solutions to problems.

CHAPTER 2

INTRODUCTION

By Sharon L. M. Duffy

The Need for This Handbook

As a professional in the field of work with the blind, and as a blind person who grew up taking advantage of both a residential school for the blind and public high school, I am interested in the education of blind children. Therefore, when I was given the opportunity to participate in writing a book on this subject, I accepted with pleasure. I hope that my perspective both as a blind person and as someone who works with the adults that blind children become, will be helpful in the context of this book.

While I worked as a rehabilitation teacher with the Iowa Commission for the Blind, I had the opportunity to work with a number of blind children in cooperation with Doris Willoughby. I also worked with a number of other blind children and their parents, primarily teaching cane travel and Braille. In Idaho, as a counselor for the Commission for the Blind, I attended IEP staffings for high school age students who were, or soon would be, on my rehabilitation caseload.

I have been teaching cane travel to adults for the past four years – first with the Guild for the Blind in Chicago, and currently with the Orientation Center of the New Mexico Commission for the Blind. Many of the adults that I have worked with were blind as children, and might have benefited greatly if a book such as this had been available then.

I hope that this *Handbook* will be of benefit to blind children by providing their teachers with accurate, practical information which will assist in the provision of the best education possible. This book is based on many years of experience dealing with blindness, not as a tragedy, but as a characteristic whose limitations are minimal when appropriate training and opportunity exist.

This book is filled with philosophy about blindness – a philosophy which runs counter to popular myth. Because it is counter to the popular myth, a few paragraphs about philosophy are necessary.

The philosophy that blindness may be reduced to a physical nuisance, and is not an unrelieved tragedy, is held by thousands of blind people; and their happy, productive lives prove the soundness of this approach. The belief that blind people can work along with their sighted peers and achieve just as much is the premise on which this book was written. Without this philosophy the reality is unlikely.

In American educational systems, as currently constituted, it is possible for blind children to compete with their sighted classmates. True, they will need to learn to do some things in a different way, but with appropriate teaching and guidance by the itinerant teacher of the blind or resource room teacher, it can be done. It may be inconvenient to learn additional skills such as Braille or cane travel, but the acquisition of such skills will greatly augment the chances of a blind child achieving a productive, normal life. Without them, a blind person generally *is* doomed to a life of dependence and tragedy.

Much time is devoted in this book to discussing the teaching of skills, but it takes more than skills to build a successful life. All the skills in the world will avail nothing if the individual does not believe in himself. The student who has learned the mechanics of cane travel, but has no faith in himself, will stay home. Therefore, it is important to understand that the teaching of skills will not, all by itself, ensure that a student will use them. A conscious effort must be made to build the student's confidence and belief in himself. Because society is forever influencing how we think, an active program to counteract negative attitudes about blindness must be engaged in by the teacher.

An easy way to start this program is by talking to all school personnel who will have contact with a blind student. Discussions about blindness will clear up many problems. The bus driver who learns that he doesn't have to put up with the misbehavior of a blind child may be teaching that child how to get along in this world, doing the child a favor in the years to come.

The obvious way to teach positive attitudes about blindness is to talk to the child, but it takes more than that. The teacher who talks to a student about how wonderful Braille is and then is overheard telling the parents what a shame it is this child has to learn Braille, defeats his own purpose. The teacher who says blind children should earn their grades like anyone else, and then advocates that they be excused from quizzes because it is easier and not very important, is telling blind children that they really don't have to do everything that others have to do.

So, it is not as simple as a chat with teachers now and then. The itinerant teacher must be aware of all actions in the context of positive attitudes about blind people. Each lesson should aim to build confidence through teaching a combination of skills and positive attitudes about the abilities of the blind. Negative attitudes are so pervasive in society, that despite best efforts, every blind person sells himself short now and then; and a teacher, believing it only reasonable that a blind student cannot do a given activity, may do the same with a student.

The best and most lasting solution to this problem is to get to know and have regular contact with capable adult blind persons, many of whom belong to the National Federation of the Blind. Parents, teachers, and blind students need a tangible reminder of the abilities of the blind to counteract society's picture of the blind as helpless and dependent. The National Federation of the Blind seeks to change attitudes about blindness and bring about equality, security, and opportunity for the blind. This book is dedicated to helping blind youth achieve these goals.

Other Publications

The "References" section of this *Handbook* lists some of the articles which I have written for the *Newsletter* of the National Association to Promote the Use of Braille (NAPUB). I am an officer of NAPUB and strongly support its endeavors.

The magazine *Future Reflections* (for parents and educators of blind children) has published my article, "A Braillewriter in My Pocket," which is reprinted in this *Handbook*.

I have also written a textbook for teaching Braille to blind adults who are in a training center. This textbook is also suitable for high school students. It is called *The McDuffy Reader* and is published and distributed by the National Federation of the Blind. Both the textbook and the Teacher's Guide are available in Braille and in inkprint.

CHAPTER 3

QUALIFICATIONS FOR ITINERANT AND RESOURCE TEACHERS

Everything in your background can be helpful in your work. Any information or skill is likely to be put to use sometime – from skiing to mushroom hunting to chess. It may help in teaching formal lessons, recreational skills, or personal skills. It may build rapport with a classroom teacher or a parent. Whenever you have a chance to learn something new, do it!

If there is an important area (such as industrial arts) in which you have no background, locate someone who can serve as a good resource, and be very positive in your own support. Better still, build yourself a background in the subject.

Everything you know about education will help you as a specialized teacher, very directly. Learn what to expect from each age group; how textbooks are structured; typical classroom procedures; discipline and motivation; methods for teaching various subjects; etc., etc. Principles are the same in teaching blind students. Gain as much actual experience in regular classrooms as possible. Observe some classes (not necessarily those where there are blind students) if you have no background with a particular subject area or age group.

Your course work should include methods and practice in teaching reading to kindergartners and first graders. Teaching a young child *how to read,* whether in Braille or in print, is not at all the same as teaching an older student the Braille code.

Most important of all, everything you know about blindness will influence your work. Meeting thoughtful blind people and thinking through the real meaning of blindness is the most important background of all. Even if you are blind yourself, the perspective of other blind people and of an organized group is vital.

Analyze

Don't fall into the trap of "scratching the surface" by teaching some skills and attacking certain problems, while failing to analyze the basic problems and solutions. A common example is teaching cane travel skills *without* demonstrating their real value and broad application, and *without* talking with the family about increased independence.

Every resource/itinerant teacher should analyze, in depth, the various approaches and philosophies about blindness. If you are not already well-acquainted with the National Federation of the Blind, you may know of only one approach, and differences may not be immediately apparent to you. Everyone, for example, says things like "Mobility is important" and "Blind people can be independent." The real differences show up in actions and in results. The chapters in this book about cane travel and Braille explain the positive approach on these important areas, and give contrast to outmoded approaches. If a person does not consciously study various philosophies, select one, and pursue it assertively, then a person drifts into a vague and ineffective approach.

Certification

Certification requirements vary from state to state. For specific information, contact state Departments of Education, and colleges and universities offering certification. Avoid programs which do not qualify you to teach all grades. Early Childhood certification (for work with infants and preschool-age children) is desirable also, although it is usually possible to share responsibility with an Early Childhood specialist.

THE GENERALIST

Some educators believe that a "general special education" background qualifies a person as a specialized teacher of the blind. This is a most unfortunate assumption. Certainly such a person can handle arrangements for a capable student who already has learned alternative techniques, or for one with a very slight visual impairment. But so can a counselor, a principal, or any other educator. But the beginner in Braille or cane travel must have someone who can actually *teach* these skills.

The "Least Restrictive Environment" provision of P.L. 94-142 (see the chapter on "The Law") is sometimes misinterpreted to justify inappropriate arrangements. This misinterpretation leads to pushing blind students (especially those with some vision) into "regular" materials and methods even when they are inappropriate and inefficient. A shortage of specialized teachers (see below) is often quoted as additional justification.

(Note: In this chapter and throughout this book, unless specifically indicated otherwise, "resource/itinerant teacher" or "specialized teacher" means a person whose *specialty* is blindness. Any educator is qualified to be a "teacher of the blind" in the sense of including blind students, with guidance from a specialized teacher.)

SPECIFIC SKILLS

Every resource or itinerant teacher of blind students should be competent with:

- Grade II Braille
- Nemeth Code (Know the more common signs thoroughly, be able to look up the less common ones easily, and understand general principles)
- Perkins Brailler
- Braille Slate
- Cane travel (at least to the point of crossing streets which have moderate traffic)
- The Cranmer Abacus
- Alternative techniques for daily living skills
- Keyboarding (Typing)
- Alternative techniques and arrangements for Physical Education

In addition, the itinerant/resource teacher of blind students should have at least a general understanding of the following, and know where to find detailed information:

- Industrial Arts
- Home Economics
- Braille Music
- Grade III Braille
- Braille Shorthand
- Optacon
- Adaptation of computers for use by the blind

SPECIFIC KNOWLEDGE

Knowledge of the skill itself (e.g., use of the Cranmer Abacus) is not enough. The resource/itinerant teacher must also know how to *teach* the skill to students of varying ages and abilities, and how to *integrate* the skill into classroom work and into life. The teacher must be able to adapt the materials and methods used in regular classes.

At the same time, the teacher must have the *attitude* that the techniques really do work well, and know how to impart this positive attitude to other adults and to the student.

The resource/itinerant teacher must understand the structure and function of the normal eye, and be knowledgeable about the medical causes of visual impairment.

The teacher also needs to know about "vision stimulation," as the term is commonly used in education today. However, this knowledge should include an understanding of the severe limitations of such programs, and the realization that such efforts are generally counterproductive. "Vision stimulation" is discussed in detail in the chapter on "The Partially-Sighted Child."

MAINTENANCE OF SKILLS AND KNOWLEDGE

Ed Carlson was a top student in his Braille class. However, his first teaching job was in a rural area with a small and far-flung population. There were only two Braille students, and they attended the residential school.

During Mr. Carlson's third year, a seventh-grader returned to the local school. Mr. Carlson eagerly helped her obtain Braille books and begin classes. But when called upon to Braille a test, he suddenly realized that many Braille signs had slipped his memory. Looking them up took time, and the rules of usage proved even more elusive. It took him five hours to transcribe a three-page English test. He shuddered to think about transcribing a math test; his college course had devoted only a brief unit to the Nemeth Code.

He also had heard that a new first-grader would soon move into his area and attend the local school. Where were his notes about materials for beginners?

If your present assignment does not include teaching a particular skill, find a way to keep in practice. Braille, cane travel, and the use of the abacus are particularly vulnerable to being forgotten.

Ask yourself also, "*Why* am I not teaching these skills?" If they are being taught by someone else, as in a special school with many students, the answer is in your job assignment. (Consider, however, whether you might do more to help students use and expand skills.) If you would be the one to teach the skill, carefully consider whether your students are instead using an inferior method–e.g., reading print laboriously instead of learning Braille, or using only the Brailler instead of also the abacus. If they must go to another placement to receive instruction (e.g., commute to a large city), consider whether you are violating P.L. 94-142.

Do not become stale. Keep up with current trends and new information. National Federation of the Blind conventions and meetings provide factual information together with guidance in evaluating and interpreting information.

Common Myths

A number of misconceptions about the education of blind students are, unfortunately, believed by a good many people. These are analyzed below:

(1) *Myth:* My college courses taught me all I need to know about blindness and blind people.
Fact: No one ever reaches *that* level–there is always more to learn. Moreover, unfortunately, often teacher-training institutions actually spread ignorance and misinformation about blindness under the guise of authority. The best source of information about effective ways of dealing with blindness is a consensus of thoughtful blind people whose training and skills allow them to live successful lives.

(2) *Myth:* Many teachers of the visually impaired have no totally blind students, and thus have no need to teach Braille or cane travel.
Fact: You will almost certainly have some students (not necessarily totally blind) who would benefit greatly from Braille and cane travel. But if you *don't know how* to teach it, you probably *won't* teach it.

(3) *Myth:* Orientation and Mobility is an exotic and very difficult field, requiring lengthy training and a very specialized degree.

Fact: Mobility is no more difficult than many other physical skills commonly taught to sighted and blind students. Of course, a person should not teach anything that he/she really knows nothing about. But a relatively short course with the proper attitudes can prepare a person to teach cane travel well. Overly detailed analysis creates problems unnecessarily.

(4) *Myth:* Braille is so complex and difficult that a teacher should not expect to be fluent with it. Students will read very slowly, anyway.
Fact: Braille is no harder than print. Large numbers of people read and write Braille fluently and quickly. Every teacher of blind students should be fluent at least in Grade II Braille and in the more common Nemeth expressions. Otherwise a teacher will hesitate to use Braille, and will hold students back by his/her own lack of confidence.

(5) *Myth:* No special preparation is needed for teaching keyboarding (typing).
Fact: A teacher of the blind should study proper stroking, posture, fingering, timing, etc. If possible, take a regular Methods course in teaching keyboarding. In addition, you should be thoroughly versed in alternative techniques for the blind, including those for tables and other special formats. It is not just a matter of moving your student along through the typing book. To begin with, you must decide *what* book (if any) to use with a particular student, and in what format.

(6) *Myth:* A very thorough knowledge of all the latest technology is vital and should receive great emphasis.
Fact: Certainly one should keep up with developments in one's field. In the education of the blind, however, there is often *over*emphasis on experimental devices, to the neglect of methods of proven worth. Be wary of devoting a great deal of your time to new, expensive devices. Be *extremely* wary of devoting your students' time.

Why Is There a Shortage of Teachers?

There are not enough competent, certified teachers of the visually impaired (especially those who are ready to teach Braille and cane travel well) to serve all the students as they should be served. The shortage varies geographically, but overall it is a serious detriment to appropriate education of blind and visually-impaired students.

To a degree, this problem is a reflection of general circumstances in the teaching profession today – low pay, criticism and complaints, lower public esteem than in the past, etc.

Furthermore, almost all jobs outside of large cities involve travel over a wide area.

The most significant reasons for the shortage of competent teachers of the visually impaired are, however, described below.

INAPPROPRIATE PREPARATION

Teachers of the blind tend to:

- be poorly prepared to teach Braille.
- have a weak knowledge of techniques in areas such as home economics, industrial arts, and science.
- have little background in dealing with public attitudes about blindness.
- have no preparation, or unsuitable preparation, regarding cane travel.

In regard to cane travel – an essential skill – there are two simultaneous problems: (a) Many teachers have no background at all, due to the false belief that lengthy specialized training at a university is required. (b) Other teachers have spent great amounts of time over-analyzing detailed and artificial procedures for mobility, thus learning an unnatural and unrealistic approach.

Details about appropriate teaching of specific skills are found in other chapters of this *Handbook*.

INAPPROPRIATE USE OF TEACHER TIME

Many teachers take too long to phase specialized skills into the regular classroom or life situation. Most Braille students can be integrated into a regular reading group by late second grade, if not before. Even earlier, when the specialized teacher presents new skills, routine practice can proceed with the help of some other adult. Abacus skills can be used in the regular classroom. Cane travel should be continued throughout school and at home, monitored by all teachers and by parents. Typewriting should be applied to some regular assignments as soon as all the letter keys are learned.

Many teachers spend fruitless time trying to "develop" vision which really is not there. It is true that all of the senses of a very young child are in the process of development. Too often, however, this is misinterpreted to justify time-consuming and futile attempts to "develop" vision which is not really there. This raises false hopes. It also lowers the self-esteem of the child who soon realizes that she cannot possibly "do better." Furthermore, valuable time is taken away from learning important alternative techniques.

Lengthy direct help in the use of low-vision aids should not be necessary. If the aid really is appropriate and helpful, the student should quickly learn to use it independently. If the teacher must spend extended amounts of time helping the child use the aid, then either the aid is completely inappropriate, or it should be tried again when the child is older.

Many teachers spend too much time working directly with partially-sighted students.

It is true that consultation, materials, and some direct contact from the itinerant/resource teacher are important for partially-sighted students.

However, most direct work with students who do not use Braille or cane travel is properly done by others:

- For regular classwork, the regular instructor should interact with the visually impaired student as with any other.
- Tutoring, if needed, can be given by a remedial reading teacher, multicategorical resource teacher, etc.
- Help with study skills and general organization can be provided by the counselor, by other regular staff, or by a multicategorical resource teacher.
- If a low-vision aid is used, the doctor should prescribe it and explain its use. The teacher may give some assistance in the school situation. However, if low-vision aids or other reading arrangements really require lengthy, continued specialized attention – then the student should also be learning Braille.

Many teachers try to take too much responsibility for developmental tasks with infants, preschoolers, and severely/profoundly retarded students. (I say "try" because usually they are not really trained in early childhood education and in the education of the retarded, and just do the best they can.) Any competent early-childhood specialist can help a blind child learn to sit up, use silverware, dress herself, etc. – if proper guidance is provided by a specialized teacher of blind children. The same is true with teachers of the severely/profoundly retarded. The special guidance need *not* include regularly scheduled direct work by the teacher of the visually impaired (until relatively formal Braille readiness and cane travel lessons begin around age 4).

Many teachers emphasize poor mobility techniques. Non-cane tactual techniques, such as trailing walls and extending the arms, are easily picked up by toddlers and should soon be discarded in favor of the cane. Human guide techniques, while useful, can easily be learned in a lesson or two. When "Orientation and Mobility" relies on low vision, it is actually a system of codified guesswork – guessing whether a spot is a shadow or a hole, or whether a white expanse is really level. Time spent on these travel methods is time taken away from effective cane use, and leads to slow and ineffective travel.

Most preparation of materials should be done by non-teachers. Brailling books and handouts is an exacting job which requires specialized skill but not a teaching certificate. Enlarging or darkening printed matter requires very little training. Organizing supplies, and checking them in and out, is a clerical job. These tasks should not be a major responsibility of the itinerant or resource teacher. Although the teacher should be a skilled Braillist, and should expect to produce various materials by himself/herself at times, the bulk of the job should be done by others.

TOO-NARROW GEOGRAPHIC AREAS

Time misspent, as above, causes artificial restriction of the teacher's territory. Braille instruction is often scarce outside of large cities-but it need not be scarce if the itinerant/resource teacher's time is used well. Neighboring jurisdictions may formally combine, either totally or for purposes of special education. An intermediate-sized special district may offer services. The residential school may provide outreach. One district may contract with another for part of a teacher's time.

SOLVING THE PROBLEM

This book and its companion volumes (*Your School Includes a Blind Student* and *A Resource Guide for Parents and Educators of Blind Children*) are filled with suggestions which can help alleviate the shortage of teachers of the visually impaired.

The National Federation of the Blind provides a setting in which dedicated and knowledgeable teachers can share ideas and methods. Each year at the banquet of the national convention, the "Distinguished Teacher of Blind Children" award is given.

Conclusion

Unfortunately, it is difficult to find a course of study which is truly adequate preparation for teachers of blind children. University courses tend to spend little time on Braille and almost none on the Nemeth code; to overemphasize cumbersome and expensive gadgets; to offer little experience in the regular classroom; to surround Orientation and Mobility with mystique; to assume that everyone knows how to teach typing; and to act as though blindness were a great tragedy which is severely limiting.

Select the best courses you can find, and supplement them as necessary. Encourage your college or university to strengthen weak areas.

CHAPTER 4

EARLY CHILDHOOD

How Soon Should I Talk with Parents of Infants?

The earlier the better.

Some say that parents must "accept" their child's blindness before they will be ready to discuss education. But what image of blindness are they accepting? They are talking with someone, if they are not talking with you, and that someone probably has much less knowledge of blindness than you do. Even medical personnel often harbor incredible misconceptions. Do everything you can so that, as soon as parents learn a child is blind, they meet competent blind people and receive accurate information. Help them contact a parent support group such as the Parents of Blind Children Division of the National Federation of the Blind.

If you do not have the main responsibility for working with very young children, keep in close touch nevertheless. Arrange to talk to parents occasionally about future schooling; it is good for them to hear it directly from you. Provide tactful consultation for preschool teachers and home teachers who may have limited knowledge about blindness.

If no agency in your area provides organized services for very young children, seek to remedy this. Meanwhile, volunteer your time if necessary to talk with parents at least briefly. Note that P.L. 99-457 expands the provisions for children under school age (see the chapter on "The Law").

Parents usually want very specific suggestions. But it is just as important to provide optimistic, accurate information about blindness in general. If we merely give detailed suggestions on readiness for independent travel, and fail to demonstrate that blind adults can hold good jobs and travel independently anywhere, then perspective will be lacking and efforts will lag.

Describe typical arrangements for elementary school. Invite parents to observe an older child. Introduce them to library services, the adult rehabilitation agency, etc. Provide the book, *A Resource Guide for Parents and Educators of Blind Children.*

GENERAL ADVICE TO PARENTS

Help parents learn, very early, to understand their child's way of reacting and learning. A blind baby, hearing a sound, may become very still while she listens intently–and this means that she is paying attention, not that she is necessarily frightened or resistant. As another example, when a parent picks up a sighted baby, the child is pleased instead of startled, because she saw the parent coming; the equivalent is true of the blind baby when the parent speaks to the child tenderly and does not approach silently.

Help the parents of young infants to think of their child as a normal baby who receives information through different channels, and who may learn things in a different sequence.

This is not at all the same thing as learning more slowly. Yet the parents will often hear or read that "blind children progress more slowly." The chapter, "Working In Partnership With Parents," contains detailed discussion about this unfortunate piece of common misinformation.

One particular blind baby may not learn to eat applesauce with a spoon as quickly and easily as her sighted sister did. It may seem that she does not learn this as quickly because she cannot see whether the food remains on the bowl of the spoon. At the same time, however, she may be delighted to use a fork which picks up the beans and keeps them speared–and may well master the use of a fork *before* the "typical age." All of this is an individual matter, since many blind children master the spoon easily and quickly. Some children, of course, have difficulty with all silverware. Again, it is an individual matter.

Do blind babies smile? Yes, indeed. Gentle tickling around the mouth (as is often done with sighted babies for this same reason) can help to bring a smile.

Working with an Early-Childhood Specialist

In many districts, the teacher of the visually impaired does not provide direct service to very young children. Instead, an early-childhood specialist, who works with many different disabilities, goes to the home or day care setting to work directly with the child.

It is highly desirable that the teacher of the visually impaired work closely with such a specialist, talking frequently, and sometimes making a home visit together. An early-childhood specialist may know little about blindness and inadvertently create problems instead of solving them. On the other hand, he/she may provide valuable background to a teacher who works primarily with older children.

The early-childhood specialist may need advice about adapting tests, lesson plans, and various procedures. You can recommend development guides such as those listed at the end of this chapter. Explain, both generally and specifically, how to adapt methods for various skills.

When tests are being given to assess a child's developmental age, see that they are administered and interpreted fairly. (Example: A typical evaluation item for an infant is, "Recognizes parent by sight." If a child with little or no vision cannot do this, does the evaluator merely score a negative? Or does he/she recognize that the question is inappropriate as worded, and instead observe whether the child can recognize the parent by listening?)

You and the early-childhood specialist should each be well-informed about the other's programs and about options available for each age group.

Concept Development

Much of the material under this heading and under the heading of "Daily Living with the Young Child" is adapted from *A Resource Guide for Parents and Educators of Blind Children*, by Doris M. Willoughby.

LEARNING BY ASSOCIATION

One mother who has raised three blind children to successful adulthood says, "Expect the blind child to learn the same things as any other child, but realize that he may need to be taught differently."

All children learn by association–that is, what goes with what, or what means what. A sighted baby learns about common household activities mainly by watching with her eyes, while a blind baby learns by listening and touching. Janie, for example, sees her father carry the towel to the bathtub, turn on the water, and fill the tub. Kim, who is blind, hears the water running, and is encouraged to feel the towel and to put her hands under the faucet. Janie and Kim can both learn to understand how the bath is prepared, and many months later they can both prepare their own baths. As they learn, however, they do need to get their information in somewhat different ways. Kim needs to feel the towel, touch the faucet, and hold her hand under the running water.

LEARNING BY IMITATION

The little child learns many things by imitation–speech, attitudes, body positions, etc. Some of these, such as speech, are essentially non-visual anyway and will not be substantially different for the blind child. But in matters such as hand coordination, you will need to arrange an alternative to visual imitation. The sighted child *sees* adults using silverware in the conventional way. Soon he is trying to imitate–often getting the food all over himself and the wall, but imitating nevertheless. Gradually his imitation becomes closer and closer to the norm. If the sighted child is reminded, "Hold your fork right," he can look around and see how the others are doing it.

Some schools of thought have stopped at this point, and concluded (wrongly) that the blind child will necessarily do poorly on such things as table manners because he cannot see what others do. We should, instead, provide a way for him to learn. We can help him to observe tactually the motions of others. We can also move his body through the motions as appropriate.

Sometimes, as you feed your infant, guide his hand to help him examine the spoon with his fingers. Help him examine how it is held in your hand, how it enters his mouth, etc. He might keep his hand on the spoon as you move it. Talk to him, too. Even long before he is able to talk, he can begin to understand words.

With this approach, through a series of gradual steps the child begins to feed himself. One day he will probably try to grab the spoon away from you. Gradually, as it is appropriate, take *his* hand and help *him* grasp the spoon to go through the motions of feeding himself.

Many situations are similar to the above, in that the child can easily be helped to observe (tactually) others performing a task, and then can be helped to begin it himself.

(Note: In some situations it is easier to guide the child's motions if the parent sits behind the child. This should only be done occasionally, however. If the parent often sits behind, the child does not learn the normal conversational position of facing the other person.)

MAKING IT MEANINGFUL

Sometimes a certain amount of planning must be done to provide meaningful learning. Suppose, for example, that the child's father boards the commuter train each morning as the family waves good-by. If one child is sighted, she sees the train and gains a reasonable understanding of how her father will travel. If some care is not taken, however, the blind sister will learn nothing except that Dad has left with something noisy called a "train." Examining a small model train may be interesting, but is not very helpful with a preschooler who has no conception of what a real train is like. Instead, arrange for the children to ride along occasionally. If possible, help the blind youngster to examine the outside of a car that is stopped. On the inside, talk to her about the seats, the doors, etc., as she examines them by touch. Walk with her from one car to another. Talk with the engineer. This kind of experience is valuable for the sighted child also, but essential for the blind child.

One need not give up if a particular experience cannot be provided in ideal form. If it is impossible for the children to ride Dad's commuter train, probably they can examine and ride in some rather similar vehicle–perhaps a subway, or at least a bus. When the child has had similar experiences, then comparison can be used: "Daddy's train is like lots of buses all hooked together in a line."

WATCH FOR GAPS

Blind children sometimes have great gaps in their understanding, such as being unsure whether certain buildings have roofs. Watch for things like this, which are seen and perceived by the sighted child but are not reached by the young blind child on his own. Lift him on your shoulders from time to time so that he may touch the ceiling and know it is there. Do this outdoors also, as you point out that there is no roof over him. He will eventually understand anyway, but you can help him learn more quickly and easily.

In teaching your child, at first you will help him become thoroughly familiar with one example, such as one particular train or bus. Move on, however, so that he learns that variety exists. Ride on another train or bus that is quite different. Look around for chances to show him examples of variety in familiar types of things, as well as things which may be totally new to him.

MODELS OR THE REAL THING

Despite all efforts to show him the "real thing," there will be times when models must be used. After all, we probably cannot have him pet a live lion. The most useful models are fairly large and very realistic.

Tiny plastic toys are usually not very meaningful, and may even have inaccuracies such as being hollow on the underside. If such models are encountered, you might say, "This toy zebra is so small that we can't feel the different parts very well. You remember what Uncle Bob's horses look like, don't you? Zebras look a lot like horses, but they always have black and white stripes."

Another situation where touching is impossible occurs with television and other pictures. With an older child, often the regular audio will be enough, and at other times a family member may explain. For the young child, you will often need to provide concrete experiences.

It is vital that a blind child learn to look with his hands skillfully. Explanation and guidance are necessary for a meaningful learning experience. Place the child's hand(s) on the object as you explain, for example, "This is a mailbox. It feels hard. It's made of metal." Help the child move his hands around on the object to look at the whole thing, and explain further: "Now we pull this handle to find the place to put the letter." Gradually teach him to examine things systematically by himself.

RELATIONSHIPS

Point out relationships and position as the child examines a new object or idea. The keyhole is *under* the doorknob; the volume control is the *last* knob on the *right;* we reach up *over* the sink to find the towels; the light switch is *down* when it is off.

VISUAL CONCEPTS

A few concepts are strictly visual – the rainbow, the blue sky, etc. As the child grows old enough that he should know about such things, explain them. Color, for example, might be loosely compared to high- and low-pitched tones. Help your child learn such ordinary associations as blue sky and green grass, so that he does not seem ignorant. In discussing color, try to avoid the two extremes of (1) never discussing it at all, or (2) dwelling on color to an extreme. For example, it is valuable to teach a totally blind five-year-old that his raincoat is blue, because he can then answer the first question that will probably be asked if his coat is lost at school. Also, at Halloween he can easily learn that pumpkins are orange, and this knowledge will be useful throughout life. However, if we tried to teach him the color of each toy he owns, he would quickly become bored – and furthermore, this knowledge would become useless as he outgrows the toys.

Some concepts which may seem entirely visual actually involve other senses as well. A good example is a shadow: the area shielded from the sun is not only darker, but cooler as well.

SOCIALLY ACCEPTABLE BEHAVIOR

As the child approaches school age, the matter of social acceptability becomes important in regard to his ways of learning. On the one hand, we should expect him to continue to examine new objects by touch. Society should accept this as a normal way of learning. On the other hand, there are certain types of touching in which the social disadvantages far outweigh any learning value. An outstanding example is feeling other people. The very young child really does need to feel other people's arms, faces, etc., in order to learn what people are like. However, the school-aged child should be long past this stage. He can become acquainted with others through conversation and through the limited physical contact that is socially acceptable. He does not need to feel faces, legs, feet, etc.

In teaching your child what he should and should not touch, consider the questions, "Does it help him learn?" *vs.* "At his age, is there any substantial disadvantage to his touching?"

Similarly, any child beyond the toddler stage should stop chewing or mouthing objects. Although all babies learn about the world in this manner, the older blind youngster has no more need for this than other children do. He can learn that mouthing toys, furniture, doorknobs, and similar objects is not socially acceptable. Thumbsucking and nailbiting can be dealt with as they would be with a sighted child.

A baby can be helped to learn to hold his head up, as we gently position his head appropriately. To the older child we can say, "We like to see your face," and guide appropriate posture.

Many people tend to allow a blind child to do things which are socially unacceptable, because "the child is blind and doesn't know it looks bad." Blind children can be taught not to do such things as twirling, rocking, jumping up and down, facing the wrong way, making noises, etc. If such habits persist, the child will become an adult who is badly limited by antisocial behavior. Many times I have met a blind adult who is very intelligent but has so many mannerisms and socially inappropriate behaviors that he meets with little success.

GETTING ACQUAINTED WITH THE WORLD

The little child learns through what we call "play." He also learns by imitating the actions of his parents and trying to "work." He learns from the speech and general behavior of adults and children. In short, he learns from all of life.

Arrange to take the child to the dentist's office *before* any uncomfortable work must be done. Let him meet the staff, touch the equipment, and listen to the new sounds. If pain occurs later, it will be easier for the child to accept if he already regards the dentist as a friend and his equipment as interesting.

READINESS FOR READING

Reading readiness is a broad topic which is dealt with specifically in the chapter, "Teaching Braille (Second Grade and Below)."

LEARNING ABOUT BLINDNESS

Give special attention to the concept of blindness itself. The little child will one day realize that others get information in ways he cannot. When he begins to ask about this, explain briefly in words he can understand. You might say, for example, "Yes, most people can see through the window with their eyes. Seeing is sort of like a different kind of hearing–you know you can hear noises through the window. But your eyes don't work. So you use listening and touching instead. Mrs. Gold's eyes don't work either, and she uses listening and touching too."

It is very important to say that blind people use other ways to do things, rather than merely explaining that blind people cannot see.

As the older child grows able to understand more, tell him more. He will need to know what can and cannot be seen by sighted people, so that he does not believe people can see through walls. He will also want an explanation of "what the doctor said." Try to give him the information he wants and needs, without burdening him with too many technicalities. Remember that it is not really kind or helpful to encourage him to expect improved sight when actually it is not likely.

Eventually the child will also raise the philosophical question, "Why did this happen to me?" This book does not presume to answer the ultimate question of why problems exist in the world; each person's individual philosophy of life will answer that. However, this book is dedicated to placing blindness in its proper perspective: it can be reduced to the level of a physical nuisance, if the blind person has the proper training and opportunity in life.

It may help to compare blindness to another physical disability. Imagine, for example, that a child must wear a leg brace, and consider how you would explain that to him.

Consider your tone of voice as well as your words; strive to sound matter-of-fact. An artificial arm, a small income, deafness, lack of musical talent, baldness–all these and many other problems can be mentioned in comparison. Avoid, however, making comparisons to real tragedies such as death–we want to show that this is *not* the category into which blindness falls.

Along with the physical explanation of blindness, the child will need to learn about public attitudes, and learn to educate other people about blindness. To the very young we can say, "Sally looks at her food with her eyes when she eats, so she doesn't know how you do it. Let's show her how you eat your lunch all by yourself." A school-aged child can discuss most of the matters of philosophy included throughout this book.

See also the chapter, "Learning About Blindness, at School and at Home."

Daily Living with the Young Child

EATING SKILLS

As explained earlier in this chapter, help your infant watch how you are feeding him. Encourage him to feel the bottle, spoon, etc., and gradually to take over the feeding job himself.

In helping your child to interpret the world, give consistent indications that food is coming. The sighted baby learns to expect a feeding when he is picked up, the bottle is in sight, the refrigerator is opened, etc. Some of these signs are the same for the blind baby. He may recognize the sound or feel the cold when the refrigerator opens. He can hear the rattle of the dishes. He recognizes his high chair when he is placed in it. Watch for ways to help this process, such as seating him near the refrigerator or the mixing counter. Let him reach inside the refrigerator sometimes. Talk to him about the food. Tell him when you are approaching his mouth with a spoonful.

This book does not go into detail on nutrition, health, or development in general. You will want to consult reliable references on these subjects as you consider what to expect at various ages. For example, it is typical for the one-year-old to develop a smaller appetite as he finishes the growth spurt of infancy; knowledge of this fact can prevent much unhappiness and misguided urging.

If the child seems slow in learning to chew, it may help to offer him more "finger foods," with various interesting textures. Place his hand on your jaw, so that he may observe how you chew. Gently move his jaw for him occasionally. Be gradual about expecting him to do a great deal of chewing, especially with meat. Many children seem "lazy" about chewing at first, but overcome this as they mature.

If learning to chew is delayed past the normal developmental stage, it becomes more and more difficult to learn. The article, "Blind Pre-Schoolers–Some Personal Experiences" (*Future Reflections,* October/November, 1982), deals with this problem.

Increased Independence

When your baby starts to feed himself, encourage him even when he gets berries all over the high chair and the floor. Large bibs and a washable floor covering help parents to survive this messy but necessary stage.

"Finger foods" are the easiest, of course. Soon the baby can also begin to use a spoon. Show him how to hold the spoon right-side up, and be sure that the upper side of the handle feels different from the under side. Move the child's hand through the correct motions. Explain and show how others are feeding themselves, so that the child does not think he is the only one expected to use silverware.

Experiment to see what foods are easiest for him. Use very stable bowls and cups at first, so that they will not slide away or tip over whenever he reaches for them. While he is learning to use silverware, the child will often need to feel with the other hand in order to find the food or the bowl, and to understand the motions involved.

Gradually the child outgrows the need for bibs and baby dishes, and can use regular adult dishes and utensils in the normal manner. He becomes more and more able to eat in a neat and socially acceptable way.

Suggestions for older boys and girls are given in the chapter, "Home Economics and Daily Living Skills."

SLEEP

Many parents of blind children are especially concerned about sleeping habits. It may seem that sleep, especially, is associated with sight, since most people sleep better if the room is fairly dark.

Again, for the blind child it is a matter of making associations which are meaningful. If the child cannot tell light from dark easily, rely on associations that are not visual. All tiny babies simply sleep when they feel like it – in the light, in the dark, in the car, wherever they happen to be when they are sleepy. (They also stay awake when they feel like it!)

As the child grows older, he should gradually be encouraged to sleep in conventional places and at conventional times. There are many non-visual associations which go with sleep – the familiar crib or bed, undressing and putting on night clothes, the bedtime story, being alone in a quiet room, hugging the teddy bear, etc. Emphasizing these kinds of things helps to bring the child into a more mature sleeping schedule. If there is difficulty getting the child to sleep, emphasize some of these things somewhat more, such as a favorite soft toy to share the nap. Also, of course, consult general references about children's sleep. At the same time, try not to let the child become too rigid about his sleep routines, or he may have great difficulty on a trip or with a babysitter. (This is not a problem peculiar to blind children.) Especially avoid making troublesome special arrangements in an effort to help the baby sleep – he can learn to ignore normal household noise, for example.

With sleeping habits, as with other behavior, expect the same level of maturity from a blind child as from any other child.

TOILET TRAINING

Use the same general approach to toilet training as for any child, but emphasize non-visual associations. When you believe the child is ready to learn, take him to the potty when he would normally need to go. Take him there also when he has had an accident – not as a punishment, but to help him associate the function with the place. Encourage him to appreciate the feeling of being dry and clean, so that he will want to stay that way.

If you use a portable potty, keep it in one location, and be sure the child knows how to get there. Be sure that the potty seat is not too similar to some other piece of furniture; help the child to recognize its characteristics. Avoid leaving him on the potty for long periods.

Praise the child when he performs as desired, but try not to shame or scold when he does not. Fear and tension make it harder for him to learn. If you use a child's seat on the regular toilet, provide a foot rest so that the child does not feel that his feet are dangling over an unknown space. If flushing frightens him, delay it until he is out of the room.

In most families, the little child is often in the bathroom when others are using the toilet, and he understands the function through observation. The blind child can do the same, through sound and odor and by noticing where the individual is.

Talk with the child about what he is learning, even if you are not sure he understands all of what you say. Teach him a simple word for each toilet function, preferably a word which everyone will understand. It is helpful for him to wear clothing he can easily pull down by himself.

The child who has just been trained may have difficulty using facilities away from home. At first parents may wish to take along a portable seat or potty. Before long, however, help the child to become used to various toilets so that this problem will not persist.

Before kindergarten, the child should become familiar with all the usual types of facilities and learn to take care of his or her needs independently. A kindergarten teacher expects to help with belts and buttons from time to time, but does not expect to give a great deal of personal help with toileting. The child can learn to use toilet paper, manage various kinds of clothing, etc., without sight.

If the child is a boy, teach him to manage his clothing, including the fly, in the standard manner. Be sure he learns how to stand up to urinate, how to hold up the seat and lid of the stool if they are unstable, and how to use a urinal. If you are a woman with the responsibility of teaching a boy, you can arrange to show him the little boys' bathroom at the elementary school.

Children need to learn that the bodies of boys and girls are different; this matter is discussed further in the chapter, "Dating, Marriage, and the Family." As you teach toilet habits, be sure that the child does not mistakenly believe that he or she should be just like someone of the opposite sex.

If the child seems to learn toilet habits much more slowly than other children, discuss the matter with the doctor and rule out physical problems. Also ask for suggestions from early childhood specialists.

SELF-CARE

The chapter, "Home Economics and Daily Living Skills," contains detailed information on skills for eating, managing clothing, doing housework, etc. Other suggestions appear throughout this book. It is vital for the preschool child to learn self-care and begin to accomplish small chores. Too many enter kindergarten expecting someone else to dress them, feed them, and pick up after them.

SPEECH DEVELOPMENT

In general, blind children learn to talk in the same way and at the same rate as other children. There may even be a bit of extra motivation: a sighted child can point to a cookie jar and demand, "Want dat!" (or even just point and wail), while the blind child must usually say "cookie" to succeed in making the specific request.

However, people sometimes assume that because the child cannot see the lip and tongue movements of others, they will have difficulty with articulation. This does not seem to be the case; listening alone seems adequate for learning to produce sounds.

The *Talk To Me* booklets from The Blind Childrens Center (see "References") provide helpful suggestions for fostering normal development and for dealing with problems if they occur. Following is a brief summary:

- Talk to the child frequently and meaningfully, from his very first days. He needs to hear and understand speech in order to learn speech.
- Help him explore the world, and talk with him about what he is doing.
- When he expresses himself in an immature or incomplete way, respond with a more mature model. For example:
  "Doggie!"
  "Yes, that's our doggie. The doggie feels soft after his bath."
- Avoid constant loud background sounds (e.g., television) which make it hard for the child to converse and to interpret other sounds.
- Although all children repeat words, there can be too much of this. If the older child is perseverating, provide different experiences and speech models to guide him into more variety. Consult a speech therapist if the problem persists.
- Although all children ask many questions, they need to learn perspective. Help children express themselves in ways other than constant questions, and to use different ways to gain information.
- Use the child's name frequently, and use pronouns in the standard manner. Some children misuse pronouns because those around them have also done so, or because the meaning is not made clear.

ORIENTATION AND MOBILITY

The four chapters on orientation and mobility contain detailed suggestions for the very young as well as for the older youngster.

Avoiding Common Traps

FEARS AND AVERSIONS

All children, sighted or blind, sometimes show fears or strong dislikes which seem puzzling to adults. A baby may cry at the sound of the vacuum cleaner. A three-year-old may suddenly refuse to talk to visitors. A six-year-old may declare that he hates first grade because "I have to use that yucky finger paint." A child of any age may cling to familiar ways and express loud dislike for new places and new activities.

Do not assume that blindness has to be the cause, or even a contributing factor. Think what you would do to help a sighted child; the same things will help the blind child as well. Introduce new experiences gradually and pleasantly, with plenty of help and support. Another youngster may be the best "teacher." Whenever possible, help the child to feel that the activity is his idea: for example, if he dislikes handling clay, leave some around so that he can find it and try it on his own.

Don't shame or scold; be supportive and understanding. At the same time, be firm when necessary.

Behavior that looks like fear may actually be a bid for attention, or a way to manipulate others. Whenever Terri was asked to try a new food or a new activity, she would scream. "I can't! It's icky! I hate it!" Soon her parents or grandparents would give in, and to quiet her screams they would provide a favorite food or activity. Terri refused to dress herself, climb on playground equipment, try new foods, walk in the snow, etc. When Terri started preschool, the teachers soon decided to ignore her screams, placing her on a chair in a quiet area if necessary until she calmed down. Whenever Terri behaved cooperatively, the teachers made a point of praising her. One day Terri voluntarily sampled green beans for the first time, and the teachers took this opportunity to invite her parents in for a conference. Terri's parents were eager to extend the school's behavior-management methods into the home. Gradually Terri came to welcome new experiences, and to seek attention through cooperative behavior.

Try to find out why the child is afraid or unhappy. Sometimes an explanation can help remove a child's fear, but this does not always work. All little children have fears which they simply outgrow. Illness and other family problems often bring about fearfulness that may seem unrelated. If you yourself fear a certain thing, or believe that it will be unpleasant, your own feelings will probably "rub off" on the child.

Sometimes the child needs more skill or experience before tackling a new or difficult task. A tragically common example is the blind youngster who is afraid to go anywhere alone because he has not had adequate cane travel training.

Sometimes the best way to deal with a fear or aversion is to wait awhile. If a toddler loudly resists your attempts to teach him to feed himself, it may be best to forget it for several days before trying again. However, do not let important learning be put off indefinitely. If learning a task is put off beyond the usual age range, it will probably become harder and harder to teach it.

If a child is extremely fearful and does not respond to reassurance, seek advice from a psychologist.

PERSEVERATIVE BEHAVIOR

Watch out for overly-repetitive behavior, often called "perseveration." Consider the child's age and general development; emphasize variety and appropriateness of activities.

All babies bang toys together. This is normal, *but* it should pass. Help the child soon to move into more mature ways of playing.

The *Talk To Me* booklets discuss the problem of a child who repeats what others say, to a degree that becomes inappropriate. The child should be exposed to widening experiences and varied speech patterns. An adult should try to respond to his or her apparent feelings and desires, and to suggest what the child might really want to say.

I recall more than one kindergartner who, if permitted, would walk endlessly around a circle of furniture. If we told him to stop but allowed him to remain there, he usually refused to do anything else. Moving the child to another location usually ended the behavior.

A similar problem can arise with toys. One child played with Lincoln Logs as though they were drumsticks, resisting all attempts to teach him to build. He had probably become discouraged when his construction fell apart easily when touched. The Lincoln Logs were put away for possible future use, and a construction set which held together tightly was successfully substituted.

OVERCOMING BAD HABITS

Another blind child refused to play with toy trucks or cars in the standard way. Instead he lay on his back, grasped a pair of wheels, and waved the toy in the air. His parents called this "twiddling," and realized it was most inappropriate for a three-year-old. They solved this problem by permitting the boy to "twiddle" only one of his toy cars. Then they gradually cut down on the time he was allowed to have that particular car.

Sometimes an acceptable habit can be substituted for a more troublesome one. If a girl twists her hair, for example, perhaps she could stroke a plush animal instead.

Feeling other people's faces, feet, etc., is a habit often tolerated because people believe it is unavoidable. But the older toddler can get away from this. Patrick not only felt other people's arms and legs at Preschool-he *licked* them. Despite his parents' objections, somehow the behavior continued. Finally the parents enrolled Patrick in a different preschool, believing that the teachers there would expect better behavior. After a few very firm "no's," this behavior disappeared completely.

PREVENTING PROBLEMS

Problems are minimized by keeping the child busy and active, and not permitting him to stay too long with one thing. Try to have something to do during long waiting periods, such as a long bus ride. Is conversation possible? Can a toy or two be brought along? A sighted child can at least look around, for some degree of amusement. A bored blind child is all too likely to nod his head, poke his eyes, and make strange noises.

The Blind Child in a Preschool Group

Should the child remain at home with some special instruction? Should she attend a special preschool? A regular preschool? How much special help (if any) should she have? A lot depends upon parent preference and the child's maturity, but you should offer advice and some direct help. Extensive suggestions on placement choices appear in the chapter on "Placement Options and Decisions."

WHY ATTEND PRESCHOOL?

Some kind of structured group situation before kindergarten is highly desirable. There are major advantages: (l) Progress and adjustment, in a group outside the home, can be reported to the kindergarten teacher as a precedent; (2) any gaps or weaknesses in the child's progress can be noted and worked on; and (3) the general setting and pacing of being with other children promotes normal expectations.

ADVISING PRESCHOOL TEACHERS

To obtain these advantages it is, of course, necessary to provide proper guidance. Carlotta became more and more unmanageable at preschool. "She won't stay seated," complained the teachers. "She's all over everywhere." Whenever the children were seated for an activity such as Show and Tell, Carlotta would run up to see the items being shown. The teachers, realizing she could not see from her seat, thought it was unreasonable to forbid this. Carlotta expanded this into running anywhere at any time. The consultant recommended the following procedure: Whenever the group was seated, Carlotta was to stay in her appointed place until dismissed. Items on display would be brought over *to her* at the teacher's discretion. This had the built-in consequence that if Carlotta began to move, the item could be withheld from her. The first two days this was tried, it became necessary to remove Carlotta from the room during some of the group sessions. By the third day she was able to remain in her seat with reasonable decorum.

Even if you do not have responsibility for young children who are still at home, you will probably do more when the child enters a preschool. Programming becomes more and more like that of kindergarten and elementary school. Formal reading readiness and beginning cane travel should be started before kindergarten.

When problems occur in elementary or secondary school, it should be a last resort to suggest a change of teachers. With a preschool child, however, a change of teachers is a more common option. After all, sighted children often change preschools. Since most preschools are private, we do not always have enough leverage to insist on appropriate programs. Look at all the options.

WHEN TO BEGIN?

When is a child mature and independent enough for a group setting? Since the advantages are so great in paving the way for kindergarten, every effort should be made to arrange group experiences for the year just before school entrance. Before that, it is a matter of individual maturity and opportunity. If a child does not seem mature enough for a regular preschool, a special preschool for the handicapped may be a good choice.

If a child seems immature, recognize that going to preschool may nevertheless be exactly what she needs. If a child, in the opposite extreme, seems exceptionally mature, do not assume she does not need a preschool experience. Some problems and weaknesses will probably show up in a group situation. And the kindergarten teacher will be much more convinced of the child's maturity if it has been demonstrated in a group setting.

WHERE TO GO?

Where can a suitable preschool be found? Must the parent be able to pay a substantial fee?

P.L. 99-457 provides many new opportunities for preschool children with disabilities. (See the chapter, "The Law and the Blind Child's Education.") Preschools supported by the public schools are becoming more available. "Headstart" classes are excellent: most of the children are non-handicapped; fees are not a problem; and regulations require the inclusion of some handicapped children. Residential schools often have preschool programs, although it is necessary to weigh the disadvantages of staying away from home overnight.

If a private preschool is desirable but the parent cannot pay, perhaps a subsidy can be provided by a private group. Many churches and service clubs offer "scholarships." Seek out a Lions Club, Delta Gamma sorority, or other organization with special interest in blind children.

Attending a *regular* preschool, whether public or private, is highly desirable in setting a precedent for regular kindergarten. When a preschool for the handicapped is attended, the kindergarten teacher is likely to say later, "That was a special situation set up for handicapped children. Just because she got along there doesn't mean she can get along in our program." Because of this, it is often desirable to attend a special preschool one year, and then a regular preschool the next.

Conclusion

Many topics relevant to early childhood are covered in great detail elsewhere in this book. The sections on Braille and cane travel, particularly, discuss development from infancy and will not be repeated here. Evaluating what a child can and cannot see is discussed under

"Assessment of Functional Vision" and elsewhere.

The young child is learning and developing in every way. Emphasize every aspect of development–hand dexterity, concept development, listening skills, everything. Although any remaining sight should be included in this encouragement, avoid an approach in which sight is overemphasized to the detriment of other skills which may in time be more useful and more important.

References

Following is a brief listing of some particularly helpful references. More complete information may be found at the end of this book.

Publications:

A Resource Guide for Parents and Educators of Blind Children
Talk To Me (two booklets)
Get A Wiggle On
Move It!!!
The Oregon Project for Visually Impaired and Blind Preschool Children
Just Enough to Know Better
Future Reflections magazine
The Blind Child in the Regular Preschool Program

Organizations and Agencies:

Parents of Blind Children, National Federation of the Blind
Blind Children's Fund (Also known as Institute for the Visually Impaired 0-7)
The Hadley School for the Blind (Offers correspondence courses for parents of blind children)

CHAPTER 5

DEALING WITH MEDICAL MATTERS

(*Note: Characteristics of particular eye conditions are discussed in the chapter, "The Partially-Sighted Child." Other references are listed at the end of this chapter.*)

"Why are you making such a fuss over getting a doctor's statement?" demanded the principal. "We can all see that Terri has a visual impairment! If we had a kid with one leg, would you insist on a doctor's statement each and every year certifying that the leg was still gone?"

"If a child has artificial eyes," replied the teacher from Educational Services, "you do have a situation like having one leg. But usually we have to assume that the eye condition will change from time to time, and that's why our department insists on having *recent* medical statements."

An Inappropriate Placement

This teacher found herself in a very unpleasant situation. She was being asked to ignore a variety of regulations and to condone an arrangement she had not recommended. Gradually she unraveled the problem which was bringing on such sarcastic questions:

(1) Six years before, when Terri was in kindergarten, Educational Services had been called for consultation. A doctor's statement–fairly current at that time–indicated an eye inflammation of unknown origin. Acuity was given as 20/30 in the better eye, 20/200 in the poorer eye; visual field was not indicated. No special services for the visually impaired were recommended, because the child appeared to see regular materials well, and because the medical report did not clearly indicate an educationally significant visual impairment. Continued medical evaluation was recommended.

(2) In second grade, Terri had more and more trouble with reading. Ultimately she was placed part-time in a Learning Disabilities room.

(3) When Terri entered fifth grade, the state regulations on Learning Disabilities were tightened, and Terri no longer qualified for the remedial room. A quick staffing was held, and she was reclassified as "visually impaired." However, no new doctor's statement was obtained. No teacher of the visually impaired was involved. No large print or other materials for the visually impaired were requested, since the print size had no effect on Terri's difficulties in sounding out words and comprehending meaning.

Preventing Inappropriate Placement

This was an extreme case, but parts of this pattern are seen more frequently than one might think. Laws and regulations require an up-to-date medical statement for three basic reasons:

(1) to provide information on the nature and extent of the disability.

(2) to qualify the student for services which are justified on the basis of disability.

(3) to ensure that the medical condition is being treated or corrected as much as possible.

Terri's principal and others were rightly concerned that she might "fall through the cracks" and lose all help with her academic problems. The remedy, however, is not to ignore all the regulations and sneak her in anyway, regardless of the true cause(s) of her problems.

Information from Terri's doctor showed that the eye inflammation had cleared up long ago, and that her good eye was now entirely normal. This and other information showed that her learning problem was *not* due to a visual impairment.

However, in other cases which might seem similar, the child may indeed qualify as visually impaired. For example, Pete's corrected visual acuity was given as 20/30. However, he had a substantially restricted field, was losing vision over time, and missed a great deal of school due to eye operations and other treatment. Pete did qualify as visually impaired.

The Doctor's Report Form

Try to ensure that when the doctor's statement arrives, it includes the information you need:

- Student's name, address, and birth date.
- Date of report.
- Date of last examination.
- Diagnosis and etiology (nature and cause of the condition).
- Prognosis (prediction of future condition).
- Visual acuity figures, with and without correction, for distance vision *and* for near vision – right eye, left eye, and together.
- Visual field.
- Instructions as to when lenses should be worn. (All the time? If not, when?)
- Instructions for the student's use of low-vision aids, if any – including information on near and far visual acuity, and on the field of vision.
- Recommendations, if any, regarding activities or environmental conditions which would harm the eyes.
- Physician's signature, printed name, and address.

It is helpful to provide a printed form which asks concisely for all this information, and which requires a parent's signature authorizing release of information to the school. If individualized questions need to be asked, they can be written onto the form or an added sheet – this is preferable to trying to make the basic form too detailed.

Emphasize the importance of reporting the near-vision acuity and the visual field. All too often these are omitted although they are extremely relevant to education.

Medicine vs. Education

Marty Novak was failing third grade. Even with his face almost touching the pages of a large-print book, he read so slowly that he only completed half of his assignments, and made many errors. Finally everyone agreed that Braille (along with some use of large print and tapes) would be best for Marty.

While studying Braille and receiving some individual help, Marty moved on into fourth grade and things got better. He learned Braille quickly and soon found that, despite his initial objections, he could already read faster and more easily in Braille than in print. His grades rose, and a timetable was set for him to start completing all of the same assignments as the others.

In February Mrs. Novak called the Braille teacher, nearly in tears. "What shall I do?" she cried. "We all thought that Braille would help Marty, and he's doing so much better. But the eye doctor says he can't have it! We just went in for a checkup, and Marty was practicing his Braille in the waiting room. The doctor was very upset. And he wrote a note saying that Marty should use large print in school. Now I don't know what to think!"

DOCTORS ARE NOT EDUCATORS

Why does this kind of thing happen? There are several reasons:

(1) *The doctor's evaluation was very short, and in a limited situation.* Using his standard chart, he observed that Marty could see print of a certain size, and thought, "Why should this child use Braille?"

Parents and educators, on the other hand, saw the child struggle day after day with long pages of print, and came to feel that Braille would be very helpful.

The doctor's test had a few isolated letters; provided no need to read quickly at a glance; was set at 20 feet; was quite short; and had some potential for memorization or guessing. Classroom materials, however, have long sentences and paragraphs closely spaced; require quick and efficient reading; are used at close range; are very long and get longer in the higher grades; and are not subject to memorizing or guessing.

An educator who sees a student only occasionally may fall into this same trap. Asking a student to read a short passage for "educational evaluation" is only a small sample. The student's total functioning over the long term should be carefully considered.

(2) *Visual acuity itself varies.* It varies for all of us, actually, although with good vision we usually don't notice. Acuity may decrease considerably as the child grows tired, if he is not feeling well, etc.

(3) *Acuity only partially reflects other problems* which interfere with the use of vision. Nystagmus, for instance, causes letters to seem to "jiggle" and blend together, especially if they are closely spaced. A field restriction may make it impossible to see even a whole word at one time.

(4) *Doctors tend to keep hoping for improvement* in vision, even when results show a clearer and clearer trend of decline. They may be less than candid about the real likelihood of improvement.

(5) *Some eye doctors seem to view a blind patient as an indication of their own failure,* and react defensively and emotionally. They may show this by resisting helpful educational measures. They may feel threatened by the presence of Braille in the waiting room.

(6) *The traditional role of doctors has placed them on a pedestal.* This view has encouraged both doctor and patient to expect the doctor to be knowledgeable about *everything,* and to see a medical component in anything the doctor says. It makes it hard to separate the educational aspects from the medical aspects of planning for a child's future.

(7) *Doctors can be subject to the common misconceptions* about blindness, since they are human and a part of the population as a whole.

EDUCATORS ARE NOT DOCTORS

Educators, in turn, must avoid the equivalent problem: practicing medicine without a license. To recommend a particular operation, medication, etc., is generally not appropriate for a teacher. At most, one might say, "I understand that [a certain treatment] is sometimes helpful. I suggest you ask your doctor about it." The school nurse may be able to be still more direct.

In fairness to doctors, it should also be emphasized that the reverse of Marty's problem occurs at times. Many times an eye doctor has spoken candidly about poor vision, and made excellent suggestions related to education–but educators or the parents have resisted due to ignorance, misconceptions, or fear of stigma.

COORDINATING EDUCATION AND MEDICINE

What Can Parents Do?

They can distinguish between medical matters and educational matters. On several previous occasions the Novaks had asked the doctor's advice about reading material, and he had always suggested large print. It would have been better for them merely to ask the doctor for a written medical report and say, "Thank you. This will help us to work with the school in planning his education." If a doctor volunteers an opinion about school programming, the wise parent will analyze how much is an actual medical statement, and how much is a personal opinion about education. They will also insist that the doctor not confuse a young child by criticizing the school when the young patient is listening. (We teachers owe the doctor the same courtesy, and should hold controversial discussions with the parent alone unless the student is mature enough to participate.)

They can ask careful questions to determine exactly what the doctor means. If a medical consideration actually is involved, is the doctor making a mild suggestion or a firm and specific statement? Exactly what is recommended, under what circumstances? If there seems to be a conflict, might there be a compromise, experimentation, or a completely different approach that will be acceptable to all parties?

They can insist that the doctor be frank even if the prognosis is unfavorable. The Novaks were fortunate in that their doctor had always said frankly that Marty's vision would slowly decline throughout life. Some doctors withhold such information on the belief that patients (or parents) will not be able to handle the news, or that they need not be faced with it until later.

It is far more helpful and kind to be frank, so that intelligent planning can be done. This is discussed in the following publications. (See "References.")

Suggested publications:

When Your Best Efforts Fail: Open Letter to Eye Specialists

Blindness and Disorders of the Eye

If an operation or other treatment is suggested, parents should insist on candid analysis of the probable results, and weigh the relative merits carefully. Sometimes a possible treatment is very uncomfortable, but will probably produce only a small or temporary improvement in vision, or even nothing more than a slight delay in loss of vision.

They can weigh each medical statement, and realize that they – the parents – are ultimately responsible for decisions. At times, getting a second medical opinion or changing doctors is a wise decision. But a tragically common and very unwise pattern is to "shop around" in a frantic attempt to find someone who will say that sight might be restored. This pattern encourages questionable treatments and approaches.

What Can a Teacher Do?

Help everyone distinguish between medical and educational considerations. The teacher can say, "This is a complex problem, with a medical aspect and an educational aspect. Let's analyze what we have on each aspect, and see what we can work out."

Conduct a careful evaluation of functional vision, from an educational standpoint. An educator should not attempt a medical evaluation; however, it is appropriate and essential to examine practical visual functioning in a normal setting over a period of time. This evaluation is discussed in detail in the chapter, "Assessment of Functional Vision for Reading."

Set a time for relaxed discussion. Arrange for a time and place where careful and reasoned analysis will be possible. It may be wise to include other parties, such as the nurse or principal.

Find out what the doctor really said. Try to reach the doctor by telephone if written reports are unclear or insufficient. If everyone seeks with good humor to find out what the other parties actually meant, major misunderstandings are usually prevented. Be humble enough to recognize that someone else may know something that you don't. Enlist the help of the school nurse, who should be an excellent intermediary.

Explain your suggestions carefully, and try to demonstrate that they do not really conflict with the doctor's medical recommendations. Talk with the parent about how he or she can handle a doctor's apparent disagreement with educators. Explain how the medical test is quite a different situation from that of schoolwork, and how issues may have both a medical aspect and an educational aspect.

In case of a serious disagreement, handle it professionally. If the parent tends to agree with you but is worried about the doctor's comments, suggest firm insistence on separation between medicine and education, and/or getting a second opinion. If the parent strongly disagrees with your ideas, it becomes a matter of handling such disagreements in a professional and appropriate way, as discussed elsewhere in this book. Avoid acting as though everyone who disagrees with you is either stupid or uncaring.

Helping the Family Choose a Doctor

Should you, if asked, recommend the name of a particular eye doctor? It is better to suggest asking the family doctor or pediatrician for a name; refer the question to the school nurse; and/or mention several doctors' names rather than just one.

Try to have names of doctors accustomed to testing children, especially if the child is very young or multiply handicapped. Some eye doctors seem to give up easily, and regularly write "too young to test" instead of a specific statement. If a child has normal communication skills, an acuity figure should be obtainable at least by age three. The National Society to Prevent Blindness offers a practice kit which explains the "E" chart used with those unable to read. With patience and with toys and other aids, it is often possible to be specific even with the very young and those with special problems.

Aids and Devices

Classroom teachers will expect you to advise about the practical management of contact lenses, low-vision aids, artificial eyes, and other devices. The itinerant or resource teacher should work with the nurse on such matters, but should have general knowledge about them. Insist that the parent or doctor provide specific directions for any prescribed aids.

Artificial eyes: My husband, who attended a residential school for the blind, tells how certain other students delighted in taking out their artificial eyes and passing them around to create excitement. This is *not* recommended! However, it is not a disaster if an artificial eye comes out. Find out how it should be cleansed and replaced.

Poorly-fitting glasses: Recently a kindergarten teacher asked if I would petition the Lions Club to get better frames for a child's glasses. They didn't fit right, she said – kept sliding off the child's nose. But the glasses were quite new, and the parents couldn't afford to buy a new pair so soon. I suggested we try other ideas before going to the Lions. The school nurse had excellent advice: (1) the parents should take the glasses back to the optician who fitted them, since he or she should be willing to alter them without charge if they really do not fit; (2) discuss the problem with the doctor who prescribed the glasses; (3) consider simple, inexpensive pads or other aids to provide cushioning and a better fit. These ideas solved the problem well.

Low-Vision Aids are generally defined as devices beyond ordinary glasses or contact lenses. Judicious use of such aids can be very helpful to some persons, both in school and in life in general. Often, however – especially with children – the aid is so cumbersome as to create problems rather than solving them.

A Year Lost

Francie had no serious trouble seeing the print used in kindergarten, but the crowded pages of the first-grade readers were a problem. The resource teacher suggested Braille, pointing out that the print would get more crowded as the work advanced. However, Francie's parents consulted a low-vision clinic and returned with a high-powered lens which attached to her eyeglasses. Each time the group began to read close work, Francie would take out her device, cover her left eye with a patch (to prevent double vision), and focus the special device. By the time all this was arranged, the group usually had finished most of the lesson. If the next activity involved distance vision (as it often did in first grade), Francie had to put everything back. The classroom teacher was distraught, trying to help Francie keep up, but the parents insisted the aid be used.

After several months, Francie's parents agreed the low-vision aid was not practical for so young a child. But by this time Francie was far behind educationally. After a second year of struggle, using large print without any special aids, she repeated second grade and began learning Braille. The low-vision clinic, however, continued to recommend this same aid for children as young as five.

The chapter on "The Partially-Sighted Child" discusses the problem of overemphasis on low-vision aids and "vision stimulation."

Advantages and disadvantages of low-vision aids are also discussed elsewhere in this book, particularly in the chapters about Braille and other modes of reading.

Interpreting "Doctor's Orders"

Interpreting a doctor's restrictions on physical activity is a touchy matter. There are two opposite dangers.

The first danger is that some activity will unwisely be permitted, causing physical harm.

The second danger, which often is more likely, is that the child will be restricted much more than is necessary or wise.

Alice had no sight in her left eye and partial sight in the right eye. When she entered junior high, the doctor's statement read, "Avoid blows to the head." The physical education teacher wondered whether Alice should be included in regular classes at all; in nearly any activity, it is conceivable that a student might receive a bump. Alice's mother was consulted, and she too was worried; she began to wonder whether Alice should be allowed to play active games at home, or even to walk to school. What would happen if she tripped or slipped?

The school nurse telephoned Alice's doctor. Then the nurse arranged a conference with Alice, her parents, and the gym teacher. She reported that the doctor had meant avoiding contact sports like football and wrestling, and certain other activities where blows to the head are *really likely.* "Sometimes we should arrange for Alice to go to another gym class," continued the nurse, "or to work alone on something like the bicycle exerciser. It is important that she gets the physical activity and doesn't just sit out. I'll go over the gym schedule and we'll talk about which things are a problem. I think we all need to be careful not to worry too much. If Alice were to avoid all normal activity, that would be just as bad a threat to her health as is the threat of possible eye damage from a sharp blow."

Thus, discussion and questioning saved Alice from severe restrictions which were unnecessary.

Medical Misinformation

From time to time you will encounter misconceptions about medical matters, and should tactfully try to correct them. The ones which I have encountered most often are:

(1) "If he reads in that light, he'll ruin his eyes." – It was indeed believed in the past that poor lighting, or lengthy close work, could be the direct cause of permanent visual impairment. However, it has been learned that such things only cause temporary tiredness, not permanent harm. Moreover, with some eye conditions it is easier to see with less light.

(2) "He shouldn't hold the book so close." –The child should hold the book in whatever position he finds most comfortable. Bringing the material close to the eyes will not cause harm (although again, it was once believed that it would), and will provide the equivalent of magnification. The further question of whether it is *efficient* for a given child to read print rather than Braille is an *educational* question, not a medical one, and is discussed elsewhere.

(3) "This child has only one eye, and so he must be visually impaired. He can only see half as much as the rest of us." –Actually, the loss of one eye leaves approximately 75-80% of the visual field intact, because the fields of the two eyes overlap. Although binocular depth perception is gone, a person can learn to perceive depth by other means, such as noting apparent size and relative position. Therefore, if the other eye is normal the youngster would not need educational services for the visually impaired, although consultation might be helpful temporarily. (And of course, anyone losing one eye should receive the very best in medical care *immediately*, to prevent the loss of the other eye through sympathetic ophthalmia.)

(4) "He'll see better when he gets older, won't he?" –This is a question I sometimes hear from younger children in talking about a blind child. They are told that they will read better, grow stronger, etc., as they get older, so they sometimes assume that better vision can be learned! I explain that blindness will continue, and that "high school books and grown-ups' books come in Braille too."

(5) "His vision is 2200."–More than once I have seen this written into a child's school records. The first time, it remained a mysterious notation with which I was not familiar. The second time I found 2200, I also found it written elsewhere for the same child as 20/200. The light dawned. If you dictate that aloud to someone not familiar with visual acuity notation..."twenty-two-hundred"...... Yes, indeed.

What Is the Real Cause?

KELLY'S EXCUSES

Kelly's grades were dropping slowly, and absences were becoming more frequent. When she missed two entire weeks, the itinerant teacher arranged a conference with the junior high principal and the parents.

"You're accusing Kelly of truancy!" cried Kelly's mother. "What's the matter? I am aware of her absences and I have always written a note excusing her."

"We know that," replied the principal. "But Kelly has been absent almost one-fifth of the time, and her grades are dropping. When this happens–even if it is due to health or other unavoidable reasons–we must examine the problem carefully."

Discussion showed that absences were correlated with musical activities. Kelly sang solos and performed with a Country-Western band. Before a performance, explained her mother, she was so intent on practicing that it was hard for her to get to school; and after a concert she was exhausted and needed extra sleep.

The teachers said that this pattern overemphasized one facet of life–however desirable–while increasingly harming Kelly's general education. The parents promised to help Kelly improve her school attendance.

After five weeks of good attendance, Kelly was again absent for several days. She returned with a note stating she had mononucleosis and should be excused from physical education and the math homework. It also explained that she would often be absent on Fridays due to tiredness at the end of the week.

Mr. Wallace, the itinerant teacher, knew that Kelly disliked physical education, math, and the Friday morning spelling tests. He also knew that solos and concerts usually were on weekends.

"May I see the doctor's statement about mononucleosis?" he asked.

"Well, we don't actually have one from the doctor yet," replied the nurse. "I've been asking for one. Kelly's mother says that she seems to have all the symptoms, and that they did talk to the doctor. But, yes, we must get a doctor's statement–for general medical reasons, and also because they are asking for changes in her school schedule."

Several weeks later, with Kelly's attendance averaging 60%, a conference was convened. The doctor had not actually diagnosed mononucleosis, admitted the parents; they had talked to him on the phone and speculated, but he had not examined Kelly. Whatever it was, Kelly was becoming more and more wrapped up in music, and less and less interested in school. "She plans to be a professional musician anyway," commented her father. "Why are you so upset? She's not actually failing her classes."

Some sighted students follow patterns similar to this one–spending so much time and energy on various outside pursuits that school suffers tremendously. Some parents go along with this and write excuses with questionable truthfulness.

With Kelly's family, the problem was intensified by these common but erroneous assumptions:

(1) Generally, blind persons cannot compete on the basis of equality.

(2) There are very few areas in which blind people may do well, and music is the main one.

(3) If a blind person finds success in one endeavor she should cling to it at all costs because it will probably be her only chance.

A Matter Of Perspective

After making some progress on the problem through the conference, Mr. Wallace contacted the National Federation of the Blind. Without revealing Kelly's immediate problem (due to confidentiality), he asked to meet some blind adults who might be role models for a blind youngster. It would be helpful, he explained, if they were interested in music, as the student was; but most of all he wanted to show that the blind could succeed in many fields of employment. A blind typist who sang in her church choir, and a blind lawyer who played the violin, responded. These and others became acquainted with Kelly and her family.

As the months went by, Kelly began to learn to schedule musical engagements to accommodate her other responsibilities. She began to understand the advice given by the counselor: "Don't limit yourself, at your age, by assuming that music will be your entire life. It may turn out to be a full career, or a sideline, or a hobby. Keep the doors open to many possible opportunities!"

Before the next IEP review, Kelly's school grades and attendance became acceptable.

WATCH FOR HIDDEN PROBLEMS

It is always important to rule out physical causes for problems.

Christie was totally blind and had done well in kindergarten except for sometimes giving silly answers. Hearing tests had been inconclusive, apparently due to the child's poor coöperation. But early in first grade, the audiologist said he finally had achieved a test that seemed valid–and it showed a very significant hearing loss.

The ear specialist recommended immediate fitting with hearing aids. However, the teachers resisted strongly, saying that Christie was doing well, had no speech impairment, and conversed normally. They said that hearing aids might confuse the child's already excellent ability to localize sounds.

The parents, however, went ahead and ordered the hearing aids on a trial basis. They conveyed the school's concern about localization of sounds, and aids were fitted to emphasize hearing with both ears. At first the teachers were relieved that Christie did not seem confused, but annoyed that there seemed to be no real benefit. Gradually, however, the child's previously good achievement grew even better, and it became apparent that she had *not* been hearing nearly as well as everyone had thought. As an intelligent and eager blind child, she had used the hearing she had to the "Nth" degree and succeeded in spite of substantial impairment. When she had been unable to understand, she covered up by silly responses.

Later Christie's mother commented, "I felt from the first day that the aids were going to help a lot. When she came home with the first trial aids, she said, 'Mom! Now I can hear my feet walking!'"

CONSIDER ALL ASPECTS

For both Kelly and Christie, once the real problem was recognized, the focus of action became clear. Kelly and her family needed to learn positive attitudes about blindness, and to keep music in perspective. Christie needed the best possible aids and arrangements to maximize her hearing. Sometimes, of course, a child's problems are so many and complex that even a general course of action is hard to plan. Bill, for instance, is a blind child who has epilepsy that is hard to control, and also has severe asthma. Helping him gain independence is very difficult because stress tends to bring on an asthma attack and/or a seizure. All of this has led to emotional problems. Deciding how much to expect of Bill is very complex indeed.

The "team approach" is essential for determining what problems and disabilities actually exist, and for dealing with multiple problems. Whenever a visually impaired student has another physical problem, it is essential that four aspects be addressed:

(1) *Medical* recommendations regarding the eyes

(2) *Educational* planning to accommodate the visual impairment

(3) *Medical* recommendations regarding the other physical problem(s)

(4) *Educational* planning to accommodate the other problem(s)

Too often it is assumed that the teacher of the blind is also knowledgeable about cerebral palsy; that the physician knows exactly what is needed in the classroom in all respects; that the educator is also a medical specialist; etc., etc.

A suitable team (including the parents) then must examine a fifth aspect: planning an appropriate course of action which takes all the problems into account, sets priorities, and handles conflicting needs.

References

The chapter in this book on "The Partially-Sighted Child" describes several specific eye conditions. See also the "References" section at the end of the book. Additional sources of information include the following:

- *Blindness and Disorders of the Eye,* from the National Federation of the Blind
- Materials from the National Society to Prevent Blindness
- Textbooks on ophthalmology
- Medical dictionaries

CHAPTER 6

PARTIAL SIGHT AND BLINDNESS

Introduction

Contrary to common belief, there is no simple division between "sighted people," who presumably can see perfectly, and "blind people," who presumably cannot see at all. There is not even a simple and obvious division between the "mostly sighted" (presumably relying on vision successfully at all times, though perhaps using magnification), and the "blind" (presumably seeing very little).

Moreover, the variations of physical vision, however complicated, are far overshadowed by the complexity and importance of *attitudes:* attitudes which determine the way a person deals with the ability or inability to see things accurately and reliably.

These complex subjects are discussed throughout this book, but the following four chapters explore them in particular detail:

"Learning About Blindness, at School and at Home" By Doris M. Willoughby
"The Partially-Sighted Child" By Sharon L. M. Duffy and Doris M. Willoughby
"Explaining the Idea of Sight and Partial Sight" By Doris M. Willoughby
"Sleepshades" By Sharon L. M. Duffy

CHAPTER 7

LEARNING ABOUT BLINDNESS: AT SCHOOL AND AT HOME

Carlotta's Problem

"Carlotta just doesn't seem interested in group activities," lamented the first-grade teacher. "We went outside and built two snowmen. Everybody was busy but Carlotta. She disappeared and we found her back in the classroom, just sitting."

Carlotta's classmates and teachers, having been cautioned that they hovered over her and gave too much help, had resolved to let her be independent. She could see where the groups were. She could feel the snow. Surely this project would go well. Yet she disappeared and sat forlornly in the classroom. Why?

As usual, there are the proverbial two extremes. Classmates and teachers may overprotect, or they may give too little help. They may misjudge the complexity of special aids and devices. The concept of partial sight seems particularly hard to grasp.

"Carlotta is still a bit shy," said the itinerant teacher the next day. "Possibly something frightened her. But next time I'd suggest a little more guidance. She could see the groups, I'm sure, but probably not well enough to tell exactly what they were doing. If she had started rolling a snowball or whatever, she could have done it easily by touch, and probably could have used her sight as well – although her sight wouldn't have been as useful as one might think since glare bothers her. But, you see, a sighted student could just look around and say to herself, 'Those two kids are rolling a really big snowball. I'll help them.' Carlotta couldn't see what was needed. And she's still to shy to ask. So, feeling bewildered, she wandered off to the security of her desk inside.... It's hard to know just how much help to give, and it won't always work out exactly right. But next time, someone could show her where to work, and explain what's needed, and then she'd probably be OK."

Direct guidance like this is often necessary. The resource/itinerant teacher should sometimes go along on a field trip, sit in on a reading group, etc., to show how to give the right kind and amount of help. Similarly, an adult may join into games and other informal activities, showing how a blind classmate can be included. Such assistance should always include teaching the blind student herself how to take more and more responsibility.

The following plan led Carlotta to independence in informal projects and activities:

(1) For the rest of first grade, the teacher directed Carlotta to a specific role each time.

(2) In second grade, Carlotta was paired with a "buddy" who helped her find a place.

(3) In third grade, a teacher helped Carlotta to anticipate the activities, walk around and ask about them, and settle into a role. Soon Carlotta required no more guidance than other students.

Give concrete suggestions. Provide copies of *Your School Includes a Blind Student* (also by Doris M. Willoughby).

How Much Help and Attention?

"If a non-disabled student had this problem, would you help?" is a good rule of thumb. Give examples:

- Suppose the blind child faces the wrong way during the flag salute. Let's compare a new (sighted) student who looks for the art supplies in the wrong place. You would tell him where they are, not leave him floundering. So, show the blind child which way to face.
- Suppose a sighted child from another classroom walks back and forth in front of your door, looking worried. You would ask if he needed something. But if he just walked by, you would say nothing (except possibly hello). Make it the same for the blind child.
- We would expect a third grader to spell "come" independently, but probably not "aggravated." Apply the usual standards to a blind student.
- If a sighted child drops two crayons, he picks them up. If he spills an entire box of crayons on the floor, other people will probably help. There is no reason for the blind child to be treated differently.

IS A "BUDDY" NEEDED?

Often another child is assigned as a "buddy." This can work out well: The "buddy" might show a new student around the playground, be a partner for a field trip, go along to lunch, etc. The blind child can receive needed help and also valuable contact with a peer. However, always consider:

(1) Does the blind child really need this help? Routine assignment of a "buddy" often retards independence.

(2) If the child really needs help, is a student able to give it? Perhaps an adult should be assisting.

(3) If the same "buddy" continually helps, the relationship almost always becomes a burden. (It may be a burden to either party.) Rotation helps to prevent this, and also gives the blind student experience in working with different people. Avoid, however, a system in which the teacher asks, "Who would like to help Billy?" and Billy cringes while waiting for reluctant volunteers.

(4) If the blind child is assisted by a student for a large share of the school day, his general arrangements are probably not appropriate.

Who Needs Education About Blindness?

Everyone needs to learn more about blindness – including teachers of the blind, agencies for the blind, organizations of the blind, and the authors of this *Handbook*. There is always more to learn. However, as the itinerant/resource teacher you are likely to be the *only* person with substantial knowledge about blindness and blind techniques. Therefore you have a special responsibility to learn and teach about the real problems of blindness and their solutions.

Unfortunately, because of the pervasiveness of negative attitudes in society, and due to a lack of contact with thoughtful blind people, resource/itinerant teachers themselves sometimes encourage undesirable attitudes. Reading the many materials available from the National Federation of the Blind is one of the best ways to prevent this serious problem. Examples of literature are discussed and listed later in this chapter and in the "References" section.

Several other chapters in this book deal with adults who have a close relationship with the blind child. This chapter will deal specifically with classmates and other children, and with the blind student himself/herself. This chapter also includes many general suggestions applicable to everyone concerned about blindness.

A Misquotation

As the National Federation of the Blind (NFB) works to build positive attitudes, one of the problems is the misunderstanding of what the NFB actually says.

Many times, someone who disagrees with some aspect of the NFB's programs and philosophy (or thinks that he/she does) misquotes as follows: "The Federation says that 'blindness is only a physical nuisance. Just a little inconvenience.' How can they say that?? We all know people for whom blindness is indeed a tragedy." ...And the speaker or writer generally goes on to list various problems.

The above is a grave misquotation. It omits a vital qualifying phrase. The Federation actually says, *"With proper training and opportunity,* blindness can *be reduced to* the level of a mere physical nuisance (inconvenience.)" This is a vital distinction. If, and only if, a person learns good attitudes and skills, and is allowed to live and compete as a regular citizen-*then* blindness can be relegated to relatively minor importance in life.

The article, "Fighting a Straw Man,"[1] discusses several typical examples of misquotations and misleading wording.

Classmates Learn About Blindness

MEETING A BLIND CLASSMATE

Teachers often wonder how the sighted students will accept a blind classmate. Generally, when their natural curiosity has been satisfied, youngsters respect the blind student's methods and accept them as a matter of course. If anything, young people tend to accept a disability more easily than do adults. Urge everyone to speak openly and truthfully about the disability, without dwelling on it unduly.

The student can introduce himself to the class in the normal manner, mentioning other characteristics as well as blindness. He can explain study methods to classmates. He can learn to explain his eye condition briefly and objectively. Help him answer the common question, "How much can you see?" (Provide him with phrases such as, "I can see general shapes in a good light.")

Coach the older child, and assist the younger child, in redirecting awkward conversations. For example, when there is too much discussion of medical matters it is appropriate to change the subject. And sometimes misconceptions should be corrected. When Zach announced an operation on his eyes, a first-grade classmate said, "Then maybe you'll be able to see this small print." The teacher, knowing that the operation was to lessen glaucoma pressure and was not expected to improve sight, said, "It's not that kind of operation. It's to keep Zach's eyes from hurting."

Specific Suggestions

Blind adults make the following suggestions about general conversation:

(1) Use the word "blind" naturally, as you would a description of any other characteristic, without dwelling on it unduly. Also use the words "look" and "see" in the usual way, although the blind person may examine the item tactually.

(2) Criticize or commend the blind student as you would anyone else.

(3) Use gestures and facial expressions normally, but supplement them verbally as necessary so the blind youngster is not left out.

(4) Introduce yourself until the blind student knows your voice, and encourage classmates to do this also. Speak to the blind student by name so that he is sure who is being addressed. Indicate when you are finished with a conversation, so that he is not left talking to the air. The blind student will also appreciate your greeting or introducing visitors and new students, so that he knows who is present.

(5) Remember that blindness affects only the eyes. Some sighted people shout at the

---

[1]Kenneth Jernigan. "Fighting a Straw Man." *The Braille Monitor,* August-September, 1986, pp. 363-370.

blind as though they could not hear, assume that a short walk would be strenuous, or otherwise seem to expect additional disabilities.

ELEMENTARY SCHOOL

When a blind child enters an elementary school, students in all grades need to learn about blindness. Provide background for teachers in talking with students. As soon as possible, arrange for someone to talk with all grades. You may do this yourself, or if possible invite a competent blind adult. Consider reading or dramatizing a book which portrays blindness in a truly positive way, such as *The Seeing Summer.* The puppet show, *Kids On the Block,* is another possibility. (Detailed suggestions for drama, literature, etc., are given later in this chapter.)

Continue to arrange programs from time to time. New students will begin school, and others will have different questions as they grow older. Following is a brief outline of a typical talk:

(1) Blind people are regular people, just like you.

(2) Blind people sometimes use different ways to do things.

(3) We have a blind student in our school.

(4) Blind people are not all the same. (Emphasize individuality, especially in a resource school.)

(5) What questions would you like to ask?

If possible, show the students some aids and devices and let them try them out. Give everyone a copy of the Braille alphabet. Also give everyone a card with just two easily-distinguished Braille letters (say, *a* and *t*), and give a "first lesson" in actually reading Braille by touch.

Adjust your talk to the maturity of the children. Younger children need a quick pace, with many objects to look at. (To avoid chaos, however, talk with the teacher about when and how things will be actually touched.) Kindergartners cannot maintain attention beyond about 20 minutes, and rarely are able to formulate real questions. Older children can be attentive longer, and ask excellent questions. Classes can be combined to save time for the speaker.

JUNIOR HIGH AND HIGH SCHOOL

Beyond grade school, it may or may not be desirable to present programs. The school may be very large, and the older student may feel self-conscious. Often it is better for the blind student and the teachers to educate students informally. Nevertheless, look for possible opportunities for structured programs. Perhaps the Health classes have a unit on disabilities. Perhaps the Literature students read about Helen Keller.

Blind Students Are Regular Students

Help the blind student to become a regular member of the class and not a curiosity. Emphasize independence, and avoid the "mother-hen syndrome."

Teach classmates to refer to the blind boy or girl by name rather than just as "the blind kid," and to speak to him/her directly.

Proper groundwork nourishes normal relationships. Occasionally, however, major problems occur and should be dealt with firmly. Barb always ate alone in the cafeteria until the counselor had some serious talks with other seventh grade girls. When Chet first went onto the playground with his cane, a large crowd grew and grew until the playground supervisor said loudly, "All right, everybody! Get back to where you were playing! Next week Mrs. Smith will show you all how Chet's cane works. Now leave him alone and let him look around our playground with Tom."

WHAT DO THE WORDS REALLY IMPLY?

There are two expressions which (with variations) a blind person is likely to encounter almost daily, and which can cause severe problems. The first is, "How marvelous that you can do that!" (Variations: "I could never find my way around as well as you do." "You read better than I do.") A compliment is intended, of course, and often one must accept it in the spirit in which it is meant. However, usually the child has not in fact done better than the speaker, or even as well as the average child of his age. Therefore, the first danger is that the youngster will believe that his own skills are greater than they really are.

A second danger from exaggerated compliments is the belief that alternative techniques really are very difficult. This belief implies that a blind person cannot work as fast or as well as others, because his methods are supposedly so complicated.

Of course, this does not mean that compliments should be avoided. Every student should be complimented for effort and/or progress, even when he is not doing as well as most children his age. However, especially as the student grows older, the wording of compliments becomes important. If he has made progress in reading but is still below his grade level, we can say, "I'm so pleased at how much you have learned," rather than "You're the best in your class." If he has learned to cross the street, the classroom teacher can say, "Good! I knew you could do it!" instead of "I'm sure I could never do as well." We can compliment effort and progress without exaggerating achievement.

A second, and even more deceptive, expression is, "You do this so well that I forget you are blind." (Variations: "You answered so well I was sure you could read the chalkboard," or "I wouldn't know that you were sightless if you didn't have that cane.") The problem here is best illustrated by comparison. If you are a woman, consider your feelings if a man were to say, "You drive so well that I forget you are a woman." (Implication: women usually drive very poorly.) Or, consider this: "You are so level-headed and easy to get along with, that I would never know you are Italian." (Implication: Italian-Americans are usually hot-headed and disagreeable.) Now examine the remark, "You crossed the street so well that I would never know you are blind." (Implication: blind people usually cannot be expected to cross the street alone.)

Again, a compliment is intended, and sometimes one must accept the intention without explaining the problem to the speaker. However, if the child believes that "I forget you are blind" is the best possible compliment, certain problems will be worsened. First, the student will be more likely to seek actively to try to hide blindness (an effort doomed to failure: people will realize that he is blind, but conclude that he does not want them to talk about it). He will resist valuable aids such as a cane or Braille. Secondly, he will be encouraged to believe that blind people in general are inferior, and that he can never be a really equal citizen as long as he *is* blind.

Therefore, try to teach sighted people to avoid this dilemma. If a youngster has just learned to fry hamburgers, we can say, "This is a great hamburger," without any implication that we had not expected a blind person to do a good job of cooking. If the speaker actually means that he did not understand how the task was done, he can say, "I'm interested in how you do that. How do you know when the meat is done?" –and thus express friendly interest without any troublesome implications.

In other words, help the youngster to think, "It's OK to be blind. Blind people can do things just as well as anybody else. I don't need to be ashamed of blindness or try to hide it." Strive to *accept* blindness as a characteristic which does not prevent normal living.

The chapter, "What Can I Tell My Child About Blindness?" in *A Resource Guide for Parents and Educators of Blind Children* offers detailed suggestions.

Classmates' Families

What about the parents of classmates? In the past it was not uncommon for a parent to complain that "the blind child is taking the teacher's time away from my child." Fortunately, this problem is now rare, as parents realize that appropriate arrangements are required by law. However, parents of sighted classmates still harbor the same stereotypes as other members of the public. If an opportunity arises for a program at the PTA, Parents Day, etc., this can be very valuable. But to preserve confidentiality, avoid detailed discussion of a particular student, and instead discuss various arrangements for blind students. Consider having speakers on other disabilities too.

Look for informal ways to help relatives and close friends, especially, learn more about blindness. Sometimes I accompany the blind child at recess and offer suggestions. Recently I included a blind girl's sister in a cane travel lesson, and showed her what Cathy could do by herself. I also explained and demonstrated how "Cathy can follow you, or walk with you, and still use her cane. That way, you don't have to help her with everything. But you can still stay together." Later I did the same with two of Cathy's neighbors.

Many youngsters greatly enjoy learning to write Braille on the slate. They may call it a "secret code" and have fun passing messages.

Blindness and Literature

THE VALUE OF GOOD LITERATURE

Good literature is a particularly effective and pleasant way to teach positive attitudes toward blindness. Below are listed several particularly good books, articles, speeches, videos, and dramatic presentations. (This is not an exhaustive list.) See the "References" section of this *Handbook* for bibliographical information. Urge agencies, school media centers, families, and libraries to acquire these.

Books for Children

- *Questions Kids Ask About Blindness*
- *The Seeing Summer* (See below in this chapter.)
- *Business Is Looking Up*
- *A Cane In Her Hand*
- *The Seeing Stick*
- *The Witch's Daughter*

For Teenagers and Adults (Including Parents and Educators)

- *The Encounter*
- *Blindness: Handicap or Characteristic*
- *Blindness: Competing on Terms of Equality*
- *Parent Tips: A Guide for Blind and Visually Impaired Parents*
- *Blindness: A Left-Handed Dissertation*
- *A Definition of Blindness*
- *To Man the Barricades*
- *Blindness: The Myth and the Image*
- *Postsecondary Education and Career Development*

For Parents and Educators

- *Future Reflections* magazine
- *Your School Includes a Blind Student*
- *A Resource Guide for Parents and Educators of Blind Children*
- *Get A Wiggle On*
- *Move It!!!*
- *Talk to Me* and *Talk to Me II*
- *Just Enough to Know Better*
- *The Blind Child In the Regular Preschool Program*

Dramatic Presentations

- *The Seeing Summer* Playlet (See below in this chapter)
- *The Kids on the Block*

Videotapes and Films

- *It's Not So Different: A Talk With Blind Parents*
- *Kids With Canes*

A Very Positive Book

Jeannette Eyerly is a widely-published author of books for young people. Now she has written a story about blindness–and it is first-rate! It is not sensational, not melodramatic, not drippy or sentimental–none of these. It is simply factual and interesting and down-to-earth. But this takes nothing away from its effectiveness. It is entitled *The Seeing Summer.*[2]

The Seeing Summer is a compelling and humorous story interesting to all ages. Although

[2]Jeannette Eyerly. *The Seeing Summer.* New York: J. B. Lippincott/Harper Row, 1981.

the reading level is third or fourth grade, the book will also be appreciated by much younger children if it is read aloud with some explanation. Stereotypes about blindness are brought out in a natural way and dealt with very well. The blind girl (Jenny) is portrayed as a normal person, appropriately competent for her age.

To quote the book jacket:

> More than anything else Carey wants a new ten-year-old playmate to replace the friend who had moved away. When she hears that the new family next door has a girl her own age, Carey straightens her room and settles down to watch and wait.
>
> She is stunned to learn that her new young neighbor is blind and carries a white cane. Not fair! Jenny will not be able to do everything Carey can do. But Carey is in for a surprise – Jenny can cook, play games, read her own books, and run outdoors like everyone else. When two thugs kidnap Jenny for a high ransom, Carey tracks them down and becomes a second captive. Together the girls keep up their courage and use their ingenuity to survive the terrifying adventure.
>
> *The Seeing Summer* is a story of capture and escape, but best of all it is a story of friendship between two ten-year-olds who are very much alike, even though one cannot see.

The Seeing Summer has been nominated in a number of states as an outstanding book for children.

The Macmillan Co. reading textbook, *Winning Moments,* includes an illustrated excerpt from *The Seeing Summer. Winning Moments* will also be published in Spanish.

A BRAND-NEW RELEASE: A short dramatization of certain scenes from *The Seeing Summer* is now available. First published in this *Handbook,* the playlet appears in its entirety as an Appendix of this *Handbook.*

NEGATIVE ATTITUDES IN LITERATURE

Is Literature Against Us?

In his speech, *Blindness: Is Literature Against Us* (See "References"), Dr. Kenneth Jernigan begins, "I would like to talk with you about the place of the blind in literature. How have we been perceived? What has been our role? How have the poets and novelists, the essayists and dramatists seen us?"

He goes on to list and analyze nine motifs from literature and popular culture:

- Blindness as compensatory or miraculous power
- Blindness as total tragedy
- Blindness as foolishness and helplessness
- Blindness as unrelieved wickedness and evil
- Blindness as perfect virtue
- Blindness as punishment for sin
- Blindness as abnormality or dehumanization
- Blindness as purification
- Blindness as symbol or parable

The Worst Book I Have Ever Seen

The Dark Princess, by Richard Kennedy,[3] has a plot as follows:

> The Princess was totally blind, but she hid her blindness from the people of the kingdom. Although she was very beautiful, no one dared to look directly at her: anyone who did so would be struck blind also.
>
> One day it was discovered that people could look at the Princess' face without being struck blind, if they looked through a colored glass. Princes began to seek her hand. But the Princess demanded a high price for her love – namely, that the suitor must look directly at her and become blind also! They all declined, and went sadly away. The Princess was deeply sorrowful, because she had no sweetheart, and because she knew that she really had

[3]Richard Kennedy. *The Dark Princess.* Holiday House, 1978.

nothing to offer a suitor–after all, she was blind. She felt that there was no real love in the world, or at least none in herself. She thought about death.

The Court Fool met the Princess as she walked near the cliffs by the sea. He talked with her and tried to make her laugh. He revealed his love for her...and revealed that he *was* willing to look directly at her and take the consequences. She wanted to feel joy, but knew that she had nothing to offer him, for she was blind. But the Fool did put down his colored glass...and in his blindness he stumbled over the cliff. She leaped in to try to save him...and they both drowned in the dark water below.

[*Summary by Doris M. Willoughby*]

All of this is told and illustrated in a style that seems romantic and has the appearance of an old folk tale. (To my knowledge it is not actually a folk tale; but even if it is, it should have been relegated to the archives instead of publicized.)

This is the *worst* children's book in regard to blindness that I have ever seen. It has no redeeming features.

Negative Attitudes Are Common

In many traditional and contemporary stories, the blind character is infirm or stereotyped.

The cartoon, *Mr. Magoo,* is particularly insidious: readers do not consciously realize that it is ridiculing the behavior of a blind person who should be using alternative techniques.

It is important for the resource/itinerant teacher to be familiar with some literature with *bad* attitudes toward blindness, learn to recognize it as such, and understand why thoughtful blind people find it offensive and harmful. Unfortunately, many agencies for the blind actually promote such literature, and some blind individuals and groups have not yet realized how they are sold short.

A Step-By-Step Guide to Personal Management for Blind Persons, from the American Foundation for the Blind (See "References"), is an example of this problem. Routine tasks, easily learned by the average blind person, are broken down into tiny steps suitable for mentally retarded learners.

Organizations of the blind are not exempt from corruption by the bad attitudes of society. One organization of the blind continues to promote artificial changes in the environment (e.g., underfoot guidance systems) despite the fact that they encourage dependence and interfere with appropriate travel methods. (See the chapter in this *Handbook,* "Travel With the Long White Cane," for a discussion of inappropriate travel aids.)

Consider the videotape, *Vision Loss: Focus on Feelings.*[4] Three well-known agencies, which distribute much literature and advice about blindness, arranged the production. Yet one blind woman says after viewing it, "It's the very worst thing I've ever seen. It features a group of blind people telling each other how awful it is to be blind–including such statements as, 'I feel like I'm in prison since I can't go anywhere,' and 'I derive my self-esteem by being known as the cake decorator's husband' and 'I get my hair fixed to make myself feel better about being blind.' It's truly depressing."

A narrator makes a few trite attempts at positive or hopeful comments, but is entirely ineffective against the background of self-pity shown.

HANDLING NEGATIVE ATTITUDES IN LITERATURE

With very young children, try to avoid literature which presents the worst attitudes. However, this problem cannot be avoided indefinitely, and as the child grows older he should understand and deal with negative attitudes.

---

[4]*Vision Loss: Focus on Feelings.* Videotape/16 mm film, 19 minutes. Venice, CA: Oracle Film and Video, 1985. Produced by Dennis Passagio, with the cooperation of the American Foundation for the Blind, the Braille Institute of America, and the Canadian National Institute for the Blind.

Ask everyone to tell you about any materials which portray blindness. Help teachers and students to recognize and counteract outmoded attitudes. For example, suppose the reading book portrays a blind piano tuner. The story says that he has a "wonderful ear for tones." He does not use a cane. Discussion could bring out these points:

- This man has a good ear for tones; that's why he is a good piano tuner. But blind people are not magically endowed with musical ability.
- Piano tuning is only one possible occupation. Blind people today work in almost every field.
- It is too bad that this man has evidently not had the opportunity to learn to travel independently with a cane or a dog.

If a particularly bad story is being used repeatedly, try to get a better one substituted.

A "Mixed Bag"

Often we find literature which includes helpful information which we want to use, but which also has some negative aspects.

This can be even more dangerous than totally bad literature such as *The Dark Princess.* Because of the natural tendency to assume that a book is either "good" or "bad," it is especially hard to analyze one which is somewhere in between. However, most books dealing with blindness are indeed of mixed quality. It is very important to recognize this, in order to decide whether (a) the book is, on the balance, worthwhile to use in a given situation, and (b) if it is, how to benefit from the helpful aspects without being misled by errors.

Counteract the Problems

Consider the following book, often used with classroom teachers:

> *When You Have a Visually Handicapped Child in Your Classroom: Suggestions for Teachers,* by Anne Lesley Corn and Iris Martinez (American Foundation for the Blind).
>
> This book offers many items of practical advice for classroom teachers. Topics include helping the visually-handicapped child feel comfortable; using special devices; working with printed materials; activities outside the classroom; and skill development. Many sources of information are listed.
>
> There is emphasis on including the child in a well-rounded life. For example, the booklet cautions against exclusion from various activities due to an unfounded belief that the child might be injured.
>
> There is, however, a glaring omission in this booklet: Not once is there even mention of a cane. The sighted guide technique is explained, and there is a general discussion of the role of an Orientation and Mobility teacher. But there is no mention of cane travel, not even as a future consideration.
>
> Also, unfortunately, the booklet recommends (as a general practice) allowing one-and-one-half the usual time span for assignments, and/or shortening assignments. This is in contrast to the excellent remarks about "Remedial Academic Assistance," which make it clear that such help is only needed for certain individuals.
>
> [*Review by Doris M. Willoughby*]

If this book is provided to classroom teachers, it is important to write in comments such as, "The student will also learn to walk independently with a cane" and "Most students do not need shortened assignments or routine time extensions."

A "Mixed Bag" For Children

Sally Can't See, by Palle Petersen, was first published in Denmark. It shows Sally as a normal, energetic twelve-year-old studying and having fun. She is "upset and cross" if people seem to feel sorry for her and think she is strange. Pictures and text are well-thought-out and interesting. The long white cane is shown and explained well.

When this book is used, I comment on certain passages which give an inappropriately negative impression. I say that although "Sally can't read as fast as her friend Pat," blind children in general can read as fast as anyone if they have a good chance to learn. (We hope Sally will get faster!) When the book says, "...a sighted person keeps close at hand to help Sally..." on a horse, I point out that actually the teacher might have been blind too: some blind people handle horses very well alone and teach other people.

I also explain that although Sally attends a residential school, most blind children in the U.S. attend public schools.

The Less Obvious Problems Are Harder

Negative attitudes mixed in with relatively good points are often the hardest to analyze and counteract. But it is vital that we do seek them out. Every story about blindness is influential.

The Blind Student Learns About Blindness

Include the blind student in programs and discussions about blindness. This may seem obvious, but too often someone talks about blindness with no participation from the blind boy or girl who is sitting right there. Worse still, the discussion is held while the blind student is out of the room. Instead, include the student in the presentation, thereby helping him learn to educate others. Even the youngest can demonstrate something he has been learning. An older student may give the entire presentation.

Unusual circumstances, of course, require good judgment. A very shy child may be unable to participate at first. If certain classmates are especially unkind, it may be best to counsel them privately.

The blind student needs a great deal of education about blindness -how to recognize what the problems really are, and how to deal with them. The chapter, "What Can I Tell My Child About Blindness?" in *A Resource Guide for Parents and Educators of Blind Children,* offers many suggestions.

MEETING OTHER BLIND PEOPLE

The single most helpful factor is meeting capable blind people. It is tragic that this happens so rarely. A single contact, while desirable, will soon be nearly forgotten. The blind youngster needs to keep in regular contact with at least one capable blind adult, and discuss new questions as they arise. Too often, a few rather *negative* contacts with a blind person set the tone. Recently I listened as a blind woman told about her own childhood, when the only blind adult she knew was a teacher who was not very independent. The speaker remembered how she (as a partially-sighted child) had often been asked to lead the *teacher* home.

Sadly, even some agencies who claim to help the blind, and even some organizations of blind people, regularly demonstrate inefficient techniques and negative attitudes. This is especially unfortunate, because the general public tends to believe that such agencies and organizations should have the right information about blindness.

The National Federation of the Blind can suggest appropriate contacts in your area or (if distances are a severe problem) people who can be reached by mail. The best way for a blind youngster to develop a positive self-image is frequent informal contact with good role models.

But how do you make this actually happen? Even if someone is readily available, transportation and scheduling are a problem. Sometimes the student resists meeting other blind people. Often the parents do not see the value. Try these ideas, alone and in combinations:

(1) Start a Parent Support Group, affiliated with the Parents of Blind Children Division of the National Federation of the Blind. See that many meetings include the children in some way.

(2) Ask a blind adult to accompany you to your regular lesson time. The "lesson" for the day is a pleasant, informal visit with the guest.

(3) When a presentation is made to a large group, invite a blind person to speak

instead of doing it yourself. Ask the blind student to join in, even if he is in a different class.

(4) Transport one of your students to spend part of the day with another student who is especially compatible.

(5) Help two families with blind children to get acquainted and visit each others' homes.

(6) Bring several students together for a group discussion. This might include a demonstration of new equipment.

(7) For any meeting, have a tentative agenda in mind. Be sure that key subjects come up. Be prepared to stimulate the conversation if it lags.

(8) Look for a situation where your knowledge is only partial. Ask a blind person with the necessary knowledge to help teach the student (either at school or elsewhere).

(9) The student might visit a blind person at work, or attend a technical meeting with him/her.

(10) An older student can participate in regular meetings of the National Federation of the Blind. A young student can attend picnics and other special functions.

(11) Encourage families to attend the Children's Seminar which often accompanies a convention of the National Federation of the Blind; ask the NFB to conduct such a seminar in your area.

(12) If a younger student seems reluctant to talk about blindness, simply proceed as planned, while seeking ways to increase interest. Watch for things unrelated to blindness which may be the real problem. Often adults assume the child is upset about discussing blindness, or about meeting other blind people, when he is really acting oddly for some irrelevant reason. Children below fourth grade hardly ever are seriously self-conscious if adults demonstrate a positive attitude.

(13) Sometimes an older student, especially in junior high or high school, really does resist meeting other blind people. This actually indicates that he has an urgent need to meet competent blind people and to feel more positive about his own blindness. Try these ideas:

a. Be matter-of-fact, and explain that this is part of your regular course of study.

b. If necessary, allow the student to take a passive role at first, just listening while you talk with the guest.

c. Look for a special area of interest.

d. Find another reason for the blind person's coming, other than just to educate this student. For example, you and a blind itinerant teacher might exchange visits to observe each other's methods. Conversation could still be worked in.

e. Seek support from the parents, counselor, etc.

f. Remember that even if a meeting appears to have been of no value, progress may have been made. The student may respond well next time.

g. Don't automatically assume that the student resists contact with blind people. A principal once said to me, "That trip to meet the blind couple really upset Carol. She's been depressed all week!"

When I talked with Carol, however, I avoided assuming anything, and she seemed genuinely enthusiastic. After awhile she confided, "Mr. Markle thinks that visiting the Schroeders upset me. But the reason I'm blue this week is not that. It's because of my boyfriend. We broke up over the weekend."

It is vital for your student to get to know other blind people as individuals, and accept himself as an individual who happens to be blind. For the young child who knows several competent blind people, this can occur very naturally and easily. For the older student or adult, however, meeting another blind person can be a major hurdle. Interaction with others who are blind is an important part of becoming comfortable with one's own blindness. If resistance (when it is present) is not overcome, and your student continues to shun other blind people, a truly positive attitude toward his own blindness cannot be achieved.

A Blind Teacher As A Role Model

The above paragraphs have assumed that the teacher is sighted. What if you yourself are blind? This is discussed in detail in the two chapters written by blind teachers. Being blind can be a great asset to the competent teacher of blind students. A sighted teacher must use a number of "alternative techniques" to accomplish what the blind teacher can do simply by example. However, the blind teacher should not presume that he/she can do everything alone. It is still important for the student to meet various blind people, of both sexes, with various interests and skills.

GUIDED DISCUSSION

However it is arranged, it is important to have frequent discussions with the student about the ramifications of blindness in everyday life. Sometimes a five-minute discussion during each lesson is best. A longer discussion, less often, is another approach. Whatever the timing, it is important to have a plan for such discussions or they may never occur.

Possibilities for topics are endless, and only a few examples will be given here. Each is followed, in parentheses, by the main point(s) to bring out.

With a Young Student

(1) "My teacher's book is in inkprint. But Miss Rasmussen, at Northview, has her teacher's book in Braille. Why do you suppose that is?"
(Miss Rasmussen is blind. Blind people can be teachers.)

(2) "When you drop a pencil, you should pick it up, and the boys and girls sitting near you should not help. Why is that?"
(The blind student can use alternative techniques to pick up dropped objects. If others pick things up for her, she won't learn to do things for herself. Other students are busy with their own work.)

(3) "What should you say if a boy or girl on the playground brings you your cane, after you set it down by the slide?"
("Please put it back. That's where it belongs when I'm up on the slide. I'll get it when I want it.")

(4) "You know that blind people don't drive cars. So how can a blind grownup get to work?"
(By walking, or by bus, train, car driven by someone else, etc.)

With a High School Student

(1) "Why bother to take notes? Why not just tape-record the class?"
(A recording is not a summary. To review a recording, one must play the entire tape. With true notes taken in Braille, one can review quickly.)

(2) "When you go to college, someone may offer you keys to special elevators for the handicapped. What would you say?"
("No, thank you. Stairs are no problem for a blind person." ... And I would realize that if I did accept the keys, this would reinforce the idea that I am very limited, and encourage people to restrict me in other ways.)

(3) "Is there any point in a blind student's buying a school yearbook?"
(Yes, indeed! Writing messages in one another's books is fun, and the blind person can dictate a message and sign it. One's own yearbook, with messages from friends, is a valued memento. There will be ways to get it read aloud. Also, one's future children will enjoy it.)

(4) "Suppose a teacher says, 'You don't have to put tables in your term paper like the

other students do.' What would you say?" ("Thank you, but I will do the regular assignment. I can type the tables or dictate them to a reader." ... And I will realize that if they "give" me a grade for doing less, then the grade won't mean much, and I won't learn much.)

Note the emphasis on the student's taking responsibility for choosing a technique, even over the objections of others. This is vital preparation for adulthood, where the entire world seems to conspire to keep the blind person helpless and dependent.

Seek out the "teachable moment" when a given point is especially easily made. Also, however, look for current topics that may not be as obvious, and anticipate the future.

BUILDING SELF-ESTEEM

A very large topic is, "Why me? Why am I blind?"

At the surface level, you may need to interpret medical information. (With a young child, be careful about things which parents may not yet wish him to know about, such as future operations.)

The deeper level of this question is one's attitude toward being blind. We want to help students and others to see blindness *not* as an all-encompassing tragedy, but as a nuisance which can be handled with proper techniques. Seek every opportunity to demonstrate that blind people in general, and your student in particular, can take a normal place in society.

Sometimes a student, trying to show the world that a blind person can get along well, is crushed whenever he has any difficulties. He feels that "being as good as everyone else" means being *perfect.* This is a common trap encountered by all minority groups as they strive toward equality. Help your student realize that *no one* is perfect, and therefore a blind person should not expect to do well all the time. Like others, he should develop and emphasize his strengths, and minimize his weaknesses, without expecting perfection. Meeting many different blind people helps to broaden perspective.

Advice From Dr. Sally Mangold

Dr. Sally Mangold, who is blind, is the author of *The Mangold Program of Tactile Perception and Braille Letter Recognition* and has produced many other educational materials. When she recently spoke at a teachers' meeting in Iowa,[5] she emphasized building self-esteem. Below are a number of important points from her excellent speech:

Don't give children the idea that we would love them more if they could see (or see better). Children often confide to Dr. Mangold, "I know my parents would love me more if I could see." Parents and teachers should avoid continually lamenting the lack of sight, and follow the suggestions below. They should not overpraise the child for *seeing* something. A teacher doing a functional-vision evaluation, for example, should say, "Thank you for giving me all this information" instead of "Good! You can see that!"

Emphasize general characteristics and normality, and avoid overemphasizing blindness. Know what to expect of each age group, to minimize blaming problems on blindness. Emphasize everyone's individuality.

Help the young person understand the world, including imperfection. The blind student who complains, "Why didn't I get an *A?*" may have no concept of what an *A* paper is like. Sighted classmates will have seen other students' papers from time to time. Get a few samples of *A* papers, as well as *C* and *F* papers, and transcribe them into Braille (probably without names).

Let the blind child know about others' imperfections. He/she will not see how classmates look when they are troubled, may not realize that someone else has spilled or dropped things, etc. Look for opportunities to describe such things tactfully.

Work on generalizations – both personal ("most

---

[5]Sally Mangold, Ph.D. Address to state-wide meeting of teachers of the visually impaired. Des Moines, Iowa, November, 1984.

people feel embarrassed when they spill something") and less personal ("most rooms have four walls").

Teach appropriate skills and techniques. Holding the paper one inch from the eyes is too close for real practicality. Writing is an important part of learning (including being able to read one's own writing). Fatigue is a very important factor. If inkprint is not really practical, then a person should learn Braille.

Closed-Circuit Television systems (CCTV's) are not a panacea. "I've seen some sad people who have been educated entirely on a CCTV," continued Dr. Mangold. They had no really practical way to take notes, she explained, and no good way to read without the CCTV. These people were bright but could not handle college because of inferior techniques. 33 words per minute is typical on a CCTV, and a person can only read in one location.

(Dr. Mangold also said that CCTV's can be helpful if they are used as a supplement to other methods which allow the student to read easily in all environments. But a student who can read *only* on a CCTV should be given instruction in Braille.)

A Braille user can be very independent. The sad case is the person caught in between, with no really functional reading medium.

There should be freedom for individual expression, within appropriate limits. Blind children are individuals. Also, in line with the thoughts about techniques (above), blind children should not be pressed into a sighted mold. One family greatly enjoyed sunset on the beach, but felt sad that their young blind daughter could not enjoy the colors. "Let her find her own enjoyment," counseled Dr. Mangold. So the family stopped describing colors at great length, and encouraged the child to look around on her own. Soon she was happily examining various shells, feeling where the sand was hot or cold, etc., and having a great time with her family every evening.

Maintain high expectations. One aspect involves appropriate limits on the child's behavior, to develop social skills. Another aspect is praising accomplishments – even small ones – in such a way that the child is continually encouraged to accomplish even more. (Note that this is not the same thing as gushing overpraise, which can actually be limiting because it implies low expectations.) A written list of accomplishments can be a great motivator.

In teaching a task, be patient and show the child over and over when necessary. After all, sighted youngsters have the opportunity to watch various people doing the task (e.g., using silverware) over and over.

Lead the child into greater and greater responsibilities. An important example at school is anticipating the need for more supplies such as Braille paper.

Be a role model to the child in explaining blindness, and help him/her gradually to take over the task. Show parents how to guide the child in dealing with salespeople, rather than simply taking over for him. Work on answering (and sometimes not answering) awkward, tiresome, and personal questions. Let the young child listen while you respond; coach the older youngster in handling more and more explanation himself/herself.

Ask the student what he/she would like to learn. Often the student knows best what has been missing.

–The address by Dr. Sally Mangold, emphasizing the development of self-esteem, was very well received by the Iowa teachers.

PROBLEMS OF IMAGE

An especially difficult problem is the matter of a blind person who actually is helpless and incompetent. Sooner or later your student will meet or hear about a beggar, a helpless elderly person, someone without social graces, etc. Help your student realize that the problems are due to something other than blindness itself, such as age, disease, or lack of training. Possibly you will be able to help the other person in some way. In any event, emphasize two important points to your student: (1) The fact that he too is blind does not mean that he must be like that other person, since everyone is an individual; and (2) even if he feels resentment toward the other person and his helplessness, he still owes him courtesy and respect.

If the less capable blind person is a classmate, relative, or other close associate, the problem is especially difficult. Resentment can occur even when both persons are actually quite competent but have differing areas of strength and weakness. Roberto and Greg were the only two blind students in North High. Greg was very popular socially, but had trouble with some academic subjects. Roberto had straight A's, but was a quiet boy with only one close friend.

"I wish Roberto didn't go to school here," said Greg. "He's such a hermit, he makes everybody think that blind people are weird."

Roberto, in turn, resented Greg. "I'm sick of people talking about that guy," he said to the counselor. "Yesterday, again, the science teacher said, 'Do you really think you can do all this? Greg had a lot of trouble with it.'"

Blind students encounter an expanded version of a problem often seen with siblings: the reputation of one tends to haunt the others. And, because of low-expectation stereotypes, the reputation tends to emphasize problems rather than successes.

Noting the boys' complaints, the counselor reminded the teachers to avoid comparison, especially in the presence of students. Since the boys were in different grades, they rarely were in the same class, and the counselor tried to arrange for different teachers as well. He talked with each boy separately and said, in effect, "People shouldn't compare you to the other boy just because he is blind. We're working on that. But you have a responsibility, too. You mustn't go around putting him down just because he happens to be blind and to have different characteristics than you do."

This example further illustrates the importance of meeting a number of blind people with a variety of interests and talents.

Simulating Blindness

One rather common method of "explaining" blindness has serious disadvantages that are often not recognized. This method involves blindfolding a fully sighted person for a short time, so that he "will understand what it's like to be blind." Unfortunately, such an experience usually results in the individual's developing *worse* attitudes about blindness than he had before. Typically the person flounders through an attempt to walk across the room (without a cane) or eat lunch (without instruction), feels totally helpless, and comes to regard blindness with even more fear than before.

On college campuses, the "trust walk" is popular. Without training in alternative techniques, some members of the group wear blindfolds, and "trust" in the help of others. This practice is especially insidious, since the instructor usually says nothing about blindness, but merely explains that the group is to learn about "trusting" one another. Nevertheless, a group of clinging and shuffling persons underlines again the worst stereotypes of blindness.

If trust is actually what is being illustrated, there are many other possible exercises, such as supporting someone who leans precariously. Covering the eyes has no relationship whatever to trust. The competent blind person need be no more and no less "trusting" or dependent than anyone else.

If you consider arranging a simulation of blindness, carefully consider what will actually be learned. If a task will really be taught, with proper instruction and pacing, and if the idea of competent blind people is emphasized, a valuable result may be accomplished. Examples include:

- Practicing actual cane travel in a setting appropriate for beginners.
- Reading and writing a few Braille letters.
- Eating a simple snack.
- Playing a table game, such as tic-tac-toe in tactual form.

Note that tasks such as these, when geared to the age of the students, can be accomplished successfully even in a brief time period. If a series of sessions is planned, one can be more ambitious. The key is to enable the sighted students actually to *learn* a task, using appropriate techniques, rather than making ineffective attempts.

There are other examples of using a blindfold as a valuable and positive tool. When a sighted person is preparing to become a teacher of the blind, he must cover his eyes in order to learn the techniques he will be teaching. For the same reason, a student with low vision should cover his eyes to practice relying on his other senses and on tools such as the cane.

If the blindfolded person actually begins to learn an alternative technique, and positive attitudes are emphasized, a desirable result can be achieved. Too often, however, all that is learned is fear.

The July, 1985, *Braille Monitor* contains the article, "They Put on Blindfolds and Play at Being Blind." In this article, discussion of a college "disability awareness day" brings out the harm that often is done, and emphasizes that one cannot really "learn what it is like to be blind" from a brief artificial experience. Another article is "'Walk a Mile in My Shoes' Gives Us Sore Feet," by Lauren L. Eckery. (*The Braille Monitor,* August, 1988, pp. 347-349.)

CHAPTER 8

THE PARTIALLY-SIGHTED CHILD

By Sharon L. M. Duffy and Doris M. Willoughby

A Positive and Realistic Approach

In recent years much has been written about children who have residual sight but are legally blind. Unfortunately, much of what is written about children with residual sight reinforces the concept that blindness or the appearance of blindness is to be avoided at all costs. These children are often told that it is better to maximize the use of their vision, however little they have and however inefficiently they perform tasks visually, because some sight is better than none. Also, according to that line of thought, the alternative techniques of blind people are necessarily inferior to those requiring sight.

In actuality, alternative techniques are efficient and sometimes superior to those used by sighted persons. Furthermore, for the blind child they are emphatically better than attempting to rely on vision. Unfortunately, children are often taught that Braille is to be avoided, and that they should not touch things to learn about their environment, because someone might discover the truth–that they are blind. They are taught essentially to pretend that they can see, and they are constantly rewarded for practicing deception.

Many adults who, as children, were conditioned in this way, say they feel in a never-never land, not sighted and not blind. Every time something cannot be seen, the child so conditioned feels like a failure, as though somehow he could have tried harder–when actually it is not his fault but, through all of this "training to see," he is led to believe that it is. In contrast, those who have accepted the fact that they are blind report that this acceptance removes enormous pressure, the pressure of pretending to be what they are not–sighted.

All of this is not to say that blind children with some remaining sight should not use it, or that they should pretend to be totally blind. That is also dishonest and harmful. But the key is that vision should be relied upon only when it is the most efficient method, and alternative techniques should be used whenever they are the most efficient. Recently a teacher told me that a student had been put back into print because he was very slow in Braille; yet he was so slow in print that this was not efficient either. And whereas in Braille he would have had the opportunity to build speed indefinitely, in print he was limited by a very low potential.

A popular myth that the "maximize vision" school of thought promotes is that these children can be taught to see more than they could before. The promoters of this theory may even feel that they have evidence to support this belief, since children realize what is wanted and learn to fake vision they do not have. Recently a blind adult said to me, "As a child, I had a piano teacher who insisted that I did better when concentrating on print music. The fact that I do not know print music, used Braille music in her presence, and told her I could not see print music did not shake her belief. I gave up and pretended to be concentrating on the print music."

Why, if it is true that blind children can be taught to see, don't we push fully-sighted children to develop even better vision? Imagine what they could achieve with a little training! .... This is obviously ridiculous, and no such classes exist, but why not? After all, it is known that certain members of the animal kingdom can see more than humans, attesting to the possibility of seeing more. Why then do these professionals, most of whom are sighted, insist that they can teach blind children to see? Could it be that they are trying to avoid facing the idea of blindness?

This is a sight-oriented world. It is unlikely that any child, sighted or blind, will not receive adequate encouragement to use vision. In contrast, however, partially-sighted children will probably need to be taught to recognize when they should use *alternatives* to sight, and specifically encouraged to use these alternatives. Sleepshades, discussed elsewhere, can encourage the best progress toward developing alternative skills which a child will need to compete with his sighted peers.

"Vision Stimulation"

THE YOUNG CHILD'S DEVELOPMENT

All the senses of infants and preschool children, along with other physical and mental abilities, are in the process of development. It may be hard to know just how much potential exists for a particular faculty such as vision or hearing. In addition to the maturation of the faculty in question, one must also consider the child's ability to communicate. For example, a very young child cannot answer a sophisticated question such as "Which lens gives a better focus?" even if the meaning is carefully explained. He/she may not even answer apparently simple questions accurately, due to fear, misunderstandings, a desire to please, etc. Tests using letters are impossible for children who cannot read; even the "E" chart is unreliable with very immature children.

Parents will naturally ask their children questions about what they see, in words they can understand. Parents will naturally teach children to recognize colors, to name the things they see in daily life, etc. Up to a point, it makes sense to say, "If they don't try to use their sight, no one will know how much vision they have."

STRETCHING TO THE BREAKING POINT

Unfortunately, a strong system of beliefs has grown up among many educators and many eye doctors (chiefly optometrists) – a system of beliefs which stretches the idea of "vision development" far beyond good sense.

Equipment, exercises, and workbooks (by Dr. Natalie Barraga and others) are promoted as "stimulating" or "developing" vision. They are promoted for older children as well as for preschoolers.

Advocates say these programs help students to make better use of existing vision. Promoters seem to imply, also, that vision will actually improve, although they avoid actually making that statement.

However, the authors of this *Handbook*, together with the National Federation of the Blind, are convinced that "vision stimulation" programs (as carried out by educators of the visually impaired) *do not* improve vision or the use of vision to any significant degree. Furthermore, overemphasis on such efforts actually does harm in a number of ways.

The appropriate thing for a teacher to do is to explore, for practical reasons, the question of how well a child can actually see. Then the teacher should proceed to teach the child efficient techniques.

FALSE HOPES

Parents of blind children, like parents of children with other disabilities, usually find it very hard to accept the fact of the disability.

They tend to consult one professional person after another, seeking someone who will tell them what they want to hear: "No, your child is not disabled." Parents, therefore, are extremely vulnerable to a promoter of "vision stimulation." False hopes are easily raised. Inappropriate expectations are easily encouraged. Development of a positive philosophy on a solid basis (including the realization that alternative techniques can be very effective) is easily destroyed.

INAPPROPRIATE EXPECTATIONS

Despite occasional remarks to the contrary, advocates of "vision stimulation" raise inappropriate expectations.

When the print-reading student who struggles with headaches, slow speed, and fatigue is given "vision stimulation" workbooks–then the viable alternative of Braille is forgotten. When a child whose eyelashes brush the page is pushed to discern huge capital letters–then the idea of reading print on a regular basis springs up. When a child walks hesitantly forward and is prodded to guess, "Is that a tree?" –then the idea of traveling without a cane is solidified.

POOR TECHNIQUES ENCOURAGED, EFFECTIVE METHODS IGNORED

"Vision stimulation" programs encourage codified guessing. Typically a few simple shapes are used and the child strains to distinguish among them–often despite the fact that she cannot see enough detail to recognize a given shape reliably. Print "reading" is applauded even when letters cannot be seen clearly, and even when only part of a word can be seen. All of this takes time which could have been used in learning to read Braille quickly, comfortably, and reliably.

"Vision stimulation" exercises for mobility teach students to guess about their environment. Examples include:

- Slowing down for shadows on the sidewalk
- Noticing blobs of light and estimating them to be doorways, windows, etc.
- Trying to see part of the traffic light if one cannot see all of it
- Watching for jagged lines which may indicate steps
- Assuming that if the head of the person in front goes down, there is probably a stairway going down

Children and adults with low vision usually figure out approaches such as these on their own. They are unreliable and unsafe methods. For an educator or an eye doctor to encourage and codify such things is unconscionable. Such approaches encourage slow and unsafe travel, and discourage effective travel with a cane.

MISLEADING, EMOTIONAL PHRASES

"The child [about five years old] walked up the steps unaided. He had never walked up steps outdoors alone before."

This remark was part of a talk promoting "vision stimulation."

Consumer education, sociology courses, etc., teach citizens to analyze statements made by merchants and politicians. The educated consumer is alert for propaganda, which may be defined as one-sided communication designed to discourage analysis. However, most consumers have little familiarity with the choices available in regard to techniques for the blind, and are not likely to analyze as they should. Popular myth holds that the use of vision is always best, however inefficient.

Consider a careful analysis of the remark about the child on the steps:

(1) How do we know that "vision stimulation" is the *cause* of his walking upstairs alone for the first time? Other possible reasons include: his parents stopped being afraid; the child stopped being afraid; he was urged and expected to do it; he had reached an appropriate maturity level (note that we do not know if he has additional disabilities); etc. It is quite possible that he does not see any better than before, and does not use his vision any better, but is succeeding because of other factors.

(2) A child of five could have learned long ago to go up and down steps safely by using a cane (or, for that matter, without one, by using other tactual techniques). Yet the speaker clearly implied that the reason this child had not done so is because he had not had "vision stimulation." It is much more likely that he simply has not been allowed to go alone before.

(3) Since the child has very little vision, he probably does not see the steps well. He may simply be holding the rail and proceeding tactually. Or, he may be using some of the visual guessing discussed above. In any event, climbing these particular steps does not necessarily mean that he can easily and safely go up and down steps everywhere by use of his vision.

Following are some other examples of emotional, slanted remarks often used in promoting "vision stimulation." Each is followed by a comment [in brackets] by the authors of this *Handbook*.

- "See how this child goes around things without a cane!" [Seeing some things visually does not prove that a cane is not desirable for efficient, speedy travel.]
- "We will help him interpret a blurry world." [Blurry vision does not need to mean "a blurry world," if proper techniques are used so that one need not rely on vision.]
- "He has greater independence and a better self-image by using vision." [The self-image of a person trying to rely on inadequate vision is indeed poor. But it cannot be raised to normal levels by trying to compete on an unequal basis. Independence and self-image can be improved only by recognizing that it is respectable to be blind, and that using alternative techniques (which do not require vision) can enable a person to compete on an equal basis. Urging a person to "improve" the use of inadequate vision is a way to *lower* self-esteem, because he realizes he cannot possibly "do better."]
- "Now this boy is walking unaided." [Unfortunately, this expression is often used to mean that a person has no cane. In contrast, we should regard the cane as one way of walking "unaided"–that is, without the assistance of another person. It is a better way than the use of inadequate vision. Here is an interesting comparison: A carpenter would not say proudly, "I did this job unaided–I didn't use any of my tools!"]
- "She is losing vision. It is important for her to have 'vision stimulation' to build up her visual memory." [A person losing vision should spend her time learning methods which will continue to work. There are other ways to learn besides through vision; one need not have a "visual memory" of something in order to understand it.]

WHAT REALLY WORKS?

If a visually-impaired person really has enough visual potential to perform up to his/her general ability by using vision alone, then this will be demonstrated in the context of regular medical attention and the regular experiences of daily life. If regular medical attention (including corrective lenses) and the experiences of daily life demonstrate that the student cannot comfortably and reliably do things as well as others do them, then alternative techniques (not requiring the use of vision) should be taught. The student will then be able to rely on vision if and when it is really best for a given situation, and use other methods when vision is not efficient.

Low-Vision Aids

Low-vision aids are generally defined as optical aids other than conventional eyeglasses or contact lenses. Examples include telescopic lenses added onto eyeglasses; separate telescopic lenses; hand magnifiers; Closed-Circuit Television (CCTV); and special lighting.

Low-vision aids can be helpful to some persons when used appropriately.

However, low-vision aids often are misused to keep blind persons from learning efficient techniques such as Braille and cane travel. As with the "vision stimulation" programs described above, low-vision aids are easily sold to vulnerable parents. Many eye doctors (encouraged by many educators) put forth high-priced low-vision aids as cure-alls, exaggerating their benefits without explaining their weaknesses.

Disadvantages include:

- The stronger the lens, the smaller the visual field. Often only one word, or part of a word, can be seen.
- When the visual field is reduced, speed of reading is reduced.
- Using a visual aid (particularly for long periods) can cause headaches, eyestrain, dizziness, and nausea.
- Fatigue and stress make it difficult to concentrate and comprehend the material. Frequent rest periods may be necessary.
- Directing a hand-held lens requires great steadiness. The slightest jiggling can cause great difficulty. This is especially hard when viewing something at a distance, such as a chalkboard.
- Time and effort are required to arrange and focus the device each time it is used. The same is true every time the gaze is shifted to a different distance (e.g., book *vs.* chalkboard).
- Especially with high-powered aids, time is required simply to get the device pointed at the right spot.
- Usually the person must move his/her head back and forth to scan an entire line. This makes fast reading impossible. Sometimes it is easier to keep the head still and move the material instead; however this is an unnatural movement which is difficult to maintain.
- Many low-vision aids give the person a most unusual appearance.

The overselling of low-vision aids tends to build up false hopes, promote inappropriate use, and discourage the use of alternative techniques which could be faster and more efficient.

Furthermore, overselling can prevent the appropriate use of low-vision aids which could be valuable if used appropriately and in conjunction with other methods. For example, some persons usually read regular print easily without aid, but find a low-vision aid helpful occasionally. Others ordinarily read Braille and recorded materials, but sometimes use a low-vision aid for brief items.

The key is *efficiency*.

Specific Eye Conditions

To aid in understanding what people with partial vision actually do see, here are a few descriptions of common varieties of partial vision. This is only a brief overview, and resources for further study are described below.

"Tunnel vision" (a severe *field restriction*) means that a person can see only in one spot, like looking at the circle of light which a flashlight makes in a dark room. If this spot, or field, subtends at an angle of 20 degrees or less, the person is considered to be legally blind regardless of the visual acuity. Many people who have this kind of vision can pass the eye test for a driver's license (if a field test is not included); yet they could not really drive safely because anything out of this narrow field is not seen at all. Retinitis pigmentosa is a common condition which often results in this kind of vision. The person may be able to look down the street and read a street sign, but not be able to see a pole near her.

Bilateral hemianopsia is the loss of half of the visual field in each eye. Brain tumors and strokes are frequent causes. The individual may see only the left half in each eye. If there is sight in only the left or right hemisphere of each eye, the eyes cannot work together normally since the fields do not overlap normally. This creates problems in print reading and in walking.

Many eye conditions result in *holes in visual fields*. Retinitis pigmentosa, cataracts, retinal hemorrhaging, colobomas, and others are common causes. Although an individual may have a visual acuity which does not meet the definition of legal blindness, functionally this person may be blind. She may see only the top of the visual field, making such things as looking at the ground for steps difficult. She may see only pieces of words on a page. Extreme tilting of the head in trying to see better may be observed; perhaps this would be encouraged by the "maximize vision" school of thought, but it looks ridiculous and is of little practical value in terms of functioning competitively. (A *mild* head tilt may be entirely acceptable if it can easily be maintained comfortably. But an awkward, unnatural position is not likely to be helpful.)

Night blindness is often associated with *retinitis pigmentosa* (R.P.) since R.P. victims often notice this as the first symptom of the disease. They may see fine in the daytime, but notice having great difficulty seeing at night or in dark places. Any change in lighting can create problems for these individuals, and the contrast can be as great as normal vision in the daytime and no vision in the dark. R.P. is a progressive condition (vision becoming poorer as time passes).

Central vision loss is characteristic of *macular degeneration*. Individuals with this kind of condition can see peripherally (to the side), but little in the central visual field. This means that reading becomes impossible, since the central vision is responsible for close viewing. For these individuals, even a visual acuity of 20/50 (which would seem relatively high) is extremely deceptive. Such an individual may not be able to read print at all, even though other persons with 20/50 acuity can usually read regular print with facility. Nevertheless, these people generally have considerable usable vision for locating landmarks, etc.

Many eye problems, of course, result in *generally less acute vision* – that is, the person can see, but does not see clearly. Vision may be relatively better or worse under certain conditions (e.g., bright light), or at certain distances. If the vision in the better eye is 20/200 or poorer with the best possible corrective lenses, the individual is legally blind – a definition which is important for funding purposes, but often not very helpful in educational decision-making. (Recall also that even a person with a high acuity is legally blind if the visual field has an angle of only 20 degrees or less.) Roughly speaking, 20/200 means that a person sees at 20 feet what a person with 20/20 ("perfect") vision would see at 200 feet.

Albinism is a hereditary condition in which there is a lack of normal pigment in part or all of the body. The hair is white, with the skin very fair, and the iris of the eye appears light colored or pinkish. The person with albinism usually has poor vision, an imperfectly developed retina, oversensitivity to light, and nystagmus (abnormal muscle movement causing constant twitching or jerking of the eyes).

Nystagmus occurs in many conditions besides albinism, and may be the only specific diagnosis listed by the doctor. This abnormal muscle movement can make it very difficult to focus, and often results in actual visual functioning which is much lower than the doctor's acuity figure would seem to indicate. Nystagmus is often less troublesome in some directions or positions than it is in others.

Lowered acuity may occur with or without a restriction in the field of vision. *Glaucoma*, for example, often causes generally poor vision as well as a restricted field.

The term *amblyopia* applies to poor vision which is not due to any observable disease and which cannot be corrected by lenses. It may be congenital (present at birth) or may develop later.

Sources of More Information

The book, *Blindness and Disorders of the Eye*, gives an overview of many common eye conditions, as well as a description of the normal eye. Portions of this chapter are adapted from that book. Literature from the National Society to Prevent Blindness, ophthalmology textbooks, and other references give detail regarding specific eye conditions. (See the "References" section at the end of this *Handbook.*)

Other chapters in this *Handbook* also give information and insights into various eye conditions. However, this *Handbook* is not intended to cover medical topics in complete detail.

Eye doctors' reports, while essential, are only somewhat useful in determining what methods will actually work best in school and in life. It is important to understand that even individuals with the same eye condition, and with the same visual acuity according to the doctor's chart, may perform visually with varying abilities. In determining practical visual functioning, observing and interviewing a child may be much more helpful than merely reading the doctor's report. (See the chapter on "Assessment of Functional Vision.")

Better than the legal definition of blindness is the functional definition, discussed in the paper, *A Definition of Blindness* (see "References"). According to this practical definition, an individual is blind if he must devise a number of alternative techniques to do efficiently those things which sighted people routinely do using vision. (Note the importance of the word, "efficiently.")

CHAPTER 9

EXPLAINING THE IDEA OF SIGHT AND PARTIAL SIGHT

Explaining Sight to the Blind Student

"I always go outside to find Mom," said Denise, a kindergartner with partial sight. "How can you see her car now?" she continued curiously as the teacher looked out the window.

Eldon stood in front of his locker in the busy hallway. After a large lunch his clothes felt too tight. He unbuckled his belt, unzipped partially, and readjusted his pants. Later when the counselor talked to him, Eldon was amazed. "But I turned my back!" he exclaimed. "I was facing the wall. I was sure no one could see me."

Very young totally blind children have no idea how sight "works." At first, young totally blind children do not even realize that such a sense exists. Those with partial sight assume that everyone sees the way they do.

Older youngsters have some understanding, but must keep refining their knowledge of what most people can and cannot see. Talk with your student about circumstances where a fully sighted person *cannot* see something – through a wall, around a corner, over a hill, etc. Compare this to hearing, and note that a person can hear around a corner. Discuss relative distances. Analyze the remark, "People look like little ants from up here on the roof," and point out that hearing has a similar relationship to distance.

As the student grows older, talk about exceptions and nuances. We cannot see clearly through translucent glass. Mirrors in the warehouse can let workers see around corners. We can "see through the wall" if there is a window; and interior walls occasionally have windows.

Talk about how much a person can see at one time, and what we mean by "I saw him out of the corner of my eye." Eldon, who adjusted his pants in the hallway, needed to understand that "turning his back" can be relative, and that students could see him from various angles. He also needed to think about what can be inferred from a partial view.

Probe your students' understanding, as by asking, "Do you think I can see [a certain object] from here?" or "If we were playing hide-and-seek, where is one place you might hide?"

HOW TO EXPLAIN

In explaining how sight is used, it is easy to overemphasize its value. Therefore, make a point of mentioning alternative techniques frequently. Also mention the names of various blind people, to emphasize that the child is not the only one using those techniques.

Denise, with low vision, was puzzled because the kindergarten teacher could recognize a car from inside the school. The teacher said, "Yes, my eyes can see farther than yours can. Since you are blind, your eyes don't see the cars from here. But there are lots of ways to find your mother, and you just use another way. You know that at 3:00 your mom will be at the corner of High Street. So you go out and look for her at the right time and place. You know the sound of your car motor. That's how Mr. Willoughby finds Mrs. Willoughby when she drives their car to his office. You will probably see the car with your eyes too. But you don't get in until you've really heard your mother's voice; you'll be careful never to get into the wrong car."

Take a matter-of-fact approach, explaining that sight can be useful, but not implying that alternative techniques are inferior. Include examples where something else is more reliable than sight, or where a given blind person succeeded and a given sighted person failed. For example, I describe a hectic moment at a wedding. The keys to the honeymoon car were misplaced. Three sighted people, including myself, had searched the interior of the car thoroughly, we thought. Then the groom, who was totally blind, came over to take a look–and found the keys immediately. They were caught in the upholstery. We all thought we had looked there, but only his practiced fingers found them quickly.

Examples of optical illusions also show that "perfect" vision is not infallible. This example is easy to demonstrate: When the cover from a Perkins Brailler is placed on a table, it may stand up by itself. More than once I have seen this and assumed the Brailler was under it. I joke with students about the "ghost Brailler," discuss why I was misled, and point out that they would not make this mistake since they would touch the cover.

(Note: avoid continually emphasizing errors made by the fully sighted, or sensationalizing the "brilliance" of a blind individual–this comes across as condescending.)

Describe the visual appearance of the eye itself. Many blind children assume that "brown eyes" are brown all over.

The general concept of color is discussed in the chapter on "Art." Methods for color coordination are explored under "Home Economics and Daily Living Skills."

WHAT DO SIGHTED PEOPLE PREFER?

Discuss the idea of visual attractiveness. Contrast this with visual annoyances–very crowded pictures, clashing colors, etc. Many things are unpleasant both visually and otherwise. Talk about things that are particularly undesirable visually, and how likely they are to be noticed.

The blind host or homeowner should maintain good lighting for the benefit of others. Lighting can also signal that a room is occupied, and this can be important in the workplace.

Explaining Partial Sight to Adults

"Andy does *not* need a cane!" declared his mother adamantly. "Why, just the other day, he was the first of the kids to see his father's car coming. He yelled to the others and *ran* down the hill to meet his dad. Andy doesn't need a cane any more than I do!"

Andy's eye condition was deteriorating. He hesitated for spots of sunlight or shade, thinking they might be steps up or down. He could not see traffic lights well, or consistently describe vehicles and their movements. Yet his parents, denying that Andy really had a problem, related the anecdote and failed to realize its irrelevance:

(1) Andy did not necessarily recognize his father's car visually. He may have recognized the sound of the motor. Alternatively, he may have relied on one conspicuous visual characteristic such as a bright color, so that he would confuse their car with others which have that characteristic.

(2) There was plenty of light.

(3) The hill in question was very familiar. There is no comparison between this situation and that of travel in unfamiliar, varied surroundings.

In many ways it is harder to deal with partial sight than total blindness. The chief reason is that public attitudes tend to push a person with some sight into trying to rely on it at all costs, while the totally blind person has no such choice. Another reason is that it is very hard for the fully sighted to understand what a partially sighted person actually sees.

WHAT DOES SHE ACTUALLY SEE?

"Doctor, a person with partial sight simply does not see the *same things* that you, or another fully sighted person, will see!" exclaimed Peggy Pinder. "You must understand that partial sight is *different* from your sight."

A prominent eye doctor was talking with members of the National Federation of the Blind at a state convention. Peggy Pinder (a blind lawyer) and others had explained why persons with low vision should use alternative techniques such as cane travel, and had urged the doctor to recommend these methods. However, the doctor – though friendly and wanting to be open-minded – found this very hard to grasp.

"But many people with low vision can see a sidewalk!" protested the doctor. "They can see a doorway. They don't need a cane!"

"OK," replied Miss Pinder, but *what* do they see when they see a sidewalk? They see a white strip, with various blurs which might be anything from holes to roller skates to shadows. A doorway may look like a spot of light, or perhaps the outline of a rectangle. Do you want your patients to step trustingly onto that strip of white, not knowing what they may be tripping over? Should they go right through that rectangular spot of light? Suppose it turns out to be a window instead of an open doorway? Or suppose there are steps going down on the other side?"

"But I *know* people with very little vision who walk around by themselves, and they get along fine!" continued the doctor.

"And what do they mean by 'fine'?" countered Miss Pinder. "Even if they are not using a cane or a guide dog, they *are* using alternative techniques! But they are using alternative *sighted* techniques – which are based on the inadequate clues we've been talking about, and therefore are slow and unsafe – instead of good alternative techniques which are not based on sight. I'll bet they don't travel alone down a street where there is construction. Travel which relies on poor vision is just *not the same* as travel with good vision. And by the way, I myself have been traveling through construction all week near my office, using my cane."

After an hour's discussion, this doctor was only beginning to grasp what the blind people were telling him. Virtually all sighted people, in all walks of life, have the same difficulty in grasping the concept of partial sight.

PREVENTING MISUNDERSTANDINGS

Too often, an adult asks a youngster, "Can you see that?" and he answers "Yes" – but neither of them realizes that he only sees a vague shape. He may say, "Yes, I can see the chalkboard," innocently taking the question literally, and having no idea that anything is *written* on the board.

Accompanied by his itinerant teacher, Dustin was touring the Middle School where he would enter fifth grade.

"How much can you see?" asked the math teacher. "For instance, can you see those boys?"

Dustin glanced in the direction indicated, and answered "yes."

However, the itinerant teacher gently helped him explain that he saw them only vaguely. "I expect you can see that there's someone there, Dustin," she said. "And perhaps you can see the colors of their shirts. But to tell exactly who they are, you'd want to talk to them, or get a lot closer – right?" Dustin agreed, and the itinerant teacher resolved to help him understand and explain his vision. She also resolved to discourage the Middle School teachers from overdoing this subject. Whenever Dustin was introduced to a teacher, the very first question tended to be the same: "How much can you see?" Normal get-acquainted remarks should receive normal emphasis: "Who is your fourth-grade teacher?" "You'll like our new gym!" "Where do you live?" etc.

When a youngster says, "Yes, I can see that," it is also quite possible that he really cannot see it at all, but is just trying to please.

Public pressure toward reliance on vision is tremendous, and children are so eager to please that they often will say what they think is expected.

It is much better to avoid asking, "Can you see [a certain object]?" Instead, if an inquiry is really necessary, ask the student to read or describe the object. Be extremely wary of assuming he can really see something accurately when he may be relying on non-visual cues – e.g., recognizing people by their footsteps. This is not necessarily a matter of conscious deception; often the child genuinely believes that he "can see it."

GAPS IN UNDERSTANDING

A third grader in rural Iowa could not describe how corn grows on the plant. "But she sees corn all the time!" protested her mother. However, the child never had walked right up to the corn plants, touched them, and examined how the ears grew. She had not been lifted up to see how high the stalk grew. She had seen only a green mass.

"Mom?" asked Tiffany one day as they sped along the highway. "How come there aren't ever any cars on our side of the road?" Her surprised mother suddenly realized that Tiffany could not see cars ahead or behind. She could only see (and hear) them as they went by – and those cars were all on the other side of the road!

Mark had quite a bit of sight. He also was very mobile and examined things well by touch. Yet at age eight he did not know what the down-spout on the corner of the house was for. He knew it only as a "pipe" of unknown purpose. He had never been close to it during a rain-storm.

These examples show how easy it is to make wrong assumptions about partial sight. The child, never having seen well, really believes that he "can see it." Adults with good vision find it very hard to imagine imperfect sight.

A Constructive Approach

The most important approach to dealing with partial sight is to recognize that often it should *not* be relied upon. With the proper attitude, we will observe a youngster and *objectively* learn what he can and cannot see. Rather than merely asking, "Can you see this workbook?" we will ask the child to *read* sample passages, and watch for errors and signs of discomfort.

We will also avoid praising a child for *seeing* something. If we are seeking information, we will thank him for giving it: "Thank you for trying out these samples so that I know what works best." When he completes a task, we will praise the achievement instead of vision – e.g., "I'm glad you can read so well," rather than, "I'm so glad you can see that."

When we already have a good idea of a child's functional vision, we will *not* keep asking, "Can you see this?" when we should realize that he cannot. Instead we will describe the item, or if possible provide the opportunity to examine it closely. It is frustrating and degrading to be continually asked whether you can see something, when you really cannot and the person inquiring should know it.

Learn the typical characteristics of various eye conditions. For example, a person with albinism prefers relatively dim light. (See the chapter, "The Partially-Sighted Child," and references mentioned there.) At the same time, do not place too much emphasis on the details of what a particular person can and cannot see. If a child cannot see the chalkboard from across the room, seat him where he will be comfortable. If he cannot see the board well even at close range, use alternative techniques such as reading aloud. Probing for the outer limits of what a person can see is uncomfortable and unproductive. If he can just barely see it, all his energy will be used for seeing rather than learning.

Even with the best attitudes and freedom to explore, a child with low vision (as well as a child with no vision) is likely to have some gaps in his/her experiences. Look around continually for learning opportunities.

Keep reminding parents and teachers, "When you show her something, encourage her to feel it as well as look with her eyes." Help the student (and others) to realize that it is really "OK" to examine by touch; too often learning is inhibited by self-consciousness about touching.

Also remember that it can be embarrassing for the student to find out what she does not know. Be sensitive, tactful, and careful about where and when you deal with misconceptions and gaps in knowledge.

CHAPTER 10

SLEEPSHADES

By Sharon L. M. Duffy

In this book, sleepshades are mentioned in each section that deals with the learning of an alternative technique of blindness. Sleepshades are a blindfold sold to the general public for use while sleeping in the daytime. They are an extremely important tool in teaching proper cane travel techniques, Braille, and other alternative techniques used by the blind.

At first glance, it would appear that their use would be counterproductive, that partially-sighted children should be encouraged to use their vision to the fullest in order to be the most able to perform tasks. Actually, most partially-sighted people tend to use their vision to the exclusion of more effective alternatives if not trained to do otherwise with the aid of sleepshades. These partially-sighted people function to some extent like the cartoon character "Mr. Magoo," relying on unreliable vision, making mistakes about what they see and generally functioning less effectively than they could.

Since blindness is generally viewed as a negative characteristic, the partially-sighted child often feels that it is better to use sighted techniques, even if they are very difficult for him and are less effective than alternative techniques not involving sight. The student may even know his inefficiency, but is socially conditioned to believe it is better to use sight.

Advantages of Sleepshades

The use of sleepshades accomplishes two things: (1) it forces the student to practice alternative techniques, and (2) it tends to help the student to accept his own blindness. When a partially-sighted student finds that he *can* function effectively without sight, accepting blindness becomes much easier. It is desirable that a blind person accept the fact so that solutions to the problems it creates can be logically worked out. If blindness is denied, the result is a great expenditure of energy in attempts to hide blindness, and less competence than is possible.

Another advantage of using sleepshades is that many, if not most, children with partial vision will lose more vision as time goes on. Retraining will be minimal or unnecessary for children trained to function without vision. Children with glaucoma, retinitis pigmentosa, optic atrophy, congenital cataracts, macular degeneration, and retinopathy of prematurity are among those who generally can expect to have very little vision by the time they are thirty years old, if not sooner. Of course, there are exceptions, but not many. However, because of the above mentioned tendency to deny blindness, there is an equal tendency to deny that vision will decrease, sometimes supported by the attending ophthalmologist. Since all students with partial vision should wear sleepshades for training purposes for the reasons given in the last paragraph, it may be wiser not to engage in the argument as to whether a child's vision will or will not deteriorate, in establishing the agreement for the student to wear sleepshades. Occasionally, parents or teachers do recognize that training with sleepshades will be useful as the child loses vision.

All of this is not to say that a partially-sighted child should not use the vision she has when this is truly the most efficient way to do something. The use of sleepshades should not be construed as an intent to deny or degrade the sight which exists. We live in a sight-oriented world and it is unlikely that any partially-sighted child will not use the vision present. Society will encourage and teach him to do so. Sleepshades are merely a vehicle to teach the alternatives in the most efficient way.

Overcoming Resistance

Because of the stigma attached to blindness, the teacher is likely to meet resistance to the use of sleepshades, from the student, the parents, or perhaps other school personnel. For this reason, it is most important that the teacher know the reasons for their use and be able to explain them with conviction. Most resistance can be eliminated by a clear explanation of their purpose coupled with a firm stand on their use. The teacher who is hesitant or doubtful about their value may encounter problems which will eventually preclude their use altogether. The teacher who handles sleepshades as a matter of course, accompanied with appropriate explanation, will have relatively few problems.

Consistency is essential in minimizing problems with students generally and the same applies to sleepshades. The teacher should *not* allow the student to make decisions regarding when not to wear sleepshades. Extra sleepshades should be available in the event of loss or damage, or the teacher may elect to keep each student's sleepshades between lessons.

Most students will not particularly like wearing sleepshades. A clear explanation of their purpose will often help. However, although it is desirable for a student to use them cheerfully, the resistant student will nevertheless learn much more with them on than off. A student will learn the skills of blindness much better and exercise more caution with sleepshades on.

A Dramatic Example

To illustrate the fact that it is actually safer for a student to wear sleepshades, consider this example. Mel disliked school and was generally regarded as rebellious and careless. With very poor vision, he often could not see well enough to perform a task accurately with vision alone. Mel handled this by bravado, rushing through the task with false confidence. In home economics (not wearing sleepshades) he nearly cut off the tip of his finger by reaching into the blender while the blades were rotating.

"We just can't have Mel in my class," said the industrial arts teacher with panic in his voice. "He'll cut off his whole hand."

The itinerant teacher, however, urged once again that sleepshades be used. "With the shades," she explained, "Mel will realize that he really cannot see things, and will be more motivated to use good techniques."

Realizing that Mel would resist, the principal called him in and made it clear that this was how it would be done. Standard safety goggles were modified to obscure vision. Mel was nervous and resentful at first, but at least he was cautious. Gradually he did learn alternative techniques for the basic power tools, and he also observed the general safety rules much better than he had in home economics. Slowly he gained some genuine confidence based on real competence. He was justly proud of his completed project. And his hands were very much intact.

MEL WAS NOT UNIQUE

Many students, if not wearing sleepshades, use an unsafe approach much like Mel's former behavior, although it is rarely quite so obvious or spectacular as in Mel's case. Realizing (consciously or unconsciously) that they cannot really see well enough to work accurately by using vision, but believing there is no good alternative, they plunge ahead by guessing and hoping.

Other students, if not wearing sleepshades, react by being overtly fearful. They too gain confidence by wearing sleepshades during all practice sessions. This seems paradoxical and needs to be repeatedly explained, but it *does work.*

"How can this be??" exclaimed Joyce in amazement after several cane travel lessons with sleepshades. "I think I actually get around *better* with my sleepshades on than without them!" As Joyce's teacher explained, she was at last learning techniques which were safer and more reliable than her inadequate vision–techniques which she had never really used during previous lessons without sleepshades. Much later, when she had learned them thoroughly, Joyce would be able to use these techniques all the time, even when not wearing shades.

Wearing sleepshades and using proper techniques is safer, more comfortable, and more efficient.

Evaluating Progress

Since resistance to sleepshades is common, it is not unusual for students to peek under their sleepshades or take them off when they become frustrated. It is possible to look under sleepshades without actually touching or removing them (by moving various facial muscles and disarranging the shades slightly, etc.) Therefore, often the only way the teacher knows about the cheating is to observe how the student is performing the task. Whether the teacher is sighted or blind, this observation of performance is the best way to know if a student is cheating. For instance, if a student veers to avoid objects without contacting them with the cane, or skips down the page without following the line tactilely, it is likely that cheating has occurred. The blind teacher will encounter the objects avoided by the student and can hear the way the hands move in the reading of Braille. Periodic discussions of the value of sleepshades also help reduce the incidence of peeking.

Also note that with younger children, the regular shades are genuinely too large, and the child may be unable to avoid peeking. Adding a small amount of fabric around the nose solves this problem.

An Exception

A word of caution: One situation in which it may not be advisable to wear sleepshades is when a student has a substantial hearing loss which results in directional hearing problems, and is traveling in an area where traffic must be dealt with. This same student should wear sleepshades while learning Braille and other skills which do not require hearing to perform–e.g., wood shop or home economics.

Conclusion

Ultimately, whether a child likes wearing sleepshades or not, they are a useful tool like any other. If a child doesn't like to work math problems by hand, for instance, we do not simply omit this from his curriculum.

After a student can travel competently and needs no more training, and after a student has learned to read and write Braille with ease, there is no more need for sleepshades when using those skills. The skills that were learned efficiently by wearing sleepshades will continue to be used.

CHAPTER 11

ASSESSMENT OF FUNCTIONAL VISION FOR READING

By Doris M. Willoughby and Caroline Rasmussen

The doctor's medical report is only a part of the picture. It is important to evaluate what the student can and cannot do well by using vision in *practical,* day-to-day situations. This is called an "assessment of functional vision," or "educational evaluation–vision." It is necessary in considering adaptations for reading print, and in considering the merits of Braille.

The resource or itinerant teacher is the logical person to do this kind of evaluation. It is generally done rather informally, partly because too much formality and structure would bring the same limitations as the doctor's exam. I have seen ready-made kits for this purpose, but have not yet found one that meets the need as I view it. Therefore Caroline Rasmussen and I have assembled a collection of books and materials, as described later in this chapter. Everything used in this kit is available from regular stores and educational suppliers, or easily produced by hand or on a typewriter.

What Are We Really Evaluating?

With a very young child, it is difficult to separate the question, "What can he recognize and name?" from "What can he see?" If a child is shown a letter he does not know, however large, he cannot name it. If he has never seen a zebra, or has not had it correctly identified, he cannot name it. I approach this by verifying that the child *can* see and name certain things correctly when very large and plain, and then showing him the same or equivalent things in a form that is harder to see. I might have him name several animals in a large and clear picture, and then see if he can do the same in a small and busy picture. Also, having determined several numerals or letters that he does know, I can then present them in various sizes.

When the student has already learned some print reading, an appropriate evaluation includes reading various samples of typical books and handouts. Note the clarity of print as well as the size; many students can read print of a particular size only if it is very dark and plain.

I recall an unfortunate error I made some time ago: I asked a high school student to read various sizes of letters, and concluded that she could read small print with ease. Much later I learned that she could read letters only in isolation; she could hardly read words and paragraphs at all. The spacing of letters, words, and paragraphs makes a great deal of difference.

With a very young child who cannot read, but who knows some numbers, this can be checked by presenting a large number such as 5244 and expecting the child to say "five-two-four-four." Similarly, if a beginner knows the alphabet but very few words, he can be asked to *spell* out words he sees. If the child easily spells any word he does not know (while looking at it), we can assume he sees the material. But if he makes errors such as the following, probably he has trouble actually seeing the print: m/n, c/e, f/t, e/a/s, w/v, F/E. (Reminder: Always be certain that a young child *knows* the letters or numerals used.) This same technique can help assess whether an older reader is having trouble *seeing* the text, or trouble knowing the vocabulary. If he can spell out the word easily (while looking at it), but cannot pronounce it, probably there is a reading problem rather than a vision problem.

Consider All Aspects

Some students have great difficulty skipping around from one place to another. Copying arithmetic problems, comparing one page with another, etc., is often difficult. Even within one page, the student may have trouble seeking answers at the top or bottom of the page. Experiment with various formats.

Consider the student's stamina for *sustained* reading. Many persons can read small print well in the doctor's office but not for a whole book or even several pages. Some can read fairly well in the morning but not later. Many report headaches, nausea, or neck strain after sustained reading. Some become restless and rub the eyes. They may say the print "gets fuzzy after awhile." If your student starts out well but seems to have a short attention span for visual tasks, consider that it may be strictly physical. Anyone who cannot read regular print comfortably and at a competitive rate for 30 minutes should learn Braille.

Furthermore, many children can see the large print used in first-grade books but will not be able to function well visually with more advanced books. These children should begin learning Braille immediately, since Braille literacy is so closely related to the age at which it was learned – the more years of practice a child has, the better he will be in general.

Who Is "Visually Impaired"?

Generally, a student clearly qualifies as "visually impaired" if the visual acuity (as measured by a doctor) is 20/70 or less in the better eye with best correction, or if there is a major restriction in visual field. For those not meeting this description, the various states and individual school districts have somewhat varying guidelines as to which students qualify. The resource or itinerant teacher should be well informed about local regulations. It is important (and sometimes difficult) to distinguish between a visual impairment as such and other reading problems.

Using an Evaluation Kit For Assessment Of Visual Functioning

General Remarks

(1) It is important to take time to establish rapport. With a young child (approximately second grade and below) this includes a "fun" activity such as briefly playing with small toys or puppets. For an older student, this includes explaining the purpose of the evaluation in a matter-of-fact and non-threatening way. Tune your approach to the maturity of the student.

(2) It is important that the test begin and end with a task which the student is able to accomplish. On the basis of information already available (school records, medical reports, conversations with teachers and parents, etc.), try to gain some idea of what the student can see. Begin with selections which are *larger* than the minimum size which you believe the student can see well.

With a younger child with low vision, it is advisable to begin with a tactual task which requires no vision, so that success is assured (e.g., use the wooden shapes, the textured circles, and/or the small toys.) Avoid ending the session with something the student cannot see; instead return to something which can be seen, and briefly re-confirm that it works well.

As discussed in the chapter, "Learning About Blindness," Dr. Sally Mangold reminds us to avoid overpraising a child for *seeing* something. Children often get the idea – very strongly – that they would receive more love and approval if they could see better. Avoid a pattern of seeming to compliment the student for the *ability to see,* as such. Instead, thank the student for cooperating and for showing you what works for him/her. "Thank you for giving me all this information," is a good phrase.

(3) Avoid a consistent progression from the largest type to the smallest type. Skip around.

(4) Type size (height) is measured in *points.* Approximately 72 points equal one inch. "Large print" is generally considered to be from 14- to 18-point. Newspaper print is about 10-point.

Point size charts may be obtained from any printer or from an agency for the blind. Note, however, that point size is often measured differently by different printers, and that characteristics such as width may vary.

(5) Distinguish, insofar as possible, between the inability to see something *vs.* the inability to understand or name it:

- Beforehand, gain some information about the student's general ability. If a high school student is a poor reader, offer reading selections from a lower grade level.
- A child in first grade or below may not have learned the names of all letters and numerals. Check with teachers. Alternatively, show him/her all the letters and numerals (out of sequence) in a very large size, and carefully determine which are known, before experimenting with smaller sizes.
- When a student cannot pronounce a certain word, it may be hard to know whether he cannot see it well, or whether he simply does not know the word. Ask him/her

to spell the word aloud. If the child can spell it easily (by looking at it), presumably he/she can see it.

- Use caution with questions such as "Which one is different?" This is a skill which which must be learned by young children. It is best to start with some very large, plain examples and be sure that the child understands the task.
- In showing pictures to younger children, consider the typical vocabulary of the age group. Rely chiefly on pictures of common things with common names. Consider whether the child may use a different name than you do – e.g., teeter-totter *vs.* seesaw.

(6) The object of the evaluation is to determine what visual materials (if any) the student can see comfortably, at least for a short period. You may also observe that some additional materials can be seen with difficulty and/or discomfort.

Keep in mind that this evaluation is, by its nature, brief. The examiner should use other means, such as interviews or classroom observation, to explore the question of fatigue over longer time periods.

(7) Make note of the conditions under which the student examined the materials:

- Lighting
- Time of day
- Head position
- Position of materials – e.g., held up to face, placed on a book rack, etc. (Note: Tell the student to place the material in any desired position, and to get as close as he/she wishes. Otherwise the student may believe you are testing his/her vision at a particular distance, as the doctor does.)
- Distance of eyes from paper
- General posture
- Squinting, etc.
- Any signs of discomfort
- Whether or not the student is wearing corrective lenses
- Any comments by the student – e.g., "I could see this better if it weren't so bright in here."

(8) Include some materials with which it is not possible to recognize a symbol or object solely from context.

- If the student is shown a picture of a child sitting at a desk and reading a book, he/she may deduce that the object is a book even without seeing it clearly. The book, *The Care Bears and The Terrible Twos,* is helpful because objects and activities appear in unexpected context. For example, a little boy is shown dunking a book into the bathtub. If the student sees the general picture well enough to determine that it is a bath scene, but does not clearly see what the boy has in his hand, the student will probably not deduce that it is a book.
- In determining exactly how well a student sees a particular size of type, numbers are often more helpful than sentences and paragraphs. In a paragraph, if a given letter cannot be seen well, it can often be inferred from the context. But if a number cannot be seen well, there is nothing to help.

(9) Often a person can read one digit or letter individually, but when two or more are grouped together they appear blurred. Therefore it is important to test words and sentences as well as individual letters, and single-spaced material as well as double-spaced. For the young child who cannot really read, this can be done by putting several numerals together unspaced, or

several other symbols close together (e.g., small circles, triangles, etc.)

(10) It is not necessary to use materials in the manner ordinarily intended. A vowel workbook may be used, not to study vowel sounds, but to evaluate the ability to see small pictures. A math workbook may be used, not for working the problems, but for reading numerals.

(11) Carefully consider the length of the session. A suggested length is given for each age group. If the student seems immature or uncomfortable, it may be wise to have more variety or more breaks than usual, and/or to have a shorter session than was planned. Continue at another time if necessary. Sometimes it is desirable to have two sessions for other reasons–for example, to check ability at the beginning of the day and the end of the day.

(12) If a student begins to read a passage and struggles severely, he or she should not be required to go on. The examiner should stop the student as soon as it becomes obvious that the passage is not suitable, and present something different.

(13) Following are examples of problems that commonly are associated with actual difficulty in seeing:

- –skipping lines
- –squinting
- –positioning the head in an unusual way, or continually moving the head
- –positioning material very close to the eyes
- –confusing symbols which a fully sighted person would typically confuse on a chart that is a little too far away–e/c, m/n, t/l, E/F, etc.

(14) Following are examples of problems that are usually *not* an indication of difficulty with vision as such:

- –reversals (for example, b/d)
- –the student cannot pronounce the word, yet is easily able to spell it out (while he/she is looking at it)

(15) This test should be given in a flexible and informal way. Include, add, or delete activities according to the individual situation. Consider presenting equivalent materials more than one time. The number of examples needed to evaluate a given kind of visual task will vary with the situation and with the student.

(16) Results of this evaluation should always be used in conjunction with other indicators of a student's visual functioning (classroom observations, interviews with various parties, medical records, etc.) No single test should ever be used as the sole method of judging special educational needs.

Children Who Cannot Read at All

The total time of one sitting should not exceed 20 minutes (less if the child seems very restless). If that is not enough time, a substantial break should be provided before resuming. It may be necessary to come back on another day.

Every session should begin with establishing rapport, followed by a task which is believed to be very easy for the child (usually examining the large, plain pictures). After that, it is *not* desirable always to proceed in the same order. Alternate between easy tasks and harder ones. Also, it may be desirable to do a few items from a given category, and then more from the same category later.

In asking the young child to identify or describe pictures, remember that vocabulary and shyness may interfere with performance. Use various approaches. Sometimes, simply show a picture and ask what it is. At other times, present more than one picture and say, "Point to the ____."

With complex pictures, it is usually necessary to elicit a full description through questioning, rather than expecting the child to explain every detail on his/her own.

If a child has difficulty with even the largest pictures, include one or more tasks which require very little vision or none at all. This will maintain rapport and help to prevent the feeling of failure. Examples include (a) identifying wooden shapes; (b) matching the textured circles according to color and/or texture; (c) playing with the toys; (d) conversing or singing.

Careful judgment and analysis may be necessary in distinguishing difficulties due to vision from difficulties due to other causes.

See also General Remarks, above.

PROCEDURE (for children who cannot read)

(1) Show the child a toy and encourage him/her to play with it briefly. Establish rapport. Explain that the toy will come back at the end of the session.

(2) Ask the child to identify several large, plain pictures (3"x3" or larger) of single objects – boat, car, dog, etc.

(3) Show line drawings of single objects, in varying sizes, as found in workbooks from the early grades. Note the size and complexity of pictures with which the child has difficulty.

(4) Show the child a very simple, large picture (e.g., apple) and ask him/her to copy it with a pencil or crayons. Ask the child to write his/her name on the back of the page. This will give an idea of what the child is seeing, and also an idea of how the child handles pencils and crayons.

(5) Show the child several pictures from a book such as *The Snowman,* a picture book with very little color contrast. Elicit discussion.

(6) Discuss complex pictures from a book such as *The Care Bears and the Terrible Twos.* Note whether the child can identify objects or situations which are unusual for the setting – e.g., the book in the bathtub.

(7) Discuss Photo Action Cards which have considerable detail and varying degrees of contrast.

(8) At the end of the session, thank the child for being cooperative. Bring out the toy again. Give the child a Scratch and Sniff sticker on a 3"x5" card.

Children Who Can Read Some of the Letters and Numbers

See General Remarks, above. The suggestions about children who cannot read at all tend to apply here also.

Total time at one sitting should not exceed 30 minutes.

Before the evaluation, ask a parent or teacher what letters and/or numerals the child already knows. Avoid trying to evaluate the child by using letters/numbers which he/she has not yet learned to recognize reliably. It may be desirable to prepare custom-made materials: e.g., if the child knows only the numerals 1, 2, 4, and 8, the examiner may wish to type up some groups of numbers in various sizes using only those numerals.

The precise shape/type font of the letter or numeral may cause confusion in beginning readers. The numeral 1, for example, typically has serifs (lines at the top and bottom) in printed matter but not in handwriting. Similarly, the lower-case *a* has several forms. Furthermore, a child may recognize a given letter in upper case (capitalized) but not in lower case (uncapitalized).

Alternate between activities involving letters/numbers, and activities which use pictures. This will help to maintain the child's interest.

PROCEDURE (with a few letters or numbers)

(1) Show the child a toy and encourage him/her to play with it briefly.

(2) Show line drawings of single objects, in varying sizes, from workbooks for the early grades. Note the size and complexity of pictures with which the child has difficulty.

(3) Show a rather simple line drawing (e.g., wedge of pie) and ask the child to copy it with a pencil or crayons. Ask the child to

write his/her name on the back of the page.

(4) Show several pictures from *The Snowman*, a picture book with very little color contrast. Elicit discussion.

(5) Discuss complex pictures from the book, *The Care Bears and the Terrible Twos.* Note whether the child can identify objects/situations which are unusual for the setting – e.g., the book in the bathtub.

(6) Discuss Photo Action Cards which have considerable detail and varying degrees of contrast.

(7) Verify that the child does indeed know the letters/numerals which it is believed that he knows. Show him all (or a substantial sample) of those symbols on individual flash cards, with heavy black letters at least 3" high. Do not present them in numerical/alphabetical order.

(8) Ask the child to identify selected numbers/letters in various sizes, including: (a) heavy black letters larger than 20-point; (b) regular 18-point; (c) regular 14-point. Work with one size at a time, but do not present symbols in numerical/alphabetical order.

(9) Show these same symbols, in similar sizes, in groups of three or more without spaces between. Do not expect the child to read words (except for any which it is known that he can recognize), or to read numbers above 10. Instead, have the child spell out a few words (while he is looking at them), and also "spell out" multidigit numbers – i.e., say "five-three-seven" rather than "five hundred thirty-seven."

(10) At the end of the session, thank the child for his/her cooperation. Bring out the toy again. Give the child a Scratch and Sniff sticker on a 3"x5" card.

Children in Grades One to Five (who can read at least 25 words)

The manner of presentation within this age group will vary with the child's maturity. The time with a first grader, or an immature older child, should include playing with a toy and giving the child a sticker. Suggestions and activities given for younger age groups may apply. With more mature children, establishing rapport should resemble the approach taken with students above fifth grade.

The session may last as long as an hour with an older child. It is vital to use sentences or paragraphs of an appropriate reading level. Sometimes it is possible to make selected use of materials at a higher reading level by asking the student only to read certain items or symbols.

See also General Remarks, above.

PROCEDURE (*for grades one to five*)

(1) Establish rapport, in a manner appropriate for the student's maturity. Explain that you want to understand what works well for the child, and to make sure he/she has the right books and materials in school.

(2) Show a vowel workbook for the early grades, and discuss line drawings of various sizes. Ask the child to identify some large letters from the same booklet, some having long or short diacritical marks. (Note: Discuss the *shape* of the mark, being sure that misunderstanding of the meaning of the mark is not confused with inability to see it.)

(3) Discuss Photo Action Cards.

(4) Present reading selections appropriate for the child's reading level. These should be several sentences long for a younger child, and several paragraphs for an older student. Listen for fluency in reading, and observe the position of the book and the child's head. Also look for words or lines skipped, and for squinting.

If a child cannot pronounce a word, he/she should be asked to spell it out.

Present appropriate selections in various type sizes. Since observing actual reading is so important, it may be desirable to present some selections early in the session and other selections later.

(5) Ask the child to read from some of the books and materials actually used in his/her own classroom.

(6) Ask the student to read from "ditto" sheets with purple ink, some of good quality and some rather faint. Note any difficulties.

(7) Ask the student to read a paragraph from a magazine that has glossy paper. Note any difficulties, especially problems with glare.

(8) Ask the child to read some math problems, with various sizes of numerals. Include numbers of several digits, but allow the youngest children to "spell them out" (i.e., name the individual digits). Since children are not asked to *work* the problems, they can be asked to read material beyond their grade level. However, keep in mind that the youngest students may not know the symbols for multiplication and division.

(9) Ask the child to write his/her name. Then ask him/her to copy selected sentences from the reading material.

(10) For children in third grade and above who have learned cursive writing, show samples of neat cursive writing in various sizes, including a normal size written in pencil. Ask the student to read several sentences aloud, and to copy at least one sentence.

(11) Dictate several numbers for the student to write. Ask the student to read them back.

(12) Using the rulers with varying graduations, ask the student to measure various lines. (Lines bordering examples in workbooks can be used.) Note behaviors such as squinting, and note how easily the student can see the small graduations. (Caution: Some children, especially younger ones, will not know how to read a ruler, especially in the smaller graduations. Younger students may be asked to "count how many little lines there are between the two and the three.")

(13) Show the small black chalkboard with several 2" numerals written in white chalk. Some numerals should be together unspaced. Ask the child to read at various distances.

The child should not be allowed to watch while numerals are being written. Also, when the same board is shown more than one time, the numerals should be changed and/or read in differing sequence.

Do the same with the green chalkboard and yellow chalk.

Optionally, ask the child to write on the chalkboard(s).

(14) Present the map. Point out various locations and ask the student to read (or spell out) the names. Note ease of reading small and irregular type, and reading against a colored background.

(15) Thank the student for cooperation. With a younger child, offer a Scratch and Sniff sticker.

(16) With relatively mature students, close with a discussion as described for grades 6-12.

Grades Six to Twelve

The evaluation will open with an informal conversation, during which time the teacher will explain briefly what will be taking place. A discussion as described in Step 12, below, will be begun.

The session should not exceed one hour without a substantial break.

It is important to present reading materials of an appropriate level for the individual student.

See also the General Remarks, above.

PROCEDURE (for grades six to twelve)

(1) Present appropriate reading selections, several paragraphs in length. Include equivalent selections in various type sizes. Note fluency and positioning.

(2) Ask the student to read a paragraph from a magazine that has glossy paper. Note any difficulties, especially problems with glare.

(3) Offer the student a newspaper (approximately 10-point type), and ask the student to read several paragraphs.

(4) Show samples of cursive writing, and ask the student to copy two or more sentences. Then dictate at least 25 numerals (some in the form of multidigit numbers) and ask the student to read them back. Take note of the kind of paper and pencil/pen preferred; the position and lighting preferred; legibility as observed by the teacher; and the ability of the student to read his/her own writing.

(5) Evaluate the ability to read numbers on a chalkboard, as described for grades 1-5.

(6) Ask the student to read a variety of math problems in various type sizes. Include decimals, fractions, and various signs of operation.

(7) Ask the student to measure several lines with a ruler marked to 1/16".

(8) Ask the student to read from "ditto" sheets with purple ink, some of good quality and some rather faint.

(9) Ask the student to read from a paper-backed book having 10-point print that is not very dark.

(10) Ask the student to read from some of the books and papers actually used in his/her own classroom.

(11) Present the map, as described for grades 1-5.

(12) The session should close with a discussion (some of which may have taken place at various times earlier). Discuss such things as sunlight/glare; steps and curbs; active games; chalkboard presentations; keeping up with reading assignments. Ask the student if his or her eyes tire quickly. Also ask about reading for pleasure: Comments such as "I used to" or "I have enough trouble getting my homework done" can be indicative of eyestrain problems.

(13) Thank the student for his/her time and cooperation.

Suggested Contents of Functional Vision Evaluation Kit

(1) LDA Photo Action Cards (color photos, approximately 4"x5", with considerable detail and often with little color contrast).

(2) Small toys or hand puppets.

(3) Small wooden shapes (circles, triangles, etc.), brightly colored.

(4) Cloth circles (approximately 4" diameter) – six pairs, each of a different color and material.

(5) Set of cards, each showing one simple, brightly-colored object approximately 3"x3", on a white background.

(6) Storybook with colorful pictures (varying sizes) showing people doing common things in an unusual setting or manner: for example, *The Care Bears and the Terrible Twos.*[1]

(7) Picture-story book in which the pictures (varying sizes) have very low contrast of colors: for example, *The Snowman.*[2]

(8) Workbook showing many pictures of simple objects, drawn with heavy black lines on white background. Size of pictures varies from one-half inch high to two or more inches high.

(9) Workbook which shows various pictures and asks student to indicate differences and similarities.

(10) Alphabet cards. Each card has one letter, approximately 1 3/4" high, which is in black ink with a broad stroke on white background. Contains upper-case cards and lower-case cards.

(11) Number cards. Each card shows one numeral 0-9, black on white. Includes a set with 3" numerals written with a broad felt-pen; a set with 10-point type; and several sets of in-between sizes.

---

[1]Ali Reich. *The Care Bears and the Terrible Twos.* New York: Random House, 1983.

[2]Raymond Briggs. *The Snowman.* New York: Random House, 1978.

(12) Workbook with an assortment of letters, pictures, and shapes drawn with heavy black lines. Includes some combinations of letters (unspaced) which do not form words.

(13) Pages showing several lines of individual numerals with spaces between. Includes 20-point type (extra dark); 20-point type (not extra dark); 16-point type; 12-point type; 10-point type.

(14) Pages showing several lines of five-digit numbers. Includes 20-point type (extra dark); 20-point type (not extra dark); 16-point type; 12-point type; 10-point type.

(15) Selections of 5-digit numbers on backgrounds of various colors. Includes 18-, 16-, and 12-point type.

(16) Math workbooks showing numbers varying in size from 2" high to 10-point type. The smallest print may be found in answer keys.

(17) Assorted "ditto" sheets with purple ink, some rather faint.

(18) Reading selections, several paragraphs in length, at various grade levels from first through twelfth. (Grade levels are not indicated on student's copy). For each grade level there are equivalent selections in 20-point, 16-point, 14-point, 12-point, and 10-point type.

(19) Magazine with glossy paper.

(20) Samples of neat cursive writing, in various sizes, including normal size written in pencil.

(21) Newspaper with approximately 10-point type.

(22) Multicolored map which includes print as small as 8 point.

(23) Three rulers, with graduations of 1/4", 1/8", and 1/16" respectively.

(24) Paperbacked book with 10-point type which is not very dark.

(25) Point-size chart, for reference.

(26) Small black chalkboard, approximately 12"x9", with white chalk.

(27) Small green chalkboard, approximately 12"x9", with yellow chalk.

(28) Chalkboard eraser.

(29) Regular pencils; bold-line pencils; crayons; ballpoint pens; felt-tipped pens of various sizes and colors.

(30) Regular lined notebook paper; dark-line notebook paper; plain paper.

(31) Scented stickers.

CHAPTER 12

MULTIPLE HANDICAPS

What Does "Multiply Handicapped" Mean?

When a student has more than one disability, it is extremely important to examine the situation *individually*. Each disability should be carefully analyzed, both separately and as it may interact with the other disability or disabilities.

Either or both of two opposite errors on the part of educators (or medical personnel) may cause unnecessary problems: (a) the assumption that anyone with a "multiple handicap" necessarily will have great difficulty in education and in life; and (b) failure to consider how two disabilities may interact and interfere with customary compensations for each. The former error is the more common.

Lori has a moderate problem with asthma. She also wears a brace on one leg, and climbs stairs slowly. If she were not blind, relatively little fuss would be made over these problems. An asthmatic child's teachers are advised of any restrictions, and medicine is kept available. The child who walks with a brace may have adapted physical education. However, if the child is also blind, some educators may immediately assume that she cannot achieve normally in any respect – an exaggeration which is unconscionable and in conflict with P.L. 94-142. Or, the student and her family may believe any and all problems are due to the various handicaps.

Michael is not so fortunate as Lori. He is barely able to walk, cannot control his hands well, and has a moderate hearing loss, in addition to blindness. Michael clearly needs a great deal of special help. Nevertheless, it should not be categorically assumed that Michael cannot do anything in a regular class at the usual pace.

EACH SITUATION IS DIFFERENT

Look for clear reasons whenever a child is not keeping up with his age group, and work hard to develop the abilities he has. Be sure that an expert in *each* disability is on the scene, working cooperatively with others. The "team approach" (with the parents always included) really shows its value with multiply handicapped children. Different specialists working alone can ruin one another's efforts. Two or more disabilities can interact in ways that may not be obvious without consultation. For example, the teacher of the blind may not realize that even mild cerebral palsy can cause much difficulty with typing. At the same time, the occupational therapist may not realize the importance of typing to a blind child, and may fail to explore ways to make it possible. If various specialists work closely with one another and with the parents, they can find an appropriate approach to each need.

Regardless of the severity of problems, expect progress and work toward it. Virtually everything in this *Handbook* (as well as in the companion books, *Your School Includes a Blind Student* and *A Resource Guide for Parents and Educators of Blind Children*) is applicable whether or not the child has other handicaps. Methods and ideas need merely to be adapted for the other disability.

Other chapters in this book explain that alternative techniques (methods which do not rely on sight at all) often are not taught to students who should have learned them. This problem may be even more common with multiply handicapped children. For example, children regarded as having low general ability are sometimes not taught Braille at all, even though they actually could benefit greatly from a vocabulary suited to their needs.

Carefully analyze priorities in working toward independence, and seek the best means available for meeting them.

When any child has a behavior or adjustment problem, it can be hard to determine the precise cause. If the child has one or more disabilities, it becomes especially complicated. Does Matt have tantrums because he is at the age of the "terrible two's," because of losing more sight, or because of the neglect he suffered before he was adopted? Does Elaine cry so easily because her heart medications need adjustment, because some classmates teased her about blindness, because of the tensions of the teen years, or for some other reason?

Knowledge about specific problems can be very helpful, but sometimes it is impossible to be sure of the cause(s). It is often best to deal with the behavioral difficulty and not worry about the cause. Whatever the cause may be, the student still needs to learn more appropriate behavior.

Beware of the tendency to blame everything on blindness. Because of public attitudes, parents and others tend to believe that blindness is more devastating than almost any other handicap. A typical result is the incorrect belief that the blind child with, say, mild mental disability, cannot succeed nearly as well as others with mild mental disability. Another common result is preoccupation with futile attempts to "develop" a very small amount of sight, to the detriment of alternative techniques and general skills which have much more potential.

Blindness and Physical Disabilities

A "physical disability" may be a problem so slight that it shows up only in certain sports, at one extreme, or near-total paralysis at the other extreme. This seems obvious, but is often ignored by unwise generalizations.

Mild orthopedic problems generally should be accommodated wherever the student would be otherwise. Consider these examples:

- A five-year-old has had surgery to straighten his foot. He has trouble running and climbing stairs. But none of this rules out his starting to use a long white cane. The cane is, in fact, increasing his confidence on stairs.
- A twelve-year-old uses leg braces and walks with difficulty. Her class schedule is arranged so that she need not walk a long distance in a short time. However, except for Adaptive Physical Education, no alterations are made in the classes themselves.
- A first grader has very little use of his right arm. He cannot read Braille with conventional two-handed motion. However, his teacher is helping him develop his own style, and he is moving right along in the *Patterns* books. His Perkins Brailler has the adaptation for one-handed use.

Any problems involving the hands will usually affect typing skill. Consult an occupational therapist. Adapted fingering patterns exist to accommodate missing or useless fingers. If a child with poor muscle control keeps striking unwanted letters, the occupational therapist can add a "keyboard shield," so that each key is in a small depression. Exercises can develop finger strength and coordination.

Although some physical disabilities affect how the hands move in reading Braille, general procedures usually need not be changed. As long as some fingers are usable, Braille can be learned. Do not assume, furthermore, that a physical disability necessarily slows down pacing – it depends on the individual. Even if the sense of touch is believed to be damaged, it may develop surprisingly well with constant practice.

Physical education is most often affected by a physical handicap. Work closely with the Adaptive P.E. specialist for the best arrangement of regular and/or modified activities. Don't let the student be left out of archery because the Adaptive P.E. teacher doesn't know about audible goal locators (devices which make a sound at the target or goal) and failed to consult you. Don't let the student be excluded from all running because you don't know how to teach him and *you* failed to ask for help. Also be sure everyone is using the same language – a bowling rail for the blind is totally different from the bowling aid for people in wheelchairs.

If the student can walk fairly well, and has the use of at least one hand, then he can learn to travel with a long white cane. A mild orthopedic handicap should have little effect on how quickly the student learns to travel well. Even some people who appear to have poor balance will walk better with a long white cane, as they no longer need to shuffle their feet and fear obstacles ahead. (Of course, the long white cane cannot actually improve balance as such.) A greater physical involvement may cause more difficulty, but need not rule out cane travel.

One student had an artificial leg. She blamed her inability to keep in step on that handicap, until the teacher explained that all students, with very few exceptions, have difficulty keeping in step at first. Once this was explained, the student mastered this aspect of travel as quickly as everyone else.

Even for people using wheelchairs, there is increasing use of white canes. One-handed steering of the chair is necessary, to leave the other hand free for the cane. A telescoping cane may be desirable for storage on the chair. Even limited independent mobility can be very important for employment and personal freedom.

Height may not be commonly thought of as a physical handicap, but it can be. Very short stature can prevent reaching drinking fountains, locker shelves, etc., and make it hard to find a suitable desk. As the student moves along in school he will have trouble with foot pedals in sewing, high tables in science, etc. Often a simple aid such as a footstool is sufficient. However, for extremely short stature a specialist (Adaptive P.E. teacher, physical therapist, etc.) should be consulted. He/she may have suggestions not readily thought of by others, and will lend weight to requests for special furniture. In the case of very tall stature, as occasionally occurs with early-maturing children, desk size is the main consideration.

With any extreme, give careful attention to the student's feeling of self-worth – teasing is common from other students and even adults. Note that abnormal growth hormones can cause early puberty, or delayed or incomplete puberty.

Blindness and Hearing Loss

A mild hearing loss need not keep a student from learning in essentially the usual ways. It is very important, however – even more so than for the sighted child with a mild hearing loss – that careful attention be given to the compensations he does need. When a sighted hard-of-hearing child (or a sighted child with normal hearing who is temporarily disadvantaged by poor acoustics) cannot hear the teacher well, he will nevertheless receive visual cues. The blind child who cannot hear the teacher well may be totally at a loss.

Work closely with the audiologist to examine the environment. Sometimes even a minor change in furnishings can make a great deal of difference. Especially helpful improvements include:

- Carpeting
- Acoustical ceiling tile
- Dropped ceiling
- Cork or other absorbent material on walls

If hearing aids are needed, urge that binaural hearing (in *both* ears together) be emphasized, even though this may mean two aids instead of one. Otherwise the child may hear a sound but not be able to tell where it is coming from – a disastrous problem for a blind child. Develop and use the hearing in each ear to the maximum extent possible. Also note that the type of aid called CROS (Contra Lateral Routing of Signals) makes it possible for one ear to hear sound as coming from two directions, thus encouraging sound localization.

Different hearing aids amplify particular frequencies to varying degrees. The importance of environmental sounds to a blind person may be relevant in the choice of an aid.

In some cases an "auditory trainer" (actually a specialized FM radio) may be worn by the child for greater amplification. Used with a special microphone worn by the classroom teacher, it helps eliminate extraneous noise. A switch selects reception for the teacher's microphone only, or reception for the classroom in general.

A hearing loss can make it difficult to orient oneself to traffic and other environmental sounds. It can interfere with using the sound of the tapping cane to locate doorways, parked cars, hallways, etc., as one passes them. Nevertheless, try to help your student develop these skills, rather than assuming it is impossible–perhaps it is possible to some extent. Also note that the identification aspect of a white cane is especially important.

Headphones may be helpful in listening to recorded material.

LEW NEEDED HELP

Lew was visually impaired; however the preschool teacher had said he could see all of their materials OK. He also had a hearing impairment, but his speech communication was good. It was expected that he would do well in regular kindergarten. However, he failed to learn the names of the alphabet letters, often ignored the teacher's directions, and generally had severe difficulty.

Ms. Pirtle, the itinerant teacher of the visually impaired, believed that not enough attention had been given to the hearing impairment. She insisted that a teacher of the hearing-impaired attend the spring IEP conference.

"I wonder if Lew should have a Phonic Ear," commented Ms. Pirtle (using the brand name for one kind of auditory trainer). "Sometimes we think he really doesn't hear the teacher's directions. And I wonder if he really hears the difference between the letter names *b*, *p*, *d*, and so on. His vision really isn't good enough to see gestures clearly or do any lip reading at all."

"We usually don't suggest a Phonic Ear for children with this much hearing," replied the teacher of the hearing-impaired. "But you may be right. Let's put it in the IEP as a trial arrangement."

In first grade with his Phonic Ear, Lew's achievement and adjustment improved rapidly. He quickly learned the letter names, now that he heard each one reliably. He no longer needed repeated explanations and reminders. Impressed with this improvement, the parents also decided to agree to include Braille in the next IEP; Lew had great difficulty seeing ink-print letters near the end of the day.

"I didn't realize," said the teacher of the hearing-impaired at the next meeting, "how much the low vision interfered with the compensations which other hearing-impaired children make almost automatically." Because Lew could see pictures and letters at close range, almost everyone had made this error. Lew himself, never having experienced good hearing, had no understanding of the problem. (If asked "Can you hear me?" he would usually answer "Yes," not realizing what he had been missing.)

DEAF-BLIND STUDENTS

If the student has very little hearing, and also little or no vision, a specialist in the education of the deaf-blind should be involved. Detail about the education of the deaf-blind is beyond the scope of this book. However, the importance of three key skills will be pointed out: Braille, typing, and mobility.

Braille is vital for all the usual reasons, plus several others. Talking books and live readers are not usable. It is difficult to keep up with the news when one cannot use the newspaper, radio, or TV; the American Brotherhood for the Blind publishes the *Hot Line for Deaf-Blind*, a weekly Braille newsmagazine.

Although manual sign language can be used by the blind (in a version contained within the hand of the listener), written language is essential for spelling, grammar, and precise meaning. Standard English may actually be a second language as compared to the sign language used.

Furthermore, for the deaf-blind Braille is a major channel for personal conversation. The Tellatouch, manufactured by the American Foundation for the Blind, enables almost anyone to communicate with a deaf-blind person. By using either the keys of a regular typing keyboard or keys like a Perkins Brailler, the "speaker" can raise pins to form Braille under the "listener's" fingertips. The Tellatouch is probably the most versatile and efficient communication aid for the deaf-blind. The keyboard can be used by almost anyone, with virtually no training necessary; the "listener" need only know standard Braille, or even just Grade I Braille; and the device is not extremely expensive.

Another device is a glove with the letters of the alphabet printed in locations which the wearer has memorized. The "speaker" touches letters in turn, to spell out a message.

Newer devices, much more complex and expensive, may enable conversation in either direction and even over the telephone.

In communicating with a sighted person who is not present, typing skill is valuable for the deaf-blind as well as others. In addition, the deaf-blind person whose speech is not easily understood will find a typewriter to be a handy, inexpensive way to communicate in person.

A person without sight and hearing may be limited in mobility. However, there is no reason why a deaf-blind person cannot use a cane at school, in the workplace, and elsewhere with appropriate arrangements.

General Health Problems

When a medical condition affects a student's general health, a primary problem is deciding how much to expect. Can tension bring on an attack or seizure? Does the health condition truly limit stamina or general ability? If so, how hard do we dare to press for achievement in school?

Solid decision-making is based on a clear medical statement from a doctor, usually with interpretation by the school nurse. Ask the nurse for *written*, specific guidelines, to be distributed to all teachers. (Example: One student was severely bothered by heat, but the school was not air conditioned. Every fall and spring there was much debate as to how much he could stand. The boy took advantage of this by avoiding assignments. Finally the nurse analyzed the temperature at which he began to have real trouble, and a thermometer was placed in each of his classrooms. When a room reached the problem level, the boy took his work to the air-conditioned office for that class period. On very hot days he worked at home. In no case was the boy excused from assignments.)

A policy of written guidelines also prevents phantom "diseases." One girl was thought to have mononucleosis, but actually was overdoing her musical activities. Another girl, after fully recovering from a severe infection, had to fight for years a reputation of being "sickly." Blind children, whom society tends to believe are frail anyway, are especially vulnerable to such misjudgments.

It is wise to check about food prohibitions for *all* students, especially those with health problems. Any child may have allergies. The diabetic child has a very strict regimen. Don't forget that small treats are "food" too.

The Emotionally Disturbed Child

Too often, the emotional problems of a blind or visually impaired person are blamed on the visual disability itself or on irrelevant factors, when the real problem is inadequate skills or incorrect assumptions about blindness.

Carol achieved excellent grades in high school, and received an award as an outstanding blind student. After graduation, however, she became more and more frightened at the prospect of college and a job. She became afraid to leave the house alone.

Carol talked with a psychiatrist, who believed that she had a "typical reaction to the trauma of blindness," and concentrated on helping her adjust to restricted circumstances. Later a second psychiatrist, while counseling Carol to build up her confidence, strongly urged her to attend the adult Orientation Center for the blind. Finally Carol agreed. She also joined the National Federation of the Blind and met successful blind people from all walks of life. Soon she was delighted with her improved practical skills, and came to realize that it is respectable to be blind. No longer feeling that blindness meant inferiority, Carol went on to college a few months later.

Carol's high school teachers had helped her to achieve well academically, but had not succeeded in teaching her real self-respect and confidence as a blind person.

Fortunately Carol lived in a state with an exceptionally good adult Orientation Center. In most states she would have received little positive help after high school. The National Federation of the Blind, however, provides a positive influence throughout the country.

Some blind children, of course, really do have emotional problems as such. Consult the psychologist or other expert if a student is destructive toward himself or others, loses or gains a great deal of weight without medical explanation, or has major behavioral changes (examples: increased withdrawal and avoidance of personal contact; increasing aggression; increased avoidance of responsibility; marked indifference to personal appearance or to things in general).

As with any other multiple disability, specialists must work together. The psychologist might be unaware of the real problems of blindness, just as you may not know how to treat serious depression.

When a blind child truly has psychological problems, it is no less important that he be taught good techniques and positive attitudes regarding blindness. He does not need the additional emotional burden of believing that blindness means inferiority. Whenever a blind child seems to have severe behavioral problems, always consider *all* of these possibilities:

(a) a true psychological disorder;
(b) low expectations due to an exaggerated view of the limitations of blindness;
(c) lack of skills (mobility, social interaction, etc.) or the opportunities to use them;
(d) two or more of these together.

Following are several examples of apparent psychological problems which turned out to be something else. In each case, if the described solution had not worked, psychological causes should have been investigated. (Caution: Often in such cases, the problem related to blindness is handled poorly, and a psychological cause is still wrongly assumed.)

- A seventh-grade girl seemed withdrawn, not talking with any of her classmates. A sympathetic classroom teacher found that she knew almost no one, and lacked experience in making friends. This teacher coached her in how to get acquainted. She also recruited three girls to go to lunch with her.
- A partially-sighted tenth grader refused to go shopping or walk to the pizza shop. If she did go out in public, she clung to someone's arm. "I'm afraid of crowds," she said, and the psychologist wondered if she had agoraphobia (extreme fear of open places). Finally her parents realized that the girl could not really tell the difference between a step-down and a mere change in pavement coloring. Also, they realized she really could not judge traffic motion. They insisted that the mobility teacher give her cane travel instruction with sleepshades, even though he had said this was unnecessary. After a few weeks the girl was shopping happily all over town, with new-found freedom and confidence.
- A third-grade boy continually poked and pushed his classmates. The counselor found that, like the seventh grade girl above, this boy did not know how to make friends. Also, some of the boys had teased him about his heavy glasses. The counselor included this student in group counseling, to help him make some real friends and to teach him social skills. This small group often

played together at recess, providing an additional opportunity for normal social interaction.

- An eighth grade girl, rather thin, never ate lunch at school. By 2:00 she was tired and listless. The nurse feared she had an eating disorder.
  "I'm just afraid I'll make a fool of myself," the girl finally confided. "Those school lunches have gravy and soup and whatever, and I know I'll make an awful mess. And don't tell me to bring a sack lunch. My mom doesn't have time to make one."
  The nurse arranged several sessions of eating hot lunch privately with coaching. She also helped the family teach the girl to pack her own sack lunch.
- "His behavior is bizarre," said the first-grade teacher. "He waves his arms in circles, just any old time. And he keeps poking his fingers in his eyes."
  The resource teacher explained that these habits, while very undesirable, are not unusual in blind children and may not mean psychological disturbance. The psychologist helped the teachers work out a behavior modification plan, with simple rewards for avoidance of these habits.
- An eleventh grade girl was very unhappy. Everyone assumed that this was because of losing more and more sight. Finally, however, her mother realized that the breakup with her first real boyfriend was the current crisis. Several heart-to-heart talks revived interest in school dances and other activities. At the same time, the counselor and the resource teacher re-examined the program of alternative techniques to cope with decreasing sight.
- A senior boy seemed deeply depressed. The psychologist found a strong fear of "spending life in a rocking chair," like an elderly blind neighbor.
  Although this boy had met some other blind people, he had never really talked with them about their jobs. It was arranged for him to visit two blind people at work, and to receive cassettes from Job Opportunities for the Blind. Soon he was happily examining several career choices at the Community College.
- "He must be autistic," said the kindergarten teacher. "If you leave him alone, all he does is whirl around and around."
  The itinerant teacher redoubled her efforts to teach the child cane travel for increased mobility. She urged the kindergarten teacher to correct him sternly whenever he started whirling. "If it's a class session, insist he sit down and pay attention, just as you would any other child. If it's free play, move him physically to something interesting, such as the clay table or the swing, and insist that he do something constructive."

"Pseudo-diagnosis" of supposed psychological problems is very common, due to the mistaken belief that blindness necessarily causes psychological difficulties, and due to inadequate teaching of techniques and skills. However, as with any student, a psychologist should be consulted if solutions such as those above do not work, or if the behavior is dangerous. Always consider also whether a medical condition (possibly undiagnosed) might be affecting behavior.

Can a Blind Student Also Have a Learning Disability?

Some students who are *not* visually impaired have a lower achievement level (in one or more areas) than their intelligence scores would lead us to expect. If there is a standard deviation of difference between the student's IQ score and his achievement, in any of several areas, that student is considered to be "learning disabled." Funding for special educational services is made available under this label.

Some students who *are* visually impaired also have a lower achievement level (in one or more areas) than their intelligence scores would lead us to expect. Yet regulations generally do not permit such a student to be served under the label of "learning disability." Nevertheless, it is possible to provide the program which the student needs.

Federal and state regulations designate which category a student's education should be *funded under.* The designation of "visually impaired" requires that funding be obtained under that name; but it does *not* prevent the provision of services appropriate for a learning disability. In other words, the student is given the services she needs, but they are funded on the basis of visual impairment.

It may be wise to get help from a teacher who has special training in working with the learning disabled. If that teacher already works with various categories of students, there should be no problem. If that teacher is presently assigned only to students whose funding is on the basis of Learning Disability, it may be necessary to apply for an exception.

If the visual impairment is so slight as not to be "educationally significant," the regulations may indeed allow funding under the designation of Learning Disability.

Remember that this kind of problem is not the same as mental disability, in which the IQ score and achievement are lowered to essentially the same degree.

Also remember that lack of opportunity can make a student appear more disabled than she really is. For example, a student who never goes shopping will naturally have difficulty understanding financial transactions. As another example, some students with partial sight spend so much effort trying to see printed matter that they have no energy left for comprehension; with the opportunity to use Braille, the apparent "learning disability" disappears.

Mental Disability

MILD MENTAL DISABILITY

Most students classified as "mildly mentally disabled" can lead an essentially normal life, and do not appear obviously "different." Regular social interaction and integration into some regular classes are appropriate. Modification is usually necessary for heavily academic work.

For the older student, emphasis is placed on vocational skills for appropriate jobs. Often high school students have a part-time job in the community, with school supervision–restaurant work, farm work, cleaning, stocking shelves, etc. These students reasonably expect to marry, to raise families, and to hold jobs in competitive employment at a level appropriate to their ability. In short, they blend into the general population.

Mild mental disability is generally defined by a score of 55 to 70 on an intelligence test. Those scoring slightly above this are often called "slow learners" and may need somewhat similar help.

There is no reason why mildly mentally disabled blind students cannot learn the same alternative techniques as others–Braille, cane travel, typing, abacus, etc. Extra explanation, practice, and repetition may be needed, but basically the education of a mildly mentally disabled blind student is similar to that for others.

The chapter on multiple handicaps in *A Resource Guide for Parents and Educators of Blind Children* (also by Doris Willoughby) includes a description of mislabeling–a common problem. Sara had always been regarded as mentally disabled. However, when a new itinerant teacher started an assertive program of alternative techniques (despite previous assumptions that Sara "could not benefit from them" because of retardation, or "did not need them" because she had some vision), Sara bloomed. By graduation, it was obviously doubtful whether Sara really was mentally disabled at all.

Blindness aside, there is much controversy as to whether intelligence tests really measure general ability. For blind students there are additional problems with such tests, as discussed in the chapter on testing. As provided in P.L. 94-142, no single test should be used to classify a student. Use more than one measure, including general behavior and achievement.

MODERATE MENTAL DISABILITY

This degree of disability is generally defined by a score of 40-55 on an intelligence test. These students have difficulty with social conventions and life skills, and have very low ability for academic work. The student generally can learn to dress himself, eat normally, and handle most self-help skills, but some supervision will probably always be needed. (For example, a person may learn to dress himself and to do laundry, but not be able to handle repairing or replacing garments.)

Typically, moderately mentally disabled persons achieve partial self-support in sheltered employment. Some, however, do hold regular competitive jobs.

Many blind students with this degree of disability read Braille with a limited vocabulary, just as their sighted counterparts do in print. If there is uncertainty whether reading instruction is appropriate, a good indicator is the degree to which the student can grasp concepts. Can he make comparisons? Draw conclusions? Carry on a logical conversation? If it seems at all reasonable, reading instruction should be attempted. Even a few symbols can be useful for labeling, for simple messages, etc.

For prereading skills, provide materials similar to those used with preschool children. If the student is really beginning to read, someone who knows Braille should work directly with him.

Most moderately disabled persons are able to learn cane travel, sometimes doing better than one might expect. Without a cane, the person is more limited than is really necessary.

For older students, independent living skills and vocational education are emphasized. Instruct the student and/or his teacher in alternative techniques for such things as:

- Personal cleanliness
- Cooking
- Laundry and very simple mending
- Housecleaning
- Shopping
- Industrial janitor work
- Sorting and assembling
- Collating, stapling, etc. (You may need to explain techniques for keeping track of which papers are which. They may be boxed, labeled, kept in a certain place, etc.)

The role of the resource/itinerant teacher of the blind will depend on the student's age and individual abilities. If a skill such as cane travel or Braille is being intensively taught, you would work directly with the student. But if much repetitive practice is needed, someone else will probably help in between your lessons. Often you will mainly provide information to other teachers and to the family.

SEVERE/PROFOUND MENTAL DISABILITY

These students have intelligence scores of under 40. Many will never walk. A sheltered living situation will be needed in adulthood.

Lessons for a Severely/Profoundly Handicapped Student

When a student is mildly mentally handicapped, working with him is basically the same as with others, but at a slower pace. Working with a school-aged student who is moderately handicapped is much like working with a preschooler or kindergartner, though there usually are complicating problems. But when a teacher is first asked to work with a severely/profoundly handicapped individual, it may be very hard to imagine how to proceed. This chapter will offer a number of suggestions.

Unless you are employed by a special school, your role probably will not usually include direct instruction. Daily contact is necessary to achieve rapport. Progress occurs at a pace so slow as to be outside many teachers' experience. "Academic" work is not appropriate. For these reasons the itinerant/resource teacher of the blind will most often provide suggestions and materials. But in order to do this, one must understand what the program for such a student is like.

"Why is it so important for that boy to shake a rattle?" I once asked a friend who worked at the State Hospital-School. "Is his hand coordination so poor?"

"That is part of it," she replied. "He can't do much with his hands yet. But our main goal on this is to get him to *sit at a table.* If we can get him to sit up and rattle something, then he'll be in a normal position instead of sprawled. This will also help him hold his head up. And if he gets used to really sitting at the table, consider all the things that can lead to – eating more normally, putting objects in containers, even starting to work a simple puzzle."

My friend was helping me think about early developmental skills. It can be hard to think in those terms when the chronological age is 12.

Following are some typical skills which (with much more specific wording) may be in the IEP:

- Turn head toward something interesting
- Reach for an object on command
- Recognize familiar objects
- Distinguish between colors
- Roll a ball
- Place a ball in a box
- Follow a simple command, such as "Stand up"
- Wash hands
- Wash face

For the severely/profoundly handicapped student, it is necessary to break skills down into very small steps, each of which must be taught by much repetition. Consider a sequence for a student learning to wash her face:

(1) Reach for washcloth

(2) Pick up washcloth

(3) Find faucet

(4) Turn on water

(5) Hold washcloth under water

(6) Wring or squeeze cloth

(7) Put cloth to face

(8) Move cloth around on face

This sequence actually is only a part of the procedure, because after each new step is learned, all steps to that point must be practiced before adding another. Also, the above sequence does not include soap. That may need to begin with "Examine soap and understand it is not to be eaten."

Teaching a severely/profoundly handicapped student to wash her face, with daily lessons, can easily take many months.

Most Blind Students Do Not Need This

Breaking a task down into small steps, as above, is necessary for students who have great difficulty. To a lesser extent, breaking a task into smaller steps is also done routinely by all teachers.

Blindness in itself does not require more of this kind of thing than is necessary for sighted students. However, unfortunately, some publications seem to make that very assumption. For example, *A Step-By-Step Guide to Personal Management for Blind Persons*[1] gives incredibly detailed directions for taking a bath – e.g., "As towel gets damp, shift to a dry section." This widely-circulated book ought to be entitled:

> *A Step-By-Step Guide to Personal Management, for Blind Persons With Special Learning Problems*

Its text should carefully explain that such detailed help is *not* needed for the vast majority of blind persons. In this way the book could be helpful for those who really need it, without

[1]American Foundation for the Blind. *A Step-By-Step Guide to Personal Management for Blind Persons.* New York, NY: American Foundation for the Blind, 1974.

encouraging the false belief that *all* blind persons are unable to follow ordinary directions or grasp general concepts.

In *To Man the Barricades* (see "References"), Kenneth Jernigan explains in detail the severe damage caused by the assumption that all blind people need the help which is appropriate for those who learn very slowly.

Helping Teachers Make Lessons Appropriate

In teaching a skill to a severely/profoundly handicapped student, it is usually necessary to move the student through it physically many times, gradually giving less and less help. For example, at first the teacher might hold the student's fingers on the washcloth and raise the student's arm to the face; later the teacher might just touch the fingers and raise the child's arms slightly as a reminder. This is called "physical prompting" and is especially important with a blind student.

Emphasis should be on skills for functioning as independently as possible in an appropriate (very sheltered) environment.

You may need to provide ideas for alternative techniques, and to help teachers realize that planning for a blind student is basically the same as planning for other students. Ask, "What is she doing now?" and "What would you be doing if she were sighted?" Teachers of the mentally disabled will know what is appropriate for each developmental level, and how to break things down into small steps. After some consultation and experience, they will usually be able to plan their own modifications for a blind student. Give plenty of encouragement and compliments for the teachers' work.

Let us return to the list of typical skills and note how they can easily be made appropriate for a blind child:

- Turn head toward something interesting: Use an interesting sound. If there is some sight, sometimes use a flashing light or a bright-colored shiny surface.
- Reach for an object on command: Associate a sound with the object, or use something very bright if that is appropriate.
- Recognize familiar objects: Make sure the objects are consistent and easily distinguished tactually.
- Distinguish colors: If the child has quite a bit of sight, this may be achieved with bright, clear colors. Distinguishing textures is an appropriate alternative.
- Roll a ball: Use a ball that makes a sound. Provide plenty of appropriate feedback (for example, the teacher might clap his hands when the child rolls the ball a certain distance.)
- Place a ball in a box: Use a stable container that will not move around easily. Help the child to examine the ball and the container with her hands, before she tries to put the ball in.
- Follow a simple command, such as "Stand up:" Use physical prompting.
- Wash hands or face: Washcloth, soap, faucet, etc., can all be found by touch. It is helpful if (at least at first) such things are always in the same place in relation to the student. Help the student examine and understand each thing (including the water itself) before starting to work on what to do with it. For example, help her to turn on the faucet with one hand while her other hand is underneath, so that she feels the stream come on.

KEEPING VISION IN PERSPECTIVE

Avoid being pushed into overemphasizing "visual development." On the one hand, especially with the younger child, it may be hard to tell how much he really can see, and therefore some effort to "develop the use of his sight" may be warranted. On the other hand, parents and teachers often overdo the visual emphasis, in a futile attempt to improve vision that is not really there, and with the erroneous idea that better vision would bring better general ability.

Encourage everyone to note what (if anything) interests the child visually. Will he turn toward a light? Does he respond to the general room lighting being turned on or off? To a flashlight? To shiny surfaces? To blinking lights? To lights of certain colors? Red and green are often favored. Also, "black light" may be especially effective (a kind of ultraviolet light which cannot itself be seen by the human eye, but which can give interesting fluorescent effects).

[*Caution: Some lighting effects, especially blinking lights, may bring on seizures in certain children.*]

If the developmental level is early infancy, remember that development of the use of vision will not exceed mental and physiological development.

For a child with very low awareness, it may help to "pair" something visual with something else to which the child already responds, and gradually encourage the child to notice the visual attraction alone. For example, if the child already responds to music, a bright red ball might be shown each time the music is started. This may help the child learn to respond just to seeing the ball.)

Keep vision in perspective by working to develop *all* senses. This approach helps to determine the child's general ability as well as his visual ability. Emphasize the integration of senses–that is, how the senses work together. Any child with useful sight (including the fully sighted) requires practice in order to know what visual information means. After he has felt a ball many times, he comes to understand when his eyes are seeing a round object.

Following are a few typical activities which help develop the sense of touch, smell, and/or taste, along with vision if it is present:

- Peanut butter is placed on the fingertip and may be licked off.
- The child examines various textures (velvet, corduroy, hay, feathers, etc.) and gently rubs his arms and legs with each.
- Corn starch is moistened to form a ball with interesting characteristics. When held in the hand it melts, but upon leaving the hand it coagulates again.
- Water play has endless possibilities.

Conclusion

"What kind of educational setting does this student need?" In answering this question, carefully consider which disability most affects education as a whole. If mental ability is essentially normal, the regular curriculum is appropriate, with only as much special help as is genuinely needed. If the student is severely mentally handicapped, then the mental disability and not the blindness is most relevant; a setting appropriate for severely mentally disabled students is preferable to one for merely blind children.

Placement should always be decided on an individual basis, however. Rigid categories are not an appropriate way to plan education.

The following chapters in this book are especially relevant for students with more than one disability: "Early Childhood," "Orientation and Mobility (Under Age 8 and Special Problems)," "Teaching Braille (Second Grade and Below)," "Dealing With Medical Matters," "Placement Options and Decisions," and "Working With Other Agencies and Organizations." See also "References."

Many people with multiple handicaps complete their education, raise families, and succeed in the vocations of their choice. Treat each student as an individual, emphasizing the strengths he has, and not permitting him to be regarded only as part of a vague lump called "the multiply handicapped."

CHAPTER 13

BRAILLE
WHAT IS IT?
WHAT DOES IT MEAN TO THE BLIND?

National Federation of the Blind

1	2	3	4	5	6	7	8	9	0
a	b	c	d	e	f	g	h	i	j
k	l	m	n	o	p	q	r	s	t
u	v	w	x	y	z				

Braille is a system of reading and writing by touch used by the blind. It consists of arrangements of dots which make up letters of the alphabet, numbers and punctuation marks. The basic Braille symbol is called the Braille cell and consists of six dots arranged in the formation of a rectangle, three dots high and two across. Other symbols consist of only some of these six dots. The six dots are commonly referred to by number according to their position in the cell:

There are no different symbols for capital letters in Braille. Capitalization is accomplished by placing a dot 6 in the cell just before the letter that is capitalized.

The first ten letters of the alphabet are used to make numbers. These are preceded by a number sign which is dots 3-4-5-6:

Thus, 1 is number sign *a*; 2 is number sign *b*; 10 is number sign *a-j* and 193 is number sign *a-i-c*:

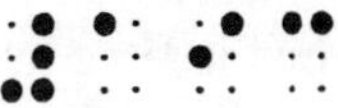

Some abbreviations are used in standard American Braille in order to reduce its bulk. These must be memorized, but most Braille readers and writers find them convenient, rather than a problem. Braille is written on heavy paper, and the raised dots prevent the pages from lying smoothly together as they would in a print book. Therefore, Braille books are quite bulky.

There are two methods of writing Braille, just as there are two methods of writing print. A Braille writing machine (comparable to a typewriter) has a keyboard of only six keys and a space bar, instead of one key for each letter of the alphabet. These keys can be pushed separately or all together. If they are all pushed at the same time they will cause six dots to be raised on the paper in the formation of a Braille cell. Pushing various combinations of the keys on the Braille writer produces different letters of the alphabet and other Braille symbols.

Writing Braille with a slate and stylus compares to writing print with a pen or pencil. The stylus is used to push dots down through the paper, while the slate serves as a guide. The Braille slate can be made of metal or plastic and is hinged so that there is a guide under the paper and on top of it. A person writing Braille with the slate and stylus begins at the right side of the paper and ends the line on the left, since the dots are being produced on the underside of the paper. Of course, the Braille reader reads from left to right, for the dots are then on the top side of the paper. Although this may seem a bit confusing, it need not be at all troublesome, since both reading and writing progress through words and sentences from beginning to end in the same manner. The speed of writing Braille with the slate and stylus is about the same as the speed of writing print with pen or pencil.

Braille was first developed about 1820 by a young Frenchman named Louis Braille. He created Braille by modifying a system of night writing which was intended for use on board ships. He did this work as a very young man and had it complete by the time he was about 18. He and his friends at the school for the blind he attended found that reading and writing dots was much faster than reading raised print letters which could not be written by hand at all. The development of this system by young Louis Braille is now recognized as the most important single development in making it possible for the blind to get a good education.

It took more than a century, however, before people would accept Braille as an excellent way for the blind to read and write. Even today many people underestimate the effectiveness of Braille. While tapes and records are enjoyable, Braille is essential for note-taking and helpful for studying such things as math, spelling and foreign languages. It is a matter of great concern to members of the National Federation of the Blind that fewer blind people now have the opportunity to become good Braille users than twenty-five years ago.

Why is this? Many professionals in work with the blind stress recorded media with blind children. Many persons who become blind do so in old age and are not encouraged to spend the time and make the effort needed to develop the new reading and writing skills that depend on feeling rather than seeing. There are even Braille teachers who do not expect speed and accuracy of blind students. The students then learn Braille as a chore and a drudgery.

Experienced Braille readers, however, read Braille at speeds comparable to print readers–200 to 400 words a minute. Such Braille readers say that the only limitation of Braille is that there isn't enough material available. They want more books produced by Braille presses, more books produced by volunteer Braillists in their homes and more advances in the computerized production of Braille.

One of the goals of the National Federation of the Blind is to help people appreciate Braille for the efficient system it is. The main difference between print and Braille is simply that print is meant to be read with the eyes, while Braille is meant to be read with the fingertips. Fingers feel dots quickly and accurately; eyes see loops and lines of ink. In both cases it is the brain that processes and reacts to the raw data sent to it by the fingers or the eyes.

This article was first written in Braille and transcribed into print to answer the questions of sighted people who cannot read Braille.

If you have further questions about Braille or blindness, write to the:

National Federation of the Blind
1800 Johnson Street
Baltimore, MD 21230

[*The above article is reprinted from the paper by the same title, also published by the National Federation of the Blind.*]

CHAPTER 14

BRAILLE:
WHAT IS IT?

Inserted just before this chapter is a reprint of a paper previously published by the National Federation of the Blind, giving a general description of the Braille system.

Literary Braille and Its "Grades"

There is a Braille symbol for each letter, numeral, and mark of punctuation. For certain special purposes, only the individual letters are used, with no short forms or contractions. This is called "Grade I Braille." The experienced Braille reader finds this a slow way of reading, and expects to find it only in special situations–notably spelling lists and dictionary entries–where there is a real reason for spelling out each individual word.

In addition, there are 190 signs which represent combinations of letters (e.g., *and* or *tion*). The use of these signs is called "Grade II Braille." The Grade designation has nothing to do with school grade level; Grade II Braille is used for the youngest children and for adults. Almost all Braille books and magazines use Grade II. The short forms and contractions save space and increase the speed of reading and writing; usage is governed by detailed rules.

Grade III Braille has many more contracted forms than does regular Grade II. It is used by college students and others for fast note-taking. (See the article by Sharon L. M. Duffy, listed in "References.") Books or magazines are *not* transcribed in Grade III.

Braille Shorthand, an even more highly contracted form, also exists. However, it is rarely used today.

Position and Context

Consider what a circle symbolizes in inkprint. It can be a capital O, a lower-case o, or a zero. It can be a degree sign. On a large poster, it might even be the dot of a fancy lower-case *i* or *j*, or a rather decorative "period." The experienced reader of inkprint does not find this confusing (in fact, rarely even thinks about it), but instead uses context, size, and positioning as clues to meaning.

The experienced Braille reader does the same kind of thing. The shape of the letter *d* is a good example (two dots across, and one dot underneath on the right). With a capital dot (dot 6) in the preceding cell, this shape becomes a capital *D*. With a number sign in the preceding cell, it becomes a *4*. At the end of a word, in a lowered position, this shape signifies a period. In other positions and other contexts, it means other things. The experienced Braille reader assumes all this and rarely even thinks about it. One factor which varies in inkprint, however, never varies in normal Braille: the *size* of the Braille cell and of the individual dot is always the same.

Related Chapters

Braille is discussed throughout this *Handbook*. The chapters which immediately follow this one, especially, offer detailed suggestions and comments.

Scope of This Handbook

A mere list of the Braille symbols is not sufficient as a guide for Braille transcription. Detailed rules of usage govern when each form should be used. Such explanation is beyond the scope of this book.

Following is an example of a rule of Braille usage (somewhat simplified): Whole-word "lower signs" (signs which appear in the lower two-thirds of the cell) may *not* be used when they are in contact with a mark of punctuation. (They may, however, be in contact with the Braille capital sign or italic sign.) For example, the word *his* uses dots 2-3-6, and thus is a "lower sign." In a sentence such as

The book is his.

the special symbol for *his* cannot be used. Instead, the three separate letters must be used with the period.

In discussing Braille rules and the teaching of Braille, this *Handbook* assumes that other sources are available for full explanation–notably the following. (See also the "References" section of this *Handbook* for complete bibliographical information.)

- *Instruction Manual for Braille Transcribing*
- *English Braille, American Edition*
- *Code of Braille Textbook Formats and Techniques*

Specialized Braille Codes

Anything which can be written with regular inkprint symbols can be written in Braille. Commonly-used specialized Braille codes are:

- *The Nemeth Code for Mathematics and Science Notation*
- *An Introduction to Braille Mathematics*
- *Introduction to Braille Music Transcription*
- *Code for Computer Braille Notation*
- *Manual on Foreign Languages to Aid Braille Transcribers*

CHAPTER 15

BRAILLE: WHY OR WHY NOT

"I'm angry that I wasn't taught Braille as a child.... Because I had some sight, I was forced to read print, but I could never read at the speed of the fully sighted students in my classes. Reading was such a chore and even though I liked to read, I stuck mainly to shorter magazine articles. I remember launching into Betty Smith's *A Tree Grows in Brooklyn;* after ten pages, I gave up. It was just too much."

We frequently encounter this – slightly sighted people not being taught Braille. They are told, "You should read print, Braille is too slow." But because of their reduced vision, they can never achieve speed in reading. In fact, reading Braille is not slow. It becomes a self-fulfilling prophecy when Braille is equated with slowness and inferiority. How many sighted people would ever have built up speed reading print if all they ever heard was how difficult and slow reading was? If Braille were taught as a reading skill in the same fashion as print, you would find no difference in reading speed abilities....

A partially blind person can...experience physical trauma when reading print – upper arm, back and neck strain are common complaints. Holding a book close to the eyes or bending and stretching the head down to the book can all lead to discomfort. Blind people who use print while making presentations before groups find it difficult to follow their notes while still facing the audience directly.

Braille, on the other hand, involves no real physical stress or awkward positions. And when making presentations, Braille allows the speaker to look out at the audience and speak much more naturally and effectively.

The above paragraphs are excerpted from "Braille for the Slightly Sighted," an article by Joyce Scanlan in the January-February, 1984, *Future Reflections.*

Many blind people read Braille at speeds of several hundred words per minute with good comprehension. (Ask the NFB to arrange personal contact with some of these people if this is new to you.) Others read Braille at an adequate speed of around 200 wpm. Others read Braille slowly and with difficulty.

Many fully sighted people read print at speeds of several hundred wpm with good comprehension; others read at an average, adequate speed of around 200 wpm; other fully sighted people read slowly and with difficulty.

What Is Our Real Goal?

Often we hear it said, "Sue can use print, but Jennifer has to use Braille." What if Jennifer, learning Braille well in spite of some negative attitudes in the atmosphere, reads easily at 250 wpm? Suppose that Sue, who has been taught to read large print laboriously with her eyes two inches from the paper, can barely manage 50 wpm, and that only for limited periods. Would it not be more accurate to say, "Jennifer can use Braille, but Sue has to use print"? For if Sue had been allowed the privilege of learning Braille (and it is a privilege – a valuable one which is often denied because of outmoded ideas), she too would probably be reading comfortably at a competitive speed. Sue "has to" use print only because misguided persons have pushed it upon her as a mainstay rather than a supplementary skill. To say that Jennifer "has to" read Braille is to take a valuable skill and label it as a last resort. In fact, learning Braille is not only a privilege but a *right* to which a student should be entitled for a good education. Carla was a good student, but reading print was slow and laborious. Her teachers "saw no need for Braille." It took Carla five years to complete a regular college course, since she had no way to read quickly or to take efficient notes.

Teaching Braille need *not* imply that the person should never, under any circumstances, read print. Many good Braille readers read print when it happens to be more convenient. However, *not* teaching Braille *does* indeed cut out an option: a person who does not know Braille cannot use it, however convenient it might have been.

The older student who learns Braille can obviously retain print-reading skills as long as enough vision is present. However, when a young beginner with low vision learns Braille from the start, the question is often raised: "She should know how to read print, even if it is useful only for short things. How will we fit print reading into the curriculum?"

It usually is not necessary to make any particular arrangements. The student will learn print reading almost by osmosis. We are surrounded by print of varying sizes – on cereal boxes, magazine covers, book covers, etc. Even if the child cannot see any standard print, he will find large letters and ask what they say. In school it will sometimes be handier to provide certain materials in large print (even feltpen letters) rather than in Braille. Most words are spelled the same, and he will eventually learn the full spelling even of the special words.

Recently I watched a six-year-old child read beginning Braille comfortably, with good comprehension and at a speed appropriate for a beginner. Later that day the same child was asked to read from a Closed Circuit Television (CCTV) screen. It was painful to watch as he struggled to keep his face at just the right distance to puzzle out the large lighted letters. He did pronounce words, although slowly, but had no energy left for comprehension or interpretation. How can any reasonable person claim that straining to make out individual letters, at a slow speed and in an uncomfortable position, is preferable to reading Braille comfortably and quickly? The CCTV may be helpful for reading relatively short passages when another alternative is less available. But how can it be claimed that the CCTV is a "better" method to be relied upon to the exclusion of Braille?

A prominent professor states that the average speed of print readers with low vision is 50 wpm, and that the average Braille speed is 90-150 wpm. Even with these figures for Braille speed, which are inaccurately low, the difference in efficiency is obvious. Yet this professor declared adamantly that print reading is much better for people with this amount of vision.

Why the Misplaced Emphasis?

There are many reasons for this overemphasis on the use of sight. One is genuine ignorance of the value and potential of a given alternative technique. For example, certain well-publicized studies have reported "average" Braille reading speeds even lower than those quoted by the professor above. But these studies are always done with a particular group of readers – usually those from residential schools, those who have not been reading Braille very long, and those who have been led to expect only minimal speed.

It is wrong to conclude that these "average" speeds, however accurate in regard to a certain group at a certain time, must be typical. Why not seek out more and better ways to improve reading speed and comprehension? Why not conduct more surveys and speed tests among strong students who have been taught truly positive attitudes and methods? With proper training and practice, most people can learn to read and write Braille at a speed which is appropriate and competitive in school and on the job. Moreover, even those who never do develop good speed will find Braille very useful; after all, sighted students are still taught to read even if they are slow.

An even deeper problem is the mistaken belief that a technique is necessarily better *just because it uses vision.* Instead of merely asking, "Can this student possibly read print?" we should also ask, "What mode of reading is likely to be most efficient?" *Efficiency* is the key to real success. To make a comparison: We generally expect visually impaired students to learn and use typing, especially for long assignments. Spending long hours working on handwriting that may be barely legible is not very efficient. If reading print is equally laborious, we should encourage Braille as a more efficient medium.

Very few books are published in large print as compared with those in Braille. Large print is generally not available at all for college texts. But even when large print is available, most students who use it read so badly that they would be far better off in Braille.

Why not use tapes? For some students they are faster to read, and often are more available than Braille.

Again, if a person learns Braille he is not prevented from using tapes when they are more convenient; but if he does not learn Braille he cannot ever use it. In many situations it is highly desirable to have things written on paper – mathematics, recipes, foreign languages, addresses, etc. In Braille one can skip almost instantly to another paragraph, item, or page – a process which is very time-consuming with tape. Furthermore, a skilled Braille reader reads much faster than is possible with tape. And general literacy (including spelling, grammar, etc.) is best developed by reading, not by listening to tapes.

One girl, forced to read print until she entered high school, had always been a poor speller. When the new resource teacher taught her Braille, her spelling ability shot up rapidly. "Oh, so *that's* how it's spelled!" she exclaimed frequently as she read along. "Now I really see the words!"

Common Misunderstandings

Some people misunderstand the enlightened approach of seeking the most efficient technique, especially the use of Braille by persons with low vision. Some people say that this philosophy forces people to be blind when they are not, and that it opposes any use of vision.

In actuality, the philosophy brought out in this book encourages the use of vision whenever it really is the best method.

In regard to "forcing people to be blind," the question actually is how the individual's blindness will be handled. Let us take the example of a person who can read large print at only 70 words per minute (much slower than the speed of speech). Let us assume that his vision cannot be improved medically, and that the slow speed is strictly because he cannot see the material any faster – not because he has trouble understanding the words. If this person relies on print as his main mode of reading, he will always be at an immense disadvantage because of reading so much more slowly than other people. He is not any less blind because of relying on print; but he is much less successful. In contrast, the competent Braille reader (with proper training and attitudes) can read at several hundred words a minute, and thus read as well and as fast as others.

If we believe that Braille is typically read only slowly, we will accept 90 wpm as the norm, and we will not use the speed exercises and other methods which are routine for sighted students. If we perceive slate writing as very difficult "mirror writing," we will introduce it in a gingerly way, and delay it past the time when an eager younger student would have found it fun and challenging. If a retarded student is capable of learning only a limited vocabulary, and we believe that "Braille is so much more difficult," we will hold back and teach him no vocabulary at all. When we approach Braille in these ways, our students *do* turn out to be slow and hesitant, thus producing more "statistics" which seem to show that Braille is slow and difficult. Keep your students out of this vicious circle.

In her article, "I Remember" (see "References"), Mary Ellen Halvorsen says:

> I had to put my face right down on the page and even then, I could only read several letters at a time. I can remember spending three hours trying to read a chemistry chapter in a large print book one evening. I imagine my fellow students read and studied the chapter in thirty minutes. Although we didn't realize it at the time, Braille would have been much more efficient and faster for me to use. Braille is not an inferior reading system, and can be easily learned.

A MISINTERPRETATION OF P.L. 94-142

Public Law 94-142 (see the chapter on "The Law") requires placement in the "Least Restrictive Environment" (that is, the most nearly "regular" placement) appropriate for each individual student. This is sometimes misinterpreted to mean that "regular" materials (e.g., inkprint) are categorically better than "special" materials (e.g., Braille). This misinterpretation persists even when students limp along slowly, unnecessarily handicapped by inappropriate methods and materials.

Transcribed materials, special equipment, and the lessons necessary for proper use, do "set the student apart" to a degree. But these special arrangements enable the student to function *normally* instead of limping along, so that in the long run he/she will be *less* set apart.

The law requires the least restrictive environment *appropriate* for a given student. It does not require pushing a student into "regular" materials when they are not suitable.

How to Decide?

THE MEDICAL REPORT

A first step always is to obtain a doctor's statement about the eye condition.

Many excellent references are available to help in interpreting the doctor's report. Enlist the help of the school nurse also. Even though you may be well informed about certain eye conditions, the nurse will have medical background which you do not. Comments on a medical subject will bear more weight if the nurse participates. (The nurse may also resent it if she is excluded.)

ASSESSMENT OF FUNCTIONAL VISION

The doctor's medical report is only a part of the picture. It is important to evaluate what the student can and cannot do well by using vision in *practical,* day-to-day situations. This is called an "assessment of functional vision," or "educational evaluation–vision." This important procedure, which typically is the responsibility of the resource/itinerant teacher, is discussed in the chapter, "Assessment of Functional Vision."

MEDICINE vs. EDUCATION

Correlating the doctor's report with educational needs is not always easy.

"Visual acuity with best correction" is of surprisingly little help in determining optimum reading mode. With the very young or multiply handicapped, the doctor may say that acuity cannot be determined. Moreover, typical eye charts are constructed so that figures of 20/100 or lower tend to be very broad categories–i.e., while the next lower acuity reading after 20/20 is usually 20/30, the next lower after 20/200 is often 20/400. For this and other reasons, an acuity figure of, say, 20/200 is only minimally helpful in indicating what the individual can do with his or her vision. A few people with 20/200 vision can read small print with ease; many can read small print to some extent; others cannot read even large print.

Often the acuity given is only for distance vision, which may be quite different from near-point acuity. Other important factors include nystagmus (continuous involuntary movements of the eye); pain; and fluctuations of vision. Braille should always be considered when corrected vision is as low as 20/200.

Furthermore, even when acuity is reported as better than 20/200, other factors may make Braille advisable. With conditions such as retinitis pigmentosa, a person may have excellent vision within a narrow field only ("tunnel vision"). He may see only part of a word at a time–hardly an efficient way to read. Also, if the doctor checks distance vision only, this may not accurately reflect difficulties at nearpoint. Problems such as nystagmus, light sensitivity, or "floaters" (particles moving across the visual field), interfering with the visual acuity which theoretically is there, may make reading laborious or erratic.

Remember that the doctor's eye test had controlled lighting; probably did not occur at the end of the day; took only a few minutes; and in most cases involved only isolated letters rather than connected text. Many persons can read very small print for a few minutes under such conditions, but cannot possibly read an entire book. Eye doctors often fail to realize these discrepancies.

A particularly touchy situation occurs when a doctor seems not to be as frank as he should be. One of my students had one retinal detachment after another; several operations with little success; almost no vision in one eye and a restricted field in the other; and glaucoma. Yet her doctor kept saying he "could not predict" how her vision would be in the future. Another doctor always told the family that the child's vision was "stable;" yet the boy had macular degeneration, and records showed a progression of 20/70 to 20/100 to 20/200. Doctors may also keep vaguely promising better operations and better lenses in the future, discouraging parents from accepting alternative techniques.

Visual acuity is sometimes given in terms such as "20/40 at two inches." Such a figure is not at all the same as the plain "20/40," which is assumed to be at a standard distance. This can be very confusing and misleading.

The chapters on "Medical Matters" and "The Partially-Sighted Child" discuss medical evaluation and terminology in greater detail.

The relationship between strength of correction and size of visual field deserves special emphasis. Doctors virtually never explain this, and its importance is rarely understood. **The higher the correction, the smaller the field.** With conventional glasses, the restricted field is usually most relevant to activities involving the whole body, though it can also affect reading. But the powerful lenses usually called "low vision aids" frequently restrict the field to a size totally unsatisfactory for regular reading–only a word or two at a time, or only a few letters at a time. Also, the aid must be moved back and forth, a tiring task which prevents real speed.

A Closed-Circuit Television (CCTV) machine, which displays lighted letters on a screen, has these same problems. Again, only part of a line is seen at a time. The reading matter itself (on a movable platform) must be moved back and forth in a precise pattern. Such aids can be very useful for shorter items, especially for the older student, but are incredibly restricting if relied upon as a main reading mode. Using them is not really "reading," but only "making out letters and words."

Furthermore, true literacy consists just as much of *writing* as reading. However, writing down class notes, phone numbers, appointments, etc., becomes impractical when a complicated machine is the only means for reading them.

Factors Which Point Toward Braille

Does the student read very slowly in print, not because of reading ability, but simply because he cannot see it any faster?

Does he see only one word–or even only part of a word–at a time?

Must he turn his head at an unusual angle, and/or keep moving his head?

Do muscles become tired and strained because of the need to stay in a very precise position?

Must the student bring his face extremely close to the page? (Note: This does not actually damage the eyes, as was once thought. But it does result in a restricted field and an awkward position, and does indicate greatly impaired vision.)

Does the student lose the meaning of the text because he must expend so much effort merely to see it?

Does he tire quickly on visual tasks – more so than his general ability and maturity would seem to indicate?

Is he unable to read standard-sized print?

Is reading mass-produced large print (usually 14-16 point type) difficult or impossible?

Is he unable to read his own handwriting?

Must he have a special lighting arrangement?

If a magnifier is used, is it bulky and cumbersome? Does it only magnify a very small area? Must it be used continuously rather than occasionally?

Does the student frequently pause or stumble over words he knows, needing to take time to bring the word into focus?

Does he read for pleasure, or is it too much work?

Efficiency Is the Key

You and the parents will want to investigate many kinds of aids, and various modes of reading. You will probably find that different methods could be useful for different situations.

In selecting the *main* mode of reading, however, *efficiency* must be the primary criterion if the student is to have equal opportunity. Braille must be regarded as a good alternative, not a last resort. The earlier in life Braille is learned, the more likely the student is to become a truly fluent reader.

The chapter, "The Partially-Sighted Child," discusses the problem of overemphasizing low vision aids and "vision stimulation" to the detriment of appropriate education.

Our ultimate goal is not to "rely on sight at any price," but to help the student attain maximum success with minimum discomfort. Don't force your student to look back on her school years and say, "I had headaches all the time. But I didn't use tapes or learn Braille. I just didn't read any more than I absolutely had to."

CHAPTER 16

TEACHING BRAILLE
TO
YOUNG CHILDREN

Second Grade and Below

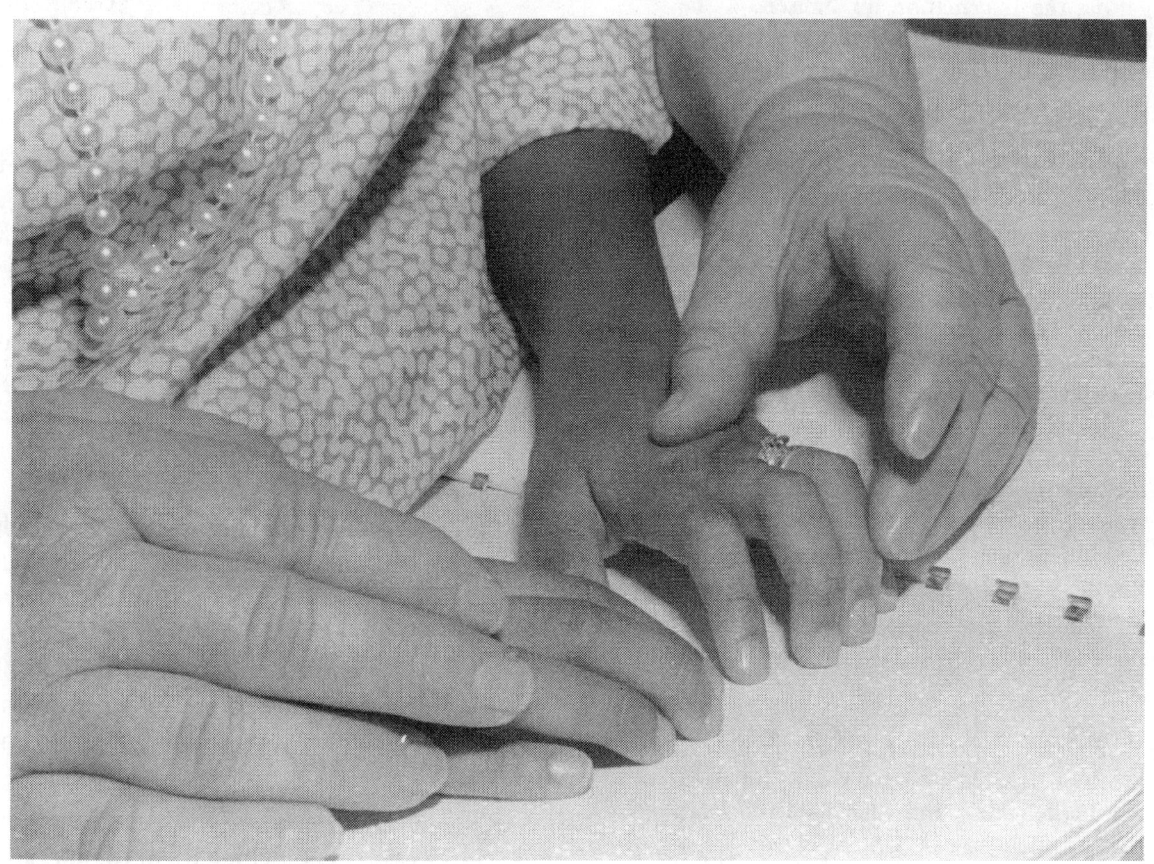

Preparation for Reading

VERY EARLY READINESS

The following is adapted from *A Resource Guide for Parents and Educators of Blind Children*, by Doris M. Willoughby.

Every experience of the infant or young child influences readiness for schoolwork.

Watch for ways to improve the child's vocabulary and understanding. Read aloud to him, being sure to describe the pictures or show him the actual objects. Discuss sounds, odors, and textures. Compare new things to familiar things, to help him understand: "This is an escalator. It is a special kind of stairway, with an electric motor to make it move. I will help you look at it with your hands, and then we will get on it." Comparisons also help him analyze the differences among things which are already familiar. ("Which of these pans is bigger?")

The ability to follow directions is important for independence. The blind child needs directions which are meaningful: "Put the book on the kitchen table," rather than, "Put it over there." At the same time, do not be too ready to help when he is already getting the information for himself. If he has almost found his pajamas by searching with his hands, do not be too ready to tell him where they are.

For the young child, everything is new. Therefore, he often needs a real, concrete experience in order to understand. If there is a TV show about icebergs, you might have your child feel some ice and discuss the size of icebergs.

When a child realizes that words can be expressed on paper, he has taken a great step. Let him feel the Braille as you read the printed equivalent in a "twin-vision" type of book, long before he can read. Provide Braille alphabet blocks and other formal readiness materials before kindergarten. Put Braille labels on furniture and other things around the house.

When you write to relatives, include a greeting dictated by your child. Relatives will be delighted, and your child will learn that his ideas can be written down. When he is in first grade, he will be able to write a simple Braille letter and have someone add a printed transcription.

Children's records – both music and story records – are fun and educational. Your child can learn to operate the record player himself. However, do not let him spend so much time in passive listening that active play is neglected. Also watch for stereotyped motions while listening – nodding, rocking, etc. If this is a problem, shorten the time spent with records, and provide a toy to play with while listening.

Modern children's television has made a great impact on the education of young children. When your blind child watches TV, look for ways to make it really meaningful to him. With *Sesame Street*, for example, show the child a Braille alphabet block or card when a particular letter is discussed, and explain the screen action as necessary. A fuzzy toy "Cookie Monster" can bring the character to life, to the great delight of your child.

Using the hands well is a vital aspect of readiness for Braille. Unfortunately, some blind children rebel at touching unfamiliar textures; generally hang back from touching things; and, when they do touch something, tend to pat it vaguely here and there rather than examining it meaningfully. Help parents learn to provide pleasant and meaningful touch experiences continually – examining raw vegetables, dogs and cats, mailboxes, architectural features, and all the other common and less common things in daily life.

FORMAL READING READINESS

Formal reading-readiness activities should begin as the child nears school age, and continue into kindergarten. (By "formal," I mean that they are structured, planned, and likely to be carried out by someone other than the parent. They should of course be quite informal in the sense of keeping the young child at ease and interested.)

Sighted children are given innumerable books and worksheets inviting them to "mark all the b's," "color the one that is different," "find all the pictures that start with *f*," etc. These kinds of things make beginning reading attractive to the young child. Blind children should have comparable activities.

A common error, however, is providing *too much* readiness work. Many kindergartners have had enough experiences already – with or without formal teaching – that they are ready to start reading and would be bored with extensive pre-reading activities. Students starting Braille after kindergarten should need very little prereading work.

Real Braille letters, numbers, and signs are used in most Braille readiness activities. However, this does not mean the child must learn the name of each sign at this time. Often he/she is simply asked to recognize similarities and differences, or other characteristics, without naming the signs. Sometimes the teacher names the symbols while the child does something with them (e.g., select the one with more dots). These activities build readiness for the time when the child does read and name the symbols.

Even at this early stage, however, it is important to start teaching the names of a few letters or numbers, at a pace and in a manner suitable for the very young child. It is *not* wise to proceed in alphabetical order. Consider the number of "confusers" in the first ten letters alone! The *d, f, h,* and *j* are exactly the same shape but rotated. The *b* and *c* are the same shape but rotated. The *e* and *i* are reversals, and also are easily confused with *b* and *c.* The child probably is not even accustomed to the idea that rotating a symbol changes its meaning. There is no reason why Braille letters need to be taught to young children in alphabetical order, and every reason why they should not be. Here is an example of a good sequence for the first few letters:

g a t l c j k m b x d r .....

This minimizes similarity. As the child gains experience, she will grow more able to distinguish between similar letters.

By the time the child has learned a few letters, the dot numbers should be taught. At first the Braille *c* might be described as having the "top dots." But soon the child will enjoy reciting the numbers of the six dots of the full cell, and can begin to analyze the dots for each letter. He will enjoy naming the holes in a large cell with removable pegs (such as the "Swing Cell" which accompanies *Patterns*). This is important for organized learning. If dot numbers are not used, it is cumbersome to discuss the shapes of letters in some other way.

It often is desirable to begin associating the single-letter contractions (but, can, do, ...) with the letters even at this early stage. Certainly there should be some association of the letter with sounds and words.

Braille Reading-Readiness Books and Materials

The *Patterns* series of Braille instruction books is described later in this chapter. The second book in the series is called *Letters and You,* and teaches the alphabet; however, it moves much too quickly to be the only instruction for this purpose. (Also, as explained below, *Go and Do* and *Letters and You* are really beginning-reading texts rather than prereading. The *Patterns Prebraille Program* is indeed at the prereading level.)

As a first introduction to the letters, I prefer various games and activities with letter cards, together with selected activities from a variety of readiness books. This should be started before kindergarten.

Besides Braille readiness books as such, many "regular" materials are suitable. An example is the book, *Alphabet Puppets* (see "References"). The songs, stories, and other activities are done orally anyway. The clever puppets may easily be made with tactual characteristics; however other objects may also be substituted. The only special materials which are essential are Braille letters.

A regular preschool or kindergarten class will have group discussions about a given letter and its sound. If the teacher has a set of Braille alphabet cards, she can show the Braille letter to the blind child.

The following are sources of ready-made materials. See "References" for more complete information.

The Mangold Developmental Program of Tactile Perception and Braille Letter Recognition. (Note: I often adapt these excellent ideas by providing shorter or simpler versions.)

Patterns Prebraille Program
Touch and Tell
A Tactual Road to Reading
Modern Methods of Teaching Braille, Book 1, from APH.

The Importance of Sleepshades

For any regular Braille instruction, it is very important for the child with some sight to use sleepshades. She will be used to bringing everything close to her eyes, a habit which will keep her from learning the proper hand motions. If sleepshades are introduced properly, the child will not be any more frightened or resistant than for anything else you might do; but it is important to go about it carefully. I approach this as follows for a very young child, and sometimes do some of this for somewhat older students:

(1) The very first session should be a get-acquainted time when the child enjoys familiar activities. Instead of beginning actual instruction, we work puzzles, talk, walk around, examine objects, etc. I do not use sleepshades during the first session with a very young beginner.

(2) If at all possible, I introduce the shades when the parent is not nearby. If the child knows the parent is near, he may be more likely to complain.

(3) The first time I use the shades, it is for a very short time–perhaps only a few seconds if the child is particularly immature. Then I increase the time rapidly, so that soon the shades are used during all intensive instruction.

(4) I set a policy that only I will take the shades off the child. This cuts down on attempts to remove them. I ask the child not even to touch the shades.

(5) The first time the shades are left on for more than a few seconds (usually this is the first time they are used), we do something that is clearly a special treat. This might be eating a raisin, smelling a flower, etc. I explain that the shades help us to use our other senses.

(6) After the shades are in regular use for Braille instruction, I continue some "pure-fun" activities as much as seems necessary. I might provide a very small treat (nut, raisin, etc.) at the end of every session, contingent upon the child's not attempting to remove the shades.

Keeping Their Interest

In working with groups of sighted four- and five-year-olds, teachers plan for plenty of variety and motivation. Quiet concentration is interspersed with opportunities for movement and relaxation. Workbooks are packed with enjoyable diversions (cartoon characters, puzzles, amusing animals, pictures to color, etc.)

Interesting variety is important for blind children as well. A few Braille pages will have raised pictures, glued-on textures, etc. Mainly, however, a teacher of young children must creatively plan interesting lessons. Several suggestions are listed below. Most young children (blind or sighted) require much repetition in learning the letters and numerals, and such lessons can become deadly dull if not planned appropriately.

Begin each session with activities which require the most concentration. Near the end, do those activities which are most active or which the child enjoys most. Provide scented stickers and other small rewards.

Avoid doing exactly the same thing in the same manner for more than five or ten minutes. For example, if you plan to work on alphabet letters, use a short worksheet with pushpins, and then sort flashcards into sets.

A Repertoire of Ideas

Build a list of activities suitable for a young child's short attention span. Following are a number of examples.

NOTE: THE YOUNG CHILD LEARNING THE ALPHABET NEEDS TO EXAMINE INDIVIDUAL LETTERS BY THEMSELVES. ALWAYS SPACE BEFORE AND AFTER EACH LETTER, AND USE DOUBLE LINE SPACING. NEVER USE THE "LETTER SIGN" (DOTS 5-6) AT THIS LEVEL. DO NOT USE THE CAPITAL SIGN UNTIL IT IS TAUGHT.

(1) Complete two or three pages in a readiness book according to the directions given.

(2) Use a Braille readiness book in creative ways. For example, suppose the directions say to follow across a row of shapes from left to right. After the child does this, have him do it again later and *name* the shapes. (Caution: Avoid becoming too analytical at the readiness stage. Following across without analysis *is* a good readiness activity.)

(3) Present flashcards with individual letters. Do something interesting with the cards that are correctly named–put them in a special container; pin them onto a bulletin board; count them and post the number on a chart; etc.

(4) Using flashcards, announce a theme such as "food." Example: "People say that goats like to eat *anything*. When you read a card right, it will go into this box with the toy goat. Then we will name a food for the goat that starts with that letter."

(5) Make a ceremony of sending something home when it has been learned. If materials are in a book, consider making extra copies which children can keep.

(6) Provide an amusing tactual picture–e.g., several birds cut from cloth or textured paper, each with its own Braille letter. As the child reads each letter, he attaches its bird to the page.

(7) Match letter cards with objects according to beginning sounds–*d* with a toy dog, etc.

(8) Provide large cards with very different textures–corduroy, sandpaper, silk, etc. Provide two of each kind and have the child match them.

(9) Read to the child from a Braille or Twin Vision book. Frequently stop and show him a letter he has learned. A beginning dictionary or alphabet book may be used, but others are suitable also. (Caution: Use of the "letter sign" in such books may make it difficult for the child to recognize the letter.)

(10) Use stories such as those in *Alphabet Puppets*, by Jill M. Coudron. Provide the child with one or more Braille letters. Each time the teacher reads a word beginning with a given letter, the child names the letter.

(11) Provide several copies of each of a few letters cards. Do this with just two different letters for a beginner, more for an experienced student. For each letter have a box with the letter fastened onto it. The child sorts all the b's into the *b* box, the d's into the *d* box, etc. (Variation: Some of each letter are capitalized, and some are lower case.)

(12) Several flashcards are punched and placed on a large notebook ring. The child attempts to read each card correctly, so that he can turn each around the ring and eventually return to the first card. (Note: If flashcards are made of paper, they may not last through a single session. Thin plastic is best for this and many other situations. It is available through sources such as Aids Unlimited. You also may be able to get some suitable plastic free from your school's media center; ask about discarded Transparencies.)

(13) When the child knows at least two Braille letters in lower case, he can begin to tell them apart in capitalized form. Work this in for variety at whatever point is most judicious. I usually start after the child has learned about ten letters, when he may be feeling somewhat bored. Matching the capital letter to the same lower-case letter offers many possibilities for activities.

(14) Find creative ways to use ready-made materials. Braille graph paper is an example: Braille a single letter in each square across a row. Cut off the row and attach a paper head. *Voila:* a caterpillar!

(15) See the ideas below for beginning-reading activities. Many can be adapted for the readiness level.

(16) As soon as he knows the first three or four letters of the alphabet, the child can begin to learn the numerals. (These *should* be taught in numerical order.) I sometimes begin by writing numbers with a space after the number sign, and then phase in the normal spacing. Many of the flashcard and worksheet activities for letters or words can also be used with numbers. Other ideas include:

- Use any of various common devices for teaching the numbers, such as flat blocks with various quantities of large holes. The child matches the Braille number card to the block with the right number of holes.
- Name an action, such as clapping or saying "meow." Each time a child reads a number, he is to do the action that many times – e.g., "meow, meow, meow" for *3.*
- Give the child several number cards in mixed order, and have him line them up in numerical order. (Caution: In this, as any activity where there may be various scattered items, plan where the child should place the cards. He might line them up on a cookie sheet, tape them down, or pin them onto a soft board.)
- Provide small objects. The child reads a number and assembles the appropriate quantity. The "Work and Play Trays" (with dividers) from APH are good for this.

(17) Following are several suggestions for worksheets that are easily teacher-made. At the readiness level, it is usually best to have only four or five lines per page. Always double- or triple-space between lines.

- "Find the ____ in each row." (At the readiness level, such rows should contain not more than five or six characters, with spaces between them. Begin by having the answers very easily distinguished – e.g., a *t* mixed in with *b, c,* and *l.* Gradually make the task more difficult – e.g., a *t* with *f, r,* and *q.*)
- "Find the one that is different in each row." (Again, the task should be easy at first – possibly having each row consisting of several a's and one full cell, but with the full cell appearing at a different location in each row.)
- "See the capital letter at the beginning of each row. Find the same lower-case letter in that row."
- "Each row is made up of several ____. Tell me how many ____ are in each row." (This is a good, easy way to reinforce letter names, if the child must say out loud, for example, "four p's," instead of merely "four." Space between the characters and use no more than six per line.)
- Provide small cards, each with a symbol on it, and with sticky tape on the back. The same symbols are written (very widely spaced) on a sheet of paper. The child sticks each card beside the same symbol. Many variations of simple matching are possible: for example, matching a lower-case letter with its capital.
- Provide several sets of two letters, each set written together unspaced – e.g., *cf, pf, ml, ws, fi,* etc. The child finds all the pairs

that contain a given letter.

- Each row consists of plain dots (e.g., dots 3-5), with one actual letter inserted at some point. The child must follow across each line with good finger motion, and also name each letter when she comes to it.

(18) Even a three-year-old can get acquainted with Braille writing equipment.

- As the child watches a blind adult write on a slate or a Perkins Brailler, she observes the motions of the hands and feels the dots.
- The child simply "makes dots" on a Perkins or a slate. After all, sighted children scribble with a crayon long before they do serious writing; why not the equivalent for a blind child?
- The child makes a few especially easy letters on the Perkins, such as *a, b, c, l.*
- The older preschooler can learn any number of symbols on the Perkins. See "Beginning Reading and Writing" (below, in this chapter) for more suggestions.

Beginning Reading and Writing – Kindergarten and First Grade

When should a child begin actual reading and writing? For most public and parochial schools in the United States, the timetable is approximately like this:

- Before kindergarten: Learn most letters and numerals.
- Kindergarten: Finish learning all letters (upper and lower case), and begin some actual reading. Read and write numbers at least to 10.
- First grade: Proceed through the Preprimers, Primer, and First Reader. Write words, sentences, and simple stories. Read and write numbers through 100.
- Second grade and above: Proceed through the materials for each grade level in turn.

The basic timetable for Braille students should be the same as for others.

Certain adjustments may be made in the *sequence* of teaching specific symbols or words. For example, wordlets like "very" and "people," written with single letters in Braille, may be learned before the alphabet is mastered and before sighted children typically study them. Conversely, since punctuation may be confusing to beginning Braille readers, its use may be delayed slightly. The *overall* timetable for Braille students, however, should be the same as for others.

If an individual student has great difficulty, his individual progress should be adjusted, but this is no more true for Braille students than for print students.

ADVANTAGES OF THE "PATTERNS" MATERIALS

Various materials may be used as the young student moves into actual reading. Special attention will be given here, however, to *Patterns,* a basal-reading series written by Hilda Caton, Eleanor Pester, and Eddy Jo Bradley. It is available from the American Printing House for the Blind (APH). (Note that Quota funds can be used.) As of this writing, no other set of beginning Braille materials can boast all the impressive problem-solving and other strengths offered by *Patterns:*

(1) The *Patterns* books introduce the Braille signs and formats in a carefully controlled sequence. In contrast, when a beginning reading book designed for the sighted is Brailled, often there will be a page which has little or nothing new for the print reader but which has many new Braille signs or formats. This is compounded by the fact that the very words usually considered easy are the ones that tend to have special signs.

(2) At the same time, *Patterns* controls the vocabulary as a whole; develops word-attack skills; teaches comprehension and interpretation; and does all the other things which any good beginning reading program does.

(3) There are no printed pictures. Instead, concepts are illustrated through planned experiences using senses other than sight. A few tactual drawings and maps appear in the books.

(4) Whereas the sighted child would not confuse punctuation marks with letters, the young Braille reader often does. The period, for example, is shaped just like a *d* and must be distinguished by its position. *Patterns* takes care of this by using no punctuation at the earliest level, instead simply placing each sentence on a separate line. Punctuation is introduced in a controlled way.

(5) A generous supply of worksheets, supplementary reading books, and other practice material makes it easy to provide variety, interest, and reinforcement.

(6) Criterion-referenced tests are available for each level.

(7) The books are interesting and challenging.

(8) Materials are conveniently labeled to facilitate comparison with other reading series:

Readiness, first book: *Go and Do*
Readiness, second book: *Letters and You*
(Note: The above two books, although called "Readiness," actually teach a reading vocabulary of 23 words, in addition to the alphabet.)
First Preprimer: *Work and Play*
Second Preprimer: *Little and Big*
Third Preprimer: *Words and Games*
Primer: *City and Farm*
Book 1: *New Friends*
Book 2: *Old and New*
Book 3: *Far Away and Long Ago*

(9) Stories about Braille and about blind people are included. They are positive, interesting, and natural in tone.

(10) The Third Reader contains a Glossary with many correlated lessons in dictionary skills.

(11) Each book is accompanied by a well-written Teacher's Edition, which provides detailed lesson guidance and can easily be used by someone who does not know Braille. Thus this series is suitable for use in almost any setting. For example, someone else can easily continue the lessons in between visits by the itinerant teacher. (Note: A convenient checklist, or other means for noting progress at a glance, is an important timesaver when two people alternate in providing instruction. See the chapter on Paraprofessionals for further suggestions.)

The *Patterns* materials are a tremendous contribution to quality education for young blind children.

SUGGESTIONS FOR OPTIMUM USE OF "PATTERNS"

Ordinarily, it is by far the best policy to provide the blind child with the very same books used by all others of his general ability level. However, the above advantages of *Patterns* are so great that many educators choose to make an exception, at least for a short time. (For suggestions about the transition to another series after using *Patterns* for a time, see the chapter, "Braille Reading and Writing–Second Grade and Above.")

Even when using *Patterns,* someone with a depth of knowledge in teaching Braille reading to young children still must take the main responsibility–and both *Braille* and *reading* must be emphasized. If too much is done by a person who does not know Braille well, unfortunate errors will crop up–e.g., using the sign for *were* adjacent to punctuation. If the instructor is not experienced in general methods for beginning reading, certain problems will crop up as with any child–e.g., instruction paced too fast or too slow.

Smoothing a Rough Place

The levels ("Second Preprimer," etc.) given for *Patterns* are generally comparable to those given on most reading books for young children. However, it is important not to assume that the comparison always applies exactly. A notable example is the first preprimer (*Work and Play*), despite its ordinary appearance and short length. Preprimers usually avoid teaching a tremendous number of new skills in one book. In contrast, the *Patterns* first preprimer is so heavily loaded with new skills that considerable extra time and extra practice is advisable. In just the first four lessons of *Work and Play,* the following new challenges appear:

- Capitals at the beginnings of sentences
- Periods
- Question marks
- Longer average sentence length
- Much longer stories
- Many more vocabulary words per story
- The word "be," with the need to distinguish it from "but"–a difficult distinction for a beginner
- Much more material per page
- Much longer words
- Multiple speakers per page
- New format with speaker's name written
- Phrases as answer choices
- *s* added to form plurals
- Detailed interpretation of complex stories

I take care of this overload by working on many of these skills while the child is in the previous book (*Letters and You,* the second "Readiness" level book). Fortunately, that book is almost too easy, and lends itself well to accommodating supplementary work. (In my opinion, the authors of *Patterns* should consider revising these two books with these ideas in mind.)

While in *Letters and You,* anticipate the heavy load to come, by practicing as follows:

- Study the vocabulary for the first three or four lessons of *Work and Play.* Incorporate this vocabulary into the other practice below.
- Match capital letters with their lower-case equivalents.
- Match capitalized words with their uncapitalized equivalents.
- Read sentences which begin with capitals.
- Introduce the period, and practice reading sentences with periods.
- Read longer sentences.
- Practice "filling in the blanks" in a typical worksheet format.
- Practice identifying two or more letters when they are written together unspaced.
- Practice distinguishing between two words which are similar in length and other characteristics (e.g., *ride* and *want.* (Until the First Preprimer level, there are relatively few words which are very similar in length and general appearance.)

When beginning *Work and Play* itself (first Preprimer), ease the transition still further during the first few stories:

- Cut long worksheets in half (or recopy in two parts) when practical, and use as two shorter assignments.
- Provide plenty of variety and short diversions. (Example: When reading about a cat, examine a toy cat.)
- Proceed slowly, with lots of practice.
- A few worksheets have *phrases* as answer choices, all on the same line and merely separated by spaces. Recopy these worksheets and place each phrase on a separate line. Alternatively, draw raised lines between choices.

Once a child is past the first few stories in *Work and Play,* the learning of new skills becomes much more even; the Preprimers, Primer, and First Reader can be completed during first grade.

Correlating Reading Textbooks

In most respects the *Patterns* books compare very favorably with other reading texts. This is particularly true with the "Readiness" books, Preprimers, and Primer. With the First Reader and beyond, however, the textbooks and worksheets have a sameness of format which can create problems.

Other reading workbooks typically have many kinds of exercises – selecting a word and underlining it; naming opposites and synonyms; filling in the blanks; matching; sequencing; adding suffixes and prefixes; working puzzles; interpreting pictures; listing rhymes; etc. The physical arrangement on the page may vary greatly.

The *Patterns* worksheets, in contrast, tend to overemphasize a format of multiple-choice fill-in-the-blanks. Also, the physical arrangement on the page tends to remain the same. Such uniformity is understandable at the very earliest levels, but for an older student it discourages flexibility and breadth of skill.

Some educators also feel that the *Patterns* series, while it does include lessons in phonics, does not emphasize phonics as much as most basal reading series.

Therefore, by late first grade the child should have occasional lessons Brailled from regular reading books. (It may be necessary to custom-Braille the selections, using only the signs which the child knows, and spelling out words which would have used signs she does not know.) Even if an actual transition to a regular reading group is not planned until much later, selected lessons can help the child become used to varied format and vocabulary. It also helps the teacher understand how the child's work compares to that of others.

Errors

Finally, as of this writing, there is one more minor problem with *Patterns*. A number of typographical errors remain – usually in the form of a slight difference between the child's copy and the teacher's copy. Also, now and then a new word slips in, a few pages before it is formally introduced, without the child's having the skills to figure it out. Be alert for these, and edit your Teacher's Edition. This problem can be made into an advantage: I make a joke about the "big mistake in the book," and my students laugh hilariously. It is good for a child to see that she is not the only one who makes mistakes.

USING OTHER MATERIALS (NOT "PATTERNS") WITH BEGINNERS

Using Grade II Braille

Why don't we simply transcribe all primary-grade books into full spelling, and teach the special signs later? In one sense the answer is that virtually no one in this country does it that way with young children. But the reasons behind this are similar to the problems with various schemes to start sighted children on phonetic spelling and then phase in standard English spelling later. That approach requires major relearning at some point, and has not been proven to help beginners greatly. The young beginner should regard regular Grade II Braille as natural and normal.

(Note: When Braille is begun with an older student who already knows how to read in inkprint, Grade I Braille *is* often used at first. This does not seem to be a problem.)

Using a Regular Text for Beginning Reading

Using a regular beginning-reading text in Braille requires careful planning.

Before the young child begins to read complete sentences in standard Braille format, she should have already learned:

- how to follow a Braille line smoothly.
- the alphabet (both lower and upper case).
- common punctuation.
- several common signs (e.g., *the*).
- several common words.

It is important for the Braille student to learn these things before starting in a regular textbook, especially with a group. Sighted children will have learned equivalent readiness skills from *Sesame Street* and elsewhere. The teacher's explanations to the group will sometimes be irrelevant to Braille:

"The *o* is round."
"The *P* is like an *R*, but it has only one leg."
"The little dot is called a period."

As the class moves along, anticipate new signs and symbols, and show them to the blind student before she meets them in class. This extra presentation will take some time which must be arranged in the schedule. Use different format, such as flashcards; do not simply expect her to read the same material an extra time, or she will become bored. It may also be necessary to provide assistance in the reading group.

Some beginning books depend heavily on pictures. In certain formats, every sentence contains a tiny picture which stands for a word, as, "Bill saw a [picture of a clown]." When the child cannot see pictures and cannot read a Brailled description, this presents a dilemma. Of course it is possible to describe illustrations aloud; however, if there is a picture in every sentence, the child cannot read any passages independently. This type of format makes an alternative book especially desirable.

Other reading texts depend on pictures less heavily. Suppose, for example, that the circus is shown and the children are to read, "Bill will come. Bill will have fun. Bill will see clowns." Often the class will discuss the illustration aloud anyway; otherwise someone can say, "The picture shows the circus." The blind child can then read the page independently.

Children with some sight may be anxious to see the pictures visually. Some planning is necessary to avoid confusion over when to use vision, arguments over sleepshades, or attempts to read inappropriate print. One approach is for the child to look at the pictures before or after the entire story (or a major portion of it) is read. Another approach is to cut up an old copy of the text, so that the pictures can be presented individually without the printed text.

Beginning reading instruction can succeed by using regular materials which have been Brailled. However, careful planning is necessary, usually with extra coaching. The advantages of using *Patterns,* at least for a short while, should be carefully considered.

Other Regular Materials In Braille

Even when *Patterns* is used as the main text, often the child also does some things from the regular reading program. For example, perhaps the school uses a "phonetic" reading program which carries over into language-arts lessons. ("Phonetic" reading programs have a very heavy emphasis on phonetic analysis, with sentences such as "Tan Cat had a hat." Other basal readers, such as *Patterns,* include work on phonetic analysis but do not give it such heavy emphasis at first.) Your student also will probably use regular materials in other subjects such as science. When regular materials are Brailled for young children, it is necessary to deal with certain problems which have been carefully circumvented in *Patterns.* Following are some suggestions about the use of regular materials:

(1) If *Patterns* is being used, look for areas of duplication which may occur under subject titles other than "Reading." For example, if the child has "phonics" or "language arts" lessons with the class, it may be possible to shorten or omit equivalent activities in *Patterns.*

(2) Deal with the problem of unknown signs. In kindergarten or first grade, selections are very short and usually read together as a group. Usually the blind child can follow along and figure it out. When more independence is expected, the itinerant/resource teacher should look for unfamiliar signs and provide a key if necessary.

Although it is usually unwise to spell out words without using the regular Braille signs, here is one situation where it may be the best solution for a time. As the child learns more and more signs, it may be possible to custom-Braille some things with only those signs, if a person is available who can keep track of this.

(3) See that Braillists observe the guidelines which apply to all materials for the first school grade and below–notably double line spacing, no italics, and no letter signs.

(4) Emphasize accurate proofreading of all materials. Errors will either stymie the beginner, or teach her that a wrong symbol

is correct. One parent found *23* errors on a single page which had been Brailled by a resource teacher and sent home with the blind child! Such carelessness is inexcusable.

(5) Oral work is often most efficient and logical. If the others are to examine pictures (cake, bat, snake) and tell which ones rhyme, name the pictures aloud for the blind student.

(6) Pencil in enough words so that the classroom teacher can tell what the blind child is reading.

(7) Consider the *purpose* of tasks such as cutting or pasting. If the purpose is to match sounds or meanings, consider using a different technique. For example, the names of the pictures might be Brailled and the child might recopy them on the Perkins Brailler under appropriate headings.

(8) Suggest various ways for the child to respond to written questions, worksheets, etc.:

- The child underlines the Braille answer with a pencil, or, better still, with a waxy crayon which she can feel.
- A worksheet can be tacked to a soft board so the child can place a pushpin on each answer.
- The child might scratch out the right answer, or use a stylus to poke a hole next to it.
- Note that with most of these methods the child can go back and check her answers. The classroom teacher can read them also, if enough print is written in; often all that is needed is the item numbers in pencil, and the rest can be inferred by the spacing.
- Answers can be given aloud to another person or into a tape recorder.
- If the child writes assignments on the Perkins, and no one but you can read Braille, the classroom teacher might (a) save papers for you to check, or (b) have the child read answers aloud.

BEGINNING BRAILLE AFTER KINDERGARTEN

The chapter, "Braille Reading and Writing, Second Grade and Above" offers detailed suggestions about beginning Braille after kindergarten.

Reading and Writing in the Classroom and at Home

BUILDING GOOD HABITS

"Lots of fingers on the page," should be a frequent reminder. Although older readers develop their own style, and a few good readers do indeed use only a couple of fingers, insist that the young beginner use both hands and several fingers. Remind her that, although only one or two fingers may seem to be really reading, the other fingers will at least help her track the line and notice where it begins and ends. Probably in time the other fingers will help with actual reading as well.

Place your hands gently over the child's hands from time to time to help maintain a good position. (I find it helpful to sit *beside* the student, rather than facing her.) Strive for a relaxed position in which each finger is slightly curved, with the soft tip against the page. Help the student develop a light touch, moving along smoothly and quickly, rather than pressing down and moving jerkily. Do not allow the wrists to become pivots. Each hand as a whole should move smoothly along.

Teach the beginner to move both hands along together. Then, after a few weeks or months, encourage separate hand movements. Experienced readers tend to finish one line with the right hand while the left hand begins the next.

The matter of tracking the lines is another reason for the use of sleepshades. Many students who cannot possibly see individual Braille dots can nevertheless see the *rows* of dots to some extent. Such an individual may try to follow the lines of Braille with her eyes, while reading the characters by touch. This is unreliable. Interpointed Braille (on both sides of the page) will seem confusing. Also, if the student later loses more vision she will then need to change.

VARIED MATERIALS

Build habits of independent recreational reading. Become familiar with local Braille library service and nationwide resources. Make a chart of books read, with a small reward for achievement. Look for contests and games, such as the "Braille Readers Are Leaders" contest conducted annually by the National Federation of the Blind.

As soon as the First Preprimer is completed, the excellent supplementary library books which accompany the *Patterns* series can be used for independent reading. They work well with any reading program, not just the *Patterns.* Unfortunately, however, the *Patterns Library Series* does not now provide an inkprint version. Many other easy-reading Braille books have the same problem. It is well worth the time to copy the earliest books into print to help parents assist the young child.

Other sources of easy recreational reading material include:

- National Braille Press "Book-of-the-Month Club"
- Twin Vision Books (American Brotherhood for the Blind)
- *Seedlings* Braille Books For Children
- *Children's Series* Braille books by Marie Porter

Parents will find it easy to help by studying *Just Enough to Know Better: A Braille Primer,* a book for parents by Eileen P. Curran.

FULL LITERACY INCLUDES WRITING

Braille writing should be taught along with reading. The preschooler can "make dots" and then form real letters on the Perkins Brailler and the slate; the beginning reader can form words and sentences. The large demonstration "Swing Cell" shows the relationship between the Braille dots as they appear on the paper *vs.* the six Perkins keys. This helpful aid is available from APH as part of the *Patterns* materials but also offered separately.

Have the young child double-space between lines at first, to make proofreading easier.

Consistent fingering on the Perkins helps prevent errors. The first three fingers of each hand should be designated for the three respective dots, with the little fingers unused; the thumb should be used on the space bar.

Following are descriptions of typical activities with the Perkins Brailler:

(1) Copy the new vocabulary words for the next story in the reading book. (Note: Do this regularly. It reinforces the reading vocabulary, and helps the child learn to write whatever he can read.)

(2) Copy a short list of letters or words. (Note that copying from a list, independently, is quite a different task than writing from dictation.)

(3) Copy a list of (uncapitalized) words, but capitalize each word.

(4) Copy a list of sentences and add one of your own.

(5) Copy sentences, inserting the word *not* into each.

(6) Write a sentence with each of the words from a list.

(7) Arrange word cards to form sentences. Then copy the sentences on the Perkins Brailler.

(8) "Here is a fuzzy toy dog. Here are a few words written to help you: dog, fuzzy, fun, bark, run. Pretend the dog is real. Write three sentences about him. If you need to write a word which you have not studied and which is not on this list, try to sound it out."

(9) Read the question and Braille the answer. (Some questions may have one certain

right answer; others may be open, as, "What food do you like?" It may or may not be required that answers be complete sentences.)

(10) Write down letters or words which have been tape-recorded by the teacher.

(11) Make a file or booklet of reading-vocabulary words.

Interesting and Well-Organized Lessons

The smallest variation in procedure or materials can spark interest. A piece of paper shaped like a heart, for example, can make a routine lesson more fun. (Note: It is possible to insert odd-shaped paper into the Perkins by placing another small piece under the sensor wheel at the left. However, this permits the paper to roll in indefinitely. Therefore, the teacher should carefully insert the odd-shaped paper and start the line spacing.)

During oral reading, some variations help speed both the lesson procedure and the child's own reading, and are discussed under "Speed." Use variations also when certain words are difficult. You might anticipate a hard word: have the child read ahead silently to find and analyze it, and then have the entire sentence or paragraph read aloud. Vary this still further by saying, "Find a word with the *gh* sign," rather than simply naming the word to be hunted. For frequently confused words, you can ask, "Does the next sentence have the word "man" or "mean"?

Time is wasted, and lessons may fail completely, if the child keeps misplacing things. Help him organize materials for maximum independence. Provide a way to keep flashcards right-side up (I prefer a raised line across the top, to promote looking "left to right and top to bottom"). Provide a work tray or other enclosed space for sorting or arranging. Use tape, pins, or elastic strips to keep small cards in place.

Be liberal with praise and encouragement, since young children are easily discouraged. At the same time, make it clear that you expect diligent work and good progress.

IDEAS FOR PRACTICE ACTIVITIES

Below is a list of ideas for materials and activities at the beginning-reading level. Most can be varied greatly in regard to difficulty; both the kind and the quantity of items will make a great difference. When introducing a new format, begin with easy content – e.g., even if the child knows a great many numbers, use only a few the first time you ask him to rearrange cards into numerical sequence.

Most of the materials described under "Readiness" continue to be suitable at the early first-grade level. The difficulty, similarity, and quantity of items can be varied according to need. Spending some time on quick and easy seatwork helps promote quick and comfortable reading; the child becomes accustomed to moving the fingers smoothly and lightly. At the same time, the difficulty of the work can be gradually increased to provide practice on specific new skills – e.g., distinguishing between letters or words that are very similar.

Many books for teachers of the sighted contain ideas which can easily be adapted for use with blind children. Following are some particularly good activities:

(1) To practice abstract or difficult words when the child cannot yet read many nouns: Provide sentences such as "I have a ___," "The ___ is here," etc. Each time a child reads a sentence correctly (saying "blank"), he may reach into a box for an interesting object to "fill in the blank." (apple, pine cone, toy horse, etc.)

(2) Use a seasonal or humorous object. Example: "This jack-o-lantern will watch you do this page. You may look at it before you start and after you finish."

(3) Pairs of identical word cards are shuffled. The child must pin them onto a soft board in pairs. (Variation: one of each pair is capitalized.)

(4) Words or letters are written on a paper, widely spaced. Others are on cards. The child must stick the cards onto the sheet, according to directions. This might be to match identical words or letters, rhymes, opposites, beginning letters, etc. Phrases or sentences can also be used.

(5) Compose an "experience story:" One or more paragraphs are composed (orally) by the child or children. The teacher takes it down in Braille, giving some guidance as to wording. Then the teacher and student(s), together, reread the resulting "experience story." Words which have not been formally taught may be used, since it is not expected that the child will read every word independently.

(6) Provide Braille labels for furniture and other things in the room. This has many possibilities, such as taking the labels off and having the child replace them.

(7) Provide sentences on strips. The child must draw out one or more strips and act them out. ("Stand up," "Go out the door," etc.)

(8) Sort word cards according to classifications such as animals, birds, furniture.

(9) With alphabet flashcards, it is easy to teach the single-letter contractions (but, can, do...) at the same time, even if the reading text has not yet introduced them.

(10) One-word answers may be matched with simple "riddles" (e.g., descriptions of three different animals).

(11) Word cards may be held in place by elastic strips or otherwise. (The "Answer Board" from Texture Touch is ideal.) Build a sentence; change a word or two to produce a different sentence.

(12) When sentences are built with cards, the teacher might copy the sentences onto regular Braille paper. Hearing the teacher write each sentence (or each word within the sentence) is enjoyable feedback for the child's oral reading. The child may then reread the set of sentences and keep them. (Alternatively, the student might copy the sentences herself.)

(13) A group of cards are to be arranged in alphabetical order (or number cards in numerical order).

(14) Set up a treasure hunt trail. For example, give the child a slip saying "Go to the sink." In the sink he finds another slip which says, "look under your chair," and so on until the trail leads to a small treat.

The following list outlines directions for typical Braille worksheet pages:

(1) Find the letter/number that is the same as the first one in the row.

(2) Find the letter/number that is different from the others in the row.

(3) Find all the words that start with the given letter.

(4) Mark *yes* or *no* according to whether the statement is true.

(5) Mark *yes, no,* or *maybe* for each statement. (Example of a "maybe" item: "A flower is red.")

(6) Look at each pair of items (letters, words, sentences, numbers, etc.), and indicate whether they are exactly the same or not.

(7) Note the two letters written together at the beginning of each row. Find another set of the same two letters. (This is helpful for the child just getting used to grouped letters.)

Pacing of Reading Instruction

Braille is *not* more difficult than print. Lest this chapter's emphasis on prereading and on careful planning seem to give the wrong impression, I will again emphasize that Braille students do not categorically need more help than print students. The advantages of Braille as a system include its uniformity in size and shape, automatic formation of the dots in writing, uniform shape for capitals and lower-case letters, etc.

Blind children as a group are ready to learn to read on the usual timetable. Some of the usual criteria for evaluating readiness, however, do not apply, and it is important to realize this. With sighted children, teachers carefully note skill in coloring, cutting, and other pencil-and-paper skills which are considered related to reading ability. This assumption may result in unwarranted delay in reading instruction, especially with a partially-sighted child.

Formal instruction before first grade is vital for two basic reasons:

(1) While opportunities for incidental learning (that is, learning without formal teaching) abound for learning print letters and words, they are usually nonexistent for learning Braille.

(2) The sequence and relative ease of learning particular beginning-reading skills vary somewhat between Braille and print, although the overall difficulty is the same.

Pacing each student, neither too fast nor too slow, is complex enough in a large classroom. The conscientious teacher observes the difficulty or ease of each child's reading, and judges whether he can handle the fastest pace provided by the curriculum, or just how much slower he should go.

With an individual blind child, receiving personalized instruction and possibly using different reading books, how do we judge this? The very same way. Even if the child is out of the classroom for reading, we can still compare his achievement with that of others. Even in a special school which has no "regular" students, we can compare children in another building. The use of a different textbook series, such as *Patterns,* is a complicating factor but manageable. After all, schools continually place transfer students. The *Patterns* books are marked for grade level. A curriculum consultant can also compare the level of difficulty. Pace instruction as for regular classes, taking into account the characteristics of the *Patterns* series as such. (See "Suggestions for Optimum Use of *Patterns,* above, in this chapter.)

If it is necessary to take a certain individual more slowly than is typical, be prepared to explain why, just as the classroom teacher must do. Pacing more slowly just because the child uses Braille is in conflict with P.L. 94-142.

THE KINDERGARTEN CURRICULUM

To provide a blind child the equal opportunity which is her right, it should be assumed that at least the First Preprimer will be completed during kindergarten. Sighted children completing kindergarten usually know the entire alphabet (upper and lower case), have acquired readiness skills such as following from left to right, and have a reading vocabulary of several words. More and more move well into formal reading.

Besides the matter of actual vocabulary, much of the earliest work in *Patterns* does involve "readiness" skills–knowing where a word begins and ends, following lines from left to right and top to bottom, etc. It is important to proceed at least this far in kindergarten.

The blind child starting first grade will be with sighted children who are very familiar with the alphabet, have completed much readiness work, and have a sizable reading vocabulary (learned from television and elsewhere if not formally taught in school). Furthermore, the blind child must learn a number of signs and symbols which have no counterpart in print. For all these reasons, even if the general curriculum does not call for formal reading instruction in kindergarten, the blind child should proceed into the preprimers before first grade.

NORMAL EXPECTATIONS

It is sometimes alleged that it is unreasonable to pace a blind child this ambitiously because "Braille is so much harder," with the special symbols and the necessity of physically moving along on the paper. None of these problems (if they are problems) are sufficient cause for a general assumption of slower pacing for a Braille student. The special signs and symbols can be learned as easily as the non-phonetic spelling of the English language. There are sighted children who read jerkily and inefficiently, just as there are blind children who do so. Moreover, some aspects of Braille are clearly easier: for example, a Braille letter always has the same dots, the same size, and the same proportions (with the universal dot 6 added for capitalization).

A parent recently asked me, "Isn't it extremely difficult for the child to tell what the symbol means, if *d* and *dd* and *4* and the period are all the same shape?"

I responded by drawing a circle. "What is this in print?" I asked. "Is it a zero, or a lower-case *o*, or a capital *O?* And furthermore," I said as I drew a vertical rectangle under the circle, "Is it perhaps the dot of a very large lower-case *i*?"

"I see what you mean," the parent laughed. "I guess we all have to figure out that sort of thing."

SET MILESTONES

To facilitate completing the First Reader during first grade, etc., set interim dates and milestones. Estimate when to complete the first unit, count the lessons, and plan your time accordingly. This helps to prevent a trap which is likely to catch the conscientious teacher – namely, working for perfect mastery of each and every task.

In the regular classroom, time may or may not be taken to help a particular child fully understand questions he missed, or to have him reread a passage where he stumbled. Often errors (or potential errors) are not observed at all because it is another child's turn to read. A student having serious trouble will probably be moved to a lower reading group, where again he receives only spotty help with errors, and again is paced along with the group. When a child is taught alone, on the other hand, often he is asked to read everything aloud, and to correct each and every error. Pacing can easily be lost completely.

Observe some regular reading groups. Make your lessons as much like a regular reading group as possible. Particularly do not have an individual child read everything aloud herself. (If no other child is present, the teacher should read part of the time. Silent reading should occur also.) At the same time, retain the flexibility for extra help when really necessary.

Increasing Reading Speed

Following are some specific ideas to help increase speed of reading.

- Be sure that dots are clear and plain. Little beginners wear down dots at a great rate. Replace Readiness and Preprimer materials frequently.
- Many readers say that Braille on paper is faster and easier to read than plastic.
- For several months after actual reading is begun, continue to provide some tasks where a line is to be followed without actual reading, and where the task is easy. A good example is seeking the one "different" character among several that are quite contrasting. This helps prevent the tendency to read slowly, character by character or even dot by dot.
- See that the experienced reader often reads easy material. This can be for recreation or otherwise, but is vital in building up speed.
- Build a smooth motion of the fingers across the page. "Don't scrub the dots," is a good admonition. "Pretend you're moving a tape along, and recording everything that is there, getting it as you go by."
- Sometimes take hold of the child's hands and physically move them along at an appropriate speed.
- The reading position for the beginner is important – pages lying flat on a solid surface, at the right height, with plenty of room. Experienced readers should usually have these advantages, although flexibility is important also.
- Provide a tape recording of a selection, at suitable speed, and have the student read along.
- From the beginning, provide much practice in following along while someone else is reading. This has many advantages, including enjoyable variety,

and develops the ability to vary speed and participate in a regular reading group.

- If the student cannot keep up when someone else is reading, alternate between two approaches: (1) start by reading very slowly while he follows, and gradually increase speed over time; (2) read along at a chosen speed, and periodically move his hands to the right place. Urge him to keep up as long as possible each time. If he drops behind, do not help him immediately; he needs to develop the ability to hurry ahead by himself.
- If no other students are available, the teacher can take turns reading. For fun and realism, the teacher might play the part of youthful readers (with fictitious names, to avoid making fun of anyone). "Matt" and "Jodi" might read quickly, "Susie" slowly, "Tommy" with mistakes, etc. Your student can help "Tommy" correct his errors.
- When the student is learning to follow someone else's oral reading, occasionally stop and ask him to show you the last phrase read (or to read the next phrase).
- Even if the student has actual reading lessons separately, have him join the class with other books in Braille–math, social studies, etc.
- Sometimes use a timer and make charts showing words per minute.
- Teach skimming and scanning. Ideas for helping a beginner include:

  Read a sentence (or word or phrase) aloud and ask the student to find it on the page. Make the task easy at first ("It's one of the first three sentences"), and gradually increase the size of the area to be searched.

  Direct the student to a story he has read before, asking for a quick review. Explain, "Let's look over this story. On page 32, you pick any sentence and read it aloud. On 33, I'll read a sentence and you find it. Now, what do you remember about this story?"
- When discussing Brailled questions, especially those which involve hunting through a passage for an answer, do not simply wait for the student to find each answer. Impose a time limit beyond which you explain the answer. If the student does poorly, repeat the lesson later rather than stretching it out interminably. Again, even with only one student you can simulate a reading group for speed, realism, and amusement: "We have ten questions. We will read each one aloud and then look on Page 17 for the answer. We'll pretend that there are five of you here; raise your hand if you have the answer, and I may call on you. I may pretend to call on somebody else, and then I will read and pretend to be that person. If you think the answer is wrong, keep your hand up."
- Balance the value of analyzing dot patterns, on the one hand, *vs.* the dangers of examining individual dots. Emphasize the shape of the whole character and the whole word.
- Speed in writing is important as well. Provide early practice in writing longer and longer selections, paced as in a regular classroom.

CHAPTER 17

BRAILLE READING AND WRITING

Second Grade and Above

Confidence and Consistency

Insist that your student write in Grade II Braille (with the contractions) as soon as he is able. Inconsistency causes confusion. Beginning in kindergarten, keep track of the signs the child has learned, and see that he uses them in writing.

Be sure that the student can describe the shape of a symbol in terms of dot numbers.

With one of my students, I found that his vocabulary of written signs was far behind his reading vocabulary. I made lists in the sequence presented by *Patterns.* I also composed dictation sentences using only those signs he knew, plus relatively easy words with no signs. We told him, "These will be a special kind of spelling lesson, where you must use the right signs. Once you have learned a list, with the words and the sentences, you will be expected to use those signs in *anything* you write in Braille."

At the same time, the student should learn where *not* to use the contractions–chiefly in spelling lists and dictionary work. It is also acceptable, if the young child has not yet learned a given sign, to write a particular word in full spelling temporarily.

Later the older student should develop his own "personal shorthand" for note-taking.

To reinforce learning the signs, use flash-cards which have a Braille sign on the front and the Grade I version on the back. (Note: Insert full cells beside signs such as *-tion* or *his,* with appropriate spacing; otherwise there really may be no way to tell the sign's position. Also note that cards with Braille on both sides tend to wear down and should be made of plastic.) Consider using a machine such as the "Language Master," with which the child can read a Braille sign and then insert the card to hear the sign named.

A touchy situation sometimes occurs when someone learns only the Braille alphabet and then wants to prepare materials for your student. Occasional labels, messages, etc., prepared in this way can be helpful. However, *lengthy* materials in Grade I Braille are very undesirable. If the student's Braille skills are shaky, he will be confused. If his Braille skills are good, he will find the material frustrating. (Compare how you would feel, as a print reader, if some reading matter were in phonetic spelling. Yes, you know how to use that mode of print, and you want it in the dictionary–but it is hardly efficient for connected reading!)

Even worse is learning *some* of the signs and rules for Grade II Braille, but not all, and then trying to prepare materials. This can result in such oddities as the word *wasn't* written with the sign for *was.* If a person really wants to prepare materials, expect him to learn the entire literary code and to have a competent proofreader available. (Note: Math problems are a somewhat different matter, as it is easier to limit the signs involved in particular materials.)

The frequency and touchiness of these situations are related to the common (often adamant) belief that *everything* should be provided in Braille. However emphatically we agree that Braille is an efficient and practical mode of reading, we must realize that it cannot be provided all the time. A student must be flexible and learn to use live readers, tape recordings, etc. The person who tries to prepare class handouts in Grade I or with incomplete knowledge would do far better simply to read it aloud.

Anticipate New Challenges

With ordinary text, a youngster properly prepared can use the help of any adult to figure out most unknown words or symbols, even when the adult does not have a copy. Teach students to spell the word aloud if possible, and otherwise to read a sentence or two aloud. If the problem is an unknown sign, often the context will provide enough clues. I sometimes tell my students that for the day I am going to have amnesia and forget all I ever knew about Braille; thus they get guided practice in having *me* work in this way.

Especially with younger readers, an unfamiliar sign or a change in format can be a major challenge. The classroom teacher may not realize that the "extra *in* signs" are actually an asterisk, or that the Braille accent sign (in dictionary pronunciation format) comes *before* the syllable. A child accustomed to vertical math problems may have no idea how to read them horizontally. Anticipate problems such as this, and practice with the format beforehand. Sometimes a judicious note of explanation to the classroom teacher will suffice. Ask teachers to save the material to show you if they cannot figure it out. Watch for the possibility that a child will continually complain of supposed "strange signs" or "mistakes," in order to avoid work.

Develop flexibility about the position of the paper for reading. The student should be able to balance a book on his lap, lie down on his stomach to read, stand up and read a page "upside down" against his stomach (i.e., with the top of the page down toward the floor), etc. Do not let your student (and other teachers) believe that he must sit at a desk when other students are elsewhere.

Skimming and scanning are important skills. Show your student how to run the hands down the page quickly (perhaps parallel, in a position different from that for detailed reading) to get the general idea or hunt for something specific. Explain that it is *not* always desirable to read every word. Look at the beginnings of paragraphs, and the first sentences of paragraphs. Read headings and consider what is covered under each. Expect your student to find things more and more quickly.

Broaden Experience and Flexibility

Be sure that you yourself know enough about the various Braille codes. Every itinerant or resource teacher should know literary Braille *thoroughly.* He/she should also know Nemeth well enough to read and write easy material with minimum use of references, and to look up less common expressions quickly.

A foreign language can be transcribed by referring to the *Manual On Foreign Languages,* from the National Braille Association.

If you do not know Music Braille and Grade III Braille, know where to find someone who does. Your regional library for the blind, or the National Library Service, should be able to help. Also note correspondence courses available from the Hadley School.

Tables, graphs, and dictionaries are as important for blind students as others. Book 3 of the *Patterns* reading texts provides an excellent glossary, with exercises, that may be used even when the rest of the book is not. Various materials from the American Printing House for the Blind and elsewhere aid in teaching tables, graphs, and maps. (See also other chapters in this book.)

Variety and interest are important for the advanced student as well as the kindergartner.

Do more and more with silent reading. However, keep track of your older students carefully even when you no longer provide direct instruction. Occasionally check oral reading. If the student does not read quickly and fluently, keep looking for a reason. Continually examine attitudes and motivation. Also examine skill: *What* words or formats give trouble? Try meaningless combinations (zn, zp, etc.) to see whether certain letters or symbols are recognized poorly. Drill on skills which are weak.

Encourage recreational reading. If the selection at your regional library for the blind is poor, try to improve it, and also look elsewhere. Other sources include your state residential school; the Twin Vision lending library of the American Brotherhood for the Blind; the *Children's Series* by Marie Porter; *Seedlings* Braille books for children; the National Braille Association Book Bank; National Braille Press "Book-of-the-Month Club;" and direct subscriptions to Braille periodicals.

Also familiarize your student with specialized Brailled items such as calendars, logarithm charts, etc.

Transition from Individualized Reading

AN UNSUCCESSFUL ATTEMPT

Denise was midway through second grade, and had finished the *Patterns* first reader. She seemed to have average ability, but had not started Braille until first grade. The second-grade teachers were pushing for transfer into the regular reading group and the books used by the district. They said it was hard to evaluate Denise's progress and to decide whether she should go on to third grade, since she had different reading lessons.

I had noted that the early *Patterns* books were very challenging–in some respects more demanding than the other textbooks in question. So, even though there were still a number of signs Denise had not yet learned, I agreed to try integration.

We looked over the stories and made lists of new Braille signs to be taught along with the regular vocabulary. But Denise read more and more slowly, and began stumbling over familiar signs as well as new ones. A month later, despite our best efforts, she showed indications of giving up altogether.

After a hurried conference, we decided to move back to *Patterns* for the rest of the year. Ultimately Denise did repeat the grade, for a variety of reasons, and the following year she did well with the regular second-grade books in Braille.

A BETTER WAY

Today, if a student begins with individualized reading and later is integrated, I insist on a gradual process. If someone pushed me for grade-placement evaluation, I would have the child try various sample lessons (Brailled) from the regular text. I might have a curriculum consultant compare the books. I would *not* assume, as I did with Denise, that the student could learn a sizable number of new signs in an uncontrolled sequence, while trying to handle many new procedures and an unaccustomed quantity of work.

Depending upon circumstances, you may choose to use the entire *Patterns* series, up through Book 3, *Far Away and Long Ago.* However, it is often advantageous to transfer the child into the regular reading group quite a bit sooner. When the student completes the second volume of *Old and New* (Book 2), she has learned the vast majority of the signs common in the early grades. From this point on, the advantages of using *Patterns* as the main series diminish rapidly.

Any transition should be done carefully. First try selections from the new materials in private, watching for problems. When this is successful, integrate the child with the regular reading group for some of the lessons–whatever kind seem easiest for a start. Gradually increase involvement. If the child works slowly, do not allow the others to sit and wait; help the child to finish individually at another time. If difficulties arise, it is possible to make changes as necessary, without fanfare.

Denise's late start in Braille contributed to her problems. Try to convince parents that Braille should be begun in kindergarten or before. Also note the suggestions later in this chapter regarding students who do begin later.

Increasing Reading Speed

For blind students, no less than the sighted, age and experience should bring increased reading speed which is comparable with that of other students.

The chapter on "Teaching Braille – Second Grade and Below" contains many suggestions about speed; most of these are also suitable for older students if made age-appropriate. Following are additional suggestions:

(1) Students above first grade should not move the lips, or they will not learn to read faster than speech.

(2) Explain that silent reading speed should vary according to the task; many sighted and blind students do not realize this. Practice reading very quickly to get the general drift; more slowly for typical study speed; and very slowly for something extremely difficult or detailed.

(3) As soon as your student can comfortably read passages of some length, encourage him to have the right hand finish a line while the left begins the next line, then bring the right hand down to meet the left hand, etc. (Ask a fluent Braille reader to demonstrate.) As the student gains experience, let him develop his own "style." Note that it is not unusual for a right-handed person to prefer reading Braille with the left hand dominant – another reason to insist that students use both hands from the start.

(4) Provide guided practice in reading two completely separate things with the two hands – reading a question on one page and its answer choices on the next page, comparing two versions of a sentence, etc.

(5) When a child reads orally, do not always interrupt to correct errors. Emphasize fluency. Sometimes work on difficult words individually, before or after connected reading.

(6) Recreational reading, at a relatively easy level, is extremely important in building real fluency.

(7) Convince the student (and his parents and teachers) that Braille readers can compete effectively, and can read as fast as anyone else, *if* they use good techniques and have good attitudes. Introduce the student to adults who read Braille well.

(8) Teach the child to turn pages very quickly. If he is not near the correct page, insist that he estimate instead of looking at every individual page number.

(9) Insist the child mark the place when he is interrupted, rather than wasting time hunting for the place when he resumes reading. Many Braille books have built-in ribbon bookmarks. A line may be marked with a pin, paper clip, magnet, etc.

(10) Be sure there are more rewards for quick reading than for slow reading. Avoid situations where the child gets much more attention if he reads slowly.

(11) Look for things which the child would enjoy if he finishes on time or early. For example, many primary-grade classrooms have "interest centers" where children may do extra activities when their work is done. Too often, individualized Braille lessons simply continue until the time is up, with no consequences for slow reading *vs.* fast reading.

(12) Determine what you believe the student can reasonably accomplish, and insist that he do it. If he is working with a group and doesn't finish with the rest, they should not wait for him; rather, he should finish alone at a less convenient time. If the lesson is individualized, keep comparing your time with the typical time for a group.

(13) Sometimes set a timer to go off when a given passage should be finished.

(14) Enter contests such as "Braille Readers Are Leaders," sponsored by the National Federation of the Blind. Create local contests.

(15) Sometimes have the student read aloud onto a tape. Strive for fluency.

(16) Sometimes count the number of successive lines which the student reads without staying on any word for three seconds or more, and without going back to look at any words. Try to set a new record each week.

(17) Avoid expecting uniform progress in all aspects of reading at once. It may be necessary to tolerate minimal comprehension while pushing for speed. As the student learns to move faster, speed and comprehension can be combined.

(18) The following procedure encourages major progress in speed. Over a period of several days, guide the student gradually through the following steps:

- Move the hands quickly and appropriately across each line, but merely *count* the lines – do not attempt any comprehension whatever.
- Move the hands quickly across each line, trying to notice a letter or symbol now and then.
- Move the hands quickly across each line, trying to notice a few words here and there.
- Move the hands quickly and get the general drift of the passage. When this is accomplished, the student is actually reading at a speed appropriate for novels, short stories, etc.
- Recognize that different purposes call for different speeds – e.g., reading for pleasure *vs.* studying a difficult text.

Mature Writing Skills

Suggestions for beginning use of the Perkins Brailler appear in the chapter, "Teaching Braille – Second Grade and Below." "A Braillewriter In My Pocket" discusses the slate and stylus.

Kindergartners and first graders should use double line spacing. Later, the student should single space most Braille writing. There are exceptions, however. For a rough draft with revisions, double spacing permits the insertion of words between lines, with some of the older wording being crossed out as needed. Blind students, like sighted students, need to be reminded to make and revise a rough draft when appropriate. On the other hand, usually a rough draft is unnecessary and time-consuming, especially in the lower grades. The student should learn to compose directly – preferably at the typing keyboard if she has learned to type. For example, suppose that the third-grade English assignment is a paragraph with one topic sentence and four detail sentences. The student should not need to write it out twice.

Unfortunately, modern technology has brought a setback, rather than an advance, for many blind students' writing skills. (Actually, it is not the technology itself, but the misuse of it.) Several years ago, it was generally assumed that blind students could write in any location – with the slate or the Perkins for Braille, and with a portable manual typewriter for inkprint. Today, unfortunately, many people assume that typing must be done near an electrical outlet. Worse yet, it is sometimes assumed that all writing must be done on a computer and be restricted to one location. Sighted people use computers and electric typewriters, but would not wish to forgo the option of pencil and paper!

I have even seen students who had lost (or never learned) the normal skills of writing Braille, due to the misuse of a computer system. The typewriter keyboard of the computer was able to produce both Braille and inkprint. These students and their instructors believed this was the only good way to produce Braille, and failed to employ the slate and stylus or even the portable Perkins. Although such a computer system can be a great boon when kept in perspective, it brought a tragic disservice to these students.

Beginning Braille After Kindergarten

This section consists of special notes for late-blinded students and those for whom the decision for Braille occurred late. The wisdom of early Braille instruction for a low-visioned student is pointed up by the scheduling difficulties of teaching Braille while the student keeps up with advanced classwork. The chapters on "Scheduling" and "Placement Decisions" contain detailed suggestions about arrangements.

ATTITUDES AND EXPECTATIONS

As discussed throughout this book, the attitudes of the student and others are the most important factor. Introduce your student and his family to competent adults who read Braille quickly. Be matter-of-fact and encouraging in your manner. If a newly-blinded student is not yet medically ready to attend school, try to start Braille instruction in the home or hospital. Learning Braille is not strenuous, and is a vital and constructive step. Help everyone to develop a positive outlook. The use of sleepshades is important with the older beginner, both to make sure the skills are learned properly and to demonstrate that achievement is possible without any sight.

As discussed previously, very young children generally need considerable prereading, or "readiness" instruction. Usually they also need plenty of fun and game-like activities as they begin actual reading. This is because of their young age, not because of blindness or because of the nature of Braille. Most students beyond kindergarten need little or no practice before working on real letters and words. A brisk and challenging beginning, besides saving time, sets a tone of mature and businesslike study. Occasional short "readiness" tasks, such as looking for the one character that is different, may be judiciously included to build smooth and speedy reading. But generalized practice at "developing the tactile sense" should not be necessary for students beyond kindergarten.

The chapter on young children emphasizes educational games and other diversions. Students of all ages do better when lessons are interesting. However, approaches which help a kindergartner may be time-wasting and even insulting for a third grader. Many ideas in the previous chapter will still apply, with modifications, when a student is in second or third grade. But the older and more mature the student, the less emphasis there should be on "fun and games" and the more there should be on businesslike, practical study. Instead of a game to provide a change of pace, vary the nature of the work: plain text, tables or other special formats, arithmetic problems, slate writing, etc. If you are unfamiliar with typical abilities and attention span for a given age level, visit a regular reading class. Also see the chapter in this book on "Motivation."

MATERIALS

What materials should be used? With a beginner who is still in the primary grades, you may prefer to use *Patterns* with some adaptations. If the student does well, you can proceed very quickly. Present more vocabulary at a time than usual, and skip some of the stories. Use only as many worksheets as are necessary to develop specific Braille skills. Skip *all* lessons which deal with reading skills which have already been covered by other classwork. If a given lesson teaches a skill already learned, but nevertheless provides needed practice in Braille itself, take time only for what your student needs. See "Teaching Braille–Second Grade and Below" for detailed suggestions about *Patterns.*

Beyond the earliest grades you will probably prefer an instruction book designed for older children or adults. Some of these, with comments, are as follows (See "References" for complete bibliographical information):

Braille for Beginners, by Pauline A. Jones. For the earliest grades. Very repetitive. May be used as a supplement to another text.

Modern Methods of Teaching Braille, Book 2, from the American Printing House for the Blind (APH). Good for later elementary school and above. (Book 1 is tactual-readiness work and not needed at this level.)

The ABC's of Braille, by Bernard Krebs. This is best used as a supplementary book. It moves through the signs very fast. At the same time, many of the stories would be unsuitable beyond grade school.

Braille In Brief, by Bernard Krebs. Late elementary school and above. This book, too, moves too quickly to be used as the only instruction book.

The McDuffy Reader: A Braille Primer for Adults, by Sharon L. M. Duffy. Suitable for high school. Presents Grade II Braille in a controlled manner and provides a great deal of practice. An inkprint copy and a teacher's edition are available.

Beginning Braille for Adults, by Nading and Walhof. Suitable for junior high and above. A self-teaching cassette is available. An inkprint copy of this book is not available, and the above cassette does not contain the entire text.

Braille: A Different Approach, from the American Printing House for the Blind (APH). Eighth grade and above. A cassette tape of the practice exercises is available.

Remember that materials from the American Printing House for the Blind generally can be obtained with Federal Quota funds.

Consider using parts of more than one text; plan supplementary lessons if needed; skip extra practice that proves unnecessary.

Beyond the primary grades it is acceptable to present the letters in alphabetical order; but skip around if reversals become a substantial problem. Teach the single-letter contractions, and possibly some short-form words, along with the alphabet itself.

It probably will not confuse the older student to read an unlimited vocabulary in full spelling, gradually phasing in signs as they are learned. Most instruction books for adults use this approach.

Build on previous knowledge whenever you can, as by comparing a Braille letter to its print equivalent. (The angle of the Braille *f,* for example, exists in a printed capital *F*).

Considering groups of signs is usually helpful. "Mother, name one part of the question right sometime!" is an amusing mnemonic for several dot 5 words.

PLENTY OF PRACTICE

Assign practice in between lessons. Sometimes the student might listen to a tape, paced just a little faster than his usual reading speed, as he reads along in Braille.

Learning should be directly helpful in daily life as soon as possible. Often it can be used almost immediately in math, with the ten numerals plus a few other symbols. As soon as the alphabet is learned on the slate, notetaking can be resumed even if it is in Grade I at first. Start a file with names and phone numbers. Use Braille labels. Look for opportunities to write spelling words or short answers, and other situations where even a limited number of symbols can be of practical use.

The many "High Interest/Low Vocabulary" books, designed for slow and reluctant readers, are helpful to the newly blinded for a different reason. Books for English as a Second Language may be good also. Transcribed into Braille, these provide short, interesting articles and stories which are not "babyish." They are helpful in the transition between individualized instruction and regular reading.

Transcribe short items of real interest to the student – riddles, newspaper articles, etc.

Keep seeking variety. When one of my students had learned most of the alphabet, I brought the flashcards for the short-form words–*ab* for *about, af* for *after,* etc. I said, "You read the letters on each card, and I'll tell you what they stand for." The second time around, *she* could tell *me* what most of them stood for.

Ideas suggested below for the student having difficulty may also provide variety for other students.

INTEGRATION

As soon as the student knows essentially all of the literary Braille code, insist that it be used more and more. Even if reading a tape is much faster at this stage, see that some classroom materials are used in Braille. For example, the following types of materials (in this order) might gradually be converted to Braille:

- Part of the spelling list
- All of the spelling list
- Math problems
- Short lists of questions in Social Studies
- Language Arts sentences for study
- Short individual paragraphs
- Short handouts (i.e., one page or less)
- Two- to three-page selections
- General use of Braille whenever available

Speed will come with time and practice.

If Learning Is Difficult

The Braille student who has continual difficulty in reading should be helped in the same general way as a sighted student similarly troubled. Provide more time and/or intensity of instruction. Be sure instruction is at an appropriate level. Consider "High Interest/Low Vocabulary" books. Depending upon job descriptions, it may not be the role of the specialized teacher of the blind to help with an ongoing problem which is not strictly a matter of Braille; consider involving a teacher who gives remedial help to sighted youngsters.

Set priorities in planning ahead for vocational needs, and emphasize basic "survival" skills. Emphasize writing on the slate for basic personal use–telephone numbers, labels, etc.

Look for mnemonic devices for symbols often confused:

"*r* has its single middle dot on the *right,* while *w* does not."

"*of* contains the dots of the letter *o,* and *with* contains the dots of the letter *w.*"

"Think about the numbers of the dots in the letter *y,* and remember the rhyme, '*you* has all but 2.'"

Many of the ideas in this chapter under "Beginning Braille After Kindergarten" are appropriate for the older student who has always used Braille. Also see suggestions in the chapter on the multiply handicapped.

Emphasize self-respect, interest, and success. I once had a seventh grader whose dismay at errors was so great that I presented flashcards in groups of two or three: instead of saying "right" or "wrong" for each individual card, I could tell him "how many right" out of the group.

Provide variety to avoid tedious sessions of oral reading. Ideas include:

(1) Take turns reading, even if there is only one student. (Besides providing variety, this gives the student valuable practice in following along while someone else is reading.) With an advanced student, each turn should consist of several paragraphs or pages. With a beginner, the teacher might read every other paragraph, or possibly every other sentence.

(2) Occasionally the teacher and student(s) might read aloud in chorus.

(3) If the student is reading a list of words, the teacher might give a sentence aloud before each word is read. For example, if the word is "weather," the teacher might say, "We had some bad *blank* yesterday."

(4) Before reading a given sentence, the student might analyze certain parts of it: find all the instances of a particular letter or sign, look for two words that rhyme, etc.

(5) If students are in groups, many more possibilities exist for varying oral reading.

Dramatization (actual or by voice only) is a good example, and often is possible even with a single student.

Although these ideas are especially important in motivating reluctant or discouraged readers, they are helpful with all students in keeping interest high.

Excuses, Excuses!

Due to traditional public attitudes which equate blindness with inferiority, many myths and misunderstandings about Braille have become ingrained. Even educators often believe them. Below are some common incorrect assumptions, with explanation of why they are incorrect:

(1) "Reading machines are replacing Braille anyway."
–Mechanical reading devices are slower and more complex to use than Braille. Searching for one particular passage is difficult to do quickly. These and other disadvantages make such devices undesirable as a main mode of reading. See the chapter on "Other Modes of Reading" for further discussion.

(2) "He will just keep trying to use his eyes. (or) "It will scare him if I try to cover his eyes."
–Use a matter-of-fact tone of voice, instead of a gingerly approach which implies that *you* think the student will be upset. Explain that sleepshades make it possible to concentrate on a new and valuable skill.
–See the chapter on "Sleepshades." Also, the chapter on Braille for young children has suggestions on helping a very young student become accustomed to sleepshades.

(3) "His hands are calloused from farm work."
–Persons with *severe* circulatory problems may indeed have trouble with the sense of touch, but even they can usually learn reasonably well. Calluses are not a substantial problem.

(4) "He has such a negative attitude that it will never work."
–Although this is a problem, it is no reason to give up. Work to improve attitudes in general. Look for ways to make Braille relevant and practical. See that other people speak positively about Braille.
–With a younger student, apply positive and negative consequences as necessary.
–With a high school student, it may indeed be impossible to proceed if he is resisting strenuously. Nevertheless, continue to look for ways to convince him of the value.
–If he had a "negative attitude" toward math (as many students do) would you simply drop it from his schedule without a peep?

(5) "But he can read print if it is very large. Braille is so much slower."
–Braille need *not* be slow if properly taught, and there is no physical limit to the speed of a good reader. The low-visioned student struggling through large print, however, certainly does have a handicap–one so great that it is unconscionable to recommend print as the main mode of reading.

(6) "If she were in first grade now, I'd consider it. But she is almost out of high school. She'll never develop any speed."
–Younger beginners do have a great advantage. However, Braille can be learned, and good speed developed, at any time in life. If the student graduates without having even started Braille, the chances of her ever learning it drop dramatically.

(7) "If she reads print she will be independent. If she uses Braille, there is always someone else between her and the printed page."
–If a person can read *regular* print with *good* speed and stamina, and the eye condition is really not expected to change, this view has merit. But if large print must be used, someone (or at least a machine) was "in between" to produce that. More important, the main issue is not whether any particular task is done "alone," but

how efficiently and effectively it is done. If we object to involving another person as a transcriber (or for that matter, as a reader), will we apply this elsewhere and produce all our own food and clothing as the pioneers did? In today's complex world we are *all* interdependent.

(8) "She has a physical handicap (cerebral palsy, use of only one hand, etc.)"
–Some physical handicaps can interfere significantly with Braille. But usually it is a matter of degree, rather than a prohibition. I know a young woman with cerebral palsy who cannot use her left hand and has considerable involvement with her right, and who nevertheless reads Braille quite well. She has developed "nonstandard" hand movements which are right for her.

(9) "Her attention span is short."
–This has no special relevance to Braille in particular. The very restless child may need a modified reading program, but should not be denied the chance to read in the most efficient mode.
–Consider the very real possibility that her attention span will be much *better* with Braille. Perhaps she is using up all her energy just trying to see the print.

(10) "This student has a low IQ, and Braille would be too difficult."
–Mentally retarded sighted students are not categorically denied the opportunity to read. Such flat categorization would violate the law. Each student, blind or sighted, is entitled to instruction appropriate for him/her as an individual. Braille is not categorically harder to learn than print. If ability is extremely limited, teach a limited vocabulary and consider using only Grade I Braille. This can be very useful for such things as labels used on the job.

(11) "Why bother with Braille when it's so easy to use tape recordings?"
–Many things are more difficult or cumbersome when not on paper. Math problems, foreign languages, recipes, and telephone numbers are particularly clear examples. It is usually much easier to skip around, as many lessons require, in Braille than on tape. All these things are true even if the Braille reader is not particularly fast. But a good Braille reader can read faster than even speeded-up speech.

(12) "Sure, there are a few *exceptional* blind persons who can read Braille quite fast. But for *ordinary* students, Braille is slow."
–This is one of the oldest excuses: belittle the evidence by claiming it is an obscure exception to the general rule. This excuse will not stand up against the large numbers of ordinary blind people who read Braille as quickly and well as the ordinary sighted citizen reads print.
–Moreover, as discussed above, Braille has many advantages even for a slow reader. After all, sighted students who read slowly are not discouraged from using any print!

Conclusion

Finally, remember that learning Braille does not rule out all use of print. But *not* learning Braille does rule out, absolutely, the option of using this effective and efficient medium.

CHAPTER 18

A BRAILLEWRITER IN MY POCKET

By Sharon L. M. Duffy
and
Doris M. Willoughby

Convenient and Portable

Yes, I do carry a Braillewriter in my pocket! And how is this possible? (They are rather larger than most pockets!) Of course, I am referring to a slate–a highly versatile Braille-writing tool. I can write a grocery list, a telephone number, a multi-page treatise, or almost anything else with it.

Yet, I have met a number of people who do not consider the use of the slate practical for children learning Braille. To the uninitiated, the prospect of punching three or four holes per letter, "backwards," and working from right to left appears complicated and tedious at best. However, in my seven years of teaching blind persons from ages 7 to 74, I have never had a student who could not master this skill.

As regards speed, I have only one thing to say–any worthwhile skill takes time to develop. Sighted children spend years learning to color, print, and handwrite. So, a blind child should not be expected to write with great speed and accuracy to begin with. It will come with practice.

The problem of having to write from right to left, letters in reverse, is a complication that many adults mistakenly believe will lead to more confusion for children learning Braille. Although this may be true initially, the marvelous human brain accommodates this problem readily–especially for children, since their thinking patterns are more flexible. When teaching Braille, I always teach the dot numbers and then explain that the numbers remain the same but horizontally change places in writing. That is, dots 1, 2, and 3 are on the right or "first" side of the cell for writing, while they are on the left side of the cell for reading. The concept of dots 1-2-3 being the first read or written, eliminates a great deal of the problem.

To say all of this is not, however, to address the real problem in teaching or encouraging the use of the slate. The real problem is the lack of faith that many people have in using the slate. They believe that, because they cannot themselves use it efficiently, it must be inefficient for others as well. So, my best advice is to sharpen personal skills to teach better. Confidence, or rather the lack of it, will undermine the best efforts of a teacher. The child will pick this up more readily than the skill itself. The hidden curriculum! So, beware of negative attitudes.

Negative attitudes regarding the use of the slate are part of the general belief that Braille itself is difficult. The fact is that the system itself is not difficult, but it does require practice, just as reading and writing print requires practice. Many factors contribute to this attitude-First, most people do not know Braille, and so assume it is difficult. Second, adults (sighted or blind) who learn Braille as adults must practice to achieve competence in reading and writing. Although the system can be learned quickly, and although they learn it much more rapidly than they learned print as children, the comparison of the new skill to the familiar one results in an unfair conclusion that Braille is difficult.

At first, the Perkins Brailler appears easier than a slate, so many teachers rely almost exclusively on the Perkins. If they teach the slate at all, they wait until junior high or high school, and they may regard it as mainly for the college-bound. I strongly advise against this practice for several reasons: first, it makes the student feel that the slate must be very difficult to use; second, it restricts opportunities to practice on the slate, thus greatly reducing speed and proficiency; third, inadequate practice with the slate discourages the use of Braille anywhere except at home and school where the Perkins is handy.

All this would not be so important if the relative competence in using Braille did not so directly bear on the ultimate success of a blind person. In college I used a slate because I am not strong enough to carry a Brailler all over campus, and because a Brailler is too noisy to use in the classroom. In one university which I attended, a blind person did use her Braillewriter in class. A very relieved professor greeted me at the close of my first day in his class. He told me of this other student and said that her Braillewriter was extremely annoying during his lectures, and that he worried that her friends were overworked from carrying her Braillewriter from class to class.

This brings up another issue, that of image. I am certain that this student's classmates viewed her as a person needing special treatment and cumbersome methods which were inconvenient both for her and for those around her. This belief does not foster equality for blind people in employment and educational pursuits. Had this student considered the slate to be a viable note-taking method, this unfortunate situation would never have occurred.

I must digress here, however, to note that she did succeed in one vital respect-at least she did produce notes which were really useful in review. An alarming number of students attempt to use a method which, though quiet, is disastrous as a study skill, namely, tape-recording lectures. This is really not "note-taking" at all. Forty hours of lecture become forty hours of tape, with no provision for quick summary or review. A rehabilitation counselor recently remarked, "Last year I knew of four students who started college expecting to tape-record lectures. Every one of them flunked out."

In emphasizing the value of the slate, I do not mean that a Braillewriter has no place. I own and use one daily. I find it more efficient for mathematical record-keeping and for editing, since what has been written is more immediately accessible for review. I also own a slate and use it daily, both at home and elsewhere, because it is more convenient. Of the two, I would say it is more important that a blind person use a slate, because it is portable, quiet, and versatile. Many blind persons function quite adequately without a Braillewriter. But those without adequate slate-writing skills must rely heavily on others for note-taking. With the slate I have a "Braillewriter in my pocket."

Note: The above article by Sharon Duffy was first published in the September-November, 1984, issue of FUTURE REFLECTIONS.

Starting Early

As an important tool for literacy, the slate should be introduced early in the child's education. Strong emphasis should be given no later than third grade. (A convenient opportunity arises during that grade to work on the slate while others are developing their cursive writing skills.)

Every newly-blinded older student should have emphasis on slate usage immediately.

Building Speed and Fluency

As suggested in the article above, emphasize dot numbers and the concept of "first side" and "second side." (The "first side"–with dots 1, 2, and 3–is always closer to the beginning of the line. The beginning of the line is on the left for reading, and on the right for slate writing.) An unfortunate common error is the misnumbering of dots on the slate: believing that *b*, for example, is called "dots 4-5" on the slate because it is on the other side while being written. This is incorrect; *b* is always called "dots 1-2."

GETTING STARTED

A very young student should first spend a few minutes merely "making dots" anywhere on the slate, to grasp the general idea without having to meet a specific standard.

A good sequence of early lessons on the slate is:

- Full cells
- Easy-to-form letters such as *a b c g l*
- The alphabet
- Combinations of letters using the top part of the cell only, such as *ab ac cd ed df gh ei ice*
- Combinations of letters in which a dot is added to make the second letter, such as *ak bl cm dn eo fp gp hr is jt ku lv mx rw ny oz mn st au* etc.
- Short words, then longer words
- Complete sentences

Letter combinations should be done with spaces between groups of letters, to establish proper patterns for spacing between words and to help build speed. Have the student do an entire line of each letter, or letter combination, as fast as possible. These exercises will help establish speed and skill, by providing plenty of practice on the letters and dot positions on the slate. They are also good confidence builders, because almost anyone can do them easily and quickly. Emphasize correct spacing.

If the student is just learning to read the alphabet, it is best not to begin slate usage until most of the letters have been learned. Starting too soon can create confusion among such combinations as *e* and *i*. However, once the basic letters have been learned, the use of the slate can reinforce learning of the Grade II signs. Some Grade II symbols are easier than some alphabet letters.

MOVING ALONG

Help your student feel with the stylus to find the six detents, or notches, in the sides of the cell frame. Too many students just poke around vaguely, hoping the dot will go through.

The stylus should be held in a vertical position, with part of the palm of the hand over the rounded top. (See Figure 18-1.) The index finger applies pressure. This position is least tiring and most helpful for speed-building. Note that it is quite different from holding a pencil.

Styluses shaped like pencils are *not* desirable. They are awkward to hold and are not good for speed.

A regular stylus with one flattened side is now available from the American Printing House for the Blind (APH)–this prevents the stylus' rolling around on the desk, a problem which has led some students to try the pencil-like type.

Strive for speed and fluency from the beginning.

Sharpen the stylus just the right amount for maximum speed. (Most of them are much too dull unless hand-sharpened with a metal file.) Experiment with weight of paper: lightweight paper generally maximizes speed, but heavy paper may help the beginner keep better control. Insist on daily practice–at first as mere practice, and later in real-life situations. Time

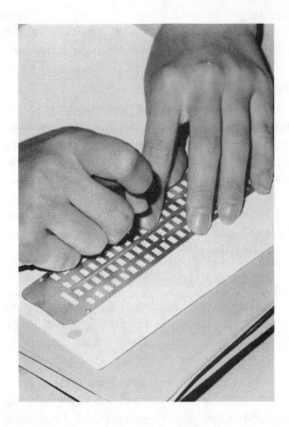

Figure 18-1
Hand Position

the characters per minute, and keep speed charts.

A good drill to help get the idea of speed is to write the same character several times rapidly – a whole row of one letter, then a row of another letter, and so on. Start with easy letters such as *a c x* and *l*.

Expect students to use all Grade II symbols. In addition, like sighted students, they should invent their own abbreviations for personal note-taking. Consider Grade III Braille (which includes the signs of regular Grade II Braille, plus other signs not used in books), especially for high school students who are college-bound. (Caution: A student with less than two years' experience with Grade II Braille should not attempt to learn Grade III.)

Class Notes

Note-taking skills must be taught. Often a student will complain, "I can't write fast enough," when actually she is attempting to write down too many things or the wrong things. Work on the art of determining main ideas and noting them down in the briefest practical form.

The slate is much quieter than the Perkins, and thus greatly preferable for taking notes during lectures.

Writing skills reinforce reading skills, for the older student as well as the younger. Some newly-blinded students become fluent in slate writing before they are fluent at reading.

See also the chapter on "Note-Taking."

Handy Hints

Ask blind adults for practical hints, such as:

- There are many sizes and types of slates. The Brown slate opens in back, so that material can be read without removing it.
- A pocket-sized notebook from the American Printing House for the Blind provides a slate of exactly the right size for its small note sheets. (The slate is placed parallel to the longer sides of this small paper – "sideways" in comparison to the usual position.)
- When using larger paper with punched holes, the holes should be on the right, and the hinge of the slate on the left. When the paper is taken out of the slate and inserted into a loose-leaf notebook, the holes will then be on the left.
- Be flexible about the writing position. Although the beginner will need a stable surface, the experienced individual can write on her knee, lean against the wall, etc.
- If writing is briefly interrupted, the place may be kept this way: Open the slate slightly. Insert the stylus gently into the next cell frame (without punching the paper), and let the stylus lean to one side. The stylus then becomes a wedge, propping the slate slightly open and marking the place.
- If the student is uncertain which cell was

used last, suggest this: Note the cell where it is believed that the last character was written. Gently feel with the stylus to determine what dots, if any, have been already made in that cell. If the cell proves to be unused, proceed in the reverse of the usual direction, until a cell is found which has dots. Check to see that it is the correct character (e.g., dots 1 and 3 if the last word written was *back*). Should you encounter a cell which is not the last character, figure out what it is and deduce where you are. (Note: Usually it is not productive to insist on this procedure whenever the student loses her place. Often it is much faster merely to go to the next line. But this technique is useful to know.)

- The slate can be used to label many things which cannot be inserted into the Perkins Braillewriter.
- Help your student plan a good way to keep track of the stylus, between writing sessions and also when briefly interrupted. Most people keep the stylus in the purse or pocket, preferably in a specific place. Some students prefer a zippered plastic envelope, punched for insertion into a regular notebook. Some people attach a string to the stylus. APH offers a regular stylus with one flat side. Howe Press offers a "tuck-away" stylus with flat sides and a screw-in point. Also note the method, above, of leaving the stylus in a partially open slate.
- If a beginner complains of tired muscles, try to make practices short but frequent at first. Emphasize correct hand position, and locating the detents in the side of the cell. With practice, "writer's cramp" should be no more of a problem than it is in using a pen.
- To demonstrate the value of Grade II Braille, occasionally write a sentence first in Grade I (full spelling) and then in Grade II. One good sentence is, "Mother and Father have very little knowledge of Braille."

Troubleshooting

Should your student have difficulty beginning to use the slate, do not assume it is impossible, any more than you would with a non-disabled student who has poor handwriting. Provide a great deal of practice, gradually increasing difficulty. Emphasize dot numbers. Try various techniques, such as pins stuck through paper, to illustrate how things come out on the other side.

Be sure that proper materials are provided. Sharpen the stylus just enough (sharp, but not too sharp). Write a few lines yourself if the student seems to be having trouble; you may discover that the slate is badly mis-aligned or bent.

Although a pocket slate is usually the most convenient, the stability of a board slate may be helpful to beginners. APH offers one with pegs to aid in moving the slate down the page.

A few students may need practice in how to find what they have written (on the back of the paper as it lies in the slate), and how to read it with the correct orientation. (Note: The student need not necessarily turn the paper over to read what he has written. A fluent Braille reader can read in various positions.)

Most students grasp the entire procedure for paper insertion almost immediately. However, if a given student has real difficulty it may be necessary to practice specific parts of the procedure (top alignment; side alignment; closing the slate; removing the paper and re-inserting in the next position). Remind the student to hold the paper with one hand as long as possible while closing the slate with the other hand. If paper alignment is poor, move the student's hands to feel where the paper does not match the slate.

Insertion practice (if needed) should not delay actual writing skills. After a few tries, adjust the slate for the student if necessary. From time to time during the writing session, take the slate off the paper (perhaps to proofread) and again work on insertion. One of my students learned to write the entire alphabet and several signs before he was able to insert the paper into the slate with good alignment. But he did succeed. A previous teacher had given up, saying that slate usage was clearly impossible for this student.

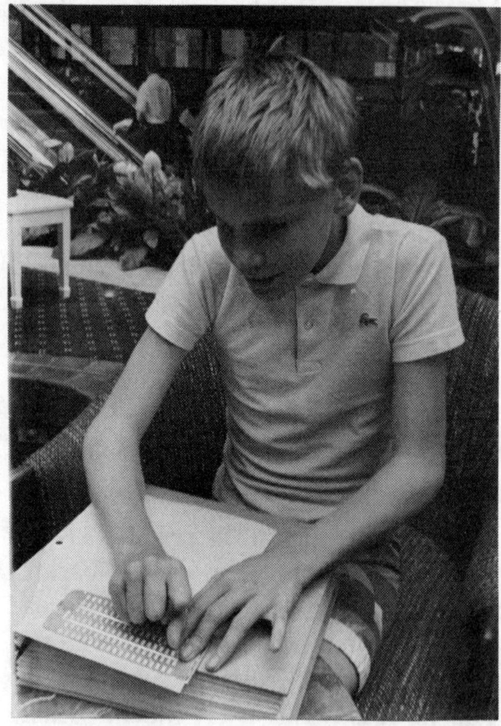

Figure 18-2
The Slate Goes Everywhere

CHAPTER 19

OTHER MODES OF READING

By Sharon L. M. Duffy and Doris M. Willoughby

(*Note: This chapter as a whole was written by Sharon Duffy. The outline, "Studying From Recorded Material," was written by Doris Willoughby.*)

If Braille were universally available in the way that print is, there would be no need for this chapter, but that isn't reality. Blind persons, in order to function effectively, must learn to use a variety of reading methods. They may include: large print, tape recordings, live readers, electronic devices such as Optacons and CCTV's, and others. These methods cannot adequately replace Braille, but these can provide written material not available in Braille or solve a particular problem better than Braille would.

Large Print

Large print was once hailed as a good alternative to Braille for partially-sighted children. It is typically produced for school age children in 16 or 18 point type, though sometimes as small as 14 point. (Type size is measured in "points.") However, any partially-sighted student who cannot comfortably read 16 point type will not be able to utilize large print reliably. Also, some producers of large print use a type font that is difficult to read, or production methods that present reading problems for certain students; therefore it is wise to try out samples of the large print material before determining whether large print will be a suitable medium.

For partially-sighted students, it has been common practice for a number of years to insist that they use print, enlarged to whatever size is necessary, no matter how slowly the student reads. This tendency is fostered by classroom teachers who are baffled by Braille, by vision specialists who either feel they are too busy or are too lazy to teach it, and by parents who are not ready to accept the fact of their children's blindness. The result is usually an inadequate education as the result of an ineffective reading method. For these children, reading is so much work that they do not do it for pleasure as do Braille readers. Therefore, they do not become good readers. Furthermore, even if a student is reasonably proficient at using large print, when he reaches adulthood he will find that large-print books are less available than Braille books. A student will find virtually no college textbooks in large print, and not many books for recreational reading either.

DECIDING WHETHER TO USE LARGE PRINT

Efficiency is the most important matter in deciding whether a child should read print or Braille. If a student can read 50 words a minute in large print for intervals of 20 minutes (not an unusual situation), that means he could only read 1000 words before resting. In many books this means he reads *two or three pages* in twenty minutes–and then has to rest because of fatigue!

Another consideration in using large print is that most eye diseases are degenerative, and Braille (to be learned in the best way) should be learned in school at the earliest opportunity. (See the chapters on Braille.) I have had a number of adult students who were taught large print as children and now request Braille, because they have either lost more sight or determined that large print was not adequate to meet their reading needs.

Nevertheless, there may be some instances when the use of large print can be helpful. The partially-sighted student may prefer enlarged graphs, maps, or diagrams difficult to reproduce in Braille. Whether using enlarged maps is useful or not will depend on the amount of vision that a student has. It is harmful to expect a student to see things when he cannot see them comfortably (or perhaps cannot accurately see them at all), because it makes the child feel inadequate and reinforces negative attitudes about the abilities of the blind.

For the above reasons, large print is not a good choice as the main reading method for most legally blind children or for those who have degenerative eye conditions.

For visually impaired students who really can make efficient use of regular print, some use of large print may be helpful at times. Examples include dictionaries and other materials which have exceptionally small print. Another use occurs where the student cannot get close enough to read small print comfortably–as with a typing text or a cookbook.

The chapter on "Braille–Why or Why Not" contains detailed suggestions about choosing the primary mode of reading.

Magnification

Magnification of regular print has many advantages over the use of large print–chiefly the fact that it can be used any time, without advance preparation of materials.

Non-prescription magnifiers are available commercially and from agencies for the blind, in great variety. The most common kinds are small hand-held magnifiers; low-power magnifiers which cover an entire page; and large "table" magnifiers which resemble gooseneck lamps and may indeed be lighted.

Magnifiers prescribed by a doctor may be even more powerful.

Trial-and-error is usually necessary in selection of a device. Analysis of the eye condition, with or without formal advice from the doctor, will be of some help. (For example, a person with albinism will probably *not* want a lighted magnifier.) Demonstrate use of the magnifier and help the student give it a reasonable trial. If the student dislikes it after a fair trial, probably the device is not sufficiently helpful to be worth using.

Full-time use of a magnifier is *not* a good idea. Most magnifiers must be moved along the line and down the page, thus limiting reading speed. Eyestrain often results as the device jiggles and provides uneven images.

Furthermore, the greater the enlargement, the *smaller* the field shown. Often it is casually assumed that once the student can see the letters, the problem is completely solved. Sadly, even many eye doctors encourage this incorrect belief. Actually, with high magnification often the student can only see a few letters at a time–hardly a satisfactory way to "read."

As with large print, the most successful use of magnification occurs with students who usually read regular print easily, but sometimes have trouble with extra-small print.

Enlargement on a screen (i.e., closed circuit TV's such as Apollo and VTEK) appears to be a wonderful idea. Now a student can read any kind of print, it seems. Unfortunately, it isn't as simple as that for most partially-sighted people. Many find that the screen gives them a headache after only a few minutes' use. Others find that reading is so slow, it would take a long time to read a few pages. Reading is very hard work under these conditions.

Closed circuit TV's (CCTV's) have many drawbacks in terms of efficiency. Because the print is enlarged, the screen can only hold a *part* of a line. This means much moving of the text, resulting in very slow reading speeds. Persons who have nystagmus or narrowed fields of vision may not be helped by the enlargement of the screen since this does not solve the focusing problems.

All of this is not to say that blind people never derive benefit from using a CCTV. Many have found it valuable in a work situation or for personal needs. Discomfort may be relieved by wearing sunglasses, reversing or otherwise altering the contrast on the screen, etc. When viewed as one tool and not a *carte blanche* solution to the reading problems of an individual, a CCTV can be valuable.

As a general rule, however, a partially-sighted student need not possess such a device in the course of a general education. Braille, tape recordings and readers will generally be more efficient and practical methods of reading. CCTV's are not very portable. I recently met a college student who was trying to rig a harness so he could carry his CCTV to his various classes. The saddest part of this situation is that this young man has an eye disease which will result in total blindness. Because of the CCTV provided him in school, he is not learning Braille and will need to do so later.

The final drawback to the CCTV is its cost – well over $1000. At that price it is unlikely that any student would have more than one; therefore the portability problem cannot be solved by buying several.

Other Aids for Print Reading

Besides magnification, various other aids and arrangements may be helpful in reading print.

Moving a strip of cardboard down the page can help prevent jumping lines and losing the place. (Some prefer to keep the strip *above* the line currently being read, to avoid blocking the next line.)

A transparent, tinted plastic overlay is favored by some readers. Especially with blue or purple print, the overlay can increase the contrast or otherwise add to visual comfort. Amber and blue are especially popular tints.

Reading racks can position books and materials to permit better posture.

The Optacon

An Optacon is a device which will transform print letters into a tactile array of vibrating pins. The shapes of the printed letters (not Braille letters) move along under the fingers. This device costs several thousand dollars, and is slightly larger than a standard cassette machine. Most people read less than 40 words a minute using it.

Reading rate is the Optacon's greatest drawback. The combination of portability and flexibility is unparalleled in reading devices for the blind, but it is simply too slow for most reading needs. Although it might be a handy skill for a blind student to have, it will not replace Braille. If young children are trained on the Optacon, they lose valuable time which could have been devoted to learning Braille.

The Optacon can be used to read textbooks, paperbacks, typed copy, dot matrix printing and graphs. Some people are able to read the newspaper, although varying type sizes and poor quality ink and paper create problems. Some people can also read the phone book and fill out forms with it. But with all of this, it is simply too slow for most purposes.

In the employment area, an Optacon has proven to be a useful device for filling out forms and reading a computer screen. However, with the advent of voice and Braille output devices on computers, the computer use is becoming obsolete. (See also the chapter entitled "Computers.")

As with the CCTV, the Optacon can be valuable when viewed as a tool. However, it is not helpful to the general education of a student unless a specific need can best be met with its use.

Other Electronic Devices

The Kurzweil Reading Machine (*KRM*) is a relatively recent invention: a printed page is read by an optical scanner and spoken aloud by a speech synthesizer. This machine can read faster than normal speech, and it was hoped that this would be the ultimate answer for print accessibility for the blind. However, this machine (especially the earlier models) will not read everything. The problem is the variety of type styles available, as well as the quality of print or paper.

This machine is significant in its development of an optical scanner which will read more type styles than any preceding scanner. Also, it is significant in its use of synthesized speech. Unfortunately, synthesized speech is not perfect and can be very distracting in the reading of difficult material. It is also not as pleasant to listen to as a person reading. It mispronounces words with enough frequency to be frustrating.

This machine has two other major problems. It is not portable, and it is very expensive – costing many thousands of dollars.

Other electronic devices are continually being invented. Manufacturers tout them as near-miracles, and glowingly describe every possible potential use. Disadvantages, though important, are rarely mentioned. The article by Curtis Chong entitled "Some Comments on Technology, Print-Reading Devices and Braille" (*Future Reflections,* January-February, 1984) analyzes this well. Following is a brief quote:

> Although it is true that technology can make life easier and more pleasant for all of us (witness the pocket calculator), it is equally true that technology can become a stumbling block that can make our lives unbearably complicated. Also, the inappropriate dependence upon certain forms of technology can cause us to neglect learning some rather basic and important skills.

Sound Recordings

THE MOST AVAILABLE MEDIUM

Tape recordings are currently the most available medium for the blind. In libraries for the blind, recorded books outnumber those in Braille and large print, with cassettes being more numerous than disc recordings. Cassette players may be borrowed from regional libraries for the blind (or the agency designated for a particular state). It is quite easy to produce books in recorded media. College texts are produced on cassette by Recording for the Blind, Inc., and by volunteers of a number of agencies for the blind. Furthermore, it requires no particular skill to operate a cassette machine.

With all of these advantages, a cassette recorder should be standard equipment for any student. Cassettes cannot replace Braille, but can be an excellent means to obtain material not available in Braille. With a recorder, a student can have a reader read materials for later review, making better use of the reader's time. Since college texts are frequently available on cassette, skill in using tapes effectively is vital.

EFFICIENT USE MUST BE LEARNED

Learning to learn from recorded media is a skill which should be developed, since Braille and large print are less available after high school. If a student receives everything in Braille (or large print) until college, he will have to learn a new skill while adjusting to college, not the best time for this. On the job, tape recordings may be the key to much needed information. If a blind person is not flexible regarding media, he may well lose out on a good job by unreasonably insisting upon Braille (or large print) for every purpose.

Efficient use of tapes is a complex skill which should be actively taught – both in regard to technical competence and in regard to study skills. The student should use all features comfortably, including four tracks and variable speed. He should be able to "troubleshoot" by checking the controls and understanding common problems. (For example, some models, despite having batteries, do not work unless they are kept plugged into an electrical outlet most of the time.)

The paper below is suitable for handing out to students, and contains many important explanations and suggestions.

Studying from Recorded Material:

Hints for Students

By Doris M. Willoughby

I. Each kind of tape should be studied in the most appropriate way. Do not read every tape the same way. (The expression "read a tape" means "listen to it and learn from it." Using a tape is one mode of reading.)

   A. You are not watching TV or listening to the radio. Keep distractions away. Watch out for habit interference if you are used to listening just for fun.

   B. Reading a novel or short story usually requires very few notes. However, it is helpful to make a few notes (in Braille or large print) describing the characters and the main outline of the plot. If you must read several selections, you won't want to re-read every selection to review for the test.

   C. Consider your own background, together with the subject. If you already know a lot about cooking but very little about biology, you will need to work harder to understand a science text-and vice versa. Also, if you are not accustomed to studying from a tape, you will need to put forth extra effort until you gain experience.

   D. Be creative in considering how best to study. Sometimes playing an entire chapter straight through is helpful-perhaps more than once. Often it is helpful to play a chapter clear through once to get the general idea, and then play it again a short piece at a time while taking notes.

   E. When you must learn many details, new ideas, etc., from a tape, do not just listen-study intensively. Examples include science, social studies, etc.

      1. If you are more accustomed to studying in Braille or in print, consider how you would study the book in that mode; this will give you helpful hints on how to study from the tape, although it will not be exactly the same.
      2. If the lesson is background for a class session-especially for something like a science lab-study the lesson *before* class. Do this even if most other students do not, and even if you need to ask the teacher to tell you the assignments ahead of time. If you have already read your taped lesson, you will be ready to get the most out of class. You will not need to be concerned about whether reading the tape takes longer than for others to read print.
      3. For concentrated study of a difficult subject, follow this pattern: play a short portion of the tape; stop and write notes as necessary; re-play the portion if it was not understood. The size of the portion you play at a time will depend on the nature of the material and on your own experience. With practice you will be able to rewind the tape to approximately the right point.
      4. The importance of taking notes cannot be emphasized too much. When the time comes to review for a test, you do not want your only choices to be re-playing the entire set of tapes *vs.* relying entirely on your memory. If you have good written notes, you can review the notes quickly and profitably.

II. Often the teacher will "skip around" in the book, instead of assigning the pages in straight numerical order.

   A. Make the most of the labels on the cassettes and on the containers. Somewhere there will be an indication as to what page is at the beginning of each track. There may be printed or Braille labels on the tapes or on the boxes. Information can also be found by playing the tape: at the beginning of the first tape there is usually a good bit of information, including where to find the table of contents on the tape; and the beginning of each track usually announces the page number. You may want to make a Braille chart of where each track begins.

B. Keep tapes organized. If you misfile a tape it may be hard to tell where it belongs.

C. Many tapes have special "beeps" (tone indexing) which can be heard at fast-forward speed. Usually there are two beeps at the beginning of each chapter, and one beep at the beginning of each new page which does not start a chapter.

D. Practice will make it easier for you to find things on a tape even when there are no beeps.

E. When there is a great deal of skipping around, or when you are spending a lot of time searching for a short passage, you would probably be better off not to use the tape at that particular time. Use a live reader instead, as it will be much faster in this case. This is one reason you should always have a regular-print copy of the book on hand.

F. Often students ask, "I'm supposed to read the chapter and answer the questions. But I don't get to the questions until I come to the end of the chapter, so I don't know what to look for. Do I have to go back and start over each time?"

1. Sometimes you may choose to go back and start over. But often it is possible to get all of the questions in Braille or large print, even when you cannot get the whole book in that mode. (The teacher may be able to arrange this for you.) Then you can look at the questions while playing the tape.
2. If there are beeps on the tape, another approach is to run the tape to the beginning of the *next* chapter; then rewind enough to play the questions for the chapter you want; then rewind to the beginning of the chapter you want.
3. Note each answer *as you come to it on the tape,* no matter what the number of that question may be. Do not insist on finding Answer #1 first, Answer #2 second, etc. Find the answers as you can and write them into their proper places on the answer sheet. Or, make a rough draft of the answers as you find them, and later recopy them in the order desired.

III. Some things may be omitted from the tape, such as pictures or diagrams. A well-made tape will either describe the item, provide a Braille/large print supplement, or at least mention that the item is omitted. Again, if something apparently important is not there, use a live reader with the regular copy of the book.

IV. In science and math, especially, be alert to the possibility that a special symbol will be read aloud as though it were a word, and that you will not know what the symbol looks like. For example, an arrow pointing to the right can mean "produces" in chemistry. If the reader simply says "produces" and you do not learn about the arrow, you may miss a test question about arrows. Be alert: learn what all symbols look like in print, and also in Braille if you read Braille.

V. Be sure that the speed selection switch is set correctly. Also, make good use of the variable-speed control if there is one.

A. At first, it may seem that the tape goes too fast. If this is a problem, you may want to slow the speed down somewhat with the variable-speed control. Also, stop the tape periodically to take notes or re-play a section, as above. Ask your teacher for hints if you still have trouble.

B. With experience you will come to prefer speech as fast as possible. Learn to listen when you have speeded up the tape with the variable-speed control. Practice listening to faster-than-average speech; it can save you a great deal of time. Remember that average speed of speech is only about 150-200 words per minute, much slower than the typical speed of silent reading in Braille or print by a skillful reader.

VI. Become thoroughly familiar with the mechanics of playing tapes.

A. Be sure you know how to find the tracks of a four-track tape:

1. Set track switch to "Tracks 1-2."
2. Track 1 is on the first side; flip tape over for Track 2.
3. Set track switch to "Tracks 3-4."
4. Track 3 is on the first side; flip tape over for Track 4.
5. Note that some tapes only have Tracks 1 and 2. Tapes from Recording for the Blind will have four tracks.

B. Ask your teacher to help you if you are having difficulty. Don't let yourself avoid using tapes just because the machine seems hard to handle. You can learn to use it confidently. Moreover, if you are having trouble, the machine may need repair.

VII. Often the question is asked, "Many students prefer to read in Braille or large print. If I prefer one of these modes, why must I use tapes (or live readers) at all?"

A. With very young children, or in a special school for the blind, it is sometimes possible to provide everything in Braille or large print. For older students in a regular school, however, this is simply not possible. There just are not enough Braillists or enlarging machines available, and/or there is not enough money to pay for this service. Also, sometimes there would not be time to transcribe an item even if someone were available.

These circumstances apply more and more as the student gets older. The Braille available to college students and other adults is much more limited than that available in high school. Large-print books are hardly available at all after high school.

Therefore, a student needs to learn to use all possible media, including tapes and live readers. Even a student in a special school, where Braille or large print may be widely available, needs to learn to use other modes because of future needs after graduation.

B. In any particular situation, ask yourself:

1. What modes are available to me?
2. Under the circumstances, what mode is most *efficient*?

VIII. Your teachers will help you when you begin something new, including the use of tapes. Until you graduate from high school, your teacher will try to provide you with extra aids (such as diagrams, questions, etc., in Braille or large print) and will help you anticipate and solve problems. As you move along in school, it is expected that you will take more and more responsibility for deciding what you need and how you can get it. Increased responsibility is an important sign of increased maturity.

THE ROLE OF RECORDED MATERIALS

Much discussion is often necessary before students, parents, and teachers fully recognize tape as a reading mode. People may say, "We don't have that book" when they really mean, "We have that book on tape, but we don't have it in Braille (or large print)." Help them to realize that when the book arrives in recorded form, they do indeed have a copy in a suitable transcribed form.

As a variation of this problem, a person may recognize that the tape is a transcribed copy, but insist that it is unsatisfactory and that Braille (or large print) should always be provided. Explain why flexibility is necessary. Work intensively on skilled and efficient use of tapes. Consider combination arrangements in which certain crucial things *are* written in Braille (or large print), while the bulk of the book is read on tape. For example, if the science text is on tape but the student needs to learn certain Nemeth-code symbols, a list of those symbols could be Brailled. Questions, tables, etc., may be Brailled even when the rest of the text is not.

When the sighted students underline passages in a booklet, the blind student should take Braille notes.

In my own college experiences, I found that I could use tapes effectively for most subjects except foreign language, math, and highly technical information. For some of this, Braille notes of the recorded information served quite well.

Unfortunately, there are some teachers who feel that if tape recordings are such a good idea, they can serve as a substitute for Braille. Sighted people would never agree to abandon print in favor of tape recordings. Neither should blind people. Again, tapes are a useful tool, and not the total solution to all of the reading needs of the blind. One itinerant teacher said she "would get the little guy some tapes" when confronted with the fact that a particular child could not read print. She resisted teaching Braille by offering tape recordings. She forgot that there are many kinds of things that exclusive use of tapes cannot teach – paragraphing, spelling, capitalization, etc. Also, some subject matter is very difficult to work with when using oral media alone.

THE TAPE MACHINE

The full-sized four-track, two-speed recorder from the American Printing House for the Blind is an excellent machine. It is portable, can be operated on battery or by being plugged in, is quite reliable, and records six hours on each "90 minute" cassette. This machine also has a built-in microphone and a tone-indexing button. To complete work quickly, this recorder also has a variable speed switch. With this feature, reading by tape becomes a fast way to get information – a critical matter in the usefulness of tapes as a learning aid.

Many models of tape machines are available commercially. However, they usually will not play the recordings made by the Library of Congress with four tracks and slow speed.

Live Readers

The live reader (i.e., a person reading aloud) is perhaps the most flexible and efficient of all methods of obtaining information for the blind student. Unfortunately, it is not always possible to have a reader for everything, because of hiring costs and scheduling. However, with a reader, a student can have access to the same material as everyone, and has the freedom to skip around easily in the book. A reader can even skip easily among various books and other materials, and therefore this is often the only practical reading mode for research and reference work. A reader can also be used to tape material for later study.

Again, it is important for blind students to learn how to direct readers while in school so that this skill will be developed to meet the challenges ahead. Using a reader well takes practice. Knowing which things should be done with a live reader is valuable, too. For instance, when doing research or getting highly technical information, it is best to use a live reader so that the student can direct the reading and take notes when necessary. Taping such material can prove ineffective: the reader may not know exactly which material should be read and which skipped and, furthermore, the reader may not read everything accurately (e.g., forgetting important spellings or punctuation and other special symbols.)

A reader also is often the most efficient means for test taking. Test taking by tape is inefficient compared to a reader who can be directed to skip or read something again quickly. Since many tests are timed, speed of completion is important.

Do not assume that because format is complex or unusual, a live reader cannot be used. Sometimes a reader is the *best* approach because large print or Braille may be unwieldy. The chapter on "General Classroom Arrangements and Study Skills" describes how dictionary entries can be read aloud even when the student himself/herself must analyze and explain the meaning of various parts of the entry.

Conclusion

Today, it is necessary for a blind student to use a variety of media to obtain written material. Too often, students and others select (or try to select) reading media solely on the basis of emotion, personal preference, and familiarity. Help your student to build flexibility so that she can use whatever is most practical in each situation. A good short-term IEP objective is, "The student will name at least two advantages and disadvantages regarding each of these modes: Braille, large print, tape, and live readers. She will also describe situations in which she might use each particular mode."

Braille, tape recordings, and readers are currently the most efficient ways to obtain information, and the development of skills in all three areas will be of great value in adult life. Using these skills, blind adults compete on terms of equality at home, in education, and on the job.

CHAPTER 20

BOOKS AND SUPPLIES

More than one blind adult has told me that when he attended public school, his large print or Braille books were often a different edition from that used by all the other students. This caused confusion and embarrassment. With modern methods and resources, your student should not need to face this problem. Speak up firmly against this if necessary.

At the same time, realize that there are situations when more than one edition, or even more than one title, may be equally appropriate. Examples include: when *all* students have a choice (as in book reports); when the student is being tutored individually anyway; and when the difference between editions is truly negligible.

Centralized Ordering

We hope you are fortunate enough to have a centralized textbook service. Much duplication of effort is saved if book requests from around the state can be sent to a single location where the staff will:

- Maintain a library of transcribed textbooks
- Send orders to other agencies around the country
- Produce books as needed
- Maintain a library of books and periodicals which may not be called "textbooks" but which are important for the total educational process
- Assist in locating materials for research, term papers, etc.
- Provide or locate specialized materials such as Braille music

If textbook service in your area is poor, search out sources yourself, and work with the National Federation of the Blind to improve service.

Ordering Materials Already Transcribed

STREAMLINE THE PROCESS

Regardless of how much searching you must do yourself, look for ways to streamline the ordering process. Set a date (probably in April) by which you expect to have orders for the following fall. Send a letter and order form to each school explaining what is needed, and send it ahead even if you plan to go there in person. Impress high school students with the importance of deciding on courses, and if necessary negotiate for early registration. Ask to be notified immediately if there is an unexpected change of text.

Older students should help assemble their own book orders, gradually increasing responsibility.

THE RIGHT EDITION

Different books often have similar titles. It is essential to have complete bibliographical information:

- Exact title (with subtitles, if any)
- Complete name of author(s) (the term *et al.* may be used after the first author if there are many names)
- Publisher
- Latest copyright date of the version desired

- Edition number, if any
- Grade level (it should not be assumed that the level listed by the publisher is the same as the student's grade in school)
- ISBN number

Ask a librarian to instruct you about common problems in locating this information. The exact title may not be obvious. Also, the grade level (e.g., English 4) is often essential. However, publishers often disguise the grade level, to avoid worrying young students who might be using a "third grade" text in fourth grade. Unfortunately for you, this disguise often hides the grade level even from the hard-working teacher trying to order a transcribed copy. Ask the local school district to tell you the level of the book. They may even be able to show you where to find it – e.g., the last digit of an obscure long number.

Usually it is desirable to get a regular copy of the desired book and take it with you, especially when the school year is ending. If you have no copy, you will be unable to answer questions from the transcribing service, and unable to provide for possible custom-transcription. If such needs arise in July, you will have great difficulty looking for a copy while the schools are closed down. Obtain copies in the spring, and store them in a central location where someone keeps track of progress throughout the summer.

COMMON PROBLEMS

"I need a good, regular-print copy of the book, so that I can send it off to be transcribed," I always say. Nevertheless sometimes I receive a used workbook (try copying *that* on an enlarging machine, without the answers!) or a Teachers Guide (again, how do you avoid copying the answers?) Explain this to the school district, and also explain that the regular-print copy may be damaged or destroyed during transcription. It may be necessary to take the book apart, either to put onto a machine or to send to various transcribers.

What if a new textbook will be used, and the school's copies have not yet been shipped? Contact the publisher's representative. Whenever I have done this, an advance copy has gladly been provided – often at no cost.

Occasionally when a student is working individually, you may locate a suitable Braille book but be unable to find an *inkprint* copy of the same book. For a young student, a sighted instructor usually must have a print copy. Even for the older student, the teacher may need an inkprint copy in order to plan lessons. If this situation occurs, inquire whether a neighboring school district uses the book. Ask curriculum laboratories, and even the field representative of the publisher. Also, experienced teachers often have personal libraries. Most people are glad to help by loaning a book for a need such as this.

SOURCES OF TRANSCRIBED MATERIALS

Following is a partial list of agencies which provide books and materials in transcribed form. See "References" for addresses.

American Brotherhood for the Blind
American Printing House for the Blind (APH) – The *Central Catalog* provides information about other agencies' production nationwide
Braille Book Bank
Exceptional Teaching Aids
The Guild for the Blind
The Hadley School for the Blind
National Braille Association (NBA)
National Braille Press
National Library Service for the Blind and Physically Handicapped (Library of Congress), and its system of regional libraries
Recording for the Blind
Royal National Institute for the Blind
Seedlings

Materials Which Have Not Already Been Transcribed

CONSIDER ALTERNATIVES

Before committing time and/or money to having a book produced especially for your student, consider other alternatives carefully.

Might the book be already available in an alternative medium which could be used, even though it is not the first choice?

If only a part of the book will be used, could only that part be produced? Similarly, if a literature anthology is needed, some or all of the selections may be already available individually or as part of a different anthology. Conversely, if one particular literature selection is desired, it may be available as a part of an anthology.

If two students will be using the same book on different dates, perhaps a single copy could be passed from one to the other. Even if they are in the same book at the same time, if one student is ahead it may be possible to move individual volumes around. (Caution: the latter approach is not desirable except in an emergency or when both students are in the same building. Students may move faster or slower than expected. A glossary may be needed by both.)

FINDING TRANSCRIBING SERVICES

Some of the above agencies will produce books on request. Develop contacts with various transcribers, both locally (if possible) and nationally. Jewish Temple Sisterhoods, the Delta Gamma sorority, and the Red Cross are examples of organizations especially interested in this kind of work. The Library of Congress catalog, *Volunteers Who Produce Books: Braille, Large Type, Tape* may help you find transcribers in your area. The NFB publication, *Beginning a Transcribing Group,* will be helpful also.

It is helpful to have access to a Thermoform machine and spiral book-binding equipment.

Computerized Braille Translation

A relatively new option is a computerized Braille translation system. Copy may be typed on a regular typing keyboard by someone who does not know Braille, and the computer will translate the material into Grade II Braille. (In most systems, it is also possible for a Braillist to use six of the keys to Braille the material manually.) The stored text has the advantages of computerization: It can be revised without complete retyping, and multiple copies can be produced.

This is, unfortunately, not a panacea. The high cost is the first barrier. Other problems arise with reliability, with maintenance, and with varying degrees of inaccuracy in the translation to Grade II Braille. Nevertheless, computerized Braille translation is a valuable option.

Note: "Computerized Braille translation" (used to produce text in Braille for use anywhere) is not the same thing as a "Braille output device" (which is used to read the screen of a particular computer). The latter is discussed in the chapter, "Computers."

Options in Large Print Production

Photocopiers are widely available today, and many of them have the capacity for enlargement. For this reason it is now rarely necessary to retype materials when large print is desired. When entire books are to be obtained in large print, it is best to use the services of an agency which has mass-production capability for large print.

DAILY HANDOUTS

When collecting book orders in the spring, try to include workbooks, worksheets, and other materials. Commercial workbooks may already be transcribed. If your textbook services will not do worksheets or handouts, you may find an individual transcriber who will–possibly a paid transcriber if you work in a large system.

Any availability of local transcribers, along with the fact that you yourself know Braille, brings the question of producing materials on short notice. New students move in; additional books are assigned; daily handouts appear. It is desirable to have some ability to transcribe materials throughout the year. On the other hand, it is never possible (except perhaps in a special school) to provide *everything* in transcribed form. There are limits, both in total capacity and in speed. And some assignments do not lend themselves to transcribing at all–for example, looking through the morning newspapers and selecting an article for Current Events study. Therefore it is always necessary to make some provision for "live" reading.

RANKING PRIORITIES

To reduce debate over what could and could not be transcribed, one large school system has the following policy:

> For Braille and large print production, we give priority to materials and subject matter difficult to use in an oral format. The *high* priorities are as follows:
>
> - Mathematics
> - Experiments and formulas, science notation, and terminology lists
> - Foreign languages
> - Copy for typing classes
> - Reading instruction materials for third grade and below
> - Materials for young students who have not developed alternative techniques
> - Materials for a newly blinded student who is still learning Braille
> - Materials for a student who, due to an unfortunate combination of circumstances, is lacking transcribed materials in *all* subjects
> - Tests
> - Recipes
> - Materials requested early (i.e., first come first served)
>
> Materials with *low* priority for Braille and large print production are as follows:
>
> - Materials which could be easily used in recorded form (for example, literature, social studies, history)
> - Complex, time-consuming formats such as maps, when a reasonable equivalent can be arranged by using ready-made materials. (An example might be detailed rainfall maps for various regions in South America. *One* Braille rainfall map – not necessarily in South America – might be provided to help the student learn how such maps are used. The various maps from South America could then be discussed orally.)
> - Pictures which would readily be described orally (for example, kindergarten worksheets where the child is to give the initial consonant for a picture)
>
> Note that taped materials often can be produced more quickly than Braille or large print. Give consideration to whether tape would be suitable.

BUILD FLEXIBILITY

With books and handouts, we face a constant tussle between the desire for "ideal" materials, on the one hand, and reality on the other. Many parents have said to me, "How can she have equal opportunity if you do not provide the same reading materials the others have? Surely she should have everything in Braille (or large print). She isn't being treated fairly!" To some extent this viewpoint is correct – if there is no good way for the blind student to read, she will not have equal opportunity; and a very young student must have materials for actually *learning* to read in Braille or print. At the same time, we live in the "real world," in two different respects. First, it simply is not always feasible to have a transcriber in the right place, working fast enough to produce the desired materials. Second, even if a school were to succeed in providing everything in the preferred mode, this could not continue in college and on the job. If a student has virtually everything provided in Braille (or large print) until she graduates from high school, and *then* must suddenly learn to use tapes and live readers, the jolt will be tremendous.

The well-prepared student will be comfortable with several modes of reading. She will read well from paper – either Braille or print. She will use tapes competently. She will make efficient use of reader time. (Note that it is important for the blind student herself always to have a copy of the regular book.) And she will have a good understanding of when each is appropriate.

Special Transcription Problems

Other sections of this book have suggestions about transcription problems in specific subject areas – for example, music, mathematics, and science. Some specific sources of materials are mentioned in subject area sections. Ideas for producing graphic aids appear under "Mathematics" and "Maps."

Other agencies and schools often will assist you with special problems. Ask the adult rehabilitation agency, the residential school, special day schools, large metropolitan districts, the Hadley correspondence school, etc.

When you or a volunteer produce tape-recorded materials, you may be stymied by specialized pronunciation. Especially if the transcriber is in a different town, the classroom teacher may not be readily available to help. Seek advice from a college professor or a person employed in the field. Also note that unusual or technical words should be spelled aloud somewhere on the tape.

Consider alternatives to transcription (e.g., learning songs by rote), and carefully balance educational value against the availability of resources. Sometimes a compromise is best. Perhaps one vocal-music selection per week could be produced in Braille, so that the student does have practice in reading the notation, and other lessons could be done by rote. Similarly, consider compromises regarding the preferred mode: if a student prefers Braille but must use a taped science text, perhaps formulas and questions could be Brailled.

Delivery and Return

At the time of ordering, plan how and where the book will be delivered. Will it go to the student's home or to the school? Will it pass through any third parties? (For example, perhaps Recording for the Blind sends the tape to the state textbook service, which sends it on to the student.) To whom will it be addressed? (counselor, student, principal, etc.)

A few itinerant teachers deliver the books themselves, but this is very inefficient if there are many students. Regardless of the delivery system, it is essential that *one* individual at each school be in charge of books and supplies. Select this person carefully. Most itinerant teachers can tell horror stories about essential volumes languishing in someone's closet.

Most districts have a delivery service with school vehicles. Make liberal use of this, as well as the U.S. Postal Service and any other systems which may be available to you.

Inform staff about the Free Matter provision, which permits special materials for the blind to be sent through the U.S. Mail postage-free. Should a U.S. Postal Service employee be misinformed or discourteous, discuss it with a postal supervisor.

Be sure to determine who will be responsible for the return of books. Send a reminder note to all schools in late April. Each transcribed volume is valuable. In case of lost volumes, urge everyone to assume that they might actually have it, however certain they are to the contrary. Ask the student to check at home and in his locker. Place a notice in the school bulletin, asking the entire staff to look.

If a book is not returned on time, the textbook service should send a reminder notice, and the itinerant/resource teacher should aid in the search.

Equipment and Supplies

The section on "Starting Anew Each Time" includes a list of basic supplies and equipment. Funds may be available from the county or joint county school district, the state department of public instruction, the state rehabilitation agency, and Federal sources. A "Quota" allotment, in the form of books and supplies from the American Printing House for the Blind, is available for every legally blind student; find out how this is administered in your state. Service organizations often will donate money for equipment.

The state library for the blind (or the agency which specifically handles machines) will lend tape players and talking book machines to individual students. Sometimes agencies or individuals will lend other equipment.

Note that "Free Matter" provides for equipment and supplies as well as books. When equipment is not available ready-made, or is too expensive, often it can be produced in a home or school workshop. Wooden geometric models, bookstands, and Braille alphabet blocks are good examples. Ask for help from industrial arts teachers and community service agencies.

Don't get carried away with assembling equipment and aids which may not be as helpful as they seem. Before purchasing or constructing a teaching aid, be sure that it really will meet a need, and that the money or effort invested is in proportion to the need.

Below is a partial listing of agencies which offer equipment and supplies. See "References" for addresses, including separate listings for computers and computer-related technology.

Aids Unlimited
American Brotherhood for the Blind
American Foundation for the Blind (AFB)
American Printing House for the Blind (APH)
American Thermoform Company
Apollo Electronic Visual Aids
Howe Press
Independent Living Aids
Learning Pillows
National Federation of the Blind (NFB)
National Library Service for the Blind and Physically Handicapped (Library of Congress)
Oakmont Visual Aids Workshop
Royal National Institute for the Blind (RNIB)
Science Products (formerly Science for the Blind)
Texture-Touch
Traylor Enterprises, Inc.
VTEK
Vis-Aids, Inc.

CHAPTER 21

TRAVEL WITH THE LONG WHITE CANE

By Sharon L. M. Duffy

Cane travel, often called mobility instruction, is one of the most important skills a blind person can learn.

Many partially-sighted people travel without using a cane; they do it at considerable hazard to themselves and with inefficiency compared to totally blind persons (and partially-sighted persons) who have learned adequate cane travel techniques. Blind persons who travel solely by using a sighted guide may travel efficiently, but less often. Although dog guides can be excellent travel aids, they are not given to children under the age of 16. Most dog guide schools expect their students to have cane travel instruction first.

Unfortunately, however, cane travel (like Braille) is considered by many persons to be a last resort – only for those who cannot possibly get around in any other way. Many also believe that cane travel is so complicated to teach that it requires a Master's degree in Orientation and Mobility. Neither of these beliefs is true.

Whether the teacher is trained by a rehabilitation agency or by a university, the most important ingredient in teaching travel well is the belief that blind people can travel independently; and the best way to instill this belief is for the teacher to know how to do it as a blind person. The best way to obtain this knowledge is an extended training course using the cane, and using sleepshades if the person has any sight.

The Cane As a Symbol

Many people resist using a cane, because they imagine that it represents dependence. They are ashamed of being blind (or of their relatives being blind, in the case of family members). However, the cane is actually a symbol of independence since it is the means for a blind person to travel safely by himself.

Most adolescents are sensitive regarding any difference that they may have from the average – weight, relative height, ethnic origin, blindness, etc. It is not surprising, then, that a junior high age student may object strongly to carrying a white cane, because she feels this advertises this difference. It does do this; however it is most unlikely that other children are unaware of a classmate's blindness anyway. It isn't a deep, dark secret, although many blind teenagers wish it were.

It is very important for a teacher to deal directly with these negative feelings about canes, and also about sleepshades (a very similar issue). It is respectable to be blind; and this must be said and expressed in every action, because society's attitudes about blindness are generally so negative.

One of the best ways to combat negative public attitudes is for the student to get to know a number of blind adults who use canes regularly, and, if possible, establish an ongoing relationship with competent blind people. The National Federation of the Blind is an excellent vehicle for this.

Ken did not think it was "macho" to carry a cane until he became friends with a blind man whom he admired. After that, he perceived other people's negative comments about the cane as ignorant, and, in fact, felt more "macho" at being able to maintain his position that carrying a cane was a good idea.

The Length of the Cane

There is some debate about the appropriate length of the cane. Blind people have found through experience that the length of the cane is an individual matter, depending upon the length of stride, walking speed, and reflexes of the student. To consider the length of the cane, hold it vertically in front of the individual: ordinarily it should reach somewhere between the armpit and the nose. Shoulder height is a good length for a first cane. A cane reaching only to the sternum (breastbone) is not long enough for the average student to assume a normal walking speed with safety. The cane must be long enough to allow a student two steps to stop.

Generally speaking, a traveler will want a longer cane as speed is developed, and this should be left up to the student who is an experienced traveler. The desire for a longer cane should be viewed as a positive sign.

One way to check whether a cane is the right length is to observe where the foot steps in relationship to the cane touch which would cover it (i.e., the place where the cane last touched on that side). If the foot touches approximately the same place the cane did, the cane is the right length. If the foot touches in front of where the cane touched, the cane is too short. If the foot touches significantly behind where the cane touched, the cane is too long.

Since children grow, it is necessary to change cane lengths periodically. Some National Federation of the Blind state affiliates have cane banks for kids, so that canes in children's sizes are available on loan and can be traded in when necessary. Since it would not be unusual for a child to change canes ten or more times from early childhood through adolescence, this is a considerable saving.

Which Cane to Use

The best cane currently on the market is called the "NFB straight cane." It is hollow fiberglass with a rubber and metal tip and plastic cylindrical handle. This cane is the most sensitive because it is light and flexible, is made in one piece, and has a metal tip which provides information both through touch and sound. It also weighs only a few ounces so that small hands do not become tired using it. Because of its construction, it can be used with either hand or switched from hand to hand when convenient. It is available in children's sizes (with handle and shank properly proportioned for small hands) from the National Federation of the Blind at the National Center for the Blind.

In my opinion, the next best cane on the market is sometimes called a Rainshine cane after the company which manufactures it, and also sometimes called the Iowa cane or the original NFB cane. It is solid fiberglass and is otherwise much like the NFB straight cane. It is not quite as sensitive or as light as the NFB straight cane. Some people prefer this cane because it is virtually indestructible.

Many other straight canes are rigid, have nylon tips which do not slide easily, and provide little information about substances touched. They wear in such a way as to make the cane either left- or right-handed. (This problem is partly due to the "golf grip" handle often used.)

Collapsible canes have one main disadvantage – they *do* collapse. They are not very sturdy because they are held together either by nylon cord or by telescoping joints. The movement of the cane shakes the pieces apart. Because they are not one solid piece, they do not telegraph information as accurately. Many blind people buy them so that they can collapse them when they don't want people to know they are blind. Use of a collapsible cane encourages avoidance of facing the real issues of blindness.

If a collapsible cane is used at all, the best use is as an extra to be kept in reserve. For example, it might be kept in the desk at work in case something happens to the regular cane.

Safe Travel for the Partially Sighted

One residential school began to insist that its students carry canes after two junior-high girls, both partially sighted, were hit and injured by a car. Prior to that time, it was believed that partially-sighted students could travel safely without canes.

Sleepshades, or blindfolds, are a must for the partially-sighted student during cane travel instruction. (See Figure 21-1)

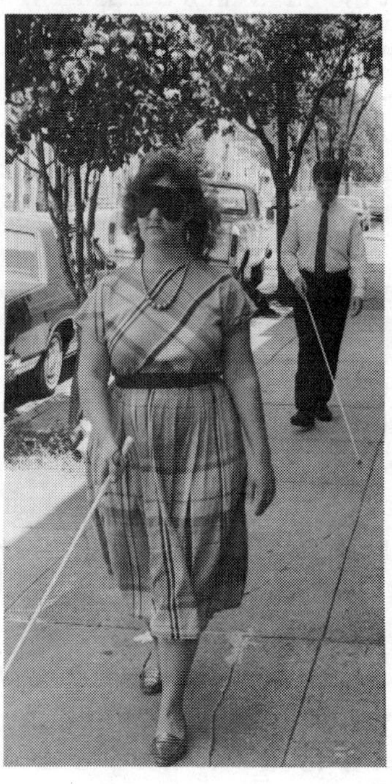

Figure 21-1
Sleepshades For
Effective Learning

In order to function in the most efficient manner, the student must learn to use alternatives to sight. Because our society is visually oriented, partially-sighted children will tend to rely on vision even when it is the least effective method to accomplish a task. Sleepshades will force the learning of alternative techniques so that the student can make an intelligent decision about when to use sight and when to use other methods. The sleepshades will dispel the idea that sight is required to perform tasks. This will also allay fears about functioning if more sight is lost – a very real probability for most partially-sighted people.

The partially-sighted person who has *not* been trained to function without sight presents a great hazard by relying almost entirely on her least acute sense, sight. To illustrate the danger, consider the student approaching an uncontrolled crossing. She will look down the street visually, see nothing coming, and begin to cross. However, since she could only see 1/4 of the way down the block, she would not see a car 1/2 block away. If she has not been trained to listen, she probably will not hear it when she begins the crossing. When she does hear the car or see it at close range, she may panic and do something unexpected, such as to run back across the street, and could then be hit. Since the pedestrian is not carrying a cane, the driver had no reason to believe that she could not see perfectly.

Some people believe that partially-sighted students should have "vision stimulation" exercises to the exclusion of learning alternative techniques. The chapter on "The Partially-Sighted Child" discusses why that approach is not constructive – and, in the case of travel, not safe.

If sleepshades are worn consistently during training, the student will listen more closely, will learn to think while traveling, and will rely on the cane as a tool more accurate than limited vision. The training with sleepshades will establish the habits of using alternatives, which will quite naturally be carried over into routine traveling. It is helpful occasionally to remind the student to continue using the same techniques when traveling without sleepshades outside of lesson times. One school of thought holds that partially-sighted children need instruction in using their vision, and that they may feel cheated if they do not receive it. In fact, however, these children receive this kind of instruction from family members, peers, and everyone else almost from the moment of birth. There simply isn't much danger that a partially-sighted person will not use vision. But there are many adults who seek out training with sleepshades in order to learn alternatives to vision.

It is not uncommon for a student to resist wearing sleepshades. To minimize resistance, consistency is essential. Begin with the understanding that this is how it will be, and resist the temptation to make exceptions regarding the wearing of shades from the beginning to the end of class. For very young students, make a rule that the teacher will do any adjusting of the shades that is necessary. If a student lifts the shades, deal directly and promptly with the problem.

Great resistance to wearing sleepshades is symptomatic of a poor attitude about blindness. The best solution may be a discussion about blindness, building positive attitudes.

Occasionally, parents or other teachers may have questions about the use of sleepshades, but if this issue is dealt with during IEP meetings and in less formal settings prior to training, most problems can be avoided.

AN EXCEPTION

One situation in which it may not be advisable to wear sleepshades is when a student has a substantial hearing loss which results in directional hearing problems, and is traveling independently in an area where traffic must be dealt with.

Human Guide Technique

The human guide technique is most easily accomplished by the blind person's grasping the elbow of the person guiding. In this way, steps can be anticipated. By putting his arm behind his body, the guide can signal the blind person to step behind him.

We call this the "human guide" rather than "sighted guide," because the guide may be another blind person using a cane or a dog.

This technique should require one short lesson. It is valuable and not difficult to learn.

If the person being guided has a cane, he should continue to use it while holding the guide's arm. Thus he can continue to take part of the responsibility for his own travel, rather than being wholly dependent on the guide. A young child traveling in this manner learns how it feels when the cane encounters various things in the environment. A competent older traveler may take someone's arm for convenience in staying together in a crowd, and continue to examine the terrain as independently as usual.

"Pre-Cane Techniques"

"Pre-cane techniques" (actually non-cane techniques) include trailing walls with the hands, shuffling along to find steps with the feet, and holding out the hands in a defensive position.

Unfortunately, some people advocate these techniques. However, they actually contribute to the image of the helpless, groping blind person. These techniques are unnecessary when the student acquires a cane. A cane can be used to follow along walls and find steps quickly, and can protect the body more efficiently than a person's hands.

"Pre-cane techniques" presuppose that a blind person should not use a cane all of the time, especially indoors. But since the cane is more efficient than non-cane techniques, it is really not reasonable to put it down when walking indoors. It makes good sense to use the cane anytime away from home.

Non-cane techniques also are sometimes taught on the assumption that a young child cannot yet learn to use a cane. The chapter on travel for younger children explains in detail why early use of the cane is in fact a far better approach.

Cane Techniques

Two things make a good cane traveler – a positive attitude about traveling, and effective techniques. Here is a list and description of time-tested techniques. When each is taught will depend upon the progress of the student and the curriculum followed.

THE TOUCH TECHNIQUE

This is sometimes called arcing the cane, or the foot cane technique. This technique is used in most situations. It is achieved by holding the cane in the dominant hand with the index finger pointing down the shaft, and the thumb and other fingers curled around the cane–a position analogous to shaking hands with the cane (Figure 21-2).

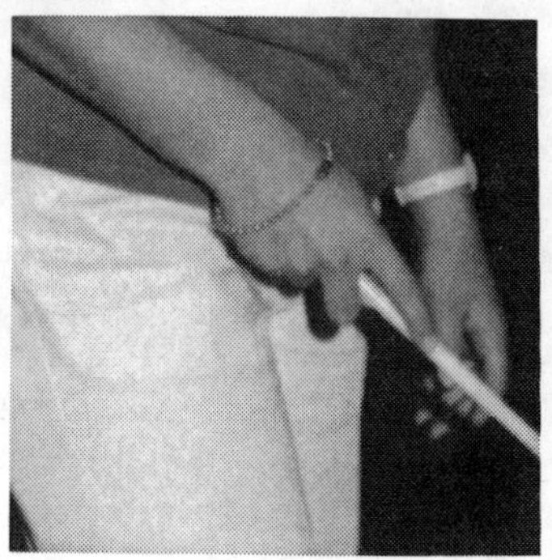

Figure 21-2
Hand Position

The cane is swung from side to side and should cover the ground approximately the width of the traveler's shoulders. When the right foot is forward, the cane should touch on the left side, and when the left foot is forward, the cane should touch on the right side–one tap per step. The hand should be centered in front of the body with the primary action in the wrist. (Keeping the forearm against the waist or hip helps to center the hand and prevent fatigue.) The elbow may be bent comfortably. (Figure 21-3).

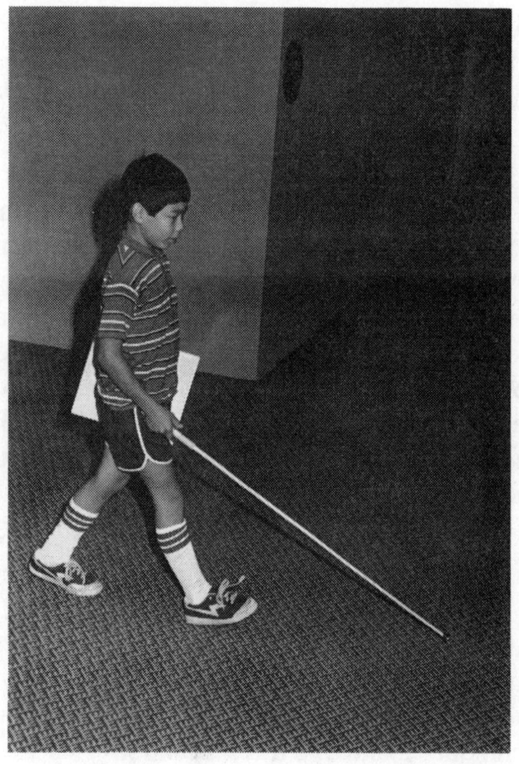

Figure 21-3
Touch Technique

The reason the cane should touch on the opposite side from the forward foot is to maintain a two-step warning for objects and steps encountered. A traveler who is out of step is clearing only one step ahead and may miss some objects altogether until they are encountered with the body.

The arc of the cane should be even on either side. If a traveler tends to drift either left or right, observe that the traveler is probably arcing farther in that direction than on the other side. Also, if the hand does not remain centered, a variation in the arc may occur, and the traveler will have more difficulty developing good distance perception with the cane. Distance perception can also be thrown off by changing the length of cane

In crowded areas, the cane can be moved into a more upright position, causing some variation in grip and slowing of walking speed. Normally, a cane traveler should be able to walk as fast as a sighted person in similar physical condition.

SLIDING TECHNIQUES

Sliding the cane rather than tapping it may occasionally be desirable. For example, when traveling next to a parking lot, there may be a substantial crack or ridge between the sidewalk and the parking lot. The cane may be slid across from one side to the other until it encounters the crack or ridge. This technique is of limited value since a crack or ridge may not be detected easily.

Ordinarily, the cane should be tapped rather than slid, to avoid sticking and the premature wearing out of cane tips. Also, the sound of the tap provides information about the surface touched and (by means of echo) the proximity of buildings, etc. Many good travelers vary cane techniques to suit the travel situation.

LANDMARK LOCATION

Locating doorways, perpendicular sidewalks, etc., can be done by arcing the cane as usual but extending the arc a little farther to one side to contact the side of the building, the side of the hallway, or the grass. The touch on the opposite side should be in the usual place. It will be necessary for the traveler to walk close to the grass or the wall. (Note that when one is *not* looking for a doorway or a perpendicular sidewalk, one should *not* hug the wall or the edge of the grass.)

THE STAIR TECHNIQUE

To go upstairs, the cane should be held in an upright position, with the tip just below the second step above the traveler, approximately in the center of the body. After a quick sweep at the start to measure the width of the stairs, the traveler should proceed with the hand held still and with the cane tip encountering each successive step. At the top of the flight of stairs, the traveler will have two steps' warning (Figure 21-4, Figure 21-5, and Figure 21-6).

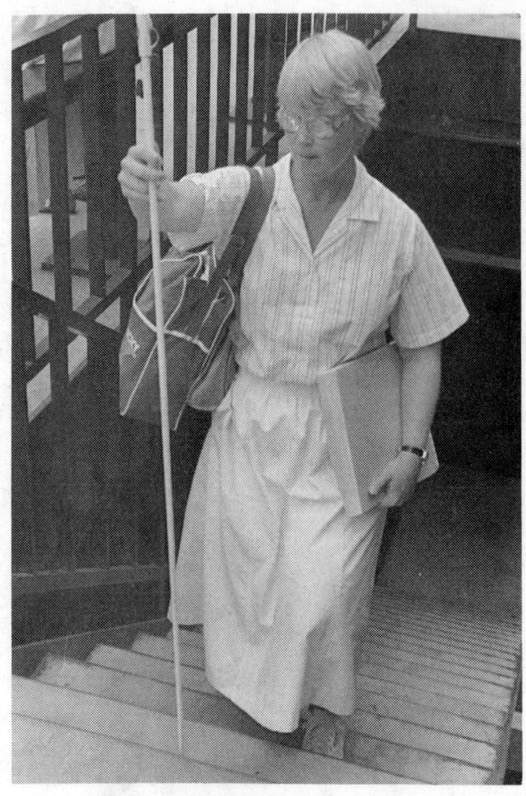

Figure 21-4
Going Up Steps

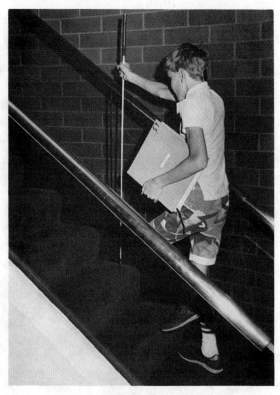

Figure 21-5
Going Up Steps

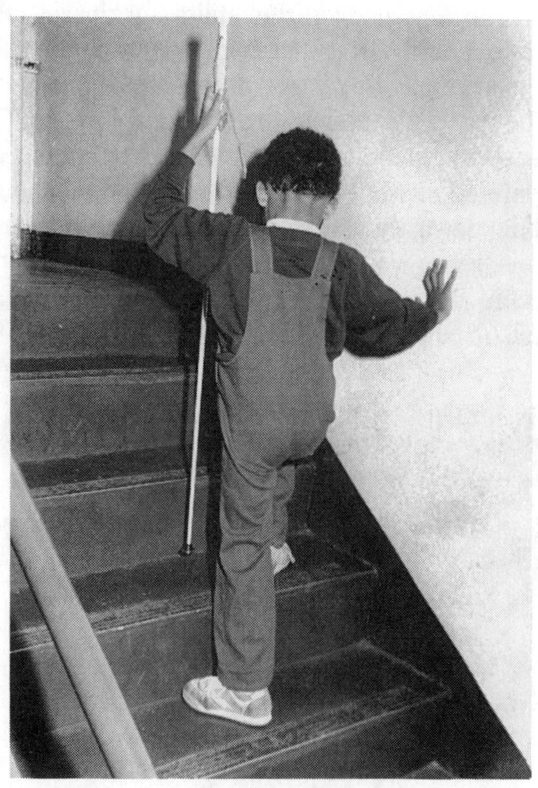

Figure 21-6
Going Up Steps

In descending the stairs, ordinarily the cane should not be tapped from side to side. The arm may be relaxed at the side of the body. The cane tip should extend just beyond the second step below the traveler, approximately centered in front of the body, and the tip should slide down each succeeding step. Again, the cane will give two steps' warning. Using this technique, it is not necessary to hold the handrail. (See Figure 21-7 and Figure 21-8)

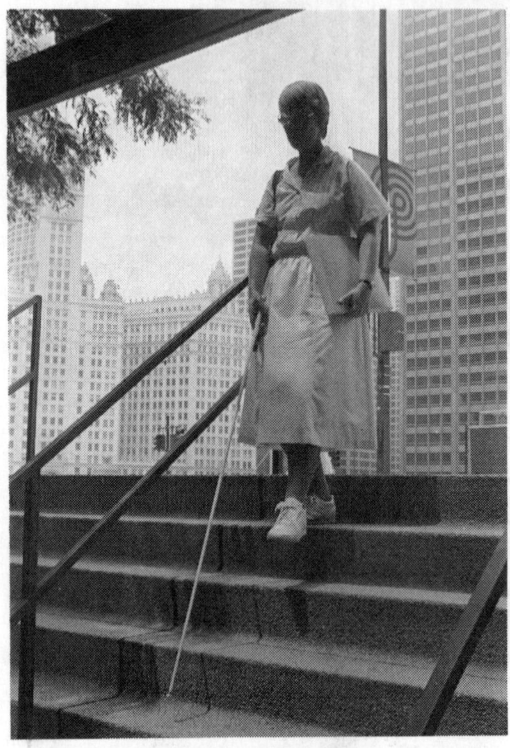

Figure 21-7
Going Down Steps

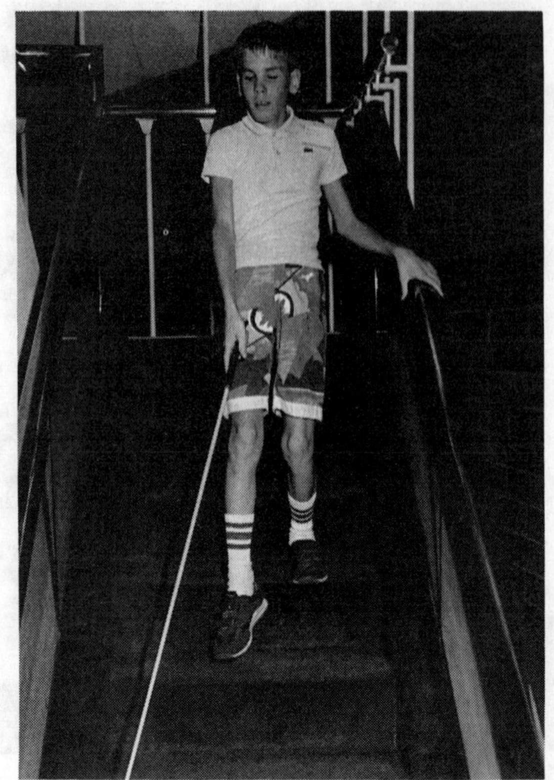

Figure 21-8
Going Down Steps

ESCALATORS

Escalators frequently make a low-pitched noise or a squeak and thus can be located by sound. The cane should contact the moving stairs and the student may put a hand on the rail before actually stepping on. Thus the direction of the escalator is easily determined.

After the traveler steps on, the cane should rest two steps ahead.

When the stairs flatten out or the cane is bumped by the stationary step, it is time to step off (Figure 21-9).

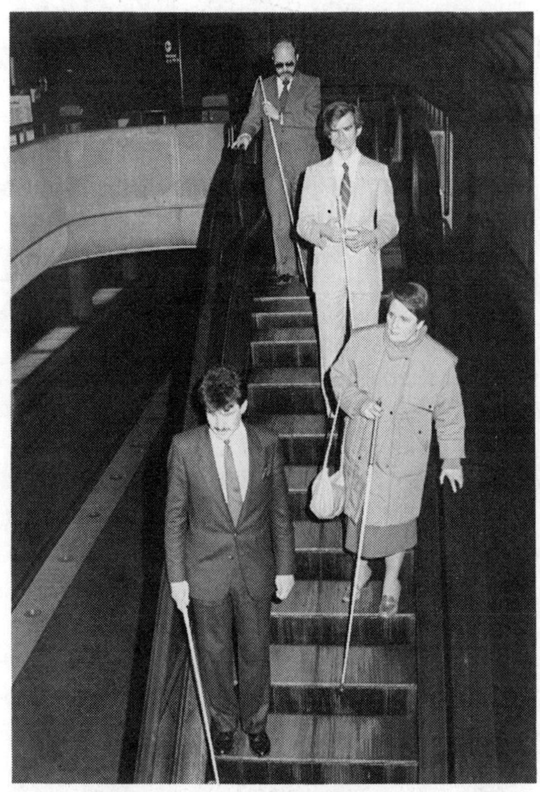

Figure 21-9
Escalator

REVOLVING DOORS

There is no right or wrong way to negotiate revolving doors. I prefer to put my cane out and make contact with the revolving door to judge where it is and step in. It may be slightly safer to approach from the left in order to minimize the likelihood of smashing the cane in the door.

Crossing Streets

UNCONTROLLED CROSSING WITH LITTLE TRAFFIC

This is a very easy crossing. The student determines that she has reached the street–noting the curb, the change in surface underfoot, and proximity of traffic. (Note that frequently there is no actual step-down at the "curb," due to wheelchair accommodations or other reasons. Therefore other clues should be noted also. In all aspects of travel, if the student becomes too dependent upon one "favorite" type of clue, she will be stymied if that clue is obscured or absent.) The student should wait if traffic is crossing in front of her, and also if a car is coming fast beside her and might turn in front of her. If no interfering traffic is heard, the student proceeds.

Upon completion of the crossing, it is important to sweep the curb with the cane before stepping up. Utility poles, fire hydrants, etc., can provide unpleasant surprises. Do not, however, permit the student to stand in the street and examine the curb area at length. Checking for obstacles should be done with one quick sweep. If it is necessary to look around to locate the sidewalk, etc., this should be done *after* stepping out of the street.

The general technique described here applies also to the other types of crossings below, with modifications according to the traffic patterns.

INTERSECTION WITH STOP SIGNS

This is somewhat similar to an uncontrolled crossing, above. However, a car crossing in front of the student should stop at the stop sign. (Note: Remind the student that stop signs may or may not be present for all four directions.) The student listens to be sure the car really is slowing to a stop, and then proceeds, listening to the idling motor.

CROSSING WITH TRAFFIC LIGHTS

Standing at the edge of the street, the student listens carefully. If she hears the traffic moving across in front of her, she knows her own light is red. If she hears traffic moving parallel to the path she plans to take, she has the green light.

If she arrives at the intersection in the middle of a green light, it is better to wait through a cycle until the light turns green again. Otherwise, she risks starting just before the light changes back to red (Figure 21-10).

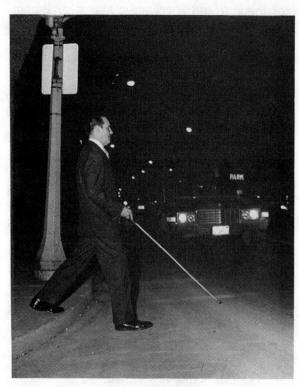

Figure 21-10
Crossing With Light

An Example

Let us assume the student wishes to cross a street which runs east and west, and that she stands on the southwest corner of the intersection, with the north-south street at her right. When she hears the traffic on the east-west street slow and stop, and the cars facing north and south begin to move, the student begins to cross. She should move briskly and assertively, to discourage north-south motorists from turning in front of her. (As a pedestrian with a white cane, she clearly should have the right of way against turning traffic. But if she is hesitant, drivers may genuinely doubt that she is really going to cross.)

In all crossings, it is important to notice all clues and keep well oriented. A particularly common error is (in this example) to veer to the right and miss the corner, proceeding to walk on ahead *in* the north-south street. The student should consciously avoid this error.

To cross correctly, the student should listen carefully to determine direction, and then cross parallel to the traffic which is moving *beside* her. She should walk as fast as possible, because she will get across faster, and also walk in a straighter path. The trick is to listen carefully and get started in the right direction. The student should listen to the sound of the cars, including idling motors, at all times.

Listening to the footsteps of other pedestrians is *not* a reliable guide. Many people cross at odd angles or against the light.

Some Differences From the Sighted Techniques

Explain to students and parents that a blind pedestrian will not always cross in exactly the same way as a sighted person, and that this is OK. For example, people may worry if the blind traveler is not *exactly* on the marked crosswalk. Actually, as long as she is crossing in essentially the right area, it is not necessary that she walk precisely on the painted lines. However, by listening to where the idling cars are, the student can have a good understanding of the location of the crosswalk.

Similarly, the blind person's crossing may not precisely coincide with the timing of the "walk" light (if present), and this too is all right. The cane gives the blind pedestrian the right to cross at a reasonable time. However, the blind person must realize that she cannot count on immunity from danger solely because she is using a cane; it is necessary to pay attention to traffic and proceed carefully.

Also, remind your student that if there is so little traffic that she cannot determine whether the lights are red or green, she should simply cross as though there were no controls. (Otherwise she might stand there forever.)

Right Turn On Red

Although the "right turn on red" traffic pattern, now legal in most localities, can be annoying to all pedestrians, usually the competent blind traveler can distinguish this from a green light. The student should learn to walk when the majority of the traffic goes, or the straight traffic, rather than when a car turns right on red. It is important to listen to *all* of the traffic, not just a single right-turning car.

Other Variations

The competent older student needs to realize that not all traffic lights have the same kind of cycle – in fact, some systems vary their timing according to the volume of traffic. For example, lights in Alamogordo, New Mexico, vary from cycle to cycle depending upon the presence or absence of cars in turning lanes, and also whether or not someone has pushed the "walk" button. Any part of the cycle may also vary in length depending on how much traffic there is. A student should learn to recognize the variations for turning traffic, and should listen to cycles of the light with and without pushing the button.

What About Audible Signals?

Learning to cross with a traffic light is *not* difficult, and should be learned in elementary school. Even a young child can understand an uncomplicated intersection.

Unfortunately, some people believe that street crossings are impossibly difficult, and advocate various special devices to "help the blind." These may include buzzers or bird calls emanating from traffic lights, and various underfoot guidance systems. Such devices actually cause difficulty rather than improving opportunities. It is impractical to install such things everywhere; yet travelers tend to become dependent on them, and become restricted to locations where they are present. If a special sound system is not properly correlated with traffic, the person dependent on it will be exposed to extra, unnecessary dangers. Furthermore, such devices interfere with more appropriate crossing methods – extra noises make it harder to listen to traffic, and extra things underfoot make it harder to observe the regular terrain.

The most important reason that audible traffic signals are a danger is that blind people are encouraged to listen only to them and forget about the traffic itself. It is more important to be aware of what the traffic is doing than whether the light is red or green. [Sighted persons, it should be noted, tend to believe that they rely on the light to tell them when to cross. But actually they observe the traffic itself at the same time, without thinking about it consciously. They notice things such as a car racing through on the end of the yellow light.] The competent blind traveler moves with the surge of traffic which comes a moment after the light actually changes. This is safer than moving exactly when the light turns green, because one can determine what the cars are intending to do (turn, go straight, etc.). If a pedestrian starts out just as the light is changing, and simultaneously a car starts to turn quickly, the pedestrian may be hit. She may also be hit if cross-traffic races through on the end of the yellow. The blind pedestrian listening to traffic is in control of what she is doing. The blind pedestrian relying on an audible signal is relinquishing control.

Moreover, audible traffic signals are different from place to place, so a blind traveler may not correctly interpret a light in a new setting. Some sound automatically when the light is green in a certain direction; others sound only when a button is pushed. Some make one noise for green and another for red. To determine what the sounds mean, a blind person must listen to traffic, which is what she should do anyway.

A BUSY UNMARKED CROSSING

Occasionally, every pedestrian must cross a fairly busy street that does not have a stop light or stop sign. If the traffic never completely lets up, this technique can be employed: When the traffic in the nearest lanes is not extremely heavy, hold the cane up and out across the first lane of traffic, and pause momentarily for the traffic to stop. Then use the touch technique to cross to the center of the street. Then hold the cane up again to stop the traffic going the other direction, and go on across when that traffic slows or stops.

Crossing a busy, unmarked intersection is an advanced skill, not to be attempted by a beginner. No one, of course (sighted or blind) should ordinarily walk across a freeway with a very high speed limit.

On the other hand, often a street will have a moderate amount of traffic, moving at a moderate speed but rarely stopping completely. Such a street can easily be crossed by a blind traveler with some experience.

Conclusion

The preceding are suggested techniques, not to be confused with absolute rules. I know a man who holds his cane in an unusual way and moves his hand continuously. However, he manages to touch his cane in the right places for optimum safety and has excellent distance perception and is overall an excellent traveler. Variation of any technique should not be discouraged unless it does not work, presents a really bad appearance, or provides unnecessary danger to others.

CHAPTER 22

PLANNING A CANE TRAVEL CURRICULUM

By Sharon L. M. Duffy

Each student will proceed at his/her own rate, but a similar sequence of training can be used for each student. The age of a student will also have some bearing upon the speed of progress. Generally speaking, an older student will progress more rapidly than a younger student because coordination and general knowledge will be better.

Indoor Travel

The first thing to be taught is the touch technique. A long, straight hallway of average width is an excellent place to begin. At this stage concentration should center on keeping in step; maintaining a comfortable, centered position of the hand; appropriate width of arc; raising confidence; and increasing walking speed. The faster a student walks, the straighter he will walk. Also, the cane provides more information if the student is walking faster, because distances can be judged more easily. Occasionally, a student will walk faster than he can respond to changes and will need to slow down a bit until his skill improves. This is fairly unusual. If, on the other hand, he appears to be off balance, and seems to be walking too slowly, he probably is.

While the student is developing good technique, he needs to learn to memorize and follow directions – left and right, compass points, turn 45 degrees, etc. Many children are not familiar with compass points and need training in how to follow directions. The concepts of parallel, perpendicular, and a right angle may need to be demonstrated and explained.

EASY BUT INTERESTING

Simple routes involving walking the halls of a building, finding a given classroom, and returning to a starting point will develop confidence and technique as well as practical experience in following directions and problem solving. Even at this stage, it is very important not to interfere too much or to allow others to do so. The student must learn to rely on himself and to suffer the consequences of inattention. The student will learn some important lessons while still in a safe environment.

To help a student cope with beginning routes, the use of landmarks should be explained – type of floor covering, the number of doors in a hallway, the noise of a drinking fountain, the different acoustical properties of halls and classrooms, etc. Using landmarks gives a traveler more confidence and should be encouraged from the beginning.

A popular myth suggests that blind people innately have a sixth sense to make up for the lack of sight. Some people do have a sense which is sometimes called "facial vision." It is the ability to sense objects and is believed to be due to changes in air pressure or sounds. It can be useful, but is not necessary for good travel. It also can be inaccurate, and thus some students will need to be told to ignore it. It is not mysterious or wonderful. A sighted person wearing sleepshades may have this sense; and some blind people do not possess it at all. It cannot be taught, but those who possess it may find it convenient in locating landmarks.

MAINTAINING AND EXTENDING SKILLS

Indoor work with the cane should continue to receive some emphasis even when the student has proceeded to working mainly outdoors. Don't let travel in the familiar school become sloppy. Have the student complete an errand in an unfamiliar building. Frequently practice with escalators, elevators, etc., even though the student has already learned to use them.

Look for new and unusual situations. Watch for bad habits or misconceptions and work to correct them. Lindsay had trouble finding Kitchen #3, her assigned station in the home economics class. She tended to find any stove and insist it was hers. "It looks just right," she would insist. "I'm sure it's mine." Lindsay's teacher showed her several stoves, all of which "looked right" because they were identical. Then Lindsay practiced orienting herself to find Kitchen #3. She also noted that in #4, the stove and sink were reversed in relation to each other. In outdoor travel, Lindsay's teacher helped her realize that she might find more than one mailbox, smell more than one bakery, etc.

Stairs

Since stairs are everywhere, stair techniques should be taught very early in training, and routes involving stairs should be included in both indoor and outdoor travel lessons. From the very first lesson in using stairs, holding the handrail should be discouraged unless the student has balance problems, gross coordination problems, or an orthopedic handicap. Having to use the handrail will erode confidence in the cane and will slow a traveler down in the long run. It will create problems when the student is carrying something or where there is no handrail.

Since learning to go upstairs usually causes less nervousness than going down, the former could be taught first by having the student walk up several flights of stairs and then down them. This technique may be taught on the first lesson.

Outdoor Travel

After the student has demonstrated some measure of competence in the touch technique and stair technique, it is time to move outside. (Note that it is usually necessary to get parental permission to take a student off the school grounds.) A route going around the block in both directions is a logical starting point. Next, routes involving residential crossings should be done, after careful instruction in using traffic as a guide to know when it is safe to cross, and some general instruction in traffic laws. Many children, blind or sighted, do not know traffic laws – things such as turning right on red after a stop; yield; the significance of 2-way and 4-way stops; and the purpose of turning arrows.

THE RIGHT AMOUNT OF HELP

A word of caution – it is very important for a student to learn on her own. That means letting a student make mistakes, correct them, and build the confidence to cope with whatever happens. Continually rescuing a student can be devastating to her self-confidence, and will lead the student to believe that independent travel is dangerous and really shouldn't be done. This clearly defeats the purpose of the training.

On the other hand, a teacher must facilitate the thinking processes necessary for solving problems as they occur. For example, a beginning outside traveler may wander up a driveway, run out of sidewalk, and have no idea what happened. If the student doesn't figure it out, explanation may be necessary. Sometimes, a few questions designed to help the student solve a problem are best.

To minimize confusion about routes, give extremely specific directions and ask the student to repeat them. Any student who is unable to do this will very likely forget the route before it is completed. For instance: "The school faces east. Go outside and turn left (north) and walk to the corner. That street is Washington. Turn left (west) on the south side of Washington and walk to the next corner, which is Pine...." etc. If there are any landmarks such as parking lots or fountains, these could be mentioned. Routes involving more and more challenge should be given–crossing streets with islands, crossing streets with stoplights, 2-way and 4-way stops, and routes with unusual traffic patterns and landmarks.

LIGHTED CROSSINGS

When teaching lighted crossings, have the student go all the way around an intersection. Ask what color the light is at each point, insist that the student only cross at the beginning of a green light, and ask her to describe the general traffic patterns as well as the paths of individual cars. Then incorporate lighted crossings into routes.

Lighted crossings should be treated as ordinary, not a major hurdle. A matter-of-fact attitude about travel will engender confidence and challenge the student to perform what she knows is expected. After all, thousands of blind people cross streets independently and safely every day.

EXPERIENCE AND CONFIDENCE

A student should be walking many blocks per route at this stage. There is no substitute for practice, and no amount of talking can replace experience. If a student becomes lost, it is her responsibility either to figure out where she is or to seek assistance to determine her location. The teacher must lay down some ground rules about acceptable types of assistance. It is not acceptable for a student to accept a ride, since that is dangerous and does not develop self-confidence. Also, a student is not to let someone escort her to a location, but merely should ask whatever questions are necessary to determine present location and how to get to the destination.

The experience of being lost and solving the problem of being lost is a most critical lesson for independent travel. Ben had had considerable training in mobility, but never ventured out alone. He was afraid of getting lost and not having a mobility instructor on hand to rescue him. Before most students will venture out independently, they must have enough confidence in themselves to believe that whatever happens, they will deal with it. Begin building this confidence during the first lesson by letting the student solve his own problems.

Since there are time limits imposed by a school schedule, it is advisable to arrange for a double class period for each lesson rather than one class period every day, at this point in training. In the beginning, one class period per lesson will be long enough.

Using Public Transportation

Two class periods will also be desirable as lessons in mass transit begin, the next step in training. This should be taught when a student can negotiate residential and downtown traffic, stairs, and escalators with ease. Of course, necessity might dictate learning mass transit earlier. The average student of junior high age is old enough to handle mass transit travel.

BUSES

Before taking the first bus ride, a verbal description of the bus (where to board, where the farebox is located, and the arrangement of seats) will be helpful if the student has not taken public transportation before. It is not necessary to spend protracted periods of time in physically showing a student these things.

Ride with the student the first few times, making sure to have the student go ahead of you to pay the fare, request the desired stop, and find a seat as he would if traveling alone. If the student follows behind the teacher, he will learn much less about how to do it alone. Then the student should be assigned routes involving independent bus travel. The teacher can meet the student at a predetermined location. (For the student to travel alone, it is necessary to secure specific permission from the parents and school. If this is not possible, ride the same bus, but sit separately from the student and do not interfere with the decisions he makes.)

URBAN RAPID TRANSIT

If a subway or elevated train system exists in the community, it is desirable to teach the use of this as well, even if the student does not presently live near the train. Someday he may live near it, and he will certainly want to use it in traveling about the city anyway. It is an excellent confidence builder as well.

To ride the rapid transit trains, specific information about routes, the stations, the types of platforms, and the design of the cars should be given in advance. It is not possible for a student to go to every station during training, so general characteristics and types of station designs will be useful for a student in feeling comfortable when traveling in unfamiliar stations. Routes involving stations of various types should be given – stations with two or four exits, stations along the expressways, underground stations, elevated stations, center platform stations, and side platform stations.

Some transit systems have pay stations with attendants. Others have machines from which tickets are purchased. Often the passenger must put the ticket into a slot, go through a turnstile, and then pick up the stub out of another slot. Ticketing procedures should be explained in advance and also practiced with the teacher at the station.

During these lessons, as with bus travel, the student should precede the instructor. On the first lesson, instructions about the stations, the trains, the platform arrangement, and how to get to the boarding area can be given on the spot to reinforce the verbal descriptions given before. The student should locate the platform edge with the cane, and trail the tip over the side edge (ahead and beside him) while walking along to the boarding area. (See Figure 22-1.) Note that this is one of the few situations where the usual arcing of the cane is not advisable. The method just described is the safest and easiest way to travel the platform, because the area near the edge is clear of obstacles and, since the student knows where the edge is, he will not walk off. If the student were to walk down the center of the platform, he would encounter many obstacles such as benches, posts, and flights of stairs, and he would not have orientation to the edge. Since underground stations and stations along the expressways are very noisy, orientation by sound is difficult.

To board the train, a student should listen for the doors opening or for people walking onto the train; or, if it is too noisy, he can trail the cane along the side of the train to the doors.

CAUTION: The student must be sure to put the cane tip on the floor of the car before entering. Spaces between cars are similar in width to door openings. (See Figures 22-2 and 22-3) Careless blind persons have fallen onto the tracks, mistaking these spaces for open car doors.

After a student becomes comfortable riding the trains, give a route and do not speak to the student again until it is completed. The teacher may ride on the same train or (if the school and parents permit) prearrange to meet somewhere to discuss how things went.

In addition to teaching how to ride the trains, it is valuable to teach where the trains go, and how to use the transit information service. A description of the train routes and a list of the stops will be useful. To familiarize the student with using the transit information service, assign a route and request him to get directions from this service. The student will need to know how to use this service for his own travel needs.

The Ultimate Test

The ultimate test of whether a cane travel course is successful is whether or not a student actually travels independently on a routine basis. If he does, it is successful. If he doesn't, it is a failure. The successful program will not only teach technical skills, but also will give the student the confidence to travel wherever and whenever he wants to go.

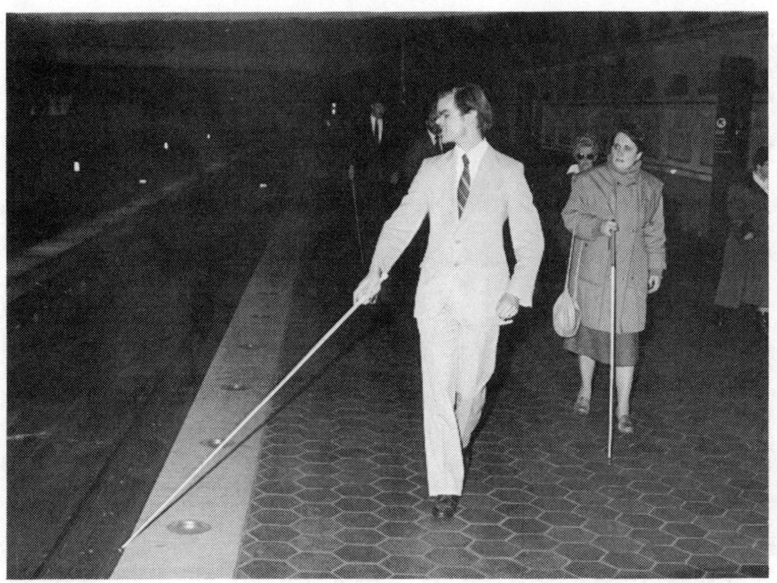

Figure 22-1
Edge Of Platform

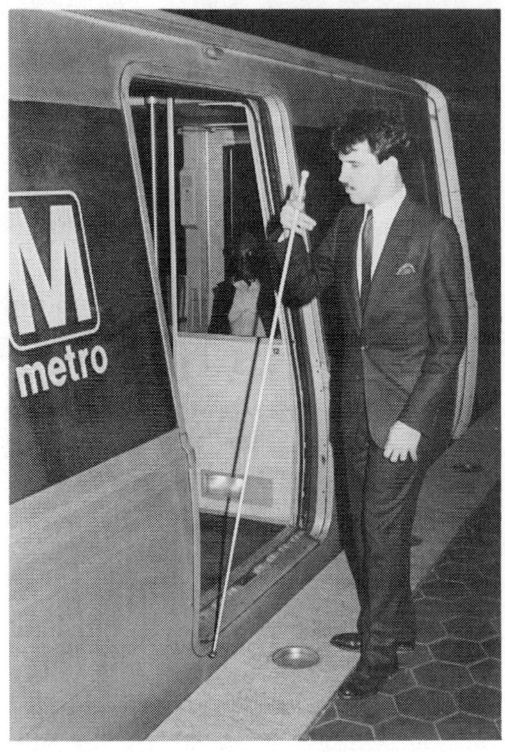

Figure 22-2
Finding Doorway

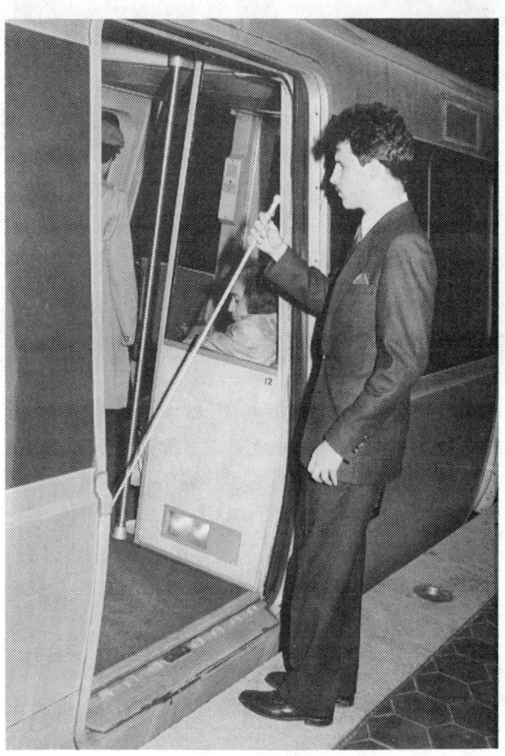

Figure 22-3
Checking For Floor

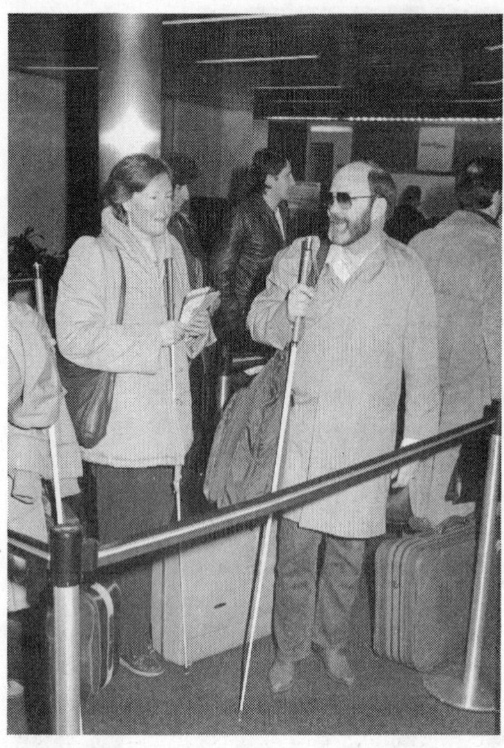

Figure 22-4
Unlimited Travel

CHAPTER 23

ORIENTATION AND MOBILITY FOR CHILDREN 8 AND UNDER, AND THOSE WITH SPECIAL PROBLEMS

These suggestions are designed to supplement, rather than replace, the remarks in the previous chapters on cane travel. For example, young children can learn to hold the cane correctly, but they may not learn it in just one or two lessons. Because previous chapters explain the standard posture and procedure for use of a cane, this chapter will not do so in detail.

Infants and Toddlers

As a resource/itinerant teacher, you may or may not work directly with infants and toddlers. Regardless, you can provide parents and early-childhood teachers with the ideas given here.

The following is adapted from *A Resource Guide for Parents and Educators of Blind Children*, by Doris M. Willoughby.

After the child learns to crawl, he will soon pull himself upright and take steps. At first, he will just follow hesitantly along a sofa or hold onto someone's hand. Calling him from a short distance away will encourage him to move toward you. Another idea is to place the child's feet on your feet as you hold his hands (with the child facing away from you) – you can then take him through the motions of walking, with you doing the work.

Actual physical support will, of course, gradually be dropped. Particularly avoid continuously holding onto *both* of the child's hands – a very unnatural position. You may need to remind friends not to carry your child around after he has learned to walk.

At the toddling stage, and even before, the baby will be developing ways to tell what is ahead of him. Each child has a different temperament, a different home, and different circumstances. One home may have two stairways, many rooms, and the toys of brothers and sisters here and there. Another home may be a two-room apartment. Each situation has its advantages and its problems. We urge you *not* to make large changes – and particularly not to move to a different home – just because a child is blind. Make temporary arrangements, such as stairway gates, as you would for any baby, and later remove them as the child no longer needs them.

Many children find it helpful to push a large object around as they begin to walk. Various types of baby walkers are on the regular market. Some toddlers like to push a kitchen chair around on the smooth floor. (A chair is very stable, and may be especially helpful for the hesitant child.) A toy lawn mower, wheelbarrow, grocery cart, etc., may be pushed also. Since such a push toy provides information about what is ahead, it is excellent readiness for cane travel. Lori used such a method even before she could walk. She pushed a toy in front of her as she crept along, in order to tell whether there was a wall or other obstacle ahead.

The tiny child may try to stand up under a table and bump his head. If this is a problem, teach him to reach up with his hand when he stands. (Later this will not be necessary, as he will stand up in more conventional places.) When an older child bends over, he similarly may need to check with his hand for potential bumps. He may choose to squat in place, without bending his head much, to avoid this problem.

Each child has his individual ways of learning. Different types of encouragement will be helpful with different children.

Remember that some children skip the crawling stage altogether and go directly to walking.

Along with learning how to move his body, the child forms a mental picture of the house or apartment so that he knows his way around. Talk with him as he is learning. You might say to the two-year-old, "Yes, there's your fuzzy chair. You went past the sofa and you found it." To the five-year-old you might say, "Remember that the door to the basement is closer to the sink, and the door to the garage is farther away. Then you won't always have to open a door to tell which is which."

The toddler is also forming a mental picture of himself. Help him name the parts of his body, through conversation and rhyming games. The bath is an especially good setting, as you say with the child, "Now we wash the left foot–can we find the toes?"

After the child learns to walk, expect him to walk by himself most of the time. He can learn his way around the house and yard at his own home and at any other homes visited regularly. Show your child any rearrangements of furniture. You may decide to keep toys and other objects off the floor in some rooms. Do not enforce such rules too rigidly, however, since the child needs experience with the real world. He can learn to go around the coffee table, and to realize that his little sister is likely to leave her blocks all over the family room.

Look for opportunities for the child to get around by himself in unfamiliar places also. Show him where the stairs are, but let him walk up and down alone. Let him explore a room without holding someone's hand.

Why Begin Cane Use Early?

Is the child bumping into things as he tries to move around? He need not find things the hard way–give him a cane. Does he hang back from moving at all? He need not fear bumps and falls–give him a cane.

Some believe that cane travel should be delayed because the young child may not be capable of perfect form and complete understanding, and because he should not enter dangerous areas alone. Some may also say that a child must walk without a cane for several years to prepare himself for using a cane later. However, with a cane the young child can find obstacles before he runs into them, and can find steps or curbs before he falls off the edge; thus he can learn to move quickly and with confidence. Learning to travel is a developmental process, like talking or reading–it begins with halting efforts and continually grows. We encourage the baby in his first imperfect words, and the beginning reader in his limited vocabulary, because that is the way he begins. It is the same with the young cane traveler. He may not use the cane perfectly or all the time at first–but he can begin.

RESULTS OF NON-USE OF THE CANE

What happens when a blind child aged two, three, four, and over does *not* begin to use a cane?

(1) To move independently at all, the child will have to devise some method of knowing what is ahead. Without a cane, this will be groping with the hands, and shuffling or sliding the feet. Often one foot becomes dominant, resulting in an uneven motion. All of this is most unnatural, inefficient, slow, and unattractive. And, once it is well established, it is very hard to change.

(2) A mobility teacher who does not teach cane travel at an early age will probably teach "pre-cane techniques" instead. Actually, these techniques (however much they are cloaked in professional dignity) are simply codified and exaggerated versions of the unnatural motions described above.

(3) If the child moves with any degree of speed without a cane or human guide, she will suffer bumps and bruises from unexpected obstacles. She also will stumble down unexpected stairs and other step-downs.

(4) Many children react to problem #3 by *not* moving with any degree of speed. They conclude (understandably) that the world is too dangerous for quick movement. Some conclude that all movement is dangerous.

(5) All life skills are more easily learned if they are begun (in an appropriately elementary manner) early in life. The three-year-old who starts to explore with a cane will quickly make it an extension of her "direct" senses. Cane use will be a natural thing, to be refined and built upon as she matures. If, on the other hand, she does not start with a cane until she is older, she will have built up a system of learning about the world without it. It will be hard to break into this and "add" the cane.

(6) The older a youngster is, the more her attitudes toward blindness and toward life have solidified. The four-year-old is eager to try new things, and probably has not learned that some people consider a white cane a stigma. The ten-year-old, however, already has definite ideas about blindness and about other people's attitudes. By the teen years, beginning cane travel involves a major emotional hurdle which could have been avoided if the cane had been introduced early.

(7) The limited mobility possible without a cane is frustrating and boring. One mother, having arranged travel instruction for her seven-year-old, became deeply concerned as week after week passed without a cane. She called the teacher, who insisted the child could not proceed until he mastered a particular "pre-cane" skill. However, the mother talked with her son and discovered he was so bored that he was deliberately doing things wrong to "spice up" his lessons. She got that straightened out fast, and he had a cane within a week.

(8) Because non-cane mobility is so limited, the child must walk with a human guide whenever speed and safety are needed. The child therefore learns that she cannot walk quickly and safely alone. Also, when walking with a human guide she does *not* learn things about the environment that she would learn when walking independently.

(9) Lack of a cane leads to the common practice of using another child as a human guide. The other child, being immature, often fails to avoid collisions. Moreover, in a special school often the "guide" is herself partially sighted and should be using a cane too. Thus the child who is guided has good reason to be fearful even when walking with others. But if the child has a cane, she has the option of taking someone else's arm while continuing to find obstacles herself.

ADVANTAGES OF CANE USE

If, in contrast to the above scenario, the child begins early to use a cane (preferably before school age):

(1) Obstacles are easily detected without bruises.

(2) Step-downs are easily detected without stumbling or falling.

(3) Unnatural shuffling and groping are avoided.

(4) Normal speed is possible and expected, without danger.

(5) Fear is minimized because there *is* a pain-

less method of detecting obstacles and step-downs.

(6) The cane is integrated naturally into the child's system of exploring the world. It becomes an extension of her own senses.

(7) The child receives the cane when she is young, eager, and unhampered by society's negative attitudes. Moving comfortably along, considering the cane as a natural part of life, she does not have to begin something unfamiliar as she enters her teens. (Should she nevertheless feel pangs of being "different" as she grows older, she will have a positive background to counteract this problem.)

(8) Since cane travel is unlimited, lessons can always be challenging and interesting.

(9) When a cane is used, a human guide is less often necessary. Even when someone assists, the child continues to use the cane while following or holding onto another person. Thus she interacts directly with the environment at all times, instead of passively depending on others.

(10) Many skills which are sometimes regarded as "pre-cane" are learned more easily *with* the cane. For example:

- Turning left and right. (With the cane, there need not be fear of what may be in the way.)
- Walking in a straight line. (It is easier to walk straight if one moves quickly rather than slowly and fearfully.)
- Walking with a normal gait. (It is hard to develop a normal gait when the feet must be used to explore the surface ahead. With a cane, the feet are freed to walk normally.)
- Finding doorways and doors. (The cane can reach farther than the hand. With it, the door or doorway can be found efficiently and deftly, while the floor surface is also being checked. The other hand is free to carry something.)

How Much to Rely on the Cane

"But he's not ready to cross streets alone!" is often heard from those who oppose early cane travel. This unfortunate excuse assumes incorrectly that a cane is useful only outdoors, and only when the blind person is alone.

On the contrary, cane travel is extremely useful indoors and in familiar situations. A very young child may even benefit from using a cane in her own home, although this is not done by older travelers. A back yard can be a threatening jungle. School hallways abound with open locker doors, bustling students, mop buckets, stairways, etc. Classrooms are crowded and changeable. The child with a cane can learn to walk confidently and painlessly while finding obstacles and steps, and while interacting directly with the environment. With a cane, he can go wherever children of his age ordinarily go.

Furthermore, when a child is accustomed to cane travel in relatively safe areas, he will merely be extending his skills when he crosses streets and goes farther alone. If cane travel is begun at a later time, there is no background and *all* skills are new.

A DEVELOPMENTAL PROCESS

There should be a gradual, natural process in which readiness leads to partial independence and then complete independence. This is what the sighted child does. First she crosses a street with her parents. Gradually she practices telling when the light is green, and may walk a little ahead of her parents. In time she is permitted to cross alone. There is no reason why the blind child cannot do the same. When she is three, adults can help her listen to traffic sounds before crossing. By age four, she should have a cane and cross with some help. During the early school years, independent crossing is learned very naturally.

Another common excuse is, "He's too young to realize that the cane is not a toy." There is a grain of truth here: the child who *uses* a cane as a toy is not benefiting from it. However, in her article, "Canes and Blind

Preschoolers" (*Future Reflections*, March-May, 1984), Barbara Cheadle says:

> Children not only learn skills gradually and at different rates, but it also takes time for them to see a particular tool as a functional object, not a "fun" plaything. My five-year-old still thinks his fork makes a fine airplane, and my six-year-old recently decided to try his penmanship on my good sheets. Again, the use of the cane is a skill which a child can acquire early, but takes time and patience to perfect, just like any other skill.

Mrs. Cheadle does not keep all forks away from her five-year-old because he sometimes tries to fly one; neither should she deprive him of a cane if he waves it around. Ordinary discipline (including a *brief* removal of the object, accompanied by loss of privileges) is applied instead. How would her son's table manners develop if he were deprived of silverware until he was ten and "old enough to use it properly at all times"? His manners would be like the mobility of a blind ten-year-old who has been deprived of a cane by similar logic.

What about the cane outside of school hours? Often I have seen a child begin to gain freedom with the cane, but falter and forget because of too little practice. I now talk with parents in detail about how to include the cane in family life. Following are examples of suggestions for parents, adapted from the article "Cane Travel," in the March-May, 1984, *Future Reflections:*

(1) DO learn the basic techniques so you can encourage and praise your child for his efforts. I know, we said that too much emphasis can be harmful, but that is only if it is done with the attitude that perfect execution of technique is essential to competent travel.

(2) DO insist that your child take her cane everywhere and that she USES it. Going to the store? Take the cane. Going to church? Take the cane. Remember the only way to become proficient in cane travel is practice, practice, practice and more practice. The cane, if used constantly and consistently, can become as natural and as comfortable to use as putting on your glasses, carrying your purse or wallet, putting on your coat in winter or any number of things we take for granted.

(3) DO NOT anticipate for your son or daughter what their cane will tell them in just a few moments anyway. For example, you do not (and should not) need to tell them when you are coming to some steps, a telephone pole, a building, etc. If you are constantly telling them everything, they will never learn to trust their cane (and neither will you). If they do miss the step or the pole, the most they will likely get is a bump or bruise (they will also remember next time to use the proper technique or pay more attention to their cane).

Of course it is only common courtesy to advise them of an overhanging branch that their cane or other senses would not detect. Use your judgment, but remember the ultimate goal is for your child to be able to travel from anyplace to anywhere independently.

(4) DO NOT teach your child to count steps. The proper use of the long white cane will allow a blind person to know when he has reached the top or the bottom of the steps or when he has arrived at a particular store, house, etc. In fact, counting steps can be a bad habit that interferes with a person's ability to concentrate on the sounds, smells, and landmarks around him that are much more valuable clues.

(5) DO NOT allow yourself or your child to be embarrassed about using the cane in public places, or anyplace at all. It is respectable to be blind, and

the long white cane is a symbol of the independence and normality of the blind. If you and your child will learn to feel and act that way, then more and more the public will take their cues from you and begin to treat the blind with respect and courtesy instead of pity and excessive helpfulness.

(6) DO help your child to learn how to properly store the cane when it is not in use. In a restaurant (movies, church, school, etc.), it can be slid under the table and chair as long as it does not stick out into an aisle where someone could trip on it. It can also be leaned in a corner or against a wall with ease. If none of these are possible, the person who is sitting can simply bring it in close to their side and rest it against their shoulder. It can be kept easily and comfortably there with little inconvenience.

In automobiles the cane can be placed in first or pulled in afterward. Even in the smallest compact car, the cane can be easily placed between or along the seat and the door or side of the vehicle. In some vehicles the person can rest the cane over the shoulder at an angle.

(7) DO expect your child–taking into consideration their age, maturity and experience–to learn and do such things as these: find a door and door handle, and open it for you; determine when to cross the street instead of waiting for you to give the go-ahead; run errands for you to the store or to the neighbor's house to borrow a cup of sugar; walk (or run) ahead of you as you walk down the street; take the bus, alone, shopping or to a school event; and any number of other things which demonstrate your confidence in their ability to travel independently.

(8) DO use sighted guide techniques SPARINGLY and only after careful consideration. Yes, it might be faster, for now, but how will it affect your child's progress? It is also faster to tie the kid's shoes, pick up the toys, make the beds, dress them, do the dishes, and all kinds of things they need to learn. Most parents finally figure out that they must take the time and let the kids learn to do by doing.

Next time you are tempted to let, or ask, your child to take your arm, ask yourself, "Am I doing this for my convenience...because I don't want to take the time, or handle the stares, or because I get tongue-tied trying to give directions...or because it is appropriate in this situation?"

Remember, if your child is to develop skill and confidence in traveling in open areas (such as parking lots), in buildings, and yes, crowds too–they need PRACTICE. They can't get that by hanging on to an arm. If the sounds you make walking are not sufficient clues for your child to follow, just remember to talk some, and you won't lose each other.

When you do go sighted guide, encourage your child to continue using the cane in the usual manner, or with modified grip. This puts your child "in-control" even when going sighted guide.

If parents do not see the value, probably the cane will never be used outside of school.

INCREASE INDEPENDENCE GRADUALLY

Sometimes parents attempt to have the child use the cane with total independence immediately. Assure them that it is often reasonable for a child to take someone's hand or arm, especially in a crowd. "Total independence" can be overdone. Among other things, eventually the parents will realize that it is impossible, and will probably conclude that *all* cane use is impractical.

More commonly, parents may assume from the beginning that the cane is of no value when the young child needs to be near an adult anyway. Often they hold the child's hand whenever they leave the house–even as the child grows to be eight or nine or older.

Recently a ninth-grade student followed me across a large parking lot to my car. "What's this?!" he exclaimed each time as his cane encountered a low concrete barrier, a grassy traffic island, and then a utility pole. He had expected to walk around parked cars, but was genuinely surprised to find any of these other things in a parking lot. His parents had always guided him completely around them. They had also encouraged him to surrender responsibility for direction. Despite the straightforward path to my car, this student had no idea how to return to the building.

Demonstrate

Demonstration must go with discussion. Walk ahead of the student across a parking lot, just as I did, while the parent watches; then ask the parent to do the same. Show how the child can take your arm and still use the cane to advantage. Demonstrate walking briskly; walking slowly in a crowd, with the cane held closer to the body but still in use; walking among obstacles. Explain about listening for traffic. Do all of this with appropriate school staff as well as parents. If possible demonstrate also with siblings, other relatives, and friends. All of this should begin at a young age so that the student does not reach ninth grade and be as inexperienced as the student above.

Another example from high school also shows the importance of integrating the cane into all of life. I complimented one of my students for an excellent talk about Braille at the citywide PTA meeting. But I was disappointed that her cane had been nowhere in sight.

"I could never have found my way around that auditorium at South High alone," she protested. "Someone had to guide me up to the podium. And I didn't know where I'd put my cane. In some theaters there's no way you can get it under the seats."

Looking around the student's own school, I located a theater-arts classroom with which she was not familiar. We found a time when it was vacant, and I (with exaggerated fanfare) simulated the PTA program: "May I show you to a seat, Miss Ainsworth?... And now it's time for the next item.... Miss KAREN AINSWORTH! Would you come on up to the podium, Miss Ainsworth? Right up here...." Thus she walked toward my voice, here and there in the large room which had unexpected step-downs. To her delight and surprise, she easily succeeded without ever taking my arm. (I explained that in a real situation, she might indeed choose to take someone's arm for a time, but this did not exclude the cane). She practiced placing the cane under her seat and by the podium. During "informal moments after the program," she walked around the room alone. Later we repeated all this while her mother watched.

With a cane one may choose to accept various degrees of help from time to time. Without a cane there is no choice but dependency.

A NATURAL SEQUENCE

Another common excuse for non-use of the cane is immature behavior. What if the young child continually drops the cane, waves it, pokes with it–everything except using it right? What if the family seems to get nothing done except to remind him what to do with his cane?

A child who is four or older should be starting to use a cane. (If he has some sight, or if he is over eight, see below for additional remarks.) However, it is sometimes wise to use the cane just part of the time at first. A good sequence might be: use the cane during actual lessons ... start bringing it back and forth to preschool each day ... start taking it to church ... explore Grandma's large back yard ... etc. Add more and more situations where it will be taken along and used. By first grade at the latest, a child should be able to use the cane wherever an adult would, indoors and outdoors, and need only a reasonable amount of reminding.

Similarly, with a very young child it may be necessary to have a gradual increase of cane use at school. In looking beyond actual lessons, first seek out the situations where this particular child will use the cane most easily and effectively. Does he enjoy walking with nothing in the way? Then start with going to the playground. Is he especially bothered by obstacles? Use the cane to avoid bumps in the crowded classroom. At first we may expect use of the cane only part of the time, and imperfect motions may be tolerated.

Students with Some Sight

In deciding whether a child with partial sight should use a cane, consider this question: "Does he walk as quickly and easily as most children his age, and with no more collisions than average?" If not, cane travel training should be provided immediately. When the child reaches school age and should be crossing streets alone, and as he becomes old enough to shop alone, other questions should be asked:

Can he safely dodge a car whose driver assumes the pedestrian can see well? (Note that a motorist will probably be wary of any *little* child, but will expect an older one to get out of the way. A white cane, however, positively requires the motorist to stop or yield.)

Can he read signs easily, or will he appear foolish by not doing so?

Can he easily interpret hand gestures from several feet away? If not, he will be often misunderstood and sometimes in physical danger.

Can he recognize individuals and interpret facial expressions at a distance, or will he seem to be ignoring people?

Many people with partial sight can see well enough to avoid tripping, but use a cane for identification, to prevent problems such as those above. They also find that walking is much less of an effort or strain when a cane is used instead of vision alone.

Barbara Cheadle comments,

> ...our son has some usable vision but he has little or no depth perception. He could never be sure if a change in shape, texture or composition of the surface he was on also meant a step-up, or a drop-down. He was also finding out that what appeared to be a smooth, flat surface – all of one color and composition – could mask unexpected drop-offs. He fell flat on his face once because he did not have his cane and he assumed that the concrete walk in front of him was flat. It was a walk-way into a church building and had several of those long steps of varying widths.
>
> – *Future Reflections,* March-May, 1984.

A blind adult recalls: "I have always had usable vision. But I couldn't tell dropoffs. I ran into poles. I fell off steps. On vacations I dreaded caves and mountains .... Now that I have a cane, I use it to supplement my vision, and I enjoy walking anywhere."

How sad for a child to dread interesting places like mountains and caves, just because cane travel instruction was not provided.

LEARNING ALTERNATIVES TO RELIANCE ON SIGHT

Sleepshades must be used or the child simply will not learn what the cane can do.

One adult commented, "I have quite a bit of sight, enough to see buildings and various landmarks. Now that I use a cane, I can make much better use of my sight, because I don't have to keep watching my feet all the time!" This man would never have stopped "watching his feet" if he had not traveled extensively with his eyes covered and learned that the cane really can tell him what is ahead.

Other parts of this book discuss the use of sleepshades in some detail – particularly the following chapters:

"The Partially-Sighted Child"
"Teaching Braille (Second Grade and Below)"
"Travel With the Long White Cane"

The chapter on "Teaching Braille (Second Grade and Below)," particularly, discusses how to introduce the sleepshades gently and pleasantly for a young child.

"Now I Understand!"

Ian had used a cane since he was seven. He seemed to have good technique, but needed continual reminders.

Mrs. Vrbek, the new resource teacher, made some changes in the Orientation and Mobility program: she provided a much longer cane, and she required sleepshades during lessons. The first time Mrs. Vrbek instructed Ian, she realized he had never really understood what the cane could do for him. He had moved it dutifully in front of him, but had not really used it for gaining information.

Mrs. Vrbek placed Ian (who was wearing sleepshades) so that he was facing a chain-link fence, and asked him to walk forward quickly. After a few steps, the cane tip encountered the fence. Ian stopped short. "Oooh!" he exclaimed softly, almost in awe. His exclamation embodied a dramatic insight: "Now I really understand what the cane can do! It can find things before I get to them. It can find them even when I can't see them, or when I can't see them well enough to tell what they are."

Mrs. Vrbek had noticed that Ian had formerly carried his cane in a gingerly manner, trying to keep it from touching anything. "He used to act as though he were carrying a box or something instead of a cane," she commented. "He would squint to try to see what was in the way, and say 'oops' if the cane did touch something. Now he realizes that the cane is supposed to touch things to give him information."

Ian soon roamed freely all over the large playground, where formerly he had played in one small area. With continued instruction under sleepshades, he crossed streets more and more confidently. Very few reminders were required to maintain good cane usage.

"He says he *enjoys* wearing those sleepshades!" exclaimed the principal incredulously. "How can that be?"

"I'm not surprised," replied the teacher. "A number of students have told me they travel better with sleepshades because they are not trying to see what they really cannot see."

ANOTHER EXAMPLE

A blind adult speaks about her childhood when she did not have a cane: "As the distance between my head and the ground increased, I used various methods to figure out the terrain. Often I would walk with one foot on the grass and one on the sidewalk. I cultivated quick reflexes to try to recover when I was jolted by unexpected step-downs. I continually guessed whether a dark spot might be a hole, a shadow, a mud puddle, or a dark-colored object. Life is so much easier now – I can easily be certain of these things with a simple sweep of my cane.

WHAT ABOUT FAMILIAR AREAS?

Often a child seems to have no trouble getting around in familiar areas, since he can see most obstacles and he remembers where the step-downs are. Thus it may appear that a cane is not needed. However, this is an unwise conclusion since the child will not be able to travel safely and independently elsewhere, and will have difficulty with changes in familiar areas.

If the child is under eight, sometimes a solution is to use the cane only part of the time – in lessons (with sleepshades) and in unfamiliar areas. This way, the child learns what the cane can do, and begins to phase it into his life. But by the time he is seven or eight, he should be using the cane at all times (excluding his own home and special situations such as sports) for the following reasons:

(1) Although a very young child rarely goes into unfamiliar situations without an adult close by, the older child does. He will roam farther in the neighborhood, walk all over the school building, run errands, etc.

(2) As the child's world expands, so does the variety of common hazards. He will encounter varied terrain, mop buckets, uneven lighting, etc.

(3) Often a need or opportunity for travel will arise unexpectedly. If the child is in the rest room without his cane and the fire alarm goes off, he cannot safely hurry out the nearest exit. If he is at the neighbor's and a trip downtown is suggested, he will not want to go home for his cane.

(4) The child of eight is forming more and more definite ideas about the world. The older he is, the harder it will be to *start* using a cane, or even to increase its use from part time to full time.

COMBINING VISION WITH ALTERNATIVE TECHNIQUES

An adult who has traveled under sleepshades will figure out an appropriate personal combination of techniques, some using sight and some not. For example, a person may see the outlines of buildings visually, but rely on the cane to find steps and doorways. Children, however, may not do this on their own. Instead they may travel increasingly well under sleepshades, but immediately revert to the old hesitations when the sleepshades are off.

Ted was terrified of crossing streets, since he did not really have enough vision to judge traffic movements. Using sleepshades, he learned to listen carefully and cross confidently. But one day after the lesson, when Ted had his cane but was not wearing sleepshades, he was asked to cross a street–and he froze! The teacher, seeing no cars coming from any direction, asked in bewilderment what was wrong. "I'm waiting for those," replied Ted as he pointed to two *parked* cars. He was relying on his eyes instead of applying what he had been taught.

It may be desirable for the travel teacher occasionally to help the child use alternative techniques when the eyes are not covered. Explain that partial sight sometimes gives such inaccurate or incomplete information that it should be disregarded. ("Never mind what you see with your eyes. That won't help. Listen with your ears, and pay attention to your cane.")

Make a clear separation between this kind of practice and the regular lessons in which sleepshades are always used. You might label the combination work as "extra practice," and possibly carry it out in a different location.

Any child who is legally blind and is crossing streets independently will be much safer with a cane.

A Regular Part of Life

Once a child has learned to use the cane well, it is important that it be regarded as a regular, normal part of his equipment for living–comparable to shoes, for example. It should be used whenever he walks around, except in his own home and in special situations such as sports. When the blind person holds someone else's arm for convenience, he should continue to use his cane, and thus avoid being completely dependent on the other person. With this approach, the blind student is always conscious of where he is and where he is going, and is always prepared for the unexpected (such as an unreliable companion or a surprise fire drill). The student should not be allowed to believe that he has memorized the school building or grounds so well that he need not use his cane. Without a cane, he must either move very slowly, receive special attention, or constantly face the likelihood of bumps from mop buckets, stairways, open locker doors, classmates standing in his path, etc.

Give classroom teachers practical hints:

- If children are walking in line, the blind child can learn to follow by sound, and by occasionally touching the child ahead. With his cane he will not need help with terrain such as steps.
- In a line moving very slowly (such as at a drinking fountain), the cane can gently touch the foot of the person ahead, to note when he/she moves.
- When the class moves in a group without lining up (as from the story corner to tables), the child can easily follow by sound, and his cane will be helpful in finding a place to sit. If he has an

assigned seat, he should have practice in finding it.

- When children are free to choose where they will go (as during free play in kindergarten), the child can learn to hunt around alone, using his cane, and then to set the cane down when he decides to stop.
- Usually we need not worry about real injury. Everyone gets occasional scrapes. The child learns by exploring on his own. If there is a special hazard, we can keep him away or teach him to remember it.
- If art projects are spread out on the floor, remember the blind child will not know this unless warned.

Cane use has been too long delayed if the child protests, "I don't need a cane to go there! I can go there myself!" He has relied too much on inefficient non-cane techniques, and is failing to integrate cane use with his "direct" senses. Such a complaint indicates need for more, not less, use of the cane. The child also needs to learn that walking with a cane *is* "going there by myself," and doing so more safely and quickly.

Many children, even preschoolers, quickly understand the value of the cane and immediately begin to use it regularly.

A variation of "using the cane only part of the time" is to supplement it in ways that would not ordinarily be desirable. If the inexperienced young child really is likely to fall down steps before realizing what his cane is telling him, his parents may decide to warn him of all steps. But they can still allow him to make mistakes with other lesser hazards. He can bump into a pole, feel discomfort, and learn to avoid it next time. Later, with experience, he will no longer need to be warned about steps.

Using a cane does not rule out direct touching. The little child may (with or without specific guidance) strike the wall with his cane, and then examine the wall with his hand; find the door with his cane, and then run his hands over it; etc. This is analogous to the way young sighted children develop their vision – they will feel or mouth a toy many times, and then gradually learn to recognize it by vision alone. The young blind child needs to practice finding something with his cane, and then examining it with his hands, in order to understand what the cane tells him. He is integrating the cane into his way of exploring the world.

CHAPTER 24

A CANE TRAVEL CURRICULUM FOR CHILDREN 8 AND UNDER, AND THOSE WITH SPECIAL PROBLEMS

Making Lessons Age-Appropriate

Be sure your student understands what you mean, and has the ability to do the task as you present it. A five-year-old has a limited vocabulary, and may need several lessons before she even remembers how to hold the cane. Some instructors get stuck at this point and conclude that the child cannot yet learn. Not so. It is just like reading or anything else–she can indeed learn, but it must be at an appropriate pace and with appropriate tasks.

A CLEAR EXPLANATION

Start by considering the spoken vocabulary. A five-year-old will not know what an "arc" is (she'll think you're talking about Noah). She may be vague about words like "posture" and "both."

Physical Demonstration

Because of the vocabulary problem, and also because children learn by doing, it is best to *show* the child most things physically. Stand behind her and move her arm into the correct position, clasp her fingers onto the cane handle, etc., as you explain how the cane should be held. Walk several steps with the child as you continue to help her hold and arc the cane. (I tend to walk a little behind and to the right, putting my left arm around her left shoulder, and keeping my right hand closed over her right hand to control the cane.) Keep doing this kind of thing frequently, rather than relying mainly on verbal explanation.

One of the best ways to get a point across is to demonstrate the *wrong* approach, sometimes in exaggerated form. Often, for example, I have a student who tends to tap the cane on one side only. I may say, "Let me show you something. I'm going to put my hand on your hand and make your cane tap in a certain way. You tell me if it's the right way or not." Then I make the cane tap for awhile on the right only; the left only; both sides correctly; in the middle only. Each time I ask, "Is this good? Why?" Younger children usually find this amusing as well as instructive. (Caution: If this idea is used with an older student, be careful not to seem sarcastic.)

Vocabulary

When you introduce a new term, demonstrate and define it. Sometimes you will not use the official term at all. Following are two expressions re-worded for a five-year-old:

(1) Poor: "The cane can detect obstacles."
Good: "This cane can keep you from getting bumped. It can find things that are in the way, *before* you bump into them."

(2) Poor: "Arc the cane evenly, tapping in front of each foot."
Good: "The cane needs to touch in front of this foot *and* that foot." (Teacher gently touches each foot as she speaks.) "Make the cane go from one side to the other side,

like this." (Teacher demonstrates by helping the child move the cane.)

Ask an experienced teacher of young children (not necessarily a specialized teacher of the blind) to watch you and make suggestions.

LENGTH OF THE CANE

Be sure the cane is an appropriate length, as discussed in the previous chapter. Children grow quickly and may need a longer one every few months. Be sure the cane is long enough to reach past the next step in going down stairs.

PREVENTING FEAR

If an older student is expected to re-orient herself when lost, and is not too quickly rescued, she will develop self-reliance. But a four-year-old (sighted or blind) can be genuinely terrified in a minute or two if she thinks she is alone and lost. Therefore, when giving a lesson to a child under six it is best to talk frequently even if you are not actually helping. You can say reassuring things such as, "I'm sure you'll find it in a minute." If a child of this age is really confused for more than a very few minutes, she should have actual help.

As the child grows older, consider her maturity and resources as you decide how quickly to help her. Until she is old enough to be really alone, assure her that you will always be nearby and watching, and that you would help in case of serious trouble.

Lesson Planning

Most students over eight, and some who are younger, can grasp the entire basic technique in a lesson or two. Lessons become a matter of keeping basic technique consistent, adding new techniques such as those for escalators, and applying the skills to an ever-widening environment.

Very young students, however, often cannot grasp very much at once. It may be necessary to spend several lessons in teaching the basic position and motion. Nevertheless, actual travel with the cane should be begun while the technique is still imperfect, with more and more elements of the standard form being gradually added.

Suppose, for example, that a beginner is still learning how to hold the cane and keep the tip down. She should nevertheless walk with the cane and find obstacles, even if she is not yet tapping in an appropriate arc. Part of the time the teacher might take hold of her and move her through the standard motions. But part of the time the child should move on her own, however imperfectly, as long as the cane is finding obstacles. If this is not done, the child probably will not understand the purpose of the cane, and lessons will also be impossibly boring.

SHE CAN'T LEARN IT ALL AT ONCE

I use the following sequence of skills when the child is too immature to learn them all at once:

(1) Begin to understand the purpose of the cane.

(2) Keep the tip down.

(3) Hold the handle with one hand. (Note: See exceptions.)

(4) Keep the cane hand centered at waist level, with the arm against the body.

(5) Use correct grip and finger position.

(6) Tap cane from side to side.

(7) Make the arc consistent on each side.

(8) Keep in step.

Note that this is a process of refining and improving techniques which are very imperfect at first. Some instructors say that this is wrong–they believe the cane should never be used except with perfect form. Their concern is inconsistent with the way other developmental tasks are handled. Recall the analogy to using silverware: The progression (for a sighted or blind baby) ordinarily is something like this:

(1) Begin to understand the purpose of silverware.

(2) Hold the handle.

(3) Insert spoon into mouth (with food having been loaded onto spoon by someone else).

(4) Lift the food to the mouth, keeping the bowl of the spoon upright (again, spoon having been loaded by someone else).

(5) Direct the bowl of the spoon into the food and proceed (receiving some help in loading the spoon).

(6) Scoop some food from the bowl and proceed independently.

(7) Consistently use correct grip and finger position.

(8) Avoid messiness.

BUILD ON EXPERIENCE

Any number of other skills are gradually refined and improved with maturity and experience: drawing, writing, walking, bathing, etc., etc. Withholding a cane completely from a young child is no more logical than totally withholding the washcloth because she flops it around.

"Improving and refining" includes developing more and more independence. At first we place the child's hand on the cane in the proper position. Later she holds the handle correctly when reminded. In time she will remember by herself.

Some beginners are better off using *two* hands on the cane for awhile. They may center the handle better, and overcome a tendency to reach out with the free hand.

Similarly, very young beginners may find it easier to slide the tip back and forth rather than tapping it.

As the child progresses, introduce new elements of technique. Simply proceed for awhile with a given level of skill, and then say, for example, "Now you're going to learn how to move the cane just the way a grownup does." Avoid waiting unduly long between refinements, lest the immature technique become too established. The ultimate example of "waiting unduly long," however, is to delay starting with the cane at all. Then the habits to be changed include shuffling feet, outstretched hands, slow motion, irregular gait, and crippling fear.

With a student in junior high or high school, the basic stance is quickly learned, and it is almost immediately possible to work on routes suitable for an adult–walking throughout the building, going up and down steps, crossing streets, etc., and proceeding into routes several blocks in length. For a youngster of nine or ten, the same is true but at a slower pace. But what about the very young child who would not be going far alone if she were sighted, and who seems to need several lessons before even crossing the room?

EXPECTATIONS BY AGE

First of all, let us consider what skills are reasonable to achieve at various ages. A rough guide for the average student is:

Under age 5:

- Use correct hand position.
- Arc the cane while walking on flat terrain. (Keeping in step may be too hard at this level.)
- Detect obstacles and go around them.
- Use cane up and down stairs. (Adult may warn of presence of stairs.)
- Cross streets with assistance (not independently), and pay attention to traffic sounds.
- Detect major differences in surface underfoot.
- Walk toward a sound, including following a person who makes a sound while walking.
- Tell left from right, with one hand marked tactually if necessary.

Ages 5-6:

- All above skills
- Detect stairs, even when unexpected, and proceed up or down.
- Keep in step when arcing.
- Begin to interpret echoes made by cane tip (when passing a side hallway, a parked car, etc.)
- Find open doorways and closed doors with cane.
- Walk independently (with cane, as always) to classroom, rest room, office, etc.

- Travel on playground, with assistance at times.
- Stay on sidewalk in non-complicated environment.
- Recognize when a street is being crossed.
- Independently cross uncontrolled intersection with little traffic.
- Cross simple intersection with traffic light (possibly with some guidance).
- Correctly identify the four compass directions, in a familiar place.
- Follow directions for a simple route of three blocks or less in relatively familiar territory.
- Attempt to correct errors or miscalculations before expecting help.
- Know left and right without aid.

Ages 7-8:

- All above skills
- Make continual use of echoes from cane tip, indoors and outdoors. Use this as one method to find open doorways.
- Follow directions to schoolrooms where student does not ordinarily go.
- Travel independently on playground, selecting play activities.
- Stay on sidewalk despite some complications.
- Independently cross simple intersection with traffic light.
- Begin to understand variations in arrangement of intersections.
- Expand ability to correct errors.
- Correctly name the intermediate compass points: NE, SE, NW, SW).
- Follow directions for a simple route of up to six blocks, in an area which may be unfamiliar but is not difficult.

WHAT IS "INDEPENDENCE"?

Let us pause to discuss the term, "independently." This has a different meaning for a young child than for an adult or even a teenager. When we say that an adult "crosses streets independently," we mean that she can choose, at any time, to proceed to any intersection and cross it. If we say that a twelve-year-old "crosses streets independently," the interpretation is not quite as broad – her parents will exert some control over where she may go and when – but she will cross without necessarily having a helper nearby.

In contrast, consider what we mean when a six-year-old "crosses a street independently." At that age, sighted or blind, parents place tight guidelines over where the child is permitted to roam. If traffic makes safety dubious, someone will watch her. This prevents the young child from attempting to cross an intersection of unknown complexity without assistance. However, there is no reason why she cannot walk to a neighbor's house alone, over a simple and safe route, while someone is prepared to look for her if she is late.

Similarly, the adult uses self-discipline to extend correct procedure outside of lessons. But the child needs to be reminded often – very firmly, if necessary. If the eight-year-old walks to the drugstore while merely carrying her cane (rather than actually using it), or crosses the street carelessly, the valued privilege of going alone can be temporarily withdrawn. The five-year-old who waves her cane around can be told, "You have to hold my hand until you keep the cane tip down."

FIT THE LESSON TO THE CHILD

Yes, the little child can learn to use a cane with great advantage. No, she can't learn just like an adult. For a five-year-old, ten minutes is usually long enough for any one activity. Change the pace frequently, with the entire travel lesson probably not exceeding 20-30 minutes. A typical lesson outline might be:

10 minutes:

Walk on sidewalk, trying to stay off the grass.

10 minutes:

Go up and down stairs.

10 minutes:

Walk around in the schoolyard. When an obstacle is found correctly with the cane, the child may examine it (and play on it, if appropriate).

In the above sequence of activities, note that the most "fun" is last.

Making Lessons Interesting

A young child has limited stamina and a short attention span. If he has a lot of difficulty, he will cry or balk. If the lesson is too easy or repetitive, he will "clown around," make irrelevant remarks, complain, etc. Since he cannot yet articulate feelings clearly, he may even say the work is "too hard," when he actually is not challenged enough.

SUGGESTED IDEAS

The following ideas provide variety and a positive approach for early lessons in cane use:

(1) Set a specific length, appropriate for the level of skill, to a given task. With a four-year-old beginner you might say: "Walk straight ahead and find the wall with your cane," or "Make the cane go from one side to the other side, for *ten* steps." A six-year-old might walk to the end of the block or to the far side of the playground.

(2) Emphasize praise over criticism. Often correction should be nonverbal – simply take hold of the child and move him into the correct position, while praising his efforts.

(3) Let the child examine or play with an especially interesting item at the end of the task – a flower, a wall with unusual texture, a swing, etc. To the four-year-old we might say, "When you walk ten steps without forgetting to tap your cane, I will show you this interesting plant." The six-year-old might be told, "At the end of each lesson, if your work is OK, we will have time to look at something especially interesting."

(4) Suggestion #3 is not only for enjoyment. Learning to examine things meaningfully by touch is crucial, yet many blind children hang back from touching things because of adults' ignorance or embarrassment. Furthermore, there are many objects which are readily available but which the child may not really understand. Does the child really know the difference between a fire hydrant and a mailbox? Does he understand where the traffic signs are? Has he ever looked at the sewer grating? Many blind adults have never examined a traffic barricade.

(5) Even when lengthy practice in a certain area is essential, do not spend all your time there. You might spend two-thirds of the time on essential practice in locating classrooms, and the other third on varied terrain outside. This alleviates boredom and provides for some progress in other techniques.

(6) The use of sounds especially lends itself to "making a game" of a lesson. For example:

- Hide and Seek: Place a beeping object within earshot. The child must use good cane technique to walk to the object and pick it up.
- Howdy Do: Direct the child to keep still while you walk away. (You may or may not choose to move silently.) Then tell the child to walk toward you, and keep on talking as he approaches. Shake hands ceremoniously when he arrives and finds your foot with his cane.

(7) Have a treasure hunt. Give a "clue" which may or may not be humorous: "Go to the stairway" or "Find something that goes up and down, yet never moves." When the child arrives there, give the clue for the next location. Provide a small treat at the end. (Variation: Braille each clue and attach it appropriately for the child to find.)

(8) Find the Teddy Bear: A teddy bear is at the end of the route to be practiced. When the activity is completed, the child is permitted to get the teddy bear and play with it briefly. (Example: Walk to the south door and out to the swings. Then come back in and go to the principal's office. The teddy bear is on the chair just inside

the office.)
(Note: directions may be given all at once, or one at a time as the child proceeds. Use a different stuffed animal periodically.)

(9) Occasionally use a stopwatch and chart speed.

(10) Personify the cane. Give it a clever name. In the videotape, *Kids With Canes,* one boy exclaims, "My cane talks to me!" and explains that its tap tells him what is ahead.

(11) Start the child where he will quickly encounter the obstacle with which he needs practice.

(12) When a child is careless in a familiar area, deliberately provide some unexpected obstacles (chairs, boxes, etc.).

(13) Take the child to a safe, interesting area and have him explore it independently.

(14) Practice locating the curb without accidentally stepping off. Have him announce, "Curb!"

(15) Have the child follow you across varied terrain. Keep talking or providing other sound clues.

(16) Walk with the child to an interesting destination, expecting him to walk independently but near you. If the child becomes careless with the cane, stop dead. Then proceed as long as he uses good technique.

(17) Work on part of a skill before expecting the child to do it all alone. For example, at first physically move the student through the motions of looking for a doorway with his cane, while he merely announces when it has been found. Later the child can move the cane himself, knowing how it feels to accomplish the task.

(18) Use a Braille map of the area.

(19) Stop and discuss orientation, as,

"Point back the way you came."
"How would we get to Mrs. Hill's room from here?"
"Have we come to the street yet?"

Such questions promote keeping track of one's location, and help avoid mere memorization.

(20) Discuss a concept, as, "Is this street one-way or two-way? How do you know? How do the drivers know?"

(21) Work on things that are closely related to mobility, and can easily be included in a route, but may be neglected if not anticipated. If necessary for practice, the travel teacher may play the roles of various other people.

- Locate the ticket line. Go to the end, move along up, and buy a ticket. (The student may need coaching to check on where the end is; to position the cane to check the feet of the person ahead as the line moves; to be attentive about reaching the ticket window; etc.).
- Go into the library and find an empty seat. Check gently with the free hand to be sure the seat is empty.
- Go to a room where class is not in session, and determine whether the teacher is there (e.g., if the room is silent, say, "Mr. Smith?")

(22) Whenever possible, have a genuine purpose for the trip:

- Buy the teacher's lunch ticket.
- Deliver a message.
- Get the art paper.

(23) For a very young beginner, sometimes say, "Walk until your cane finds something ahead. Then reach out and look it over with your hands and tell me what it is." This is important in helping the very young child understand what the cane is telling him. However, do not do this too much, lest the child form the habit of always doing it. Alternate it with the opposite idea: "Keep walking until I tell you to stop. Use your cane to find *space to walk.* Don't touch anything with your hands."

(24) Explore a place where children rarely go. For example, the tornado shelter may be a basement area with steep steps and low ceilings. Children would always be accompanied, but the blind child need not be helpless.

(25) Watch for interesting features temporarily present, such as scaffolding, and examine them if possible. (Caution: Check with an authority before touching anything which could possibly be hazardous.)

(26) Walk the child through something which he is clearly not ready to do independently, but for which readiness work and anticipation would be beneficial:

- Cross a busy intersection with a four-year-old.
- Cross a controlled intersection with a five-year-old and help him listen to the traffic change direction (even if the IEP does not yet call for his learning to cross such a street independently).
- Ride the city bus with a six-year-old. (Note: Many families use the automobile exclusively, so that the blind child has no background in using public transportation. Urge parents to take the child on buses, taxis, subways, etc.)

(27) Work with two students together. If one is more advanced, he can help teach the other one. Two students who are equal in skill will pick up ideas from each other. Everyone will be stimulated by the change of pace.

(28) Go to something unusual or unexpected, with or without warning the student. For example: a very high step; the edge of a stage or platform; a swimming pool; a tree in the middle of a sidewalk; a tiered classroom or theater; etc. Besides being interesting, such things help show why a cane is valuable. An "ordinary classroom door" may actually lead onto a stage, with a dropoff a few feet inside.

(29) Often the desired area for practice is some distance away, and the child takes a long time to walk there independently. Take the child's hand and walk briskly to the area desired.

(30) Do not assume that the young child should practice only near the school or home. Get appropriate permission and transport the child elsewhere.

(31) Practice telling left from right:

- At first, use a ring or rubber band on one arm or hand. Mark a doll in a similar way.
- Find right ear, left foot, etc.
- "Look on your right. What is there?"
- "Turn left and find the wall."
- Play "Simon Says."
- "I will place a toy car on the left side of your desk. See how fast you find it." (Teacher taps *both* sides of desk when placing the car.)

(32) Practice finding things inside the classroom, particularly the child's own desk. (Try to practice when the class is not present.)

(33) Some things that might be considered "physical education" may be included in mobility lessons:

- Using playground equipment, including climbing
- Hiking in rough terrain
- Ice skating
- Roller skating
- Sliding on ice without skates
- Sledding on snowy hills
- Clambering up and down a steep embankment
- Wading through deep snow

Putting It All Together

BLINDNESS IS RESPECTABLE

Condition yourself, your student, and others to assume that the primary goal is to travel successfully and independently–*not* to be as inconspicuous as possible. The cane has to make some sound in order to be useful, and the beginner may be rather noisy. A more experienced traveler will be quieter and more deft, but still should not expect to be silent. Teach your student and his family that blindness is respectable, and that the sound of the cane is respectable.

Help parents, especially, to confront the tendency to leave the cane at home because people may stare. For one thing, as the child grows older people will stare at him *without* a cane and think, "Is he retarded? Ill? Drunk?" If, instead, the cane is used regularly, people will understand and respect its use. They will soon take it for granted and stare much less. Also, the family will soon become much less self-conscious.

It can be very hard to discuss this because there is so much rationalization ("He doesn't really need the cane when he's with me.") Help parents to get past the initial feelings of embarrassment, to realize it is respectable to be blind, and to avoid letting personal discomfort deny independence to their children.

A major reason for children's fearfulness is the tendency of adults to gasp in horror at the slightest bump or jostle – even the *anticipation* of the slightest bump or jostle. Parents and teachers must observe competent blind travelers and realize that cane travel is safe and effective. When a parent says, "He doesn't need a cane when he's with me," one implication is, "It wouldn't help him much anyway." Show parents that a competent blind person traveling with a cane *is* safe and independent.

GOOD EXAMPLES AND HIGH EXPECTATIONS

In an article in the March-May, 1984, issue of *Future Reflections,* Barbara Cheadle writes:

> We gave Chaz the cane and took him on some walks. He quickly learned how to use the cane to probe the area in front of him. With it he learned some general spatial concepts and such practical things as how deep curbs are and where you can expect them. We showed him how to use the cane and what it could do for him. However, he did not fully understand (as much as a two-year-old can understand, anyway) until he had some exposure to blind adults who use canes. What really made it click for him was spending a day with a blind couple. My husband and I had a day-long meeting to attend, so some friends of ours (the blind couple) offered to babysit our two sons. They played outside, took them for a ride in a wagon, and walked to an ice cream shop about five blocks away from their home. All the while, they used their long white canes. They did not give our son any formal instructions in its use (though I believe they answered some questions he had). The results, however, were dramatic. He obviously had a much better grasp of the cane's function and usefulness to him after that experience.

Watch for things which need to be changed as the child grows older – especially things which sighted children may pick up by watching. Zach, at six, was still going up and down stairs "baby fashion" by placing both feet on each step. When the cane travel teacher helped him learn the alternating pattern, Zach asked, "Does everybody do it that way?" It should be noted that he had quite a bit of useful sight.

From the beginning, help the child to take responsibility for the cane. Expect him to keep track of it and use it properly.

Teach Flexibility

Avoid simple memorization. Instead, emphasize real understanding of where a person is in relation to surroundings. When the child practices going from the first grade room to the rest room, avoid having the path exactly the same every time. Occasionally force him to walk on the other side of the hall. Practice when the area is crowded and when it is deserted. See that doors are sometimes open and sometimes closed.

Frequently analyze how a particular route relates to other locations or routes. Ask questions such as,

"If we turned left here, where would we be

going?"
"Are we closer to the rest room or to the principal's office?"
"How could we get outdoors from here?"

Practice "changing your mind"–e.g., proceeding part way to the principal's office and then going to the gym instead.

Help the student to develop an integrated mental map of everything he knows, rather than a set of self-contained, unrelated paths. An important example appears when a junior high student learns to follow his class schedule. He should also be able to walk from his first-period classroom to his last-period classroom *without* having to go to all the others in the usual sequence! The competent traveler goes wherever he wants, keeping oriented to his surroundings, rather than memorizing limited and self-contained routes.

WHAT IS THE REAL GOAL?

The goal should *not* be a "perfect" walk every time, without any hesitation or variation. For one thing, this would assume that there would never be any changes or obstructions in a familiar route. It assumes that no exploring should be necessary on an unfamiliar route. It assumes that the student will always have exactly the same stride. All of this is unrealistic. It also is unnecessary for efficient travel.

Instead, it *is* reasonable to expect the student to:

- Grasp the idea of the route (e.g., proceed east in the hallway, and enter the second door past the drinking fountain).
- Realize that there may be variations which do *not* necessarily mean he is in the wrong place (e.g., if he does not hear the refrigerated drinking fountain humming as usual, it may be turned off).
- Quickly recognize when he is really in the wrong place (e.g., he reaches the end of the hall or enters the wrong room).
- Figure out how to correct his path if necessary.

The goal should be to reach the destination with satisfactory speed and efficiency.

One way to get this across, and also to promote confidence, is to avoid calling deviations "errors." One ninth grader was very nervous about "mistakes" until her teacher started saying, "That was just a little detour. A detour is OK." Soon the student was saying cheerfully, "Well, I got here OK, with a little detour on Cherry Street."

Another student, Lindsay, was completely stymied when she found a large table (much too heavy for her to move) blocking the way to her bookshelf. Climbing over or under never occurred to her. When climbing under was finally suggested, she insisted it was impossible until the teacher helped her. See that your student practices climbing over, under, and around various obstacles from time to time.

A STRAIGHT LINE?

Help your student learn to walk in a reasonably straight line without constantly caning the wall, the curb, or some other edge.

There are, of course, times when it makes sense to keep caning the wall–chiefly when one is imminently searching for a particular doorway. Similarly, on the sidewalk there are times to cane the edge continually, as when searching for a driveway or a branch path. Also, a three-year-old beginner may need to keep in touch with the wall to understand that it is there.

However, one school of thought overemphasizes this (sometimes called "shorelining"), and encourages its routine use as the means for walking in a straight line. Actually, this is not a reliable method for maintaining a straight path. The wall may bend; the sidewalk may widen or disappear. The competent traveler realizes that following an edge is only one possible means for maintaining a straight path, and mainly relies upon walking speedily and consistently while keeping oriented to the environment. The sound of parallel traffic is a superb guide. Strenuously avoid teaching your student to cane the wall or the edge of the sidewalk, etc., with each and every arc. Instead teach him to move ahead and simply *notice* whenever he naturally encounters an edge or barrier. If he continually runs into the grass on his right, then he should keep a bit more to the left. If he bounces back and forth from one side to the other, he is correcting too much.

Another question arises in crossing an open area such as a playground. The blind traveler should not expect to walk "straight as an arrow" toward a precise point (say, the gate on the other side of the grassy play yard). Some correction should be expected. In this case, if the student reaches the fence and does not immediately find the gate, he should follow the fence for a few feet to the left or right, and then try the opposite direction if necessary. It *is* reasonable, however, for the blind traveler to learn to walk in a fairly straight line so that the correction is relatively minor. Walking quickly and confidently is important; the slow and hesitant traveler wobbles and has no clear direction.

Orientation to a New School Setting

When a sighted child enters a new schoolroom, he will look with his eyes to see where things are. The blind child needs to walk around and touch things, and this cannot easily be done while class is in session. Provide the child a chance to explore before school starts. Walk through typical routes while discussing such things as right and left turns. Help the child to examine things by touch, and to explore with his cane. As you walk along with a kindergartner, you might say, "Feel the rough brick on this wall.... Now, here's a sink; let's turn the water on and off once.... Here we go through a big door. Notice that your cane makes a different sound when it hits the door instead of the wall. Let's open and close the door. Look at this bar that opens it from the inside; it's a lot different from a doorknob, isn't it?.... Now, this wall feels smooth; it's made of plaster and it's painted green.... We're walking through a doorway and into the coat room. We'll walk along this wall and look at all these hooks. You and the other children will hang your coats on these hooks...."

As the older child moves on to a new grade, do not omit this. Besides knowing how to get around inside the new classroom, he should know the way to the bathroom and playground. Phase out help as follows:

(1) Show the child the route.

(2) Give continual guidance, as he tries it with less help.

(3) The child tries it alone, but someone is close by for guidance if needed. At this point, if there are difficult places, you may have much discussion of how to recognize and correct errors.

(4) The child goes alone, but someone watches unobtrusively at a distance.

(5) The child has no more supervision than is usual for his age.

If the path is easy and/or the child is experienced, he may be ready for step #5 after one lesson.

Special Problems

The above suggestions are not restricted to very young students. Many remarks in this chapter actually apply to various ages. Others apply to older students having difficulty because of multiple handicaps or other problems.

The chapter on "Multiple Handicaps" has many suggestions on adapting procedures for various handicaps, including some specific comments on mobility.

Don't sell your student short by saying, "He's not ready for cane travel," when you should have said, "He needs some modifications in the cane travel program."

SELECTED PROBLEMS AND SUGGESTIONS

Following are some comments (examples only, not exhaustive) on selected problems:

(1) Gait (the movement of the legs and feet) is uneven or inappropriate.
  - Emphasize even arcing.
  - Consult an Adaptive P.E. teacher or physical therapist if problem is severe.
  - Be sure student understands how well the cane explores the path ahead. He may

still be relying on one foot to find obstacles and step-downs.

(2) Overall posture is inappropriate.
-Discuss and demonstrate good posture.
-Sometimes have the student take hold of you as you walk briskly with him.
-If the problem is severe and continuing, consult a physical therapist or other specialist.

(3) When looking for something on the right side (assuming the cane is in the right hand), the student extends his entire arm out to the right, thus reaching a great distance and tripping others.
-This is one of the best reasons *not* to do as one school of thought advises: use a short cane and make the stiff, extended arm a part of the reach. Instead, insist that the student keep the forearm against his waist, centering his hand and using only hand and wrist movements to direct the cane. Then the arm cannot be flailed out to the side. Tell the student, "If you need to reach farther than your cane can reach, then turn and *walk* in that direction. People expect you to move forward, not sideways."

(4) The student is very fearful. (This may be general, or in certain situations such as stairs or streets).
-Don't expect too much too fast. If necessary, let the student hold onto you until he is accustomed to a new experience. Provide plenty of successful practice, often familiar, rather than too much variety. (At the same time, do not let progress remain at a standstill.)
-Have the student observe other blind travelers. This will help convince him that cane travel is practical and safe.
-Consider whether someone else is extremely fearful about the child's safety. Such fear "rubs off" on the child.
-Realize that sometimes behavior which looks like fear is actually an attempt to manipulate others. Kindly firmness may be necessary.
-Consider whether something unrelated (e.g., serious illness in the family) may be bothering the student and showing up as fear during lessons.

(5) The student objects to the cane, or continually loses/forgets it.
-If he leaves the cane at home, consider providing another at school.
-Mainly, however, work on the cause of the problem. Probably he does not appreciate the value of the cane. His family and other adults may see the cane as a stigma rather than a tool for independence. Through contacts with other blind people and by general attitude development, help everyone realize that the cane is respectable and helpful.
-Also, valued privileges should be conditioned upon having the cane ready.

(6) The student continually gropes with his free hand instead of finding things with the cane.
-See suggestions above for teaching the very young child how to interpret what the cane tells him. Consider using both hands on the cane. An older student should carry something in the free hand.

(7) The student runs right into things even when the cane has already contacted them.
-Isolate the task of *detecting* the object. For example, sometimes have the child stop dead whenever the cane touches an obstacle. You might say, "Walk through the park here. When your cane finds something in your way, you must freeze *before* you touch it with any part of your body, and count out loud. That is, say 'one' for the first time you do this, and then go around the thing and find something else. Then say 'two' for the second thing you find, and so on. When you have found eight different things, we will go swing on the swing." (A young child will need to have this explained and demonstrated more than once, but should be able to understand.)
-A child may want to touch and explore the object. In this sense, he may be rewarded by *not* responding to the cane's

warning. You may decide to forbid him to pause and examine the object unless he first finds it with the cane in a controlled way. (Note: Be sure to see that there *are* some times when he is encouraged to examine objects.)

(8) The student gets lost easily and cannot seem to re-orient himself.
-See the above suggestions on teaching flexibility rather than mere memorization. Also extend the length of time before help is provided. Sometimes interrupt with a deliberate "distraction" (e.g., pull the student out of the way of an imaginary janitor's cart, and face him in an indeterminate direction) and expect him to recover. Gradually make distractions more challenging.
-See also the above suggestions for orienting a student to a new classroom and phasing out help gradually.

(9) The student seems to pay no attention to his surroundings. He does not notice landmarks. He does not use sounds well.
-Be sure that hearing has been checked.
-For generally poor attention to surroundings, consider whether too much help is being provided, and/or too little reward for taking responsibility. Practice in varied and interesting surroundings.

(10) The student adds extra motions, such as swinging the head or waving the free hand.
-See suggestions on "gait" and "overall posture," above. Also see "Fitting In Socially" for ideas on overcoming mannerisms.

(11) Although the student can use the cane well when reminded, his technique is usually very sloppy.
-Consider the child's age and experience, and be careful not to expect too much. But if the student is unreasonably careless during lessons, structure them to reward good technique in creative ways. If he is careless outside of lessons, ask others to remind him. If technique is so poor as to amount to non-use, it may be approached as described for students who "lose" the cane.
-See also the chapter on "Motivation."
-Do not expect to achieve uniformly good technique instantly. Gradually increase the amount of time during which you require it.

CHAPTER 25

THE LAW

THE IEP

AND THE BLIND CHILD'S EDUCATION

Until relatively recently, a school system had almost total discretion regarding placement of handicapped students. Many children were simply excluded. When a child with a disability did attend public school, often it was with little or no suitable provision for dealing with the disability.

Public Law 94-142, the *Education for All Handicapped Children Act* of 1975, as amended, has brought vast changes in this respect for all public schools in the United States. It provides a system by which states can get Federal funds to provide appropriate opportunities for handicapped children.

This law is often called the "mainstreaming" law, and has in many cases helped to place a handicapped child in the regular educational "stream" when he/she might not have been otherwise. However, the common belief that this law flatly requires *all* handicapped children to be placed in regular classes is not correct. (The word "mainstreaming" does not even appear in the law.) Rather, a formal written agreement, signed by the parent and the school, is required by law and sets forth in detail the arrangements for the education of a particular handicapped student. The agreement is called the "Individualized Education Plan," (IEP), and the process for developing it is described in this chapter.

Two closely related laws – P.L. 99-457 (dealing with very young children) and "Section 504" of the Civil Rights Act – are discussed near the end of this chapter.

This chapter does *not*, however, purport to analyze the law in complete detail. Every educator should study the law continually, as changes are constantly being made both in the laws themselves and in the regulations which put them into practice. Local policies, also, can make a great difference in how a law is applied.

Every educator should keep well-informed for another reason also: to influence the development and revision of legislation and policy, for optimum education for blind students.

Public Law 94-142

A FREE, APPROPRIATE EDUCATION

A free, appropriate education must be made available to *all* handicapped children. In the past, a school district could simply declare a student "not eligible" and disclaim all responsibility. This is no longer the case; and even if there is an agreement to place the student in a special school outside the district, the home district still retains responsibility for appropriateness of program.

This applies to ages 3-21, with strong incentives to provide programs for children under 3 also.

It is possible for a state to decline to comply with P.L. 94-142; however substantial Federal funds will be withheld.

Non-Public Schools

If the formal agreement involves placing a child in a location other than his/her own regular public school, because the parties agreed that this is the best placement for the child, this must be done at no cost to the parent. The home district retains responsibility for the student, and is expected to follow his/her progress by participating in annual reviews. The home district also must pay expenses such as tuition and transportation. All of this is true whether the IEP provides that the student will be sent to another school in the same district, to another district, to a state residential school, or to a private school. The placement may even be in another state.

Generally, a "parochial school" is defined as one having a religious orientation, while a "private school" is not a religious school. Generally, tuition from public funds may not be paid to a parochial school; however it may be paid to a private school if the IEP so provides. When a private school receives tuition under an IEP, or receives Federal funds in any other way, it is bound by the rules of P.L. 94-142. Otherwise, private and parochial schools are not necessarily bound by this law.

If a parent places the child in a private or parochial school (or in another district) because of personal preference, the home district would not necessarily have the responsibility for paying expenses. State laws, which vary considerably, affect the amount of responsibility retained by the local public school in such instances. Often the public school must still provide such things as diagnostic services, consultation, and special materials. Typically it is possible for an itinerant or resource teacher of the blind to serve a private or parochial school student at a "neutral" location. For example, the itinerant teacher might meet the student in the public library across the street from the parochial school. As another example, the student might come to the resource room in the public school for an hour a day, and work in his own school the rest of the day.

Provisions for serving private and parochial schools vary from state to state. Always the public school would be expected to assume its complete mandated responsibility under P.L. 94-142 in the event that the parent decided to transfer the child back to public school.

LEAST RESTRICTIVE ENVIRONMENT

Handicapped children are to be educated in the "least restrictive environment" appropriate for each student. This important phrase means that, *to the maximum extent appropriate,* handicapped children must be in a normal setting with non-handicapped children, in the same school they would attend if not handicapped. Students are to be placed in separate classes or schools only when the separate arrangements afford the least restrictive means to provide an appropriate program that meets the child's needs.

This does not mean that all handicapped children must be placed in regular classes. It does mean that there must be a good reason for special placement. All placement decisions must be made on an *individual* basis. The IEP process determines what is deemed "appropriate" for each particular student at that particular time. Reviews held annually (if not sooner) may adjust program placement.

A common belief holds that, if P.L. 94-142 has not served a particular student well, it is because the child was set apart too much from the "regular" environment. However, with blind children in recent years, the opposite has more often been true: the student has been left in regular classes without being taught the techniques needed for success. Too often, students have been given magnification devices and expected to read print (however slowly and laboriously) when instead they should have been taught Braille. Too often, students have shuffled their way around, or depended on sighted guides, when they should have been taught cane travel. Too often they have fended for themselves in an environment where no one knows anything about blindness, appropriate techniques, or overcoming poor attitudes and wrong ideas. Blind students should receive the specialized programming required by their specific needs, instead of having "mainstreaming" in and of itself overemphasized.

A Misinterpretation

A number of people, including some educators of the visually impaired, tend to assume that "regular" materials and methods (e.g., inkprint) are categorically more appropriate than "special" materials and methods (e.g., Braille). This error persists even when students achieve below their ability solely because of methods and materials which are not suitable for their needs.

Transcribed materials, special equipment, and the lessons necessary for proper use, do "set the student apart" to a degree. But when special arrangements and materials enable the student to function *normally* instead of at a disadvantage, they are part of the Least Restrictive Environment for that individual.

The National Federation of the Blind is working to counteract misinterpretation of the "Least Restrictive Environment" concept.

Extracurricular Activities

Extracurricular and non-academic activities (when sponsored by the school) are included under the law.

PARENTS MUST BE INFORMED AND INCLUDED

When special education is first introduced for a given student, parental permission must be obtained for the initial evaluation and the initial placement. Thereafter, the school must notify the parents if there are plans for additional testing, if a change in placement is contemplated, or if termination of special services is being considered. The timing of the notice must allow parents sufficient time to respond and participate in decisions.

The intention of the law is that the parents be fully involved in deciding what is indicated by testing, and in deciding what special programming (if any) should be provided. It is a great temptation, however, for the evaluators to talk with one another (without the parent) and essentially decide what the programming should be. Too often the professional staff decide this among themselves, write up a detailed recommendation, and in effect say to the parent, "Sign this or else! This is what we know is best for your child!" Such an approach is condescending and in violation of the law. Each staff member may (and should) make recommendations about programming; but the parent has the right to participate in decisions. Every IEP conference should have more than one possible outcome.

ACCESS TO RECORDS

Parents have the right to examine all written records concerning their child, and to obtain copies at reasonable cost. The parent may ask questions and must receive a clear explanation (in the language used by the parent, even if that is not English). Should the parent disagree with any portion of the records, he/she may seek to have it removed or altered, and/or may place the parent's own comments in the official file.

Records may also be accessed by a professional who is with the local school district and has a reason to see them in planning the child's program. If anyone else wishes to see the records, this can be done only with the parent's specific permission.

Personal notes written by one staff member solely for his/her own use are generally not considered "records" for this purpose.

THE IEP PROCESS

Parental Participation

If it appears that special services may be needed, a formal agreement must be reached between the parents and the school to determine the student's individual program. The parents must be included for direct participation, as must a representative of the school's administration and an educator having knowledge of the child. Parents must be given the opportunity to be present in all official meetings. They may bring any representatives they wish, although the representative may have limited participation unless authorized to act for the parent.

If the student is 18 or over, the rights and responsibilities under the law fall upon the student. Throughout this description of the IEP procedure, it should be assumed that the term "parent" refers instead to the student if he/she is 18 or over. It should also be assumed that the term "parent" may refer to a legal guardian who is not the natural parent, or to a surrogate parent authorized to act for the parent in educational planning.

Many additional persons may take part in an IEP meeting, depending on circumstances – the student (even if under 18); classroom teachers; administrators; counselors; various individuals who have done testing and evaluation; representatives of a regional, intermediate, or state educational unit; etc. Parents have the right to know in advance who will be present.

What Is the IEP?

The formal written agreement is called the "Individualized Education Plan" (IEP). (Note: The "P" in "IEP" is also often considered to stand for "Program." Frequently the written description is called the "Individualized Education Plan," while putting it into practice is called the "Individualized Education Program.")

The IEP sets out in detail:

- the child's present level of performance
- educational goals
- objective evaluative criteria for determining whether goals are being met
- a description of the special education and related services to be provided
- the extent to which the student will participate in regular programs
- expected duration of services

Both long- and short-term plans must be agreed upon in writing. They must be updated at least annually, and oftener upon request.

The IEP applies only to the special arrangements or modifications for the individual student. It does *not* set a curriculum for the class as a whole (although it does state the extent to which the student will participate in the regular curriculum).

Writing and implementing the IEP is a dynamic and ongoing matter, both in regard to curriculum detail and in regard to general placement. In a sense no placement is final, because it can always be changed by a meeting to draw up a new agreement.

The policy of "least restrictive environment" prevents arbitrarily providing a more specialized setting than is really needed. It also means that the student must not be kept in a specialized setting which he/she no longer needs. For example, if a blind first grader needs three hours daily from a resource teacher in order that he/she may learn Braille well, this individual help should decrease as the child grows older and more independent. Similarly, if a young child is sent to a special school, as he/she grows older it may become possible for him or her to succeed in the regular public school (with individual help there as appropriate). At the same time, it is important to realize that a change to a more restrictive setting, with *more* special help, is sometimes the best solution to an educational problem.

The IEP requires educators to provide the services as described, until a new IEP is agreed upon and signed. It does not, however, guarantee that the child will actually attain the goals described.

Consider the example of an IEP which says that a kindergartner shall have "instruction from the itinerant teacher of the visually impaired 5 hours per week." Assume also that a goal for this child is to learn to "read and write the Braille alphabet." If the itinerant teacher does *not* in fact work with the child for 5 hours per week, a violation has occurred. However, if the teacher *does* work with the child for the indicated amount of time, and the child nevertheless learns only ten letters, there is no violation. (This assumes that the teacher's time was spent on instruction related to learning the Braille alphabet. It also assumes that if there are other goals (e.g., cane travel), the teacher's total time was allotted in the manner agreed upon. Sometimes there is a dispute over whether the teacher's time was spent appropriately as directed by the IEP. Such a dispute would be relevant to the question of whether a violation had occurred.)

Evaluation of Current Level of Performance

As a basis for planning the IEP, the child's present level of performance must be evaluated and described objectively. This is accomplished through medical reports, formal and informal observations of behavior, school reports, academic testing, and testing by specialists in various fields (e.g., a speech therapist).

This subject is explored further in the chapters, "Testing and Evaluation" and "Assessment Of Functional Vision For Reading."

Testing and Evaluation

A free, complete, and individualized evaluation must be provided as a basis for planning the IEP. Tests must be administered by trained personnel using standardized procedures that reflect the child's aptitude and achievement. No single test, and no single person giving tests, may be used as the sole criterion for a placement decision. Testing must be in the child's native language and not culturally discriminatory.

A comprehensive, multi-disciplinary re-evaluation must be conducted at least every three years.

An Independent Evaluation

If the parent desires, he/she must be informed how to obtain an independent evaluation (that is, an evaluation by an "outside" party separate from the local school district). Under certain circumstances the local school must pay the cost of such an evaluation. In any event, the parent may have the results of an independent evaluation entered into the records and considered in the IEP process.

Goals and Objectives

Educational goals must be stated in both long-term form (applicable for at least one year) and short-term form.

Examples of *long-term goals* include:

- Learn to read and write Braille
- Broaden cane travel skills
- Build arithmetic skills
- Improve self-help skills

Short-Term Objectives: Let us assume that the long-term goals above have been written for a first grader. Following is an example of a short-term objective for each respective long-term goal [with the long-term goal given in brackets]. (Note, however, that actually several short-term objectives would probably be written for each. The teacher would then proceed through each set of short-term objectives in reasonable sequence, according to a timetable stated or implied).

- [Learn to read and write Braille] Write the entire alphabet (both upper and lower case) on the Perkins Brailler.
- [Broaden cane travel skills] Cross a lightly-traveled street independently.
- [Build arithmetic skills] Set numbers 1-30 on the abacus.
- [Improve self-help skills] Put on coat, hat, boots, and mittens, with help required not more than once a day on the average.

Note that goals and objectives are written in terms of what the *student* will do, not what the instructor will do.

Objectives may specify precisely what materials will be used (e.g., *Patterns* Preprimers). The date by which the objective should be reached may also be specified.

Long-term goals may be rather general. Short-term objectives must be specific and measurable.

Objectives for Abstract Goals: Even things which may seem abstract can often be written down and measured. Suppose, for example, that a seventh grader reads Braille well but resists ever using tapes or live readers. Suppose also that, despite being a good student, she is very shy, and she seems to believe that she never will be able to hold a good job. The following goals and objectives might be agreed upon:

GOAL: Increase flexibility in modes of reading.

Objective: The student will state at least two advantages and disadvantages in using each of these modes of reading: Braille, recordings, reading machines, and live readers.

GOAL: Increase social contact and assertiveness.

Objective: The student will initiate conversation with someone else at least three times daily. At least one of these contacts must be with another student.

GOAL: Recognize that blind people succeed in a variety of regular occupations.

Objective: The student will name at least five blind persons who are successful in regular full-time work outside the home, and describe methods used by each.

Criteria for Meeting Goals: Long-term goals may be rather general, while short-term goals must be specific and *measurable.* The short-term objectives serve as criteria for whether long-term goals are being met. In addition, whenever the IEP is reviewed, various other kinds of evaluations are included in the process. For example, with a three-year-old, a developmental checklist might be presented. With a tenth-grader, school grades would be considered.

Every three years the student must be thoroughly re-evaluated to re-determine disabilities, abilities, and program needs. The evaluation should be comparable to that done as an initial evaluation. This is to ensure that the child is not retained in a special situation beyond the need, nor denied help for a problem which may have arisen or worsened.

Special Education Services

The service model – that is, the general outline of how the special services are to be provided – must be written carefully into the IEP. Time allotment must be specified.

The chapter on "Placement Options and Decisions" describes in detail several common models of service to visually impaired students – residential school, special day school, special class, resource room, itinerant teacher, and teacher aide. If individual help from an aide is to be provided, this too is part of the service model, and the amount of time must be spelled out. Many other models, and combinations involving these, are also possible.

The law requires that a continuum of services be made available, rather than only a rigid set of discrete choices. It is particularly inappropriate for educators to say, "We will provide this program because this is what we have available." Instead, individualized arrangements and modifications must be made as necessary, based on the *needs of the student.* Similarly, it is inappropriate to misquote the law and make total "mainstreaming" the unqualified criterion for desirability of programming. Blind students do need some specialized services – particularly Braille and cane travel lessons – which usually are best provided individually or in a special group. Specialized lessons prepare the student so that he/she can then use the skill in a regular setting.

Related Services

P.L. 94-142 gives the following definitions in Section 602:

> (16) The term 'special education' means specially designed instruction, at no cost to parents or guardians, to meet the unique needs of a handicapped child, including classroom instruction, instruction in

physical education, home instruction, and instruction in hospitals and institutions.

(17) The term 'related services' means transportation, and such developmental, corrective, and other supportive services (including speech pathology and audiology, psychological services, physical and occupational therapy, recreation, and medical and counseling services, except that such medical services shall be for diagnostic and evaluation purposes only) as may be required to assist a handicapped child to benefit from special education, and includes the early identification and assessment of handicapping conditions in children.

Sometimes it is hard to determine whether something is a "Related Service" or a "Special Education Service." It is even possible that a given educator may provide each of these at different times.

However, the distinction between Related Services and Special Services is not the major concern. More relevant is the following distinction: Special Education Services and Related Services, both of which *are* provided by educational agencies, *vs.* medical services which are not provided by the educational agency.

Time In Regular Classes

The IEP must also spell out the amount of time spent with the regular class (if any). Ordinarily a blind student in public or private school, even when just starting to learn Braille, will spend at least part time in a regular class.

If a first grader is having individualized reading and math, the IEP might say, "all regular classes except reading and arithmetic," or it might name the specific classes to be attended. If a ninth grader receives individual help during study hall and after school, it is necessary to add "attend all regular classes."

The student must have the opportunity to participate in all activities that the school provides to other students, using special services assistance only to the extent specified by the IEP as necessary.

Duration Of Services

"Duration of services" estimates how many years (or months) it is expected that special services will continue to be provided with the same general arrangements. This estimate can be revised at any review of the program.

Due Process

When parents disagree with the school staff's proposals or performance, and the disagreement is not resolved in IEP conferences, P.L. 94-142 provides for an impartial Due Process hearing. Mediation may be available to try to resolve differences and/or clarify issues, and attempt to prevent the need for a hearing. Civil court action may occur as a last resort if a party wishes to carry the matter further after a hearing. However, Due Process administrative reviews (mediation, hearings, etc.) ordinarily will be attempted before court action may occur.

The article, "Lessening the Trauma of Due Process," by Patricia Edmister and Richard E. Ekstrand, appeared in the Spring, 1987, issue of *Teaching Exceptional Children*. This helpful article describes in detail how an educator should prepare for a possible hearing, and conduct himself/herself if called upon to testify.

Every educator should keep the possibility of a hearing in the back of his/her mind at all times. Sometimes Due Process is necessary in order to determine the best course of action in meeting the needs of the child. Meeting the needs of the child is, after all, the primary goal of both parent and educator; but honest people can have honest differences.

Keep informed of local policies. Consult your supervisor immediately if you have reason to believe that a hearing might transpire.

Preventing the need for a hearing: Keep records current and appropriate even when it is tedious. Listen to parents and respect their opinions. Be rigorous about providing the services mandated by each IEP. Do not add any significant course of instruction without its being approved in the IEP meeting.

If it appears that you will not be able to provide the services as required, or that they are really not appropriate, call for a review and work on changing the IEP. Do the same if someone seems to be interfering with your performing your duties. An excessive delay in providing services is a violation.

One itinerant teacher made many attempts to set up a schedule for Keith's Braille lessons. At first the principal told her, "Our schedule is not finalized yet. We're not ready for you to start." Other excuses followed, and the principal asked her not to come to the building at all. Early in October she wrote the principal a letter (carefully dated, with copies to her supervisor and the parent), to document the fact that she was attempting to carry out her assignment. In November her supervisor helped her insist on a meeting to review the IEP. As the situation unfolded, it appeared that Keith's parents had changed their minds about Braille, but neither they nor the principal had wanted to face the issue and change the IEP. It was very important for the teacher to protect herself against possible accusations of undue delay in providing services (a violation).

Differing Terminology

P.L. 94-142 speaks of the Individualized Education Program (or Plan) as the entire plan, especially the written plan. The IEP encompasses the following:

- Evaluation, determination of need, and selection of resolutions
- The service model (e.g., resource room)
- Related Services
- The amount of time each service will be provided
- Long-term goals
- Short-term objectives
- Amount of time to be spent in regular classes
- All revisions (periodic, annual, or three-year)

Local usage, however, varies in regard to what is commonly called the "IEP" and what transpires at an "IEP meeting." In one district, for example, a conference to decide upon the service model is called a "Staffing;" the general review which occurs at least once a year is called a "Program Review;" and the short-term objectives are discussed at an "IEP meeting." Parents and educators in this district often fail to realize that actually the IEP is the entire formal plan, rather than just one part such as the short-term objectives.

Examples Where An IEP May Not Be Written

If no services are required: When a child has a slight visual impairment, sometimes it is decided that no special services are needed at the time. It is wise to keep in touch with such a child, since the visual condition may change.

Private arrangements: Another reason why an IEP may not be written is that arrangements may be made privately or informally. When the Redlens realized that their son John should be learning Braille, they did not wish to transfer him from their religiously-oriented school to the public school. One alternative would have been for John to spend part of the day at a public location for Braille lessons. However, the Redlens sought out a different arrangement. They hired a retired teacher of blind adults to work with Johnny at their expense, at the parochial school. Thus they chose not to go through the IEP procedure at all. Some parochial schools regularly provide special help.

Sometimes private arrangements are made to supplement the work of a *public* school. This should be written up in IEP form (even if virtually nothing special is to be done by the public school itself) to protect all parties. "Integration into regular program" should be specified.

Resolving Disagreements

Sometimes one party (either the parent or the school) asks that special services be provided, and the other party says they are unnecessary. This is a matter for resolution through the IEP procedure, and one of the following should result:

- By mutual agreement, it is decided that services are not needed at this time.

- It is agreed that services *are* needed and will be provided.
- If the school suggests services but the parent declines, this is documented.
- If agreement cannot be reached, steps begin toward a Due Process hearing.

Note that one alternative is missing from this list: "The parent wishes to have services but the school declines." If the parent comes to agree that it is appropriate to have no special services, then one of the other options has occurred. If the parent really wants services and the school refuses, this is a matter for Due Process.

The Law Extended to Very Young Children

A particularly important extension of P.L. 94-142 has occurred with the *Education of the Handicapped Act Amendments of 1986* (P.L. 99-457). This legislation relates to children under six.

As of 1991, if a state does not provide a free, appropriate public education for all handicapped children ages 3-5, that state may not count its 3-5-year-old handicapped children for P.L. 94-142 funds. Such a state will also lose its eligibility for certain preschool grants.

Also, a new provision (Section 672 of P.L. 99-457) strongly encourages making early intervention services available to children from birth through age two.

Following is a quotation from a summary outline by the federal Office of Special Education:

> Handicapped infants and toddlers ages birth through two years are eligible for early intervention services as currently defined in the law if:
>
> (1) They are experiencing developmental delays.
>
> (2) They have a physical or mental condition that may result in a developmental delay.
>
> (3) They qualify, according to a state definition, as being 'at risk of having substantial developmental delay.'[1]

This phrasing tends to provoke discussion about what constitutes "a high probability of resulting in developmental delay." In regard to blind infants and toddlers, this produces a kind of "Catch-22" situation. For a child to be eligible for services, it must be shown that the fact of visual impairment "has a high probability of resulting in developmental delay." However, intervention service, if well done, helps to assure that blind children are *not* necessarily behind developmentally. Furthermore, many well-informed and positive parents, without formal professional assistance, have guided young blind children through normal development. If a given child does experience developmental delay, often it is not obvious for several months or years. Furthermore, in the case of children so young it is often hard to assess just how much the child sees. Other abilities (particularly intelligence) can be very hard to judge. For all of these reasons, visual impairment should be included in a list of conditions that *automatically* guarantee eligibility for early intervention services.

Note that this new provision does not actually require services to children ages 0-2 in the same way that they are required for those 3 and over.

Other Laws

"SECTION 504"

Other laws complement P.L. 94-142. Especially relevant is Section 504 of the *Rehabilitation Act of 1973* as amended, with its accompanying regulations. This declares that agencies receiving Federal funds must not discriminate solely on the basis of a handicap, and are required to make "reasonable accommodation" for a handicapped individual. School districts receive Federal funds. So do some preschools,

---

[1]Alana M. Zambone, Ph.D., Barbara McCarry, and Alan Dinsmore. "Your Response Is Needed: Early Childhood, P.L. 99-457." *DVH Quarterly*, June, 1987.

notably Headstart.

If a school, for example, excluded a student from science classes solely because he/she was blind, this would be unlawful discrimination. If the class admitted the student but refused to allow any alternative methods in using a microscope (such as learning to describe verbally the important features of each item studied), this would be a failure to make "reasonable accommodation." The analysis of what is "reasonable" takes into account such factors as the money, time, and effort which must be expended in order to provide the arrangement. Also, an exclusion is not considered "discrimination" if it is based on genuine evidence that the handicap *per se* precludes the activity (e.g., a blind teenager is not allowed to drive a car). Note, however, that the agency bears the burden of proof that the exclusion is based on real evidence and not mere belief.

"Section 504" has many of the same provisions as P.L. 94-142. But remember that even if a situation is not covered under "Section 504," it probably is covered by P.L. 94-142.

THE "BUCKLEY AMENDMENT"

Teachers who began their careers prior to 1974 will remember that formerly parents (all parents, not just parents of handicapped children) could be denied access to records about their sons and daughters. Teacher comments, descriptions of misbehavior, etc., could be kept from parents. However, in 1974 the *Family Educational Rights and Privacy Act* (often called the "Buckley Amendment") provided that school records were to be open to parents, and to students 18 or over. Within certain guidelines, a parent (or student) is now permitted to review all teacher comments, and may also file his/her own written comments and/or insist that certain items be removed from the file.

P.L. 94-142 explicitly extends these types of provisions to handicapped children.

GENERAL EDUCATION AND THE LAW

Special education is a part of general education. Legal risks which affect classroom teachers apply also to special teachers, sometimes in a concentrated fashion.

Permission for Excursions or Publicity

If the first grade goes on a field trip to the zoo, every child must have a signed permission paper from the parent or guardian. Without this, the teacher (and his/her superiors) would be extremely vulnerable in case of an injury or problem on the trip.

Special teachers must apply this rule rigorously also. Avoid the temptation to think, "This is just very informal," or "We are not going far," or "His mother said OK on the phone." If you are taking the student beyond the schoolyard, you should have written permission. Spell out transportation, or state that you will walk. For a series of outings, arrange permission describing the kinds of activities and the locations, at least in a general way. Indicate whether the teacher will stay right with the student, follow at a distance, or send the student alone on independent activities. Have an updated permission form signed each year.

Written permission is also required if the child's name or photograph will be used in any way other than within the school's educational program.

Preventing the Appearance of Misconduct

Sad to say, even a kind and helpful teacher may be accused of sinister motives. Protect yourself by maintaining a dignified demeanor, and by working at times and places which are obviously appropriate. If you work in the student's home, avoid going there when no other adult is present, especially if you are a man. At school try to avoid lengthy sessions behind a closed door and without windows.

Physical contact is necessary in showing blind students how to do things. Also, it can be appropriate to hug a three-year-old child, or to touch an older student on the shoulder to show approval. But watch yourself, especially if you tend toward displays of physical affection–you could be misinterpreted. It is also possible to belittle a student with gestures which are commonly used with younger children – e.g., patting a short seventh-grader on the head.

Teachers should be well-informed also in regard to physical discipline or restraint, including "time-out" procedures with young children. Check local guidelines.

Personal Influence

Despite the First Amendment, there are limitations to what a teacher may say on the job. Religion is a good example. It can be difficult to draw the line with a blind student, since it *is* appropriate to help the family locate religious materials in transcribed form if desired (without public-school funds being used to obtain them).

Ask the *parents* if they would like to have any religious materials (e.g., Sunday School papers in Braille). Rather than making the arrangements yourself, tell the parents how they can get in touch with a suitable transcribing service. Although it may be desirable (with parent approval) to talk briefly with students about obtaining religious materials, be careful not to seem to urge anyone to do anything of a religious nature.

Additional Information

The chapters on "Placement Options and Decisions" and "Paperwork" extend this discussion of the law and the IEP. "Working In Partnership With Parents" is closely related also.

A complete copy of each applicable law, with its accompanying regulations, may be obtained from your U.S. Senator or Representative or from:

Assistant Secretary For
Special Education and Rehabilitation
Room 3006
Mary E. Switzer Bldg.
330 C Street SW
Washington, DC 20202

The "References" section at the end of this book gives sources of further information. The following were used as sources for this chapter:

- P.L. 94-142
- P.L. 99-457
- Coalition In Oregon for Parent Education, *Parents Rights Card*
- "Lessening the Trauma of Due Process," by Patricia Edmister and Richard K. Ekstrand
- "Your Response Is Needed: Early Childhood, P.L. 99-457," by Alana M. Zambone, *et al.*
- Materials from Closer Look

CHAPTER 26

PLACEMENT OPTIONS AND DECISIONS

Putting P.L. 94-142 Into Practice

Chet struggled along for five years at the special school. "He still doesn't know the entire Braille code," complained his teachers. "He requires a lot of individual help. He's nowhere near ready for a regular school." Chet's parents, however, insisted on a transfer to public school. Chet was thrilled to be with his neighborhood friends, felt challenged by the regular classes, and worked diligently. Whereas Braille lessons had formerly been disliked, his new itinerant teacher emphasized speed and efficiency in a way that captured his attention. Three months after transferring, he easily passed a test on the entire Braille code. His grades in regular classes were above average.

Denise was in second grade at Northview Elementary. She was reading well in her individualized Braille lessons, and a transfer to the regular reading group was arranged. But the quantity and speed of work soon overwhelmed her. She not only stumbled over new words and signs, but even over those she had already learned. Soon a hurried conference was called, and Denise returned to individualized reading.

How can we decide what is best for any individual student? How do we know when the time has come to change placement?

Six Typical Options

The first five placement options below are listed from most restrictive to least restrictive. This is also the sequence in which, historically, they became available in this country.

Local custom may use names which differ from terms used here.

THE RESIDENTIAL SCHOOL

For many years the residential school, where students stay overnight, was the only option available for blind children.

Every aspect of the curriculum can be tailor-made for the particular students in attendance. Houseparents continue the students' training outside of school hours. With modern transportation, it is often possible to send students home every weekend. The disadvantages, of course, result from taking the child away from his home and the regular world. When the student leaves the residential school, it is a major adjustment.

THE SPECIAL DAY SCHOOL

Like the residential school, the special day school can tailor all lessons to individual needs. Since students do not stay overnight, they need not be separated from their families. However, there is little or no time spent in regular classes with non-handicapped children.

THE SPECIAL CLASS

Special classes often are located in regular schools. Typically, the students spend some of their time with non-handicapped students–perhaps only for things like recess and lunch, or perhaps for certain classes.

The *amount of time* spent in the special class distinguishes this option from the resource room, below.

THE RESOURCE ROOM

The resource room represents a major historical change in educational arrangements. Blind children are placed in a regular school, and spend the majority of their time in classes with non-handicapped students.

A "resource" teacher with special training spends a certain amount of time with each student (individually or in small groups) as directed by the student's IEP. The resource teacher helps by (1) direct instruction, especially in such skills as Braille and cane travel; (2) helping classroom teachers include the blind child in regular lessons; (3) providing transcribed books and other materials; (4) helping everyone to maintain positive attitudes; (5) providing extra help with lessons the child may not understand; and (6) "troubleshooting" any unforeseen problems.

Since one school is designated as the resource school for a given area, that building may not be the child's own neighborhood school.

THE ITINERANT TEACHER

Education with an "itinerant teacher" is similar to that with a "resource teacher," with one difference: the itinerant teacher travels around to several schools. This provides the child with the advantage of attending his own neighborhood school. It also brings a disadvantage in that the special teacher is available only at certain times, and usually has less time for a given student than would be the case in a resource program.

A PARAPROFESSIONAL (AIDE)

This option is ordinarily used in combination with one of the above options. In an itinerant program, usually the aide is assigned to one particular student, and provides individual attention when the itinerant teacher is not present. If there are several blind children in one building, an aide may work with various children.

A major portion of the aide's responsibilities usually is the preparation of materials.

The chapter on "Paraprofessionals and Volunteers" discusses this option in detail.

No Single "Ideal Placement"

A common misconception asserts that some placements are categorically "better" than others, in the abstract. The usual assertion is that the itinerant program is "ideal," the resource room is better than the special day school, etc.

This idea is false, because what is appropriate for one child is unsuitable for another. Furthermore, the concept of one particular "ideal" placement is an illusion even for one particular student. P.L. 94-142 recognizes this by using the term "appropriate" rather than the term "best." For any particular student, there would be a variety of ways to plan an appropriate education.

Special Schools Can Be Valuable

Is a special school for the blind–especially a residential school–*ever* a good placement? Certainly it is.

A STUDENT WITH PERSISTENT PROBLEMS

Jamie had struggled through grade school and junior high with much help from aides and remedial teachers. Teachers hated to give him an "F," but his achievement was below passing, and placement with the class for the mentally retarded did not seem appropriate. The itinerant teacher of the blind had worked diligently on Braille and cane travel skills, but continual reteaching was necessary. Jamie was older than his classmates but far less mature, and had no real friends. Virtually all his lessons were individualized.

His parents felt trapped in a worsening cycle of dependence. Jamie complained that his parents did too much for him; yet he resisted doing things for himself.

In ninth grade, Jamie transferred to the residential school. For him it was a great step toward independence. In a practical sense, the residential placement was actually "less restrictive" for Jamie, since tailor-made situations let him succeed with much less one-on-one help. Houseparents helped him learn living skills without the conflict his parents had. He soon had several friends whose maturity and interests were similar to his.

Jamie's problems were unusually great and had not responded to long-term strenuous efforts in his home community. For most students, a successful local placement *is* possible. But special placement should not be ruled out arbitrarily.

HIGH-ACHIEVING STUDENTS IN SPECIAL SCHOOLS

When a special school program (residential, special day school, resource, or other) has several blind students, those students can gain a great deal from being together. Any particular individual is less likely to be coddled. Each realizes that he/she is not the only blind student. *If* (and only if) proper attitudes are taught and demonstrated, the staff can more easily teach good techniques and attitudes to a group of blind students than to scattered individuals.

Unfortunately, today many special schools (especially residential schools) are almost entirely populated with the multiply handicapped and those with severe adjustment problems. This can make it difficult to challenge the average or superior student to work up to his/her capacity. It is especially difficult to challenge the student who is multiply handicapped or has special problems and is nevertheless capable of normal achievement; too often such a student is pressed into a stereotype of far-below-average expectations.

With proper arrangements, however–including the opportunity to attend some classes in a regular school–a special school can have a great deal to offer. Competent blind adults as role models can have close and continual contact with students. Positive attitudes can be taught, lived, and discussed in a variety of settings. Especially in a residential school, many things that parents may fail to arrange can readily be practiced–cane travel throughout the community, independent shopping trips, varied recreation, self-help skills, home chores, etc.

Ideas and challenges are passed on from one student to another. Camaraderie discourages the feeling of being "different" and "alone."

The value of the well-run special school is especially obvious in remote rural areas where specialized help is scarce; but it should be considered elsewhere also.

As with all placements, a special school may be right for some years and not for others. Many students attend a special school for a while until specialized skills have been well established. Others find the special school valuable at an older age when independence is increasing.

The quality of a school, however, depends on the beliefs and practices of the staff. Too many special schools actually discourage appropriate alternative techniques, and encourage low expectations. Often this is true in actions and policies, despite glowing words.

A Wide Spectrum of Services

VARIATIONS OF COMMON OPTIONS

Possible variations and overlaps in the above options are numerous. One student might be on the roll of the residential school, yet be extremely independent and attend most classes at a nearby public school. Another might be served by an itinerant teacher in his neighborhood school, yet have a much simplified curriculum due to special problems. Always the guiding principle should be, "What is appropriate for this student at this time?" Consider variations and combinations; be creative. Do not assume that certain settings are categorically "better" or "worse." It all depends on the individual. On the one hand, the burden of proof is on us to show why the student should not be in a regular setting with regular students. On the other hand, a more restrictive setting may provide needed help and actually let the student be more independent.

ADDITIONAL OPTIONS AND COMBINATIONS

Build a repertoire of options for enabling success in the neighborhood school.

Enhancing the Itinerant Option

Although the itinerant/resource teacher should take the main responsibility for direct teaching of specialized skills, often someone else can handle routine practice with those skills. And certainly someone else can work with things not specific to blindness, such as a general deficit in mathematics, weakness in general study skills, etc.

Most schools have staff who give individual help. They may be called remedial-reading teachers, multicategorical resource teachers, etc. (If the help desired is ordinarily outside that teacher's assignment, often it can be arranged anyway through a rule exception.)

Often the blind student's difficulties are really the same as those with which these teachers are accustomed to working. For example, although the itinerant teacher should teach the Nemeth Code as such, a remedial teacher can work on deficits in mathematics itself (just as a classroom teacher can include a blind student in a regular math class). The itinerant teacher should suggest methods for using Braille, tapes, readers, and visual aids. But a remedial teacher can help the student organize her belongings, take appropriate notes, study for tests, etc. (just as the classroom teachers can explain the regular assignments, make general recommendations about study, and so on).

Also, an aide may help a student with many kinds of things.

Often it is practical to have individual help from different people at different times.

Priorities for the Itinerant/Resource Teacher

One reason for the shortage of teachers of the visually impaired is inappropriate time usage. Too often, itinerant or resource teachers help students in situations where other staff could take over – multicategorical resource teachers, remedial teachers, paraprofessionals, etc., as just described. Another problem is time spent on things that are not really helpful and should not be taught – notably non-cane mobility (discussed in the chapters on cane travel) and "vision stimulation" (discussed in the chapter on "The Partially-Sighted Child." If these errors are avoided, the specialized teacher of the visually impaired can devote his/her time to the initial teaching of valuable skills which other teachers really do not know – Braille, cane travel, and other alternative techniques.

Continual Re-Evaluation

No placement should be considered final. Always expect progress and change. If the child is in a special school, perhaps today she can make friends in her home neighborhood and join a regular Scout troop. Perhaps next year she can attend one or more classes at a regular school. With preparation, probably someday she will be able to succeed in a regular school full time. Every teacher of the blind should constantly strive to "work himself out of a job," so the student will no longer need special help.

Grade and Classroom Placement

"Next year would be much better," said the principal firmly. "By that time we will be in the new building and we won't have to worry about stairs. I'm sure she'll be much better off if we just wait."

This child had no physical handicap and easily climbed stairs. She was five years old, bright and eager, and almost everyone agreed she was ready for regular kindergarten. But the principal kept asking, "Why can't she go to the school for the blind?" When he realized that the parents would not agree to that, he began pushing for a year's delay.

Upon insistence by the parents and the joint county school district, the child entered kindergarten and did well. In April, however, the principal said, "Surely we can't pass her on to first grade! Our curriculum is very demanding. The class is large. Why can't she go to the school for the blind? Or at least, let's keep her in kindergarten another year so she'll be better prepared for a full day of school."

This principal had one all-consuming thought: any excuse to avoid including a blind student. He disregarded evidence of past successes; denied that the child met the regular criteria for grade placement; ignored the concept of the least restrictive appropriate placement. Such blatant discrimination still occurs, although it is becoming less common. More subtle versions, however, still occur continually. Are blind students routinely tracked into the easier math classes? Are science labs avoided in favor of lecture courses? Is Adapted P.E. automatically arranged? All of these things should be individual matters.

EQUAL OPPORTUNITY

Grade placement should be on the same basis as for non-disabled students. If the youngster is of the appropriate age, and there is no clear and relevant reason for lower grade placement, then he/she should be in the usual grade. For the young beginner, readiness tests can be adapted, and other characteristics can be assessed in alternative ways. For the older child, academic achievement should be the main criterion.

There are two sides to the coin: sometimes equal opportunity directs that the child *should* repeat a grade. As always, ask the question, "What would be done if this child were not blind?" In the earliest grades, it is common for a child to repeat if he falls far behind but is believed have the capacity for satisfactory work. The blind child should have this chance also. Too often, a very weak student is passed on, with the unspoken assumption that a blind student could not be expected to do well. More subtle, and even more common, is the tendency to give so much individual attention that one cannot tell what the student can do on his own. Repeating a grade, under appropriate circumstances, is a *less* restrictive alternative than continued tutoring and simplified assignments. It can give the student the opportunity to compete normally the following year.

COMPARING INDIVIDUALIZED LESSONS

A special problem occurs when the child receives individual lessons which are hard to compare to the group lessons. This is discussed in detail in the chapter on teaching Braille. Use the same materials whenever possible, or ask a curriculum consultant to help with comparison. Minimize individualization as much as possible. Experiment with selected group lessons.

Be especially careful with grade placement during transfers to a much less restrictive setting. Standards for grade placement and achievement may be vastly different. The example of Allan's transfer from a "first grade" placement in a residential school, described later in this chapter, illustrates this.

STUDENTS WITH GENERAL ACADEMIC DIFFICULTY

There are some blind students, as well as some sighted students, who really do not have the intellectual capacity to handle the regular academic curriculum. They have great difficulty if asked to read advanced material independently, select main ideas, answer complex questions, etc.

Ask, "What would be done to help this student if she were sighted?" Often there are special classes for students who are mentally handicapped, for those who are learning disabled, etc. Look into this kind of placement even if it would require a rule exception. For the older student, vocational training is especially important, including on-the-job practice in the community. School classes should emphasize "survival" skills for realistic situations – income tax, budgeting, job application forms and interviews, etc.

Level of Achievement

If this student were not blind, what would be expected of him/her? The answer should be basically the same if the student is blind. Sometimes there is a *temporary* need for shortening or simplifying the general curriculum – chiefly while the student is learning a new specific skill such as Braille. In the long run, however, blindness in itself does not justify lowering the quantity or quality of expectations. The student should carry a normal load of classes, complete all work, etc., at the same level of difficulty where he would have been if he could see.

Sadly, blind students often do not achieve according to this standard, because (a) it is believed that they could not, and (b) they are not taught techniques to enable them to work efficiently. Inefficient techniques are discussed throughout this book. Some of the most widespread and serious are:

- Reading print slowly and laboriously, when Braille would be much faster.
- Tape-recording lectures instead of taking real notes in Braille.
- Weak typing skills, learned much too late.
- Cane travel taught too late and too little.
- Inadequate personal management skills.
- Lack of organization of possessions and study materials.

The only class in which a blind student really cannot participate fully is Drivers Education. And even there, he/she may audit the class for the theory portion.

It's Not a Perfect World

We live in an untidy world. Lack of money or personnel may interfere with a good plan; various parties may disagree on what constitutes a good plan. Be creative and keep looking for solutions. For example:

- Consider variations and combinations of the more obvious options.
- Look for summer programs which can supplement yours. Ask private agencies, the public agency which serves blind adults, etc. Residential schools often have summer programs which are appropriate even if the year-round setting is not.
- Watch for problems apart from vision.
- Look at the schedules of all service providers *together.* Be flexible in planning who will do what.
- Other chapters in this book, particularly "Scheduling," have many ideas.
- Explore cooperative arrangements with nearby school districts. Either the student or the teacher might travel.
- Consider an aide, volunteer, or part-time teacher.
- Look for new sources of funding, including private sources.
- Ask the residential school, the adult agency, the state department of education, etc., about consultation or itinerant service.
- Be innovative. Real integration of blind students is a new and still-developing field. You may think up an excellent idea that has never been used before.
- If disagreements among various parties are the problem, look for compromises and ways to help people "save face."
- Beware of the trap of planning for the convenience of the staff or administration. "This teacher has a full load already" is *not* an adequate excuse for ignoring P.L. 94-142.

Transitions

In the examples at the beginning of this chapter, why did Chet rise to the challenge of a regular class while Denise foundered?

A more gradual approach would have helped Denise greatly. Her teachers were so anxious for placement in a "regular" reading group that they moved her suddenly on an arbitrary date.

It is hard to make the procedures and pace of individualized lessons comparable to group lessons. However, even when a transition seems years away, we should work to prepare for it. Even when alone with the teacher, the student can take turns reading aloud; do worksheets independently; raise her hand; etc. The teacher can compare the progress of a reading group in comparable material, and set timelines. (Detailed suggestions appear in the chapters on teaching Braille.)

PLAN AHEAD AND COMMUNICATE

When a transition nears, provide some introductory experiences in the new situation or one similar to it. Look for "bugs" and work on them before making the complete transition.

Two different educators may speak the same words and yet seem to be on two different planets.

A Very Bad Transition

"Eldon is in all regular classes," said the principal of the city school. "Our resource teacher works with him only three hours a week now. And this year Eldon has learned to type. He should have no trouble in the suburban junior high."

Three weeks into the new school year, the suburban teachers tried to avoid bitterness. "Eldon says he never did *any* art before. He has no idea even how to make a ball out of clay."

"In science he can recite some of the information, but he doesn't really understand a bit of it. He just verbalizes. It's the same way in social studies."

"What was the matter with that resource teacher, saying he only needed three hours a week from her? He can't do *anything*. He can't hang up his coat...take notes...keep track of his papers...find his desk.... When he takes a drink, he gets water all over his shirt."

"And they said he could type. But he only knows the letter keys. And he can't put the paper in by himself."

"The only things he really can do well are reading and writing Braille. Oh, yes, and the music teacher says he sings beautifully."

Why Did This Happen?

Did the city school staff really believe that blind students could not participate in art? Did they think that basic concepts in science and social studies were too difficult? Did they believe there was no need to type numerals or punctuation, or insert the paper independently? Or were they ashamed to admit how little progress they had made with Eldon? Whatever it was, the suburban teachers were forced to conclude that reports from the city school were meaningless. (Note: Failing to document important problems with the curriculum, and failing to address these problems in the IEP, is in violation of P.L. 94-142.)

Possessiveness and egotism can affect anyone. Eldon's transition to the suburban district might have been easier a year or two earlier, when he would have had fewer teachers and less responsibility; but the city school wanted to keep him as long as possible. Chet's residential school teachers, their feelings colored by declining enrollment, had avoided placing Chet in trial classes at a nearby public school; thus they risked a difficult transition (although fortunately Chet did well anyway). Denise's teachers tended to see separation from the regular class as categorically bad, and subjected her to an abrupt transition.

Lack of information, also, can occur anywhere. The county itinerant teacher had believed her colleagues at the city school, since another student had transferred smoothly, and since she herself had not observed Eldon. The city teacher had never visited the suburban junior highs, and had little idea of what was really expected there.

PREPARING FOR A MAJOR CHANGE IN PLACEMENT

Moving To a Much Less Restrictive Placement

If planning is done carefully and all parties work together, a reasonably smooth transition can be accomplished even when there is a major change in placement. The greater the change, however, the more aspects there are to consider. (Avoiding any need for a major transition is one of the advantages of placing the child in the local school from the beginning.) Following are a few examples.

When the parents of Allan, who was totally blind, decided to transfer him to public school at midyear, the residential school staff said he was doing well in first grade. But as the public school analyzed Allan's skills, they learned he had a Braille reading vocabulary of just four words! He recognized only six letters of the alphabet. Unaccustomed to raising his hand, he shouted for the teacher when he wanted help.

At the residential school, all the other young students had very serious difficulties. Allan, with strong average ability, was far ahead of all the "kindergartners" and most of the "first graders;" therefore the residential school had actually moved him up a year ahead of his age group. But the public school expected much more than this level of skill, even at kindergarten entrance. After much discussion, it was decided that Allan would attend kindergarten in the mornings and receive special supplementary help in the afternoons.

With an older transfer student, the problem may be more subtle. The student may be working on grade level, but be accustomed to short assignments with much individual help. He may be unaccustomed to ordinary classroom procedures and to independent study. He may lack important skills such as note-taking or typing. A severe emotional jolt occurs when a student who has always been "outstanding" at the special school suddenly finds himself competing with many others of equal and greater ability.

One student insisted that he should be excused from the regular high school industrial arts requirement. At the residential school, he said, he had done many advanced projects. But when the public-school teacher offered to test him, it became apparent that he lacked many elementary skills. At the residential school he had always worked with someone else, with many things simplified.

Transition from a special school to a regular school can be quite traumatic. Careful planning and communication among all parties is very important. If at all possible, teachers from the new school should observe the student in his former setting, and talk with his teachers there. A strong support system–both academic and personal–should be provided in the new setting, with extra-careful troubleshooting for many months. Talk with other families who have recently completed such a transition, and with successful adults who can provide perspective.

Many smooth transitions do occur. The above examples are not meant to imply that all transfers from a residential school are fraught with difficulty.

Many residential school students follow a demanding curriculum which is very much the equal of the curriculum in a public school. Often a student who lives at the residential school actually attends some classes at a nearby regular school. In any event, careful planning and good communication can prevent most disasters.

Moving To a More Restrictive Placement

In a transfer to a *more* restrictive placement, it is less likely that the student will have serious problems. After all, more individual help will presumably be available. Watch carefully, however, to see that neither too much nor too little individual attention is added.

If the change is to a residential school, anticipate that the child may harbor many worries about living away from home. Assure the younger child that she may take along her favorite toys. Even with an older student, anticipate possible fears such as, "What if I feel sick in the middle of the night?"

If at all possible, get acquainted with some staff and students ahead of time. Visit classes and dormitories. Read the Student Handbook and talk about daily routine. Often the greatest problem is fear of the unknown.

Help the student and parents not to feel that the change to a more restrictive setting constitutes a "failure."

Maintaining Skills

DURING THE SUMMER

Most beginning readers tend to forget a great deal over the summer, but inkprint is seen everywhere and is never totally absent. A beginning Braille student may forget virtually everything; Braille may be totally absent from the environment if proper arrangements are not made.

Summer school programs are sometimes available – perhaps a special program, or perhaps a regular program which is appropriate for a given need.

Under some circumstances it is possible to mandate summer instruction in the IEP. Usually, however, it becomes a matter of searching creatively for ideas.

During the first two or three years of Braille instruction, plan very carefully for summer maintenance. Will the parents help if you send materials home? Might a community volunteer give some time? Could you or another paid staff member help for even a short time? Perhaps a combination can be worked out – e.g., the parents will help the child practice, and you will come to the home once in July. Even a few short practice sessions, spaced throughout the summer, can make an enormous difference to a beginner whose skills are very tenuous. Note that maintenance help of this nature, which involves skills already learned, can be done by almost anyone. An older brother or sister may be ideal. Be sure, however, that print copies of all materials are provided if the helper is sighted.

DURING THE SCHOOL YEAR

During the year, the itinerant or resource teacher must keep checking on skills "already taught." Especially if you are no longer in regular contact with the student, check on such things as typing, cane travel, Braille reading, and the Braille slate. Is the student really using his typing skills? Is he really using the Braille slate, or has he slipped into using a tape recorder, thus having no true notes? Does he really travel independently, or does he merely carry the cane and rely on sighted assistance?

Regular checking is vital to the maintenance of skills in your older students, but is neglected by many teachers in two opposite ways. It may be blithely assumed that the skill is being used, when in fact it is not. This can occur even when the student is seen daily in another context. In the opposite extreme, the resource/itinerant teacher may spend too much time working on artificial lessons when the skill should now be used in practical situations. Instead monitor, check, and assist as needed. At this stage, it becomes easier and easier to maintain a good program in a distant location where you cannot go often.

What Is the Real Problem?

MARCIE'S LOW GRADES

Marcie was failing all her classes. Her mother called the itinerant teacher and exclaimed, "Why haven't you been here? The principal says he hasn't seen you since October! We signed that paper to have you help Marcie in school, and what help are you? She's failing everything!"

"I'll see what I can do," responded the teacher. "Our written agreement specified that I would see her twice a year, and I have been doing that. But if more help is needed, I'll join you right now in looking into what we can do. Let's emphasize trying to figure out just *why* she is failing, because last October she was doing average work."

People often blame vision for every problem, and expect teachers of the visually impaired to solve all problems. (They may also expect them to do it without anyone's telling them the problems exist!) Marcie had 20/50 vision with a full visual field. Her eye condition was not degenerative. She could see most small print easily at normal reading distance, and only needed magnification occasionally. There was no problem of headaches, tired eyes, etc. She always sat where she could see the chalkboard easily.

The psychologist, however, found evidence of severe personal problems. Also, a physical checkup revealed severe anemia. With advice from the itinerant teacher, the school counselor and the nurse helped Marcie get the kind of help she needed.

DARYL'S SUDDEN "F"

Daryl, usually a good student, was failing tenth grade science. "We shouldn't have placed him in that lab course," said the counselor. "After all, he is totally blind." The itinerant teacher, however, believed that Daryl had the capacity to succeed. He found that Daryl had a poor grasp of how to make and interpret graphs; lacked scientific vocabulary; did not understand scientific measurement well; and was afraid of the gas jets. Individual help was arranged to strengthen the missing skills. Also, Daryl visited a blind scientist and discussed techniques. The gas jets were examined carefully at leisure. Within three weeks Daryl's grades were average and rising.

BE A DETECTIVE

Avoid blaming vision for a problem unless the evidence is clear. However, it may require detective work and considerable tact to sort out the causes. Blindness is commonly viewed as a great tragedy and the cause of all sorts of difficulties. Teachers are reluctant to admit that they are not expecting enough. Students and parents are embarrassed to recognize problems of a personal nature, and find it easier to blame vision.

It is especially tricky to distinguish problems of vision *per se* from a reading difficulty due to other causes. From time to time you may be urged to help students who are not really "visually impaired" (as we define it) at all. Be prepared to describe your local guidelines, and to explain that other disabilities and problems may appear to be a physical vision problem.

A seventh grader may have trouble adjusting to adolescence and to a large junior high. At the same time, it is possible that longer assignments and smaller print intensify a vision problem which had seemed slight. Again, look carefully for the real cause(s) of each problem.

Beware of a vicious circle in which a student has difficulty, the classroom teacher handles it poorly, the student has more difficulty, etc., and a more restrictive placement is sought. Try to prevent problems, nip them when they are small, and work assertively to help others do likewise. If a classroom teacher is doing a poor job, seek to change that – through administrative help and an IEP meeting if necessary – instead of immediately urging a change of placement.

AN UNNECESSARY BARRIER

There is one final category of "problems not truly due to blindness itself," which, sadly, may be the most common one of all. This is the problem of not teaching efficient alternative techniques, or teaching them poorly.

Too many blind students receive mediocre grades because they struggle with print instead of reading Braille rapidly. Too many are poorly adjusted because they have not learned independent travel and daily living skills, and have a generally low self-image. Too many have difficulty in lecture classes because they lack slate skills. Too many receive simplified or shortened assignments because teachers believe this is usually best. Don't sell your students short.

Related Chapters

Three chapters closely related to this one are "The Law, the IEP, and the Blind Child's Education," "Paperwork, Ouch" and "Early Childhood."

CHAPTER 27

PAPERWORK, OUCH

Putting P.L. 94-142 Into Practice

What Is Really Needed?

A common failing among resource and itinerant teachers is to keep far too many records in our heads. Remember, there are reasons why paperwork is kept.

I recently met an itinerant teacher who had no organized file or list of students – despite being responsible for 20 students scattered around a large school system. The legally required records were at the Administration Building, where access was limited. The itinerant teacher (whose office was not in the Administration Building) explained that she simply kept a few informal notes and remembered where the students were.

Classroom teachers always realize they might wake up with the flu and face the principal's wrath over lack of plans for the substitute. Specialized teachers get the flu too, but often there is no substitute teacher. Therefore we easily fall behind in the required records, and are tempted to keep no others. Remember that you too could face a major family emergency/ have a heart attack/ find your spouse has been transferred/ be hit by a wild driver. If one of these things happens to you, you won't want to spend a week creating better student records. Also, important details that you thought were etched firmly into your brain may simply be forgotten – especially over the summer. Keep up on the paperwork which your employer expects of you, and when necessary supplement it so that the basic facts on each student are always available.

Besides the possibility of sudden personal absence, there is another urgent reason for good written records. You too could learn that the parents of one of your students have requested a hearing, asserting that you have behaved inappropriately. In this case there is probably no way to hurry around and write up what is needed, because the necessary records should have been dated and approved long ago. Backdating would be fraudulent and make things still worse.

VITAL INFORMATION

Your employer should provide for at least the following records, constituting the IEP and various other legal obligations:

(1) Each student's full name, birth date, address, telephone, school, school district, and names of parent(s) or guardian(s). (The resident school district may be different from the district attended.)

(2) Up-to-date statements from eye doctors

(3) Other medical records, when relevant

(4) Parent permission for evaluation

(5) Copies of recommendations from multidisciplinary team members

(6) Lists of transcribed books or specialized materials recommended

(7) Records of all evaluations relevant to the decision

(8) Each student's IEP:
- Current level of performance
- Long-term educational goals
- Short-term educational goals
- Special education and related services to be provided
- Extent of participation in regular programs
- Expected duration of services
- Specific educational objectives, putting the goals into practice

TOO MANY FORMS

Probably you will sometimes feel that your employer requires too many forms and too much detail. When this is a serious problem, work with your colleagues, your supervisors, and your teachers' organization to streamline procedures and cut out nonessentials. Simply to omit paperwork which has been assigned to you, however, is to court various disasters.

Characteristics of Good Records

Maintain objectivity in written records. It's so easy to slip into personal comments and opinions. As a Rehabilitation Supervisor once put it, "Paperwork is not designed to be a record of your feelings – it is designed to be a record of events."

Remember that records are open to parents. Avoid writing vague or judgmental remarks such as, "Billy never finishes anything." Instead be specific and objective, as, "During the month of March, Billy has completed an average of 30% of his math problems. Accuracy is satisfactory, but he does not do all of the problems. A checklist of assignments is being kept for the IEP meeting."

Particularly avoid speculation without documentation. If you do speculate in writing, give specific reasons. Also try to find out how the situation actually does turn out, and then write that down too.

Often what may seem like a minor incident will later be very helpful in planning. When Jerry was ill on a seemingly random basis, a careful record compared to his class schedule revealed that he missed days when his gym class was working on sports he disliked.

There are some items so touchy and subjective that it is best not to write them down even in the most informal summary.

RECORDS READILY AT HAND

If you work in a single building, you may be fortunate enough to have all the original records handy. Many itinerant teachers, however, travel considerable distances and rarely are in their "home office." Besides making sure that required records are in the place designated by your employer, arrange also to keep working files with you – copies of any file information needed in your day-to-day work, and also essential notes. (Be careful to avoid having confidential records in an exposed location.)

For example, I travel to several towns up to 80 miles away. Each school has copies of the IEP for its particular student(s), and another copy is filed at our agency's office for that county. In addition, our department keeps a file of the basic information about each student. However, since sometimes I only go to our main office once a week, I often find myself in (for example) Longview District while making a phone call or doing paperwork related to a student elsewhere. Therefore I need to carry some records with me.

My co-workers and I have also worked out a valuable supplement to the official documents. At least once a year, each itinerant teacher writes an informal summary of the work with each particular student. We include the name and title of the local staff member coordinating special services; grade level and classroom/homeroom teacher; reasons behind various arrangements; suggestions for the following year; and an easy-to-read summary of events during the year. We have found this invaluable when someone takes over a new territory, and very helpful even when resuming work with the same students in the fall. We are careful to write objectively so that parents may read even these informal records.

PERSONAL NOTES

Brief personal notes, recorded daily or weekly as appropriate, make required reports an easy task at the end of the term. This kind of notetaking need not be carefully worded, or readable by others. The purpose is to remind you of events and details easily forgotten. Examples include page numbers within Braille texts; cane travel routes taken; contacts with parents, classroom teachers, and others; directions for finding new locations; and any unusual situations or problems.

Notes must be kept up regularly to be meaningful. The fact of great importance this week will have blurred within a month; circumstances will have changed enough that you will not remember accurately what happened. This might be all right if everyone else were to forget in exactly the same way that you did. Unfortunately, a parent is bound to remember an unpleasant conversation, or an administrator will hold up an error for scrutiny. If you know precisely what occurred, you will be in a better position to explain what happened.

The Right Form Can Save You Effort

My husband, a blind electrical engineer, saves dictation time by running off fill-in-the-blanks forms for certain routine messages. Taking a tip from him, I use a form whenever I can.

Also, when I find myself writing two similar letters, I save effort by copying. (If I'm lucky, a computer is available to do this.)

At the end of the school year, for instance, we send out a form letter asking that books be returned to the appropriate agencies. We attach individualized lists, and often make personal visits, but the form letter saves a great deal of effort.

Use a written form for parent consent for field trips and outings, as described in the chapter on "The Law."

Conclusion

This chapter is closely related to the chapters on "The Law" and "Placement Options and Decisions."

A final caution: A paperwork lover can easily invent enough paperwork to avoid a lot of real work. Keep paperwork only when there really is a purpose for it.

CHAPTER 28

GENERAL CLASSROOM ARRANGEMENTS AND STUDY SKILLS

Classroom teachers sometimes assume that someone must always act as an intermediary for the blind student. Whenever I asked a certain fourth-grade teacher to explain the regular assignment to me, so that I might help solve a problem for the blind girl, she would say, "Why do you ask that? I leave the plans for Denise up to you and the aide." It took a long time for this teacher to see Denise as *her* student. She tended to think of Denise as someone else's student who just happened to be sitting in her room.

It is vital to overcome this barrier. The blind youngster is a regular student who uses alternative methods and may receive some individual help. She is not an irrelevant outsider who is merely physically present.

Written Assignments

THE BEGINNER

What about the very young student who can write only in Braille? For a time it will probably be necessary for someone who knows Braille to go over written assignments. Even here, however, it is important to focus on interaction between the student and the classroom teacher. The Braille teacher, for example, need not actually evaluate the papers – he/she might simply transcribe them into print for the classroom teacher.

When I find an error, I try to transcribe it to show what kind of mistake was made. For example, if the student writes a Braille *d* when he means *f* (a reversal in Braille), I will copy it as a backwards *f* in print. If he writes a Braille *d* when he means a period (placing the symbol too high), I will print it as a dot which is high instead of low.

To maintain excellence in Braille, someone who really knows Braille must continue to read samples of the student's writing. Many students write sloppy Braille because no one ever notices. One residential-school student, who had above-average ability but average laziness, wrote more and more carelessly. However, the ninth-grade English teacher was blind herself and an excellent Braille reader. For the first time since fifth grade, Braille papers were closely analyzed. The improvement in this student's Braille writing (and that of her classmates) was phenomenal.

Oral alternatives can be used by any student. Provided it is not used to displace typing or Braille, this is an excellent possibility. The young child can read his Braille answers aloud to the teacher. (Caution: this should not be the *only* method of handing in work for the young student. He may use incorrect signs and misread his answers. An adult who knows Braille well must check his work some of the time.) Sometimes the student might give his answers orally without Brailling them – perhaps dictating them to someone who will write them down, or perhaps using a tape recorder. These methods are available also to the newly blinded older student.

Furthermore, an oral alternative is sometimes best, regardless of the student's age and experience. Always analyze the nature and purpose of the task. Dictating a few short answers may be faster than arranging for a typewriter. Instead of transcribing a worksheet into Braille, it may be simplest for someone to read it aloud and mark the student's answers. On the other hand, sometimes it is essential to have the student's own spelling and punctuation down on paper, as with an English assignment.

HANDWRITING

The student with considerable useful sight will use handwriting (cursive and/or manuscript) for many assignments. As the student gets older, however, typing long assignments can make a great difference in time, effort, and neatness.

Conversely, students who usually do not use handwriting may nevertheless find it helpful for certain activities. It may be simpler to print short answers (possibly with a heavy feltpen) than to get out the typewriter. A totally blind student can mark a Braille answer sheet with a pen or pencil, and probably can make two distinguishable marks for "true" and "false." (+ and 0 may be easier than T and F.) Be creative. At the same time, do not allow these ideas to displace typing, which is almost always best for longer assignments.

TYPING–A NECESSITY

Typing is by far the most versatile and essential skill for doing written assignments. (See the separate chapter on "Keyboarding.") Do not let a student "slip by" by using oral reports or poor handwriting. Often one must speak very frankly about illegible handwriting, and bluntly refuse to accept papers that are hard to read.

The student must be provided with the means to type anywhere, anytime. Unfortunately, this is a situation where modern technology (or, more properly, the misuse of modern technology) has made some blind students *less* competent. When manual typewriters were standard, most blind students did readily type anywhere, anytime. But today some educators believe that a computer with Braille (or speech) output is the only appropriate means of typing. Their students are forced to work only in one place. These students also fail to learn to recognize and correct errors as they occur, and instead spend great amounts of time finding errors and going back to fix them. Speed, efficiency, and flexibility are sacrificed in the name of "modern technology." In contrast, the properly-taught student may use a specialized computer for lengthy reports and whenever else it is convenient, but will also type confidently on a portable machine.

After a blind student learns to type, she should nevertheless continue to write Braille when it is appropriate. Explain to the student: "If the material is for *you* to read, then it should be in Braille. If it is for the sighted teacher to look at, then it should be typed." Typically notes, drafts, and computation should be done in Braille, while only the final copy or final answer is typed up and handed in. (Note: Sometimes the teacher wishes to evaluate such things as study notes and partial answers. In this case the student should use Braille notes but also read them aloud or type them up for the teacher.)

MARKING AND GRADING PAPERS

Classroom teachers commonly mark or correct papers with red pencil to indicate misspellings, incorrect answers, etc., and also to give a letter grade. When the student cannot see such marks, the teacher often feels perplexed as to how to communicate corrections. If the teacher were to discuss each paper individually with the student, time would be hard to arrange, and there might be no written record of the marks.

"Just use your red pencil as usual," I urge. "We will teach the student to expect this, and make it his responsibility to find out what the marks say. If you have time, go ahead and explain them. If you don't, he can get someone else to read the corrections – a friend, the teacher aide, myself, or someone at home."

THE IMPORTANCE OF FLEXIBILITY

If the obvious or customary way of doing an assignment is cumbersome or unsuccessful in a given case, look for alternatives.

What about diagraming sentences? Instead of using an actual diagram, might the student type the words and phrases under column headings? Could the sentences be typed with creative use of symbols – such as underlining the prepositions, enclosing clauses in parentheses, and stating what modifies what? Or, consider simply using a reader and having the student dictate how to diagram the sentence. For a student having difficulty, consider providing Braille words on cards which the student can move around physically to form a tactual diagram.

If the classroom teacher says, "Turn in your notes on 3x5" cards," it is foolish to struggle to accommodate this literally. Why not use 5x8" cards if that is easier? Depending on the task, it might not be necessary to use cards at all. Size and shape are usually unimportant to the nature of the task. The overall quantity and quality of the work *is* essential to the task, however, and should not be altered solely because of blindness.

At the other extreme, caution teachers against *too much* flexibility. One high school student, assigned to write a 30-page term paper, negotiated for three ten-page papers instead. She offered many "reasons," none of which were really relevant to the fact of blindness, and which boiled down to avoiding a new and difficult task.

Meeting New Challenges

Now and then someone may ask, "Why does he need to do this assignment at all? What will he get out of it, anyway?" Following are two examples, and this problem is addressed throughout this book.

Tom was enjoying the theater arts course, but saw no value in learning to apply stage makeup. "My folks and I decided I should sit this one out," he declared. "I know I'd put it on all wrong. And I can't see it anyway, so it wouldn't mean anything to me." Unfortunately, the teacher did not insist, and Tom missed a valuable experience. He could have learned concepts about visual appearances and color; improved his understanding of facial features; and avoided reinforcing the idea that he "couldn't get anything out of" experiences such as this. With proper guidance he need not have worried about putting the makeup on badly. (Unfortunately, one reason for hesitation was that this teacher avoided using tactual guidance, and tended to rely solely on verbalization.)

Another student was excluded from learning to operate various projectors and other audio-visual equipment. Despite her plans to become a teacher, and despite the fact that many blind teachers do operate such equipment (perhaps asking students to tell when the material is focused), everyone believed that "she couldn't really run those machines, so the class would be a waste of time."

Try to anticipate activities which you have not already discussed with that particular teacher. If Speech students will be interviewing persons outside the school, you may need to do some coaching about travel, about note-taking, and about explaining blindness to a stranger.

In many classes, students "exchange papers." Answers are given aloud, and each student marks his/her partner's paper. If papers are traded frequently, work out a way to include the blind student. If he is always excluded, he will miss valuable experience, and everyone will become accustomed to his being "left out."

Blind adults often check the accuracy of various things, generally using sighted assistance in various ways, and the blind student can do the same. Perhaps the partner could read his own answers aloud, and mark them as the blind student directs.

When a sighted partner reads his answers aloud, he may not have time to check the blind student's paper. Instead, another student might check two papers, or the teacher might check one.

If the blind student's paper is in Braille, he might read his answers aloud to a partner, or check his own paper.

Contingencies

PROBLEMS WITH MATERIALS OR EQUIPMENT

Classroom teachers worry, justifiably, about what might go wrong. Suppose the Brailled materials are misplaced? Suppose the child can't figure out the Braille, and no one can read it? What if the Braillewriter or typewriter breaks down, and the child cannot write? Such things are trouble enough in individual lessons, but can be disastrous in a class of 28.

Help the older student build a repertoire of ideas. Even a younger child can learn to explain what seems to be wrong–e.g., "I think this is the spelling book instead of the math book," or, "I can only find ten problems."

Mention alternative ways that assignments could be accomplished, and be sure everyone realizes they are OK, at least for use in a pinch. Chief among these is the use of a live reader. If the Braille cannot be found, probably someone can be found to read the material aloud. If the Braillewriter or typewriter will not function, the student might dictate his answers.

For younger students, especially, it is important to have "standing assignments" which can be used any time. This is not only because things may go wrong, but also because it is hard to judge how long a given assignment will take, and young children cannot just sit until all classmates finish. Give the first-grade teacher several extra Braille worksheets, suggestions for practicing Braille signs, etc.

Sometimes tomorrow's assignment can be done today, and vice versa, if there is difficulty in getting today's materials ready. Completing work at home is another possibility.

Primary-grade teachers commonly provide "interest centers" or other optional activities for children who finish before everyone is done. These may be puzzles, art, library books, etc. Unfortunately, blind students often miss out for various reasons: (1) the child is struggling to learn alternative study methods, and is slow to finish the regular assignment; (2) the child has a different assignment, and is asked to "use all the time available" rather than doing a fixed amount of work; (3) no one has planned how the interest centers might be used by a blind child; (4) the centers are used during the reading period, and that is when the child leaves for individual instruction. It is important to overcome these barriers and see that the blind student gets to do these kinds of things at least occasionally.

Another common problem is a misplaced or broken cane. Sometimes an extra cane can be kept at school. A good rule is that the student must not leave the classroom alone without the cane because the cane enables safe and independent travel. The "Travel" chapters in this *Handbook* discuss various ramifications of this problem.

ABSENCES

If a student's absence is anticipated ahead of time, assignments should be completed beforehand if possible. Otherwise, appropriate staff member(s) should help him get caught up when he returns.

What if the aide or the resource/itinerant teacher is late or absent? For short absences, ideas such as those above usually enable the student to get along in the regular classroom. Perhaps the student could participate in some activities he usually misses. If you are teaching individualized reading, leave enough "standing assignments" so that the child could work independently for awhile.

A special problem arises if the student leaves class to meet the itinerant teacher in an extra room, but he/she is not there. This illustrates the importance of calling ahead about schedule changes; but emergencies or errors sometimes occur. Tell older students they should practice slate writing, or another suitable task, if you are a few minutes late. You might say, "If I am more than ten minutes late, something is wrong, and go back to your regular class." With a very young student who cannot judge time, say, "If you ever come to look for me and I am not here, go back and ask Mrs. Green what's wrong. If something big has gone wrong and you can't find your own class either (maybe they went to the gym), remember that the secretary in the office would always help."

When a person who gives a great deal of individual help is gone for more than a day or two, a substitute should be found. If the aide is ill, the district should transfer someone temporarily, or possibly seek a PTA volunteer. For a resource teacher in just one building, a substitute should be provided on the same basis as for a classroom teacher. (Or, if the teacher is assisted by a competent aide, the aide might be able to take over for awhile.) For an itinerant teacher it may be more complicated because of the wide territory. If no actual substitute is available, perhaps a neighboring itinerant teacher or a Braillist could help those in most need of attention, while the simpler situations might "run on their own" for awhile.

Reassure classroom teachers that no serious damage will be done if occasionally the schedule is ruined or a lesson is botched. See that advice is always available within a few hours. If a particular student or teacher continually has severe problems, general program planning should be carefully re-examined.

Spelling

Good spelling is essential for every educated person, and the blind student is no exception. If the proper tools and materials are provided, and if good performance is expected, the blind student can be a good speller.

In almost all Braille books, even those for kindergarten, the contractions of regular Grade II Braille are used at all times. Examples are the use of *nec* for *necessary,* and a special symbol for the word *with.* However, in Braille dictionaries and spelling books, words being defined or studied are spelled out completely. Thus the blind student has several ways to learn and practice the complete spelling of a word: (1) reading it in the spelling book and dictionary; (2) working on spelling lists; and (3) typing various lessons on the regular typewriter.

Braille abbreviations can be confusing for only a few words. As a resource or itinerant teacher, you should know what these words are, and watch for problems.

Sighted first graders commonly study spelling words appropriate for their level. The blind first grader can readily practice ten or more Braille words per week, writing them both with signs *and* without signs. (Most children, even at this level, can understand the idea of "two ways to write it" and are not unduly confused. Should a child be confused, the work on full spelling could be carefully separated; for example, it might be done orally at a time well removed from the Braille writing lesson.) Lists may easily be taken from the child's reading instruction book, if not already compiled by the school's curriculum.

A good exercise at any age is to give a list of Grade II Braille signs, and ask the student to give the full spelling.

A classroom teacher should be aware that spelling confusion due to Braille signs could exist, but should not assume it does very often. The beginning Braille reader will learn that the *of* sign stands for the letters o-f wherever it appears, and will read it as such. Therefore, just because a word has a Braille abbreviation in it does not mean that spelling is confusing or difficult. It is vital that the blind student's spelling be evaluated and improved in the same general manner as for anyone else.

When a student first begins to type class lessons, should errors in typing be counted as spelling errors? During a short transition period, the student might be permitted to correct mistyped words by spelling them aloud. Before long, however, typing errors should be considered spelling errors. Otherwise the student will have little motivation to develop accuracy.

Jeremy "got by" for years reading large print. His grades were generally above average, though he read slowly and his spelling was poor. In eighth grade Jeremy began to learn Braille. Within a year, his grades were rising and his spelling had improved dramatically. Now he could examine words accurately and comfortably.

Foreign Languages

When a book written in English contains a foreign word or passage, that portion is transcribed in Grade I Braille (full spelling, no contractions). Any letter with an accent or other mark is preceded by a dot 4. Braille code references explain this and list special symbols such as Greek letters.

An exception occurs with "Anglicized words" – those which have been borrowed from a foreign language but are in such common usage as to be considered part of the English language. With Anglicized words in English context, contractions should be used, but accented letters (preceded by dot 4) must not form part of a contraction.

For a foreign-language textbook, or any other book actually in a foreign language, consult the following (see "References" at the end of this book for complete information):

- *Manual on Foreign Languages To Aid Braille Transcribers*
- *Code of Braille Textbook Formats and Techniques*
- *Instruction Manual for Braille Transcribing*

In a foreign language book, unaccented letters which are like English letters are transcribed in Grade I Braille. Accented or marked letters are handled in a completely different manner. Special Braille symbols represent the letter and the accent together – that is, a single Braille symbol represents the letter *and* its accent. For example, in French when the letter *a* is written with a "grave" accent (which in inkprint slants from upper left toward lower right), the letter and its accent *together* are represented by dots 1-2-3-5-6.

There are special symbols and conventions for each particular language. Punctuation may be different also. A complete listing of special symbols should be included in the preliminary pages of each transcribed volume.

For textbooks in languages using a completely different alphabet, such as Russian, the above references give a Braille symbol for each letter. For these languages, do *not* assume that because a letter visually resembles a familiar letter, the English-Braille letter should be used.

The above applies to materials produced in the United States. Braille produced in other countries may use yet a different set of symbols. However, foreign-produced Braille is not normally used in this country except for college postgraduate work.

Since many Braille transcribers are not familiar with foreign language symbols, specialized help may need to be sought if the use of references is not sufficient. If local sources cannot be found, help may be obtained through the American Printing House for the Blind, the Braille Book Bank, or the National Library Service for the Blind and Physically Handicapped. (See also the chapter on "Books and Supplies.")

With the key to special symbols, the blind student should be able to interpret the materials by following the regular class instruction. Also note that individualized Braille instruction in foreign languages is available through the Hadley correspondence school.

If other students are expected to write in the foreign language, the blind student should do so also, in Braille and/or print according to the situation. Otherwise the student would be omitting a vital part of the course, and would probably fail to learn spelling also. For languages with a completely different alphabet, a typewriter with special keys is desirable. Special keys also are helpful for any language student planning a career in the subject. However, usually it is possible to invent a readable system using the standard keyboard. In Spanish, for example, one might use the apostrophe for the accent, and the underscore in place of the tilde. The English question mark and exclamation point could be used at both the beginning and end of a sentence. If such substitution is used, the blind student should also learn what the inkprint symbols look like – e.g., upside-down question mark.

Where to Put Things

An amazing amount of hassle can revolve around storage and organization. Many people assume, unfortunately, that the blind student needs a cart and/or a personal assistant to move things between classes. At the other extreme, the student may be unable to work because of cramped space and inadequate materials.

IN THE CLASSROOM

It is important that the blind student sit where she can hear well. If there is a separate typing table, or a shelf for specialized materials, she also needs to be able to get there easily. However, do not rigidly assume that the blind student must always sit in the front row and next to the special materials. Also avoid the assumption that she must sit in the seat nearest the door because of presumed limited mobility. Several blind adults have said to me, "I got so tired of sitting by the door! Every teacher I ever had, made me sit right by the door, in the first row. Always the very same seat."

The student should be part of the regular group, near other students and facing the normal direction. If it is necessary to place a typing table at the back of the room facing the wall, then the student should sit there only when actually typing; she could also be assigned a regular desk for other activities.

The teacher should use the student's name in speaking to her, so she knows when she is being spoken to. (If there are two students with the same first name, this should include the last name or initial.) This is important for partially-sighted students as well as the totally blind.

If an aide assists the student, insist that he or she *not* sit with the student except when absolutely necessary.

Use of the typewriter, Brailler, recordings, and live readers can produce noise, and the student should be considerate. Headphones render a recording silent to others. The Braille slate, which produces very little noise, is preferable to the Perkins Brailler. If classmates are distracted by the reader's voice, the work can be done in a far corner of the room or even outside the classroom. Actually, noise almost always proves to be much less of a problem than might be anticipated, since the class quickly becomes used to the blind student's methods.

In a classroom which is largely self-contained, a shelf or extra desk is usually necessary. This will accommodate the volumes of Braille or large print, and also tape recorders and other equipment. Enough table or desk space must be available so that the student can spread out a book and still have room for a typewriter. If both typewriter and Braillewriter will be used, it is helpful if both can be set up at the same time in the self-contained classroom.

MOVING AROUND

Older students, however, usually move from classroom to classroom. How do we provide materials in several locations? This question emphasizes the need for flexibility and good alternative techniques. The student who takes notes with the Perkins must move a heavy piece of equipment (or provide several of them); but the Braille slate is slipped into pocket or purse. The student who reads with a CCTV screen is tied to a heavy, delicate, and expensive piece of equipment; but Braille and tapes are easily portable.

As a compromise for personal preference or inexperience, a large piece of equipment may be kept in the room where it is most desired, while other alternatives are used elsewhere.

Typewriters and tape players may indeed be essential in several different rooms. Perhaps two typewriters could be placed where they are most used, and carried occasionally to other classes. Alternatively, the student might go to a central location such as the resource room, and type there. Tape machines are easily carried. However, the student should avoid unnecessary carrying, by anticipating what will actually be needed. Ask classroom teachers to help with this.

Tina was constantly weighted down by many Braille volumes. A classmate carried her tape machine and typewriter. The new resource teacher helped her change this: In the centrally-located Media Center, a large cupboard was provided. There Tina stored her portable typewriter and tape machine, along with all tapes or Braille volumes which were not in *current* use. Her locker, at the north end of the building, provided additional storage space, as did the resource room at the south. An extra typewriter was provided for English class. At any particular time, Tina would carry only her notebook and the current volumes for two classes.

Be creative in solving logistics problems. Remember that it is usually not necessary or desirable to make the *same* arrangements for *all* classes. Mix and match ideas such as:

- Look for storage space in various locations: library, resource room, administrative office, miscellaneous closets, etc.
- Provide two lockers, in different parts of the building.
- If two or more blind students are in the same building, try to share some equipment.
- For any particular textbook, the volumes not in current use might be kept almost anywhere.
- If it would be tremendously helpful to have two of something, look for ways to provide two. However, if you seek a great many pieces of expensive equipment, you encourage unrealistic expectations.
- For very small amounts of writing, consider alternatives to the typewriter. For example, for a short pretest the student might write her answers in Braille and read them aloud as necessary.
- Equipment might be shared between two classrooms which are near each other.
- Provide a Perkins Brailler, if desired, in the room where the most Braille is written. Use the slate in other rooms.

"But why not just carry things around?" your student may ask. "My friends like to help."

The appropriate role of the blind student does *not* include a heavy load of special equipment, constant assistance, and endless special arrangements. The independent blind student is easily mobile on her own, without fuss and bother, fitting in as a normal participant wherever the work is done. Friendship can wear thin when constant service is required. If this is not yet seen as a problem, it will be in the future.

LOCKERS

Student lockers bring the question of combination locks. Sometimes an existing lock can be made accessible by tactual markings, but usually that provides obvious clues to the combination. A regular padlock with a key is one satisfactory solution. So is a combination lock especially designed for the blind, with levers that "click" into position. Some commercial companies offer a combination padlock with wheels which will not turn backwards through zero–thus the blind student can turn the wheels to zero and then count the "clicks." This type offers good security, since it is possible to change the combination.

The school custodian should easily be able to remove the school's padlock and accommodate an alternative. (Caution: "Go through channels" and consult the principal or counselor first, before talking to the custodian.) Alternative locks are one of the most universally helpful devices. Many students who read print well have difficulty seeing small, closely-spaced marks in a poorly-lighted hallway. Several times I have had a conversation like this:

> "I really think this lock would be helpful. Why not try it?"
>
> "I don't need it. It looks funny."
>
> "Let's go to your locker, and you show me how you open it. It's hard for me to understand how you could see all those little marks."
>
> "Well... lots of the time I can see the marks. But if I can't, I get my friend to open it."

"But your friend isn't always there. And other people open their lockers by themselves–don't you want to? I think it looks funny to have to get somebody to open your locker for you. People won't pay much attention to a lock that's a little different shape."

"Well, OK... I'll try it."

Dictionary Skills

If a student cannot use extra-small print easily, he/she should have access to a suitable dictionary in large print or Braille. Since dictionary work is usually done individually, and since dictionaries are very long and detailed, this is one situation where it often is not practical to provide the very same dictionary that classmates use. However, it should be possible to provide one which is reasonably comparable.

Sometimes it is sufficient to provide a Braille copy of *20,000 Words,* which is immensely shorter than an actual dictionary. This book provides spelling and syllabication, and is sufficient information for many purposes. The *Vest Pocket Dictionary,* which is an actual dictionary, is also considerably shorter than most dictionaries.

Discuss how to handle any inconveniences due to the use of a different dictionary. If younger classes have group lessons using a few specific pages, it should be possible to provide those particular pages in Braille or large print. When a different Braille dictionary is used with a younger child, try to provide an identical inkprint copy for the teacher.

Also note that a lengthy "glossary," such as that in the third-grade *Patterns* reading book, can be used for instruction in dictionary work.

The *Code of Braille Textbook Formats and Techniques* (commonly called the "Textbook Code") includes an explanation of Braille dictionary usage. Provide teachers with some basic information from this book–notably a key to the symbols for syllable division and accent; the fact that the accent mark goes *before* the syllable; a key to the phonetic symbols; and the fact that Grade II Braille is never used in the syllabized entry or the phonetic spelling.

FLEXIBILITY

An experienced student should be able to read a Braille dictionary independently, so that it is no longer necessary to have an identical inkprint copy. Should she have difficulty with a given entry, she could read it aloud well enough so that any teacher could help her interpret it.

Sometimes it is asked, "Why must the blind student learn to use a dictionary, anyway? Braille dictionaries aren't available in the workplace." One answer is that many other skills are taught along with dictionary skills: alphabetization, pronunciation, word meaning, library reference use, parts of speech, etc. Just as important, even if the blind person has no Braille dictionary at a given time, he can use an inkprint dictionary with a reader. If the blind person understands dictionary entries better than the reader does (as is often the case), the reader can simply read the *entire* entry, leaving interpretation up to the blind person. For example, the reader can simply read the letters "v.i.," instead of being expected to figure out that this means "verb, intransitive." If the reader has trouble with the pronunciation of an uncommon word, he can describe the marks (straight line, two dots, etc.) and read part of the key aloud. This way of reading the dictionary aloud can also be used when a young student is to analyze the entry independently, and it is only available in small print.

Tape-recorded dictionaries are increasingly available. Often, however, use of a live reader is much faster than searching through a tape. Braille (if available) also is much faster. For the young student just learning dictionary skills, it is important to have a dictionary on paper.

Quantity vs. Time

"But he can't do all that!" complained Phil's parents. "His eyes get tired. And so many of those worksheets are just busywork."

There are some legitimate reasons for cutting quantity–basically (1) if a student is spending great amounts of time with *initial* learning of a major skill such as Braille, or (2) if there is a strong, specific reason apart from vision (such as mental disability). If shortening is really necessary, be specific so that the student will not just lazily do less and less. (e.g., "She will do every other problem" *vs.* "She doesn't have to do all the problems.")

To shorten or omit assignments solely because of visual impairment or blindness is to shortchange the student. However, this is one of the most common errors. If it is really Phil's eyesight that is keeping him from doing all the work, then he should be using alternative techniques - Braille, tapes, and live readers.

Too often, quantity of work is simply reduced routinely, on the assumption that the visually impaired or blind student cannot work as fast as others, or will get too tired. Remember the old maxim, "Work expands to fill the time allowed." If a student is assigned only half as many themes as the others, he will learn habits to accommodate that level of work. He will not learn the efficiencies which would have allowed him to do the usual level of work. Thus we have a self-fulfilling prophecy.

"But why does it matter?" someone may ask. "If he knows *how* to do the work, why does he have to do it over and over? It's just busy-work!" Part of the answer is that such accommodations cannot go on forever if a person expects to be in the "mainstream" of life. Teachers in the higher grades will be less and less likely to allow an adjusted quantity when giving regular credit. Post-secondary institutions are even less likely to tolerate this. And an employer is most unlikely to accept the excuse, "I can do only half as many reports as the others, because I can't see."

Furthermore, quantity actually is an integral part of the task.

ARITHMETIC

Working a few examples of arithmetic problems is *not* equivalent to working two pages - even if the sample is analyzed to contain all the main points of the lesson. The normal two pages will contain many review elements, nuances, and variations not present in the smaller sample. Often a student learns a new principle and then becomes confused on related principles; a large and varied quantity helps to overcome this. Moreover, speed and stamina are part of what is to be learned. Again, an employer will not agree to an employee's doing a "small representative sample" of the tasks at hand.

TERM PAPERS

With lengthy research projects, it is especially true that "work expands to fill the time allowed." If the student is permitted more time than others have, he may easily be able to search at leisure, read everything he can find, get it in the reading mode he prefers, and compose at leisure. He will not be well motivated to learn things such as using indexes; quickly analyzing what is most relevant; scanning for needed information; taking efficient notes; using various reading modes, including readers; composing and revising efficiently; etc. He will stay with the methods he is already comfortable with, even when they are slow.

EXCEPTIONAL SITUATIONS

There are times when it is reasonable to arrange some extra time. This may occur with a test or other in-class assignment, when materials are only available in a form much more cumbersome than that used by others. For example, if sighted students are allowed to do mathematical computations right on the test paper, but the blind student must copy each example, work it on the abacus, and then retype it in print, it may be reasonable to allow extra time.

However, the student and the staff should constantly strive for greater efficiency to minimize the need for extended time. The math student, above, may realize that he need not recopy problems, but can refer directly to the book while using the abacus. Also, the teacher may realize that she does not need to see how the student sets up the problem, but only his final answer.

When the time extends beyond one school day anyway, the blind student should be able to work within the limits even with less-than-optimum materials.

See also the chapter on "Testing and Evaluation."

IDEAS FOR INCREASED EFFICIENCY

The following suggestions are especially relevant for a student learning to handle increased quantity of work:

- The student who reads print slowly or with difficulty, or tires easily when reading print, should also use Braille and tapes. Be flexible about the reading mode.
- Instead of asking for a time extension to obtain Braille or large print, use a reader.
- Plan efficient use of reader time. Use the reader for the things where it is most helpful to have him/her.
- Have the reader use a tape recorder at times. This can solve scheduling problems and avoid repeated readings.
- Become competent in the use of reference aids, such as the *Readers' Guide to Periodical Literature,* the card file and/or computerized files, the Dewey Decimal system, etc. Learn to use them efficiently with a reader, regardless of whether the reader himself/herself is skilled in their use. The reader is not the one doing the research.
- Develop various styles of reading: skimming and scanning; quick reading for the general drift; detailed study; etc. This can be done with Braille, recordings, and live readers, as well as with inkprint.
- Good notes are vital. Select the key items and write them down in the briefest appropriate form. If print does not work well, use Braille. Develop ways, such as 5x8" cards, to move notes around during organization and composition.
- Develop at least one good method for composing and revising rough drafts. Braille may be double-spaced to facilitate correction and insertion. Find creative ways to combine modes of reading/writing (e.g., make a draft in Braille. Then read it onto tape while making revisions. Then type the final copy from the tape.)
- Polish up typing accuracy and speed, for preparing the final copy.
- Avoid putting work off until the last minute. For long-term assignments, make a schedule.

The chapter on "Note-Taking" offers additional suggestions.

Grading

REGULAR GRADING

Classroom teachers should grade the blind student according to his or her performance, applying the same standards that are used with the rest of the class. This point cannot be emphasized too strongly.

(Note: With a *newly blinded* student, it may be desirable to use a non-competitive evaluation, such as satisfactory-unsatisfactory, for a few months. It should be clearly understood that this is only temporary.)

The student who is given "sympathy grades" and allowed to get by with sub-standard work will pay a tremendous price at some future time. As he/she grows older, teachers or professors will be less and less likely to accept poor work, and certainly no employer will hire and keep an employee with inadequate skills.

If papers are penalized for spelling errors, the same policy should apply to the blind student. If ten book reports are normally required during the semester, the blind student should meet the requirement in quantity and quality.

There are some circumstances where special grading and assignment policies may be appropriate with very young children, the newly blinded, and others in special situations. In general, however, the blind student having difficulty should be graded in the same manner as any other student having difficulty. The blind student whose work is average or above should receive the grade which he or she earned and no more.

INDIVIDUALIZED GRADES WHEN APPROPRIATE

Usually grades are given by classroom teachers, with advice and input from itinerant/resource teachers. Individualized special lessons are usually not graded. Sometimes, however, the resource or itinerant teacher is indeed the "teacher of record" for a given subject, and does have the responsibility for grading. The most common example is reading instruction in the primary grades, when the child is actually *learning to read* (as distinguished from an older student who already knows how to read and is only learning Braille as such). And resource teachers, especially, often take over the basic responsibility for any subject when the student needs much individual help.

An individualized grade should be tied as closely as possible to the regular grading system. If the student is able to grasp the content, and is working alone to learn alternative methods, it is usually possible to grade him according to regular standards (with the possible exception of speed expectations). For example, if the child understands arithmetic but you are working alone to teach him the Nemeth Code, find out how the classroom teacher grades, and use the same standard.

If the child works alone because of difficulty with the actual *content* of the regular course, the matter of grading should be covered in the IEP. Consult resource teachers who work with other disabilities and discuss policies on grading special students.

NARRATIVE DESCRIPTION OF PROGRESS

Many school districts do not give letter grades at all for the youngest students, but instead give descriptive reports. For a student working individually, look at sample reports and follow the usual format.

Occasionally narrative reporting is desirable as an alternative to another format. Consider this example for a first-grader:

> Zach has completed 39 of 75 pages in the Braille Primer, *City and Farm.* Phonics, comprehension, and oral reading are satisfactory. We continue to work to improve finger motion. On the test preceding this book, Zach scored 87, well above the "mastery" level of 69.
>
> Zach practices writing all vocabulary words on the Brailler, and is beginning to write sentences independently. We will begin creative writing soon.

The customary grading at this level consisted of a check list. Zach's Braille teacher felt that his achievement would be better explained by actual description. However, she carefully included every point from the usual checklist. She also gave the level of the instruction ("Primer" is a customary designation for "early first-grade level") and the results of objective testing.

THE IEP

When Zach was in second grade, he began the transition to using the same textbooks as his classmates (in Braille). By the middle of third grade Zach was completing all the regular assignments. Narrative reports were discontinued and Zach was graded in exactly the same manner as his classmates.

The narrative style should not be substituted for another format unless there is a very good reason.

If an alternative method of grading is used, the reason and the plan should be stated in the IEP, along with the duration of its use. If a newly-blinded student is learning the Nemeth Code, it may be reasonable not to give him a letter grade in math for a year or so. However, it is not reasonable to slip into a permanent pattern of pass/fail or narrative grades.

The Real World

Recently my husband and I looked forward to meeting a young woman who was graduating in electrical engineering. We recalled that my husband had pioneered as a blind person in this field, and also noted that engineering was formerly closed to women.

However, our delight quickly turned to dismay as she talked about her university studies. She did not take notes in lecture classes – she did not even *attend* most technical classes. Instead, she had a tutor who went over the material with her individually. She needed a tutor, she explained, because she couldn't follow the class presentation. Did she read the textbook assignment before class? No, she didn't read the textbook at all; again, the tutor summarized it. Soon my husband and I were nearly speechless. What could we say to this young woman, who eagerly anticipated graduation and entry into a prestigious technical field? By using all this special help, and by *not* doing the usual things, she had deprived herself of most of the background expected of an engineering graduate.

"I'm having a little trouble understanding how you study," my husband finally said tactfully. "Let's see – how would you work a problem like this? `Given: a circuit consisting of a 100-volt voltage source with its positive terminal going through a 40-ohm resistor and thence through a second 40-ohm resistor to the positive output terminal, with the negative output terminal going to the negative side of the voltage source, and with a 60-ohm resistor going from the junction of the two 40-ohm resistors to the negative terminal of the voltage source. Convert this circuit to an equivalent circuit consisting of just one voltage source and one resistor.'"

"Well, I can't work that here," she replied. "I'm used to working with my tutor. He goes over the problem with me, and we discuss it together. I dictate my work, and he reads it back. I don't always do all the problems, you know – I don't remember doing one quite like that."

That was a very basic type of electrical engineering problem, my husband told me later, and should be mastered by the end of the sophomore year. A major part of solving it is *recognizing* that it is a "Thevenin equivalent" problem. My husband works easier ones (such as this example) in his head. For harder ones he uses Braille notes and/or a talking calculator. In college he occasionally used raised or bold-line diagrams.

A TRAGIC LACK

This young woman not only lacked the necessary depth of knowledge and wide experience which is needed for success in engineering. She had even been deprived of the screening process which weeds out those who are unsuited for a particular profession. Many young persons start out in engineering (or any other field), only to find that the work is too hard for them, or that they greatly dislike it. They are forced to seek another field – a change which may be very disappointing, but which in the long run channels them where they can succeed. But when this young woman seemed unable to comprehend the textbook on her own, and to take notes from the regular lectures, special help was arranged instead.

Did she really have the ability to be an electrical engineer? Who could tell? She said that she always passed tests; but we hesitated to inquire further. We could guess how the tutor would "read" the tests.

In high school, if a student really needs help with the content of a course, that fact should be made plain to everyone, and she should be guided into the less difficult classes in that subject. In college, if a student really needs a tutor (as distinguished from a reader) for a particular course, then that subject should not be her major field.

This young engineering student could not use print, and yet did not know Braille. She had very little experience with tape recordings. She had no way to take effective notes. Simple techniques and approaches, such as asking the professor to speak formulas aloud, were foreign to her. She had almost no experience with using a real reader, as distinguished from a tutor. If she had had these methods during high school and college, she might have been able to succeed at independently reading scientific textbooks and taking class notes. If she had not succeeded, a positive attitude would have led her toward success in another field.

This student's tragic lack of preparation epitomizes the problems which this chapter (along with this entire book) seeks to prevent.

Conclusion

"But he just can't keep up!" classroom teachers may protest.

Throughout this chapter and this book are ideas to increase efficiency and speed, and (most important) foster the attitude that normal speed and efficiency are to be expected of blind persons. Analyze just where speed is lost. Consider providing some help at times (e.g., the aide helps the first grader find the right page). Provide directed practice (e.g., when alone with the student, name various page numbers and see how fast he can find them. Help him estimate where the page will be, rather than painstakingly reading every page number.) Be creative with incentives, such as charting how many seconds it takes to find the page. For the older student who should be able to do better, apply the same standards as for others: if he does not complete the assignment, he must do it at recess or as homework.

Work with the classroom teacher and the student to seek creative and practical solutions to specific problems.

Waiting for transcribed materials is a common cause of unnecessary delay. For the first grader, daily worksheets are an essential part of learning to read, and many of them should be in Braille. But for the older student it is often more practical to have daily handouts read aloud, and this also provides valuable experience in working with a reader. Similarly, the very young student needs real objects and Braille diagrams, to build understanding. But often the older student needs only a verbal description. Avoid assuming that the nearest possible equivalent in tactual form is always the best. Consider instead, "What is the most practical and efficient way to accomplish the real goal(s) of this lesson, given the ability and background of this particular student?"

CHAPTER 29

KEYBOARDING (TYPING)

The greatest problem with keyboarding is the belief (often unrecognized) that it is not possible for a blind person to become really competent and versatile. This belief is false, because with proper training the person will succeed according to his or her general ability. If this major problem of attitude is overcome, other problems will tend to disappear, because teachers and students will seek to solve problems rather than considering them insoluble.

Many blind people are employed as keyboard operators, in varied settings.

Since good typing is always done by touch anyway, the methods for teaching blind students are really not very different from those used with others. Even starting in elementary school is now common.

Benefits

The *value* of typing skill to a blind person is especially high. The student can submit written work directly to any teacher. Differences between Braille and inkprint usage are learned and practiced (e.g., spacing twice after a period instead of once). Meaningful practice is provided in spelling out words which are abbreviated in Braille.

Because of the great practical value, blind students typically begin learning keyboarding in third or fourth grade.

Typing remains a vital skill for blind adults regardless of occupation. The salesman types orders into the computer; the homemaker types notes to her child's teacher; the engineer types specifications; the maintenance worker orders parts and supplies. Everyone appreciates the ability to write personal notes without involving a third party.

Computers are now used in almost every place of business, in virtually all schools (even elementary schools), and in many homes. The chapter on "Computers" contains many suggestions about typing (now often called "keyboarding," probably because of the influence of computers).

Typing is important even for a visually-impaired individual who reads inkprint and uses handwriting regularly. Lengthy handwritten assignments are likely to be laborious to write and/or difficult to read.

Since typing is important to the totally blind, to the legally blind, and even to those with a relatively slight visual impairment, it is the skill which you will probably most often teach directly. Unfortunately, some courses for teachers of the visually impaired tend to assume that you already know how to type and how to teach typing. They may or may not give you adequate instruction in how to adapt techniques as necessary. If at all possible, take a course in Business Education. (If something major which you do not need is included, such as shorthand, audit the class or register for Pass/Fail.) Analyze posture and stroking. Learn the instructional methods used by teachers of general typing. Become thoroughly familiar with the uses of various parts of the machine; various formats; spaces per inch and per line; etc. If you are uncertain, you will tend to rationalize a reason not to teach these things.

Because of computers, most students today readily appreciate the value of typing. However, some discussion of the immediate value to the individual is always wise. A totally blind fourth-grader once asked me, after several weeks of lessons, "You know I can't see this, don't you?" I suddenly realized he meant, "Why am I doing this, anyway?" Now I always explain the value at the beginning. I also make sure that partially-sighted students realize that they can use regular typewriters and computers even if they cannot read small print.

Techniques

INSERTING THE PAPER

The student should use his fingers to find the place for inserting the paper, trying not to move the paper guide accidentally.

The paper should then be lined up evenly with the top of the erasure table or platen cover – that is, with the solid surface which is above the platen (roller) and immediately behind the paper. Alternatively, the paper may be aligned with the paper bail (the horizontal rod which holds the upper part of the paper against the platen). Various models may have other straight edges near the top of the paper. However, the unfortunately-common idea of touching the top and bottom of the paper itself together is *not* efficient – it is time-consuming and unreliable.

Strive, of course, for straight insertion the first time.

WHERE IS WHAT?

Take the beginner's hands and show him the various parts of the keyboard (with the power turned off). Rather than analyzing all the parts of the machine immediately, it is better to give a general overview and then go on to actual typing. Later, the discussion of a new part of the machine can bring pleasant variety.

Describe the keyboard overall as the student examines it: "At the bottom of the keyboard you find a wide, thin bar called the space bar. This makes a blank space, just like the spacer on the Brailler. Above that, find a row of small keys. The next higher row of keys is called the home row. So far most of these are letters of the alphabet. The third row up is also letters. The very top row has the numbers and some other symbols that are not letters."

Then help the student find the home row independently, and show him the fingering pattern there. The little finger of the left hand can observe the differences between the shift lock and the *a* key – differences in height, shape, and/or distance from surrounding keys. When starting to type, the two forefingers can be brought together to check that only *g* and *h* are not covered by resting fingers. (This can also be done after each use of a manual carriage return).

It might appear desirable to label the keys in Braille, especially for the beginner. However, this would interfere with normal stroking, and discourage the memorization which is essential for speed. It is much better to explain verbally, drill for memorization, and use a separate Braille chart of the keyboard for reference.

If a beginner has real difficulty keeping track of the home row position, or if a computer has many extra keys surrounding the letters, the problem can be solved by bits of tape on just two keys. The *f* and *j* keys are often used. Another possibility is *d* and *k*. Either of these pairs of letters provides a convenient guide for each hand on the home row. In selecting which keys to mark, check whether there might be tactual markings already on a computer which the student may use; be consistent if possible.

POSTURE AND FINGER ACTION

Standard Fingering

Use of standard fingering is essential. If the student is allowed to be inconsistent, he or she will never develop maximum accuracy and speed, and will have trouble in a formal typing class. If a younger child with a small hand seems really unable to manage standard fingering for certain keys, work out a compromise that is as close as possible to the standard fingering, and plan to reteach in the standard way later. For example, the child might move his entire hand to the top row when striking numerals, but nevertheless use the correct fingers. Make sure the student understands *why* standard fingering is so important: it is essential for consistency, speed, and efficiency.

After teaching the eight keys of the basic home row position, explain each reach as you come to it during your course of instruction. Have the student gently touch back and forth with the correct finger–*juj, ded,* etc. For the more distant reaches it is desirable to touch another key on the way–e.g., *ju7.* Encourage the student to touch that intermediate key each time until he no longer needs the extra guide. Emphasize staying in touch with the home row position, keeping at least one finger on each hand there as much as possible.

The fully- or partially-sighted student who types from print should keep his eyes on the copy. With the totally blind student there is no question of looking at the fingers visually. But when the student does not use print as typing copy, yet can see his fingers and perhaps the printed labels on the keys (especially if he bends over), how do we make sure that he memorizes and develops real touch-typing techniques? The best solution is to use sleepshades during lessons, and insist that everything be done by touch. As discussed elsewhere in this book, this is the only really effective way to teach alternative techniques.

General Posture and Arrangements

If the forearms are not approximately parallel to the slant of the keyboard, and if the student must reach upward, typing becomes unnecessarily tiring and it is difficult to use the correct touch. Most school desks are poor because a storage space raises the top surface. Computer keyboards are often much too high. Look for a regular typing stand, adjustable seating, or a plain table which is the right height. Watch the student from the side as he sits in the typing position, and see that his forearms are parallel with the keyboard. With suitable seating, you can insist on proper posture and touch. The student should sit up straight, leaning forward slightly. He should be attentive but relaxed, with elbows near the body. Action should be in the fingers, with little movement in the hands and arms.

The wrists and forearms should be kept just *above* the keyboard and the table, never touching. Most students need to be reminded of this frequently.

The beginning student who is blind needs to touch the keys to know where they are, and at first he will not have a light and quick stroking pattern. Therefore, with electric keyboards he will tend to get many unwanted letters at first. In an effort to keep control, he tends to rest his wrists on the typewriter, and has difficulty using proper stroking technique. This is one of the reasons I prefer manual machines at first (if available) for beginners. Another reason is flexibility –sometimes, especially in a home, a manual typewriter may be the only one available.

(Note: For convenience, this chapter will sometimes use the term "electric" to include electric typewriters, electronic machines, and computer keyboards.)

Stroking

Ask the student to listen while you demonstrate correct stroking. Since the touch is quite different from that on a Braillewriter, and since many youngsters experiment with a keyboard informally, you may need to devote considerable emphasis to the correct finger action. Show how fingers should be curved, not flat. Take hold of the student's hands and shape them into position; also let the student feel your fingers.

When starting on an electric keyboard, first have the student examine the machine while it is off; a very young or nervous student may benefit from some "dry-run" stroking practice with the power off. Help the student relax and get over a possible fear that the machine will "run away with him," typing in an uncontrolled manner. Help him to check the home row position (the shift key at the left is a good reference point), and to keep in gentle touch with keys which are not to be struck. Appropriate stroking consists of a gentle tap rather than a push.

Be sure that the little finger is used for the "return" key.

On a manual typewriter, instruct the student to strike each key with a sharp, staccato touch. Explain that one should lift the finger ever so slightly and *strike* rather than push the key. Then one should immediately snap the finger off the key, curving the fingertip more toward the palm as this occurs. If the student has previously used an electric keyboard, give special attention to the shift key; he may have "raised" capitals, since he is used to touching the shift key very lightly. Also instruct him on throwing the carriage manually, and assure him that a vigorous motion won't break anything.

Note differences in key placement between electric keyboards and manual typewriters–notably the underscore, apostrophe, and quotation marks. Late-model keyboards have a numeral "one" at the top left, but on some older models (especially manual typewriters) the lower-case letter *l* is used for the "one." Note that computers do *not* treat the lower-case letter *l* as interchangeable with the "one" key.

CONTROLS, SPACING, AND FORMAT

The blind typist should always check such things as the ribbon control, the line-space regulator, and the margins. Occasional carelessness here would rarely be serious for a sighted typist, but the careless blind person could type many pages with an inappropriate setting.

Margins

To change margins by hand, first move the settings outward as far as they will go. Move the carriage or carrier to a position at the extreme left edge of the paper. (Examine the position of the paper by touch, and look for "card holders" or tabs surrounding the location where the type will strike.) Then space the appropriate distance to the right using the space bar, and set the desired left margin. A similar procedure, in reverse and using the backspacer, is used for setting the right margin; however, five fewer spaces are counted inward, to allow for the bell.

It is not essential that the zero on the printed scale (found on the paper bail and elsewhere) be used as the reference point for the margins used by a blind typist. Suppose, for example, that the paper guide is at *5* on the printed scale, but the blind typist uses that location as zero. It does not really matter, so long as the typist counts correctly from the reference point used. It does matter, of course, if the reference point is so far to the right that normal alignment is impossible, or if the reference point is inadvertently moved during typing.

For most school assignments, a margin of approximately 1" or 1-1/2" on each side is appropriate, and precise counting may be unnecessary.

Tabs

To set tabs, first clear out all old tabs, then count spaces as desired.

Columns may be typed as described in any good typing textbook. Count the longest word or phrase in each column and add the spaces desired between columns (usually six). Having set the left margin as desired, use the space bar to proceed forward according to the number of spaces in the longest line of the first column plus the number of spaces between columns; then set a tab. Count similarly for each succeeding column. Set the bell to ring while the last column is being typed, as a reminder that it is the last.

To center a heading or other single item, use a center tab; backspace once for every two characters (including spaces) in the heading. The Braille reader must remember that this means inkprint characters, not Braille characters. The beginner may use a center tab which has already been placed by the teacher.

Alignment of Various Formats

The advanced student should memorize the spacing characteristics of both elite and pica typewriters, and handle all aspects of centering and spacing. Elite type has 12 letters to the inch, with 102 characters to the line; thus the center point is 51 (usually considered as 50 for convenience). Pica type has 10 letters to the inch, with 85 characters to the line; the center is 42.

If the blind typist is not certain whether the type is pica or elite, this can be checked by placing the card holders at the left edge of the paper and then counting across to see whether there are 102 or 85 spaces. Such counting can also be used to establish a center point for a tab – note that this can be done even on nonstandard-sized paper, cards, or envelopes. It can also be used if variations in type font cause the regular line to be neither 102 nor 85 spaces.

An outline may be typed by setting appropriate tabs. In this, as in all matters of spacing, the blind student must have specific spacing methods, although the sighted teacher may be accustomed to judging "what looks right" visually. Vertically, there are 6 line spaces to the inch on all pica and elite machines, with 66 lines to the 8-1/2" x 11" sheet. On most models, typing would occur on line #3 if the top edge of the paper were even with the top of the card holders, and on line #6 if the paper were even with the paper bail. By understanding this kind of thing, it is possible to plan vertical centering and arrangements. If the typist begins on line #6 and ends at line #60, there will be one-inch vertical margins. It is important to remember whether the line spacer is set on single or double spacing, and to realize that on many models we may hear *two* "clicks" for each line space.

End of Page

There are many ways to anticipate the end of a page.

Look for a way to compare the top of the paper with some part of the machine. Perhaps as the typist nears the end, the top of the paper will touch the table or reach a certain place on the back of the typewriter. Tape can be placed on the back of the machine at the appropriate place. On a portable typewriter, the top of the page may touch the table long before the page is full; but it is also possible to check length by pulling the top of the paper *forward* to see how far it reaches in front.

Another approach is to use a sturdy backing sheet with a tag of paper extending out to one side for approximately the bottom two inches. The student can then check for the tag when he nears the end. He must understand how the paper feeds, in order to avoid typing on the backing sheet.

Many late-model typewriters have an automatic end-of-page warning.

Footnotes, Superscripts, and Subscripts

When the blind student has a method for determining where the page should end, he can also learn to type footnotes at the bottom of the page if desired. As explained in any typing textbook, one should allow approximately three lines for each footnote, and three lines for the divider with its surrounding blank lines. The blind student, as well as the sighted, must keep track and anticipate this; when the one-inch bottom margin is reached, it is too late to type a footnote. If there are a great many footnotes, it may be worthwhile to place more than one tape guide on the back of the typewriter. If a backing sheet with a tag is used, there might be a longer tag, perhaps with raised guidelines at intervals.

Today "run-in" references within the text, and end-note pages at the end of a chapter, are often used as alternatives to traditional footnotes. Nevertheless, the blind student should learn all methods that the other students learn. If a given format is preferred by a college professor or a business establishment, the blind typist should be prepared to use it.

If the machine has two definite "clicks" per line of typing as the paper rolls, this makes typing superscripts and subscripts easy. The typist simply moves the paper one "click" up or down, as appropriate, and then moves it back after typing the superscript or subscript. Another method is to make careful use of the control which temporarily releases the line spacing and then returns it to the same position.

THE IMPORTANCE OF FLEXIBILITY

Computers and late-model typewriters will do many things automatically. However, even if your student has a model with all the latest devices and indicators, he should also learn alternatives which will work on an older model. The latest model will not always be readily available. Also, sometimes an automatic feature cannot be used by a blind person independently (especially a beginner).

Handling Materials

The beginner must have at least enough organization to avoid reusing the same sheet and typing over his own work. (He should sort papers appropriately and also realize that it is possible to feel whether or not a sheet has been typed on.) The advanced student can keep track of several kinds of paper; type envelopes; align letterhead paper; use multicopy paper; fill in blanks in printed forms; etc.

Note the way the paper feeds in – the reverse of the way it feeds into the Brailler. Show the beginner where the top front of the paper is when it is first inserted, and how it travels until the paper is removed. Although reinserting to continue typing is to be avoided if possible, it is desirable to know how it can be done: Stop at a good stopping place – the end of a paragraph or section. Remove the paper by turning the knob or indexing slowly enough to count the lines to the top of the page. Keep track of the top front of the paper. Then upon reinsertion, be sure that the margins are the same; count lines down to the stopping place; and line space appropriately.

See that your student understands the orientation of such things as letterhead paper and envelopes, and that he is organized to find clean paper reliably and efficiently. Labeled file folders, boxes, drawers, etc., can be used. The spacing of letterhead paper and of envelopes can be analyzed. If there is a need to fill in blanks, the student can use sighted assistance to make Braille notes or memorize the horizontal and vertical spacing for each blank, and thereafter can work independently.

If the student keeps track of the orientation of printed matter, there should be no problem with using a photocopier. Bits of tape or other simple tactual guides may be placed on the copier if necessary for correct alignment of copy.

Accuracy and Speed

According to keyboarding textbooks, common causes for inaccuracies are faulty stroking (including inconsistent fingering); uneven rhythm; tiredness and tension; incorrect use of controls and devices; poor understanding of the location of keys; and typing too fast for one's skill. The best way to build accuracy for any typist, blind or sighted, is to *prevent* errors by building good habits.

The beginner should ignore errors completely, or merely retype the word. When the more advanced typist is pushing hard to develop higher speed, it is desirable to ignore errors for a time as well. Most learners experience "plateaus" – that is, (1) the student raises his speed (e.g., to 40 wpm), but errors rise with it; (2) the student is unable to type faster, but does improve his accuracy at 40 wpm; (3) after some time on this "plateau," the student again raises his speed, again with accompanying increased errors at first.

Computers make corrections with a simple keystroke. Late-model typewriters have a "delete" key or a white correction ribbon. (The blind typist needs to anticipate when the correction cartridge will run out, and know how to replace it.)

However, it is also important to know a correction method which can be used even with older models. When the young beginner has learned most of the letters, he can start to cross out errors with x's on a typewriter. A more advanced student can remove errors with correction paper such as Ko-Rec-Type. Insert a piece of correction paper behind the card holders, backspace, and type the wrong letter again – now in white to cover the error. (It may be wise to strike the wrong letter twice, moving the correction paper slightly between times, to ensure a neat correction.) Then remove the correction paper, backspace again, and type the right letter. It is often wise to backspace once more and type the right letter an extra time to be sure it is dark enough.

The blind typist should keep correction paper available by placing it in a pocket on the typewriter or by carrying it in notebook or bag. The student must keep track of which side has the white powder, rotate it to avoid reusing the same spot, and discard each piece before it becomes badly worn.

"But how will I know when the letter is wrong?" your student may ask. Again, the most important factor is *prevention* of errors by building good habits. In addition, most errors are conscious ones–i.e., immediately after the wrong key has been struck, the typist realizes that an error has been made. The blind typist must develop this sensitivity to the fullest.

Especially at first, a sighted person will proofread the work. But help your student to decrease dependence on this as a method for correction. Too often the student is actually rewarded for not catching errors as he makes them: if they are still there when the paper is done, someone else makes the corrections in ink!

One way out of this trap is requiring the student to retype the paper if there are more than a certain number of errors.

If this is too demanding for a young beginner, a standard might be applied to each paragraph separately. If only certain paragraphs need to be retyped, the page could be cut and patched. However, this piecemeal approach is not appropriate for an older, experienced student.

I recall many a student whose improvement was truly phenomenal when required to retype a paper.

Some electronic models will "beep" when an internal computer recognizes a word as "possibly" misspelled. This is a mixed blessing. It may help a student overcome constant dependence on a sighted proofreader. On the other hand, there often are "beeps" for things which are not actually misspelled–proper names, compound words, animal sounds, etc. There are many errors which are not caught–substituting "there" for "their," omitting a word, etc. See that your student works without this feature much of the time.

If a device is available which speaks each word or letter aloud, use it only occasionally. It may be helpful (though not essential) to a beginner first learning the letters. The advanced student will sometimes use it for checking. But to use such a device continually is to prevent normal stroking and normal speed. Dependence will prevent the student from using other models.

Similarly, do not let your student assume that he can only prepare accurate copy if there is a Braille printout. While computer systems which provide both print and Braille can be valuable, they are not necessary for accurate work. If overused, they are very restricting: the student believes he can work only in one place and with one kind of equipment.

Typing from Copy

INKPRINT COPY

If the student usually reads print, it is very important that the copy be easily seen while typing. The student who usually reads small print will probably need large print. Be creative if a large-print book will not fit into a standard book holder; in a pinch, a metal cookie sheet from the kitchen will often do for holding the book.

If large print cannot be seen in the standard position, there are various special stands with extensions to bring it closer to the eyes.

USING RECORDED COPY

If it is difficult for the student to read printed copy even with special arrangements, he should learn to type from recordings. Outside the school setting, large-print copy will rarely be available.

Recorded copy, of course, is also suitable for totally blind typists. Recorded copies of regular typing texts are increasingly available, as are various dictating machines.

It is vital that the machine have a foot pedal, so that the hands need not be taken off the keyboard to operate the tape machine. The foot pedal *must not cause any words to be lost,* and must play the tape both forward and backward. Variable speed is also important. (I have seen some foot pedals which were designed for use with special tape machines for the blind and which did not have these features which are essential for use in typing.) Any regular dictating machine should be appropriate.

Today most dictating machines use regular cassette tapes.

In individualized lessons, you may often dictate "live." But an older student should also learn to type from printed copy or from recordings, as these skills are different from those used with live dictation. In using a tape, the student must adjust the speed, stop or repeat if necessary, etc. When a taped lesson is interrupted, the student must make a note of where he left off, and should stop at the end of a sentence if possible–preferably the end of a paragraph or the end of a page.

You may find it helpful to make a simplified recording to help your student get started: spell out many words; repeat sentences so the student need not do any rewinding; dictate slowly; use very easy copy; etc. Gradually increase the difficulty until the student can use regular recorded copy.

If you prepare regular recorded copy, observe these conventions:

- Spell out all proper names and unusual words.
- Indicate capitalization if it is not obvious.
- Pronounce each mark of punctuation. (Especially in repetitive drill, consider saying "sem" for "semicolon," and "open paren" for "open parenthesis.")
- Enunciate very carefully.
- Speak as quickly as is practical for clear enunciation. Beginners' material should be read more slowly.
- If the drill specifies where a new line begins, say "return."
- Watch for context where an actual word might be misunderstood as a command or a mark of punctuation–e.g., "The students will *return* for the last class *period.*" One solution is to spell out any such words instead of pronouncing them.
- Format is often illustrated visually in the text. Explain clearly and concisely on the tape.

USING BRAILLE COPY

Beginners may need directed practice in typing from Braille copy. Although this is not a fast way of typing, it is necessary when working from Braille notes or Braille rough drafts.

However, it is *not* appropriate to provide a Brailled typing textbook, since moving the hands off the keyboard prevents speed and fluency. (An exception occurs with a deaf-blind student who cannot use recorded copy.)

Planning Individualized Lessons

APPROPRIATE LESSONS FOR YOUNGER STUDENTS

For students with little or no vision, typing should usually be started in the third or fourth grade, and customarily is taught by the itinerant/resource teacher. With the availability of computers, many children are learning the keyboard as early as first grade.

If you have no textbook designed for elementary school, a junior high text may be used if you go slowly and adapt it.

Twenty- to thirty-minute lessons, at least twice a week, are usually about right for elementary children. If you can only get there once a week, arrange for someone else to drill the child in between times. Although the "home row" may be memorized very quickly, after that a pace of one new letter per week is suggested. Avoid teaching in quick succession any pair of letters which have the same fingering pattern on opposite hands (e.g., *e* and *i* or *q* and *p*).

Do not use up too much time and patience on any one task, such as inserting the paper. If it seems difficult, spend just a few minutes per period on this and then proceed to work on actual typing–even if you must insert the paper for the child. Also work on various parts of the skill, rather than immediately tackling the whole task. For example, at first the child might work on *recognizing* when the paper is straight. The teacher might insert the paper with varying degrees of crookedness, as the youngster evaluates them.

CONTENT OF AN INDIVIDUALIZED COURSE

How much should the individualized course include? Most students at junior high level or younger need all the letters and numerals; the more common punctuation marks and symbols; centering of titles; paragraph indentation; and insertion of the paper. The youngest students can be aware of margins and use a tabulator which is set by the teacher, and later they can learn to set their own. This much instruction enables the student to complete classroom assignments independently.

If your student will soon be taking a regular typing class, *avoid* using the very same text which that class will use.

COMPOSITION AT THE KEYBOARD

Since the blind student will often type words, sentences, and paragraphs directly from his own ideas rather than from copy, it is important to teach composition at the keyboard. Begin by requiring one-word answers to questions. Next, dictate a word and have the student type it in a complete sentence. These kinds of things are typical of regular classroom lessons in spelling and other subjects, and such lessons can often be used for typing practice. Gradually work up to where the student can compose complete paragraphs at the keyboard. (There are times, of course, when a Braille rough draft should be made. But often it is appropriate to compose directly into print.)

The Regular Typing Class

An amazing number of "bugs" can show up when the blind or visually impaired student starts a regular typing class. The large print book may be the wrong edition; it may not fit on the typing stand; it may fit but be too floppy to stay up. A tape-recorded book may neglect to spell difficult words and proper names; may be on a tape incompatible with all available machines; may be the wrong edition. Even if your student usually needs no direct help from you, do some planning for the typing class. The student who ordinarily reads small print may find large print necessary. A student who usually reads print may not be able to read it while sitting in typing posture: in this case, experiment with stands which bring the material up closer, but consider seriously whether recordings would be more efficient.

If tapes will be used, plan carefully with the student and the classroom teacher. During initial lessons when practice selections are short, it may be more efficient to provide an aide to dictate rather than to keep hunting the place on the tape. Go over the tape beforehand yourself so that you can explain how it has been transcribed. You may discover that some of it is unsuitable for your student, and may need to do some alternative taping.

Try out the specific dictating machine that will be used. How do all the controls work? Is the machine compatible with the tapes you have? If not, can they be dubbed into the needed format?

The best way to check for "bugs" is for you to give the student at least one practice lesson before the class starts. Set everything up, with the exact machine, type of copy, location, etc., and proceed as though class were in session.

What keyboard should be used? Usually the same kind that others use. This would include a computer keyboard if it is normally provided. It should be noted that a large-print typewriter has different spacing, and is therefore undesirable for a typing class.

TRANSITION FROM INDIVIDUALIZED TYPING

For those students whom you have already taught individually, it is just as important to plan carefully when he or she approaches the age for regular typing courses. I recall a student, very weak in many skills, who needed all the typing instruction he could get. He almost was excluded from the compulsory introductory course because the counselor assumed I had already covered "everything." Even a student who has done well in individualized typing will find that the regular course is more demanding and covers more material.

Sometimes a student who started typing at a young age asks to be excused from the first few weeks of the regular class, saying it will be too easy. Explain that the class will move at a pace that is unfamiliar, and may use unfamiliar methods. Typing from taped copy may be a new skill. Suggest that the student begin with the class for a few days to see if he is indeed bored–he may be surprised and find himself challenged instead. If he really is bored and doing well, then the teacher could assign some advanced extra-credit work until the class reaches a point which challenges the student. Even in this case the student should continue to do some of the lessons with the class–perhaps every third lesson.

Typing for Other Classes

As soon as the student has learned the alphabet, he should begin using the skill to type some lessons in other subjects. The high school student usually will immediately find it convenient to type term papers, book reports, etc. The college-bound student will see the value especially clearly. However, for the younger student who writes fairly well with pen and pencil, it may take more planning. Explain that typing can be much faster and easier, especially as assignments get longer in the higher grades. Computer use is a great motivator. Look for a logical place in the curriculum for regular use of keyboarding.

Students with little or no vision usually find typing an immediate boon, as they learn to communicate directly with sighted teachers who do not know Braille; they usually need little urging to make extensive use of typing. However, if all the teachers know Braille, or if a Braillist constantly transcribes the child's Braille into print, the student may wonder, "Why should I bother to type it myself?" The IEP should include gradually broadening expectations for typing regular class lessons. The school day should provide rewarding opportunities for direct written communication with people who do not know Braille.

Even with the student who does not read print, discuss situations where typing is *not* the most efficient mode. For instance, although it might be possible to diagram sentences on the typewriter, it would be so complex that it is far more sensible to dictate answers to a sighted person who will draw the diagram. Another alternative is to type the lesson in another format: e.g., use tabular format with headings for the parts of speech, and with an explanation of what modifies what.

Also, in making a rough draft or study guide for the student's *own use,* Braille or tape is called for.

Note that making a final copy from a rough draft is one of the situations where typing from Braille copy can be a good idea. Another is in doing assignments from a Braille textbook–using spelling words in sentences, listing all the nouns in a paragraph, or otherwise answering questions. A magnet, paper clip, or other method to keep the place on the Braille page is often helpful.

PHASING IN TYPING FOR YOUNGER STUDENTS

When a third- or fourth-grade child who has previously used only Braille is ready to start typing, it is a cause for celebration. No longer need his answers be transcribed or read aloud. They can be directly read by any teacher. Without careful planning, however, enthusiasm can easily become misery.

The classroom teacher may despair at continual technical problems. The child may feel overwhelmed and balk at assignments which he did easily in Braille. These problems are minimized by a carefully planned approach. The paper below describes such a transition, and is written in a form to be distributed to teachers:

STARTING TYPING FOR NED

Ned has now learned the alphabet on the typewriter. He is eager to begin using this skill in his class assignments, but there will be some things he is not yet able to handle on the typewriter. I have written these remarks which I hope will be helpful as he gets started.

(1) The Language lesson, with its short answers, seems to be a good place for the first typing experience. When he is comfortable with typing the entire Language lesson regularly, let's talk about where to start next. I would like to have him do a sample lesson with me before he starts in the classroom.

(2) Ned cannot yet type numerals. Therefore he should not type any math as yet. When numbers appear in other assignments, try these ideas to avoid asking him to type numerals:

- He might spell out the number.
- If there are two or more short answers for one item, he might keep them all on the same line.
- He could use extra line spaces to indicate a major break in format.

(3) If you run into something else Ned cannot yet type, work out a way to handle it temporarily and ask me to teach him as soon as possible.

(4) He can cross out errors with x's. Later he will learn another method for correction.

(5) In Braille, certain words are ordinarily written in a shorter form rather than being fully spelled out. However, Ned understands this difference and uses standard inkprint spelling on the typewriter.

(6) With the keyboard at the correct height, Ned's forearms should be approximately parallel to the slant of the keyboard, and his elbows should be approximately at his waist. He should *not* let his wrists or arms lean on the typewriter or the table while typing.

(7) If the present location of the typewriter in the classroom does not work out, let me know. We may need to figure out a different arrangement.

(8) There is a supply of paper in the drawer in the typing table.

(9) When working from a Braille copy, have him use the magnet on the Braille (with the metal sheet under the page) to keep the place.

(10) Be liberal at first with help when he makes mistakes. Give him hints as he goes along ("You're forgetting your capitals.") It may be appropriate to give him a second chance at accuracy, and for the teacher to pencil in some corrections ("I think you forgot about capitals. I will reread these sentences aloud, and you tell me which words should have capitals.") In time we will tighten our standards.

(11) If a lesson is long, have him type only part of it. (Later we will expect more.) The rest could be completed in Braille or done orally.

(12) Please keep me advised of problems. I will be glad to sit with Ned in the classroom from time to time if that is helpful.

Common Weak Spots and How to Prevent Them

Recently two sixth-grade students, from two different highly-regarded programs for blind children, transferred to their neighborhood schools. Both had records stating that they knew how to type. But both had the same incredible lacks: They used non-standard fingering on the numerals, and they could not type any punctuation except apostrophe, period, and comma. What had they been doing with questions and with quotes? What about hyphenated words? How had they underlined? Why were they not expected to learn standard fingering for numerals?

These limitations on typing instruction for blind youngsters are unnecessary and inexcusable, but widespread. Both of the above students had been typing for at least two years, could easily reach all the keys, and believed that they knew all they needed to know. Apparently they had only been expected to type limited kinds of material–again, a matter of attitudes about what blind students are capable of doing.

Another common weak spot is overemphasis on one kind of copy, regardless of suitability for the individual. An adjustable stand for large print is fine for students who merely need to have the copy somewhat higher and closer and then can read it easily. However, I have seen students trying to type from large print they could barely make out, placed awkwardly a couple of inches in front of their faces. They spent so much effort in keeping the copy in just the right position, and in trying to make it out, that they had little energy left for good typing. They should have been using recordings.

BAD HABITS

Another common weak spot is the toleration of bad habits which would never be permitted in a regular typing class. This need not occur if the teacher expects blind students to achieve as well as others, and makes only *appropriate* and *temporary* allowances for small hands.

Start out by *preventing* bad habits, through teaching good technique:

- Use correct fingering.
- Adjust seating so that the keyboard is at the proper height (arms parallel to the slant of the keyboard, student not reaching far up).
- Sit up straight, leaning forward slightly.
- Keep arms close to the sides of the body, elbows in.
- Keep feet flat on the floor.
- Do not rest wrists on the machine or table.
- Develop a clear, crisp touch.

Ask the high-school typing instructor to explain how he/she helps students build correct posture and stroking. Observe some sessions of the beginning typing class.

Place no emphasis on speed at first. Speed will come with experience, confidence, and good habits. Similarly, at first make no corrections of errors, except to retype as necessary. As you later begin to time certain selections and to teach how to make corrections, emphasize either speed *or* accuracy in any particular assignment. Still later the advanced student will be able to "put it all together."

Since typing is such an advantage to the young blind child, we are sometimes faced with the dilemma of adapting standard fingering for a small hand. If the child uses a position other than the standard "home row" position–e.g., moving the hands entirely up onto the top row when typing a number–insist that he use the correct fingering. This will minimize the difficulty of converting to a standard reach later. Similarly, if a student insists he cannot strike certain letters without curling up other fingers, insist that he use the standard finger, and gradually work him into the standard hand position.

OVERDEPENDENCE ON ONE MODEL

Always give a beginner experience on at least two different keyboards, even if the differences are slight. Flexibility is vital. An advanced student should know how to use electric typewriters, electronic typewriters, and computer keyboards – both "bare-bones" models and those with special features. Too many blind students (and their teachers and parents) assume they will have great difficulty using a model without features of automatic delete, centering, spelling check, end-of-page indication, etc. Worse still is dependence on a computer system which provides simultaneous copy in Braille and inkprint.

Partially-sighted students may not realize they can use a small-print typewriter.

There are some special features which are not only nonessential but actually undesirable. Braille labels on all keys, for example, interfere with normal stroking and full memorization. Worse still is a feature which always speaks each letter or word aloud as it is typed. Features such as these can be useful under certain circumstances, but should *not* become routine.

Multiply Handicapped Students

Don't give up if your student has other disabilities besides blindness. Talk with someone knowledgeable about the other problem(s) – probably an occupational therapist. Be sure that *each* of you corrects any misconceptions about the limitations of each disability. Be creative. Ask about keyboard shields (which make the keys recessed rather than raised), adaptations for missing fingers, etc.

Problems in Motivation

Most students enjoy typing as a "grown-up" skill and a welcome diversion. Braille students are excited at communicating directly in print. However, there are of course some students who resist learning, and others who want to rush along without concentrating on proper technique.

When I taught second grade, the student teachers who worked with me tended to say, "Jimmy, be quiet ... Jimmy, stop talking ... Jimmy, I've asked you to quit that ... Jimmy ..." on and on and on. I learned to insist that they *act* (as opposed to merely talking) on the second or third warning, as: "Jimmy, no more talking....Jimmy....Jimmy, take your book to the side table and work there, please." The difference in response, for both Jimmy and the other students, was striking.

We need to take the same approach in teaching individualized typing. It is not productive to nag endlessly, "Don't rest your wrist on the keyboard ... wrist up ... don't lean ... remember ... don't lean ..." Instead we can say, "Wrists up ... Don't rest your wrist on the keyboard surface ... Retype that line, please, until I see that your wrists do not touch anything." Or, the teacher may simply tap the student's arm gently.

For general motivation, try to find results that matter to the student. Would typing a book report be faster? Is there a routine assignment that might seem more interesting if typed? Would he like to visit the high-school typing class? How would typing be helpful in his chosen vocational goal?

Make use of "the carrot and the stick," with advice from a counselor or psychologist in difficult cases. Two of my students, for very different reasons, have responded well to the simple device of playing a short table game each time they learned five new letters. One was a low achiever who detested all schoolwork. The other was bored and frustrated because a previous teacher had taught him half the keyboard, and then, due to scheduling problems, allowed him to forget so much that I had to start all over.

Related Chapters

The chapter on "Computers" is closely related to this one. Also, "General Classroom Arrangements and Study Skills" discusses how the student can select a mode in which to prepare a written assignment, proceed independently, and receive feedback.

The Importance of Monitoring

Remember those transfer students who could type correctly only on the letter keys? It is possible that they *were* taught the numerals and punctuation marks, and then were promptly allowed to forget. After completing regular typing lessons for a particular student, plan in some detail how skill will be maintained. See that the Braille student uses typing in all appropriate situations (working up to it gradually). Watch for new formats such as tables. For the student who uses handwriting, make sure that certain assignments will be typed. Continue to observe both the accuracy of the typed material and the maintenance of proper technique. Occasional "brush-up" lessons are important.

CHAPTER 30

NOTE-TAKING

Class Notes

AN EFFICIENT METHOD IS ESSENTIAL

By the intermediate grades, the student should be proficient in using the slate and stylus, which can be carried in the pocket or purse and used as the equivalent of pencil and paper. The advanced student may wish to learn a form of Braille with many added contractions, such as Grade III. (Note, however, that this is not advisable until the student has been using Grade II comfortably for at least two years; otherwise confusion will result.) Courses in condensed Braille are available free from the Hadley correspondence school.

If a partially sighted student complains that she cannot read notes taken with a dark pen or pencil, this indicates she should be learning Braille.

It might appear that tape-recording lectures would be ideal for blind students, but actually this is *extremely* inefficient. Twenty hours of lectures, tape recorded, become 20 hours of tape–no summarizing has been done–and studying for a test would require going through all 20 hours again. The blind student should be given regular instruction in note-taking, learning how to take down the key points in brief form. Then the blind student can refer to efficient notes.

Learning How

Students often complain, "I can't write fast enough," when actually they are trying to write too many things or the wrong things. Give your student plenty of instruction in *how* to take notes.

This is the same skill for blind students as for the sighted, but too often it is assumed to exist without real instruction. In the early grades youngsters are constantly chided to spell every word correctly, be neat, use correct punctuation, etc. Suddenly in the higher grades we expect them to know (by osmosis?) that note-taking is best done by writing only essential words, with abbreviated spelling and only as much neatness as it takes to read one's own notes.

Every student should be able to recognize main ideas, note them down in the briefest appropriate form, and do so while the speaker continues to talk. (In taking notes from a tape, there is the option to stop the tape, but the student must be taught when to do that also.)

Seek out books or lessons which teach various aspects of note-taking–finding the main ideas, finding topic sentences, writing summaries, etc. Invent your own exercises. Simulate a classroom situation in your individual lessons: for example, give a brief talk (or read a brief selection) without stopping, while the student takes notes. Start by using selections which have very obvious main ideas.

Condensing

A ninth-grade student wrote fairly well on the slate but could not seem to take class notes. "Let's see a sample of how you take notes," said the itinerant teacher. "I'll pretend I am your French teacher, and I'll explain a homework assignment."

Several minutes later, the student had written:

French assignment: Read pages 13 through 20. Answer all the questions on page 20. This is due Friday, April 15. Be careful of spelling.

All of this was written in perfect Grade II Braille, with complete capitalization and punctuation.

"There are many kinds of writing," began the Braille teacher as she discussed the difference between verbatim transcription and personal note-taking. Tactfully she pointed out:

- It is, of course, necessary to indicate the subject or book title. However, a short abbreviation should be enough. When there is no formal Braille short form, make one up.
- The page numbers can be abbreviated to "13-20" by using the hyphen. The word "pages" can be abbreviated as "pp" or even omitted.
- If every chapter has questions on the last page, the word "questions" will suffice. Even that word may be unnecessary if it is customary to answer the questions.
- The date due is essential. However, why write *both* the day of the week and the calendar date? And why write the word *due?*
- Normally it is not necessary to write down routine cautions such as "Be careful of spelling." That should be assumed.
- Do not write complete sentences. Use only enough punctuation and capitalization to make the note clear. Note that Braille capitalization adds a dot.

Eventually a reduced note was developed:

---

fch 13-20 with questions, 15th

This second note is even shorter in Braille than it appears in print, because *with* and *question* have special signs.

The Classroom Teacher's Presentation

To make explanations clear to the blind boy or girl, the classroom teacher may verbalize things which otherwise might have been presented visually only. For example, one might say, "This worm is usually about four inches long," rather than, "It's about this long." One may speak a formula aloud as well as writing it on the board. This often has the pleasant result of making explanations clearer or more compelling to the sighted students as well. The classroom teacher should *not* feel, however, that he/she must overhaul the entire vocabulary and make sweeping changes in the manner of presentation.

Material on the Chalkboard

Although telescopic lenses are sometimes suggested for seeing the chalkboard, these rarely are very helpful. Usually the individual can see only a few letters at a time, with considerable effort, so that the method is far less efficient than those described below.

If important material appears on the chalkboard and is not discussed aloud, several alternatives exist. Sometimes the teacher or an aide can provide a printed copy to be read aloud at a suitable time. A reliable classmate may be supplied with self-carboning paper and asked to make a duplicate copy. If the item is very short, a congenial classmate might read it aloud during class. Longer presentations might be read aloud before or after class. In certain situations, the material might be Brailled beforehand so that the blind student may follow her own copy in class. (A word of caution: The blind student should need sighted assistance only for reading or copying *written* material. With oral lectures, there is no reason for the blind student to use someone else's notes.)

As the student matures, she should take more and more responsibility for making arrangements and for asking appropriate questions if she does not understand.

Research Notes

When notes are taken from a book (print, Braille, tape, or read aloud), the tendency is to copy complete sentences or phrases. Many students (blind or sighted) have no idea how else to do it. When cautioned not to "copy," they simply take sentences or phrases here and there, and move them around.

Below is the procedure which I teach my students. (I often write this formula down and ask aides to see that students follow it.)

(1) Read a passage that is not too short. For a beginner, an adult should give specific guidance on the length. The passage should be long enough to contain one or two main ideas, but not too many.

(2) Close the book or stop the tape, and *do not* look back while summarizing.

(3) (For beginners only) Summarize the main point(s) aloud to the satisfaction of the adult who is helping. (This step should be dropped as soon as possible, but can be important at first.)

(4) Write the main point(s).

   a. Use condensed note format rather than whole sentences. This greatly cuts the likelihood of using the author's exact wording.

   b. With a beginner, the teacher may need to set an arbitrary limit of one or two notes per passage. Otherwise the student may write down everything he can remember instead of just the main ideas.

   c. Particularly avoid a habit of routinely writing down the last sentence of the passage, since it probably can be remembered verbatim and is especially tempting.

(5) It *is* all right to copy the *spelling* of key terms or proper names. However, the student should make the notes for the passage *before* looking up any specialized spelling. Avoid expanding into copying many words and phrases.

(6) Repeat the above steps until the entire selection has been read.

(7) Follow the above procedure for as many references as desired, *without* starting to compose the research paper.

(8) Make an outline, still without any actual composition. Decide which notes go with which outline points. (Notes on cards are good, since they can be physically moved around.) Emphasize combining notes which came from different sources but relate to the same point.

(9) Using the notes and one's own general understanding, compose a rough draft. Consciously avoid trying to remember the exact wording in an original source. Concentrate on ideas.

(10) Revise as necessary.

(11) Prepare the final copy to hand in.

As each student gains experience, of course, the procedure is modified. As soon as possible, drop the step of summarizing aloud to someone else (or use it only occasionally).

As time goes on, the student will develop her own style and methods for research.

The Notebook

Tina's notebook was always too full. She hunted through many Braille pages to find the one she wanted. Typed assignments were often late because she could not find them.

The new resource teacher helped Tina make notebook dividers with Brailled tabs. A separate folder was carried for algebra, where notes and papers were especially copious. All inkprint papers were to be labeled in Braille and sorted carefully. Each Friday Tina was required to sort through her notebook, remove any papers no longer current, and discard or store them appropriately. Teachers were asked not to give Tina any more time extensions for misplaced papers.

Following is a partial summary of ideas for notebook organization:

- Divider tabs, manila folders, etc., can be easily Brailled. If the item cannot be placed in the Braillewriter, use the slate, or stick a label on.
- Typed assignments, inkprint handouts, etc., can be labeled in Braille. Simply insert the page (or several pages together) into the Braillewriter or slate. Write the simplest label that will suffice (often a letter or two), preferably where it will not distort the inkprint. Alternatively, attach a 3x5" card which is labeled in Braille. If the student routinely does this when she receives or types a paper, she can identify each easily. There are, of course, situations where such labels are unnecessary, but too many blind students never use labels.
- If an inexperienced student has great difficulty with a loose-leaf notebook, consider enlarging the holes at first. This should not be necessary indefinitely unless there is a physical handicap.
- A small notebook can be a helpful supplement to a larger one. For example, the American Printing House for the Blind (APH) offers a pocket notebook which contains a small Braille slate and is just the right size for short, current notes.
- Notebooks for 11" x 11-1/2" Braille paper are available from APH. However, consider using 8-1/2" x 11" Braille paper, which fits into a standard, smaller notebook.
- Many students prefer folders rather than a divided notebook. For each class, only the appropriate labeled folder need be used. For this system, one must have a bag or briefcase of suitable size to accommodate the folders without their slipping around. Folders should be kept in a certain order for easy selection.
- There are many ways to label folders. Partially sighted students may find color-coding convenient. Different textures are also a possibility. Finding a folder quickly can make a great difference in efficiency.
- Use pockets to maximize the sorting potential of folders. For example, Braille papers might be kept on one side of a pocket folder and print on the other.
- Remember that materials for different classes may be organized in different ways.
- For loose items such as stylus and pen, consider a zippered plastic pouch in the notebook.

A strong necessity for organization may not be apparent until junior high. However, that is much too late to begin. Even a first grader can get the right book, label her papers, and keep track of most materials.

If the student is blind and disorganized, don't let everyone assume she is disorganized *because* she is blind. Think, "How would we help this student become more organized if she were not blind?"

CHAPTER 31

MAPS
PICTURES
AND OTHER
"VISUAL AIDS"

How Helpful Would It Be?

When I first started teaching blind children, I collected toy animals and other models avidly. "The sighted children see pictures," I thought, "and my blind students should have the same thing in three dimensions."

Some of those models have been very helpful. There are other tactual aids which I wish I had. But I now realize that I was a bit carried away in acquiring objects that I never use, and some that are really hard to learn from by touch. Small, delicate items are hard to show to a young child, and the older student probably no longer needs the experience. I now collect only the models most often used–items featured in the curriculum for the primary grades (e.g., birds for the *Patterns* preprimers), and hard-to-find items which can readily be appreciated by touch (e.g., a starfish). I also keep track of where collections of touchables may be found: media centers, children's museums, universities, etc.

Emphasize to classroom teachers that it is *not* necessary to provide everything in tactual form. The younger the child, and the newer the concept, the more important it is to have something concrete. But frequently it is not only unnecessary, but undesirably time-consuming, to try to show everything tactually. If the child understands what birds are like in general, an eagle can be described verbally.

Blind students do need to learn the concepts that others learn through vision. But judgment must be used regarding the importance of each visual aid. Do not automatically assume that the best plan always is for the Braille student to have a tactual model, and for the partially-sighted student to examine the item visually at close range.

A kindergartner may want to climb on the teacher's lap whenever a story is read. On the other hand, a teenager may vehemently prefer to sit with his class in the auditorium, even though he could see the performers from the front row. The same teenager may want to sit at the back of the classroom where he cannot see the chalkboard well. We suggest that the student be permitted to sit with his class in the auditorium if he prefers, where the program is not a detailed academic lesson, but be required to sit at the front in the classroom if he can see the board well there. The kindergartner should remain in her place (near the teacher but not on her lap), whether she has little vision or none at all, and should wait for the book to be shown to her.

Films, Pictures, Displays

Often a visual presentation becomes an oral presentation in the process of discussion, and there is no problem. Also, many times it does not really matter whether the blind student examines a display which reinforces a concept already taught.

When it is important that a student learn from a particular picture, then a model, raised diagram, or live specimen may be provided if practical. Three-dimensional representations are often available from the regular school media center. However, often the best way is for a sighted person (possibly a classmate) to describe the picture, with explanation or comparison to develop concepts if necessary.

Usually a film or filmstrip will be well narrated. If not, someone should be available to provide a quiet description. A student above grade school should be consulted about whether additional narration is wanted.

Tell the blind student the location of such things as the movie screen or the Flag, so that he/she may face the right way. Many a blind person has been embarrassed by carefully facing toward the source of the sound, only to learn later that it was a loudspeaker at the back of the room!

Tables, Graphs, and Mathematical Diagrams

The chapter on "Mathematics" contains suggestions about the construction and use of tables and graphs. Mathematical diagrams are also discussed in that chapter. Those suggestions, however, can be used for any class.

Presentations on the chalkboard or Overhead Projector often can be handled orally; see the chapter on "Note-Taking" for additional suggestions. The chapters on "Art" and "Science" also contain comments about visual displays.

The *Tactile Graphics Guidebook*, by John L. Barth, is a valuable reference.

Using Maps

PARTIALLY-SIGHTED STUDENTS

The student with some useful sight will probably make maximum use of it in map work. Use large, clear maps and keep them as uncluttered as possible. Experiment with magnifiers and various kinds of markers. If a closed-circuit television is available (see "Other Modes of Reading"), this may be one of its best uses. The student may be able to use sight profitably for map work even though he/she does not ordinarily read inkprint.

At the same time, students who ordinarily use regular print may have trouble reading detailed maps, and find magnification helpful.

THE BEGINNER

The young student who is forming concepts of geography must have maps and globes he/she can use. If print is not appropriate, Braille maps and globes should be provided. Some are available from the American Printing House for the Blind (APH) and other sources.

APH has recently developed a number of helpful kits and booklets for teaching map reading. However, as of this writing, APH seems actually to be *decreasing* its production of regular Braille maps of actual places – despite the importance of these materials and despite the fact that few are available elsewhere. This is a most unfortunate trend, to which consumers should object strongly.

Do not assume that when a geography book is transcribed, the maps will be included in usable form. Tapes generally omit maps altogether. A large print book will have the maps, but they will be black-and-white and often of very poor quality. A book ordered in Braille (even one actually entitled "Map Study") may or may not contain real, usable maps. Often only the text will have been transcribed. Until better technology and/or greater attention to the importance of maps solves this problem, you will often need to compensate for this problem.

An ordinary relief map may be satisfactory for some purposes.

Among the many advantages of the *Patterns* Braille reading series is its beginning map work. Map-skills workbooks for the sighted can also be transcribed into Braille.

The regular reading-readiness activities may be helpful to the student with poor skills in using his/her hands. After all, if the student cannot easily tell a triangle from a square, or determine which symbol is smaller, then he will not do well with a regular Braille map. Even good Braille readers may do poorly in these skills, and these ideas may be used at any age level.

Consider using selections from Braille reading-readiness books. These usually have many pages of simple raised shapes of various sizes – circles, squares, triangles, etc. There may be several on a page, in various positions. Often these can be used for elementary map practice. Using simple pages of this type, devise basic map-skills lessons, designating symbols as you see fit:

(1) (Several circles in a row horizontally): "These are cities. Show me the city that is farthest east; west."

(2) (Circle, triangle, and square): "This is a map of a park. The circle is a fountain, the triangle an evergreen tree, and the square a flower garden. Look them over and then show me how to walk from the tree to the flower bed *without* getting wet."

(3) (Three triangles of graduated sizes): "The larger the symbol, the larger the city. Show me the largest city; the smallest city."

(4) Attach letter labels to certain shapes, and explain, "*A* is Apple City," etc. Make a Braille key.

Two readiness books I have found especially suitable for this kind of thing are:

A Tactual Road to Reading, Skill Books, Kurzhals and Caton, APH. (Some volumes are better than others for this purpose).

Modern Methods of Teaching Braille, Book 1 (Kansas Braille Reading Readiness Book), Stocker, APH.

THE VALUE OF MAP SKILLS

Map work sometimes prompts the question, "What will she get out of it, anyway?"

Explain that maps teach important concepts which are part of a basic education. Give practical examples. Many jobs require a basic grasp of distances and geographical relationships – a travel agency or an airline; a traveling sales job; a supervisor over a wide area. As a close-to-home example, consider the blind itinerant teacher: he/she must hire and instruct a driver, who may have limited education and be inept at reading a map and using the scale of miles.

APPROPRIATE MAPS

Keeping the map uncluttered is very important. It may be necessary to provide two maps, each with some of the information, instead of one cluttered one. Another useful technique is to provide a very basic Braille or large print map (for instance, just the state boundaries, abbreviated state names, and marks for the capitals), and give other information in a key.

It is often helpful to explain orally while moving the student's hand over a simple political map. ("Look here at the western states. Now, the Rocky Mountains extend all along here .... Actually they start 'way up north in Alaska and Canada, which are clear off the map here ... they extend through Idaho, Montana, Wyoming, Utah, and Colorado ... and on into Arizona and New Mexico, here .... This is the southern border of the United States .... The mountains don't cover *all* of each of those states, and there are valleys in between mountains, but this is the area where the Rockies are. .... Now, I'll show you that once more, and then I'd like you to take your hands clear off the map for a moment and then *you* show *me* the general area where we find the Rockies.")

This same general approach can be used with a very simple large print map if the student cannot see much detail. Because of frequent need for various explanations, some individual attention is usually needed for map work.

CREATIVE IDEAS

For the older student who has already acquired basic geographical concepts, oral discussion alone may be sufficient. ("As you know, the Rocky Mountains appear in the western part of the United States. This chapter expects you to know rather precisely where they are. I will describe the map on Page 35. They begin in Alaska and extend through western Canada, and on through Idaho, Montana....")

What if the assignment is to mark up a map–say, insert the state names and draw rivers? Just as the sighted student will essentially copy the information from a ready-made map, the blind student can examine a Braille map and dictate to a sighted assistant. He might indicate position on a simple, unlabeled raised-outline map, "marking off" each state as he names it, by placing a pin or a bit of tape. (After all, sighted students can easily tell which answers have been given.) An adult might "check off" each answer as it is given, with or without actual transcription onto a printed map. ("I will name several states, and you show me where they are on this raised outline map. Then show me where the Mississippi River runs. You may refer to the Braille atlas.")

More ideas for making and using maps include:

(1) Make a floor plan of the school and a simple map of the student's immediate home neighborhood.

(2) Try to provide a selection of map-skills sheets, plus maps of continents and regions. With a little adaptation and explanation, a basic political map of France can be used for almost any map work about France.

(3) For a general map-skills unit, consider using a ready-made package which is equivalent but not exactly the same. Custom-producing Braille maps for one student is so time-consuming as to warrant the strongest consideration of other alternatives.

(4) For the partially sighted, laminate bold-line outline maps of countries and regions. These can be written or drawn on with china marker or crayon, then wiped off and used again.

(5) Temporary labels can be attached in many ways. Form a short segment of masking tape into a loop, or buy double-stick tape, and apply to the back of a label. Or, attach small "flags" to pins, and tack the map to a soft board. For practice or testing purposes, remove one or more labels and have the student put them back. Or, replace keyed labels with simple numbered labels, and ask the student to tell what each represents.

(6) Braille maps are usually not as precise or uniform as print maps. Often it is unfair to practice with one map and then give a test with a different one. Changing or removing labels, as above, is one way to give a test fairly.

(7) Maps and globes can be obtained from APH or libraries for the blind. They can also be constructed with Plaster of Paris, clay, or papier mache.

(8) Certain maps are so detailed that it is hardly ever worthwhile to custom-produce them in Braille. An example would be topographical maps showing altitude delineations within a small area. If the student does not understand the concept of such a map, try to get a previously-made one of *any* area, to demonstrate the general idea. Then verbally discuss the maps the class is using. Include whatever specific concepts are being taught by the classroom teacher.

(9) Sometimes a complex map is more meaningful if broken down into two or more simpler maps. For example, a state map with a great deal of information might be reproduced as three Braille maps: counties; major cities and highways; and rivers.

(10) Ways to make various kinds of dots include:

- The Perkins Brailler or the slate
- Pushing with either end of a pen or pencil, or with the stylus from a Braille slate, into paper that is on a soft surface
- Gluing on seeds, beads, or other objects

- The Swail Dot Inverter from APH (makes a large dot)

(11) Tactually different lines must be used to show different things (e.g., county lines, roads, rivers). Otherwise, when lines cross on a tactile map, it will be hard to know which line goes where. Various ways to make lines include:
- Any of the above dots in series
- A tracing wheel or wheels – steady or interrupted
- Gluing on string or yarn, cutting the ends with a razor blade for precision

(12) There is a common method of making lines which I have *not* found very satisfactory: trailing "Elmer's Glue," or a similar product, on a line and allowing it to dry. This is difficult to follow by touch, and not very durable. It is far better, and not much more work, to trail the glue into a line and then apply string or yarn.

(13) The Tactile Graphics Kit, from APH, has special symbols such as a print v-shape in raised form. These are applied like Notary seals.

(14) A very durable map, especially suitable for Thermoform, may be made from the special heavy aluminum foil from APH. Any of the above methods, including gluing objects on, can be used with this. Some things are much easier to do with this medium, especially making a "flat" line (comparable to a pencil line, with no interruptions).

(15) Except on the very simplest and most uncluttered maps, labels should be abbreviated and keyed. Try to make the abbreviations logical. For example, *sw* for *swimming pool* and *gf* for *golf course* would be much more easily remembered than an arbitrary *a* and *b*. Save space by using no capital dots.

(16) Graph paper (available from APH with raised lines or bold lines) can be used for practice with latitude and longitude.

(17) Look for easy ways to enlarge a map. A photocopier with enlarging capabilities may produce a suitable map for a large-print user. The enlarged copy may also be traced with feltpen or a tracing wheel (using carbon paper to compensate for reversal with the latter). Alternatively, tape a large piece of paper onto the wall, and use an Opaque Projector to create a very large image. Trace over the image with pencil. Then the paper can be taken down and used to make a bold-line map or a Braille map.

(18) Use reference books such as the *Tactile Graphics Guidebook* from APH. This book gives practical suggestions and shows good and poor examples of Braille maps and tables.

(19) Especially for the beginner, it is helpful for the student actually to face north while studying a map.

When the Blind Student Prepares Visual Aids

"I can give a speech all right, but how on earth can I draw a picture? The teacher says everybody has to have a visual aid!"

This question need not be perplexing if good attitudes and techniques are present. The blind student should, first of all, *decide* herself what display will be prepared.

Then she might work with a sighted assistant to complete the actual preparation – with the blind student continuing to be the one making decisions. The assistant might be directed to cut out and mount pictures, do lettering, draw pictures, etc. Computer graphics may be an alternative also. (Note: If the *purpose* of the activity is the art rather than the oral presentation, an alternative medium should be substituted instead of drawing, and the blind student should be the artist.)

Braille labels will enable the blind speaker to point to things while talking. If the speaker will be holding a chart in front of her, she may prefer upside-down labels just above the corresponding visual item, so that she can read them while pointing to the item in a natural manner.

Mechanical and technical drawing is another situation where the blind student will not be producing a perfect product with his/her own hand. Instead, the blind student should expect (1) to learn the concepts taught by the course, and (2) to know the standard appearance and form of each symbol. This will enable him/her to use a sighted reader (who may have no technical knowledge) to interpret or produce diagrams.

CHAPTER 32

ARTS AND CRAFTS

The student with some useful sight will probably make maximum use of it in art. Even if sight is not efficient for reading print, the student may find it possible to enjoy art visually by using a magnifier or bringing the paper quite close to the eyes. It may be necessary to work to a larger scale than others do, and avoid fine detail.

Making Art Lessons Appropriate

Many good alternatives exist when sight is not used. Clay is an especially obvious one, appropriate for any age. In fact, it is sometimes overused to the point of boredom. Do not make it the only medium for art, and introduce new techniques as the student grows older – glazing, firing, the potter's wheel, etc. Show the blind child techniques which others may pick up by imitation: rolling a ball or snake; decorating with a toothpick; using various tools; etc. Show her how to use her hands.

With paint or glaze, teach the student to apply it in an organized pattern to cover the surface.

Children sometimes fuss about touching certain textures such as paste, clay, or fingerpaint. Try to prevent this problem through early pleasant experiences, or to deal with it through gradual and pleasant conditioning.

Older blind youngsters often become very self-conscious about their art products looking strange or different. Teachers should recognize this as a real problem and avoid embarrassing the young person. In the very earliest grades this is rarely much of a concern. But by the upper grades, the blind student's product may indeed appear quite unusual, depending on the nature of the project and the skill of the individual. It would be most unfortunate if a sensitive junior high student were forced to make a sculptured head independently even though she would have great difficulty aligning the facial features. I would suggest two possible alternatives: (a) someone might work with the student individually, frankly guiding her hands into making a sculpture that is similar to the others; or (b) the student might work on some completely different project which does not involve reproducing a face.

These two alternatives suggest the general ways to prevent embarrassment. If the student cannot make a realistic picture or sculpture on her own, then sometimes the teacher should guide her hand and help her get the concept. But much of the time she should work on her own in media which produce designs or stylized objects rather than realistic pictures.

Usually it is not essential that the blind student's project be as similar as possible to that done by others. If the others are sketching outdoor scenes, there is probably no great need to have the blind student also work with outdoor scenes. One exception to this, however, is the matter of concepts. If the main thrust of the outdoor sketching is to balance the elements of a picture and make a pleasing scene, the blind student might make a collage with good balance. If perspective drawing is being studied, show this to the blind student in raised-line form.

A List of Ideas

There are many especially suitable media – string art, metal sculpture, macrame, leather work, pipe cleaner sculpture, weaving, soap carving, etc. Build a list of clever projects, such as making creatures out of rocks or pebbles, and offer the list to art teachers along with your general suggestions.

Collage (gluing things onto a surface to make a picture or design) is a very good medium. Use things that are really three-dimensional, especially with a young child. A very flat work, with very similar textures (such as different kinds of paper) may not be meaningful. Sort objects into containers for ease of use if they are not easily distinguished by touch. Rolled-up bits of tape can attach things temporarily while the art work is being composed.

Sometimes students draw a picture of a bird or animal, and then cover each part of its body with a different kind of seed. Raised lines between areas enable the blind student to do this independently. The best lines are made with yarn which has been cut with a razor blade, soaked in glue, and allowed to dry in place.

The article, "Craft-Sewing Idea," in the March-May, 1984, issue of *Future Reflections,* describes the use of "plastic canvas." This material, used with yarn, has many possibilities for students of all ability levels.

Be Organized

Avoid letting loose objects roll around on the desk or table. Keep crayons or chalk in a box. Have another box for scraps when cutting. Avoid confusing clutter. Can some parts of the project be placed inside the desk while the student is working on other parts?

Crayons, paints, etc., may be labeled in Braille. Sometimes a rubber band or a bit of tape can serve as a "label."

Help the student be independent and organized.

Can a Blind Child Understand Color?

Color theory can be learned by rote, and this involves important practical knowledge for coordinating clothing and household furnishings. If you have a student with good sight for most purposes but a significant deficiency in color vision, this is one situation where he/she may need considerable help. The color-blind child may need to discuss a color wheel or other illustration with someone else in order to understand what is there. Remind the art teacher, also, that the color-blind child will need to have paints or other media labeled or explained so that he/she can choose the color wanted.

"But how can colors *mean* anything to her?" is often asked in regard to the totally blind. The young child can learn by discussion and rote learning, to make many standard color associations – snow is white, grass is green, etc. This is important for understanding everyday conversation and comparisons. As the child grows older, he needs to refine these basic associations – dirty snow is gray or black, dead grass is brown, etc. She also needs to learn about the transparency of air and glass.

Sighted people tend to become too absorbed in the question of "How can she really understand?" Actually, all of us must deal with concepts we cannot fully understand – infinity, for example – and work with them as necessary. Only astronauts and a few others have personally experienced weightlessness; yet all of us can grasp the concept and discuss it intelligently. The young blind child will probably not find colors especially puzzling, but will just accept them as one more thing to learn about. It may be helpful to compare color variations to texture variations. To explain transparency, we might liken it to listening through a curtain, as opposed to listening through a brick wall.

The blind student should choose the colors for her projects, even if she says she does not care. As an adult she will need to decide about colors in clothing and household furnishings.

Drawing and Painting

Realistic Pictures and Sculpture: Blind students, including those with some useful sight, may need to be taught concepts and conventions which others learn by general observation. Examples include:

- Body proportions
- How to show a sky
- Filling the entire space
- Relationships of size and distance
- Perspective drawing

Beyond the early grades, if the student's pictures look greatly different from those of others, it is best to use the alternatives mentioned above – either give considerable direct help to achieve the customary form, or else substitute an abstract design.

Abstract Designs: Expect the student to fill the space and make a real art work rather than just "taking a stab at it." The blind student should learn principles of proportion in space, color, size, etc.

Coloring, Cutting, and Pasting

Coloring: In preschool and the early grades, children are often asked to color a picture – that is, crayon inside the lines of a picture that is already drawn. Often they are also expected to cut out a shape, and perhaps assemble it into a basket or other object. Unfortunately, although this is easy and pleasant for most sighted children, it is often difficult for blind children.

It is possible to make raised-line pictures, label the crayons in Braille, and ask the blind child to do the same task as the others. Raised lines can be made with a tracing wheel, or by gluing on string or yarn, etc. Some raised-line picture books are now available ready-made. One can also make a line with glue and allow it to dry; however, I have found this less satisfactory because the lines are harder to feel.

These activities for the blind child have their place. The child learns what others are doing when they "color." She learns to cover a surface – valuable preparation for painting sculptures in art class, and for finishing furniture in Industrial Arts. She can choose a crayon and cover an entire surface within lines.

Waxy crayon is easiest to feel. Another possibility is to place the paper on a wire screen, so that a roughened texture results during coloring.

A few simple, medium-sized shapes are more satisfactory than a complex picture or a very large surface.

Cutting is, if anything, a more valuable skill, since it will certainly be useful in daily life. One blind adult says, "Because I never learned to wrap packages as a kid, I found myself being embarrassed as a young adult at having to learn to do this. I finally got my mother to teach me when I was in college. She had just always done it for me, until I educated her enough that she understood how ridiculous it was for me not to know how to do such a rudimentary thing."

If a child has some sight, a heavy feltpen line may be satisfactory for cutting. However, for safety reasons, avoid letting the child bring the scissors close to the eyes. If she really would need to do that in order to cut on a bold line, a raised line would be preferable.

Consider simplifying the shape to be cut – e.g., rounding off tricky places.

When using raised lines, the kind made with a tracing wheel is generally the most practical. The younger child can follow a raised line as the fingers of her left hand move just ahead of the scissors in her right hand (or vice versa for left-handed children). In the chapter on "Home Economics and Daily Living Skills," another method of cutting is described. That method is highly desirable for precision in sewing, and may work well for younger children as well.

At first the child will, of course, have to be shown how to hold the scissors. This should be done during the preschool years, but unfortunately often is not. A good first activity is simply snipping at the edge of a firm piece of paper, with the object being merely to place the scissors correctly at right angles to the paper and make a snip. Slightly more difficult steps are (a) to make a snip at or near a raised mark, and (b) to cut a narrow strip of firm paper in two.

One kind of starter scissors has four finger holes so that the teacher's hand can be placed over the child's hand. These are similar to standard scissors, and thus are preferable to the type with a flexible squeeze-type handle. Experiment with different types of scissors. Especially good are the beginning scissors which are plastic except for metal cutting surfaces.

Give attention to position. Almost always (especially if a tactual line is used) it is much better to place the paper on the desk rather than hold it up in the air. Remind the child that turning the paper in various directions can make cutting easier.

Pasting may be difficult at first, partly because paste on the fingers interferes with the sense of touch. Experiment with different types of paste and glue, and try to let the child use the type she prefers. Library paste may be applied with a wooden stick, with fingers wrapped in a paper towel, etc., as well as with fingers alone. Also consider glue dispensers such as Elmer's or a "glue stick."

A Matter of Perspective

In looking at a youngster's total education, it is worthwhile that she learn to cut and to paste, and that she learn to cover a surface with crayon or paint. This is a foundation for industrial arts, home repairs, etc.

However, in considering any one lesson or activity, always look at the purpose and at the child's ability and needs. Often in the early grades, a picture is to be colored as part of a reading lesson – as, "Color all the pictures that have the long *a* sound." In such situations it probably makes more sense for the blind child to work orally or with Braille words. (For example, we could provide the Braille words for the pictures, and she could mark the long *a* words. Alternatively, we could give her the choices orally.) If variety and enjoyment are the point, it may make more sense to provide a different activity.

In subjects such as social studies, students often give reports which include "visual aids" such as a scene from life in South America. It may not be appropriate for the blind student to attempt to produce these with her own hand. Instead she might direct someone else, telling that person just what is to be drawn and where. Using pictures from a magazine would be another alternative.

When an "art appreciation" class studies famous paintings, this can be handled by verbal discussion in the same way as any other presentation involving pictures.

To those who may say, "She won't get anything out of it anyway," mention the learning of concepts, the value of learning to use the hands in various ways, and the general importance of being in class with others. Blind adults select clothing and household furnishings. Scissors are used to cut string, open packages, etc. Blind parents and teachers direct sighted children in all kinds of art projects.

CHAPTER 33

COMPUTERS

By Curtis Chong
D. Curtis Willoughby
and
Doris M. Willoughby

Note: Curtis Chong is a blind computer analyst, and president of the National Federation of the Blind in Computer Science (NFBCS). D. Curtis Willoughby is a blind electrical engineer, and past president of the NFBCS. In addition to his regular employment with a telephone company, he is also president of Willoughby Enterprises, Inc., a company specializing in computer aids for the blind.

The third grade at Eastridge School eagerly anticipated a six-week "Introduction to Computers." A fund drive was launched to buy a speech-output device for Ashley, a blind student. However, by the time the device was purchased, installed, and working, the project was half over. Furthermore, the device proved impractical for most of the activities because every time Ashley wanted to check any part of the display, she had to listen to the entire screenful. Soon the expensive piece of equipment was gathering dust as the third grade moved on to other units and the computers were used by other grades.

Be sure the device will do what is desired. This problem is discussed in detail throughout this chapter. Since Ashley could not make the computer speak just the desired information, she needed a sighted assistant for most activities anyway. Little was gained.

Be sure you have all the elements needed to make the device work. Is all necessary hardware and software available and compatible? Do you have written references/documentation about each? Is a knowledgeable person available for "trouble-shooting" possible difficulties? Will the same (or compatible) equipment remain available for the foreseeable future? Does your student have the ability to use the equipment independently?

Consider the age of the student and the length/depth of the course. For a young student who will have only short and limited contact with computers anyway, it is usually more practical simply to have a person read the screen aloud to her.

When Ashley reached junior high and registered for a semester of computer science, the old speech device was dusted off. However, it was totally incompatible with the school's new computers.

General Background

The computer has poked its terminal into so many corners of our lives that all of us, including blind citizens, need a basic understanding of computer use. However, this chapter does not attempt to provide a complete education about computers as such. Neither does it go into detail about specific products and brands, since technology changes so rapidly. Rather, the purpose of this chapter is to discuss general principles in the selection and use of computers and computer-related devices for blind students.

Following are definitions of a few basic terms:

Software (also called *programs*): The sequence of instructions needed to make a computer do something.

Hardware: The physical computer, its parts and accessories (usually not including removable disks or tapes on which software is stored).

Input: Information going into a computer or other device.

Output: Information coming from a computer or other device.

Output Device: A piece of equipment which provides the computer output in a particular form (e.g., video screen, speech synthesizer, Braille device, printer).

Speech Synthesizer: A device that converts text transmitted electronically from a computer into speech. This is accomplished by converting a string of text characters into "phonemes" (basic speech sounds) which are then combined to form more or less natural-sounding speech.

Terminal: A device through which a person can both enter data into a computer and receive data from a computer. Typically this is a keyboard and a screen, although it can be a keyboard with either a Braille display or a speech synthesizer.

Display: This term usually refers to the lighted screen which displays the communications of the computer. May also be called CRT (Cathode Ray Tube); monitor; video display or screen; VDT (Video Display Terminal); "tube." It is also possible to have a Braille display.

Cursor: A symbol on a computer video screen, indicating the current position for the next entry or output character. It is usually a small lighted box or underline, blinking or steady. The non-visual equivalent which is maintained by a Braille or speech output device may also be called the "cursor."

Screen Review: The ability, after a screenful of information is displayed visually, for a blind person to have small portions of the screen spoken or displayed in Braille, at will. This feature may include options about whether material is to be pronounced or spelled, and how much is to be spoken at a time.

Spreadsheet: A paper or computer display in which figures are arranged in rows and columns. A "spreadsheet program" makes it possible to create a spreadsheet on a computer. This is done by entering formulas so that changing one figure will automatically alter other figures. Examples include budgets, ledgers, cost estimates, etc.

Manuals and Study Materials

Suggestions for reading technical materials aloud appear under "Live Readers" (below in this chapter), as well as elsewhere in this book.

If advanced study materials explaining actual computer programming are to be Brailled, it is important to use the appropriate notation. Refer to the *Code for Computer Braille Notation*, from the American Printing House for the Blind.

Very elementary materials, of course, may not contain any technical material. Also, the need for a special reference does not apply to reading the regular output of the computer, as discussed throughout most of this chapter. If a Braille output device is purchased, the Braille representation for each computer character will already be set, and the user must simply learn that system.

The Computer Keyboard

The letters, numerals, period, comma, and question mark are usually in the same positions as on a typewriter keyboard. (Note, however, that the computer will *not* treat the "zero" as being the same as the capital O, or the "one" as interchangeable with a lower-case L.) Other symbols may be in any of several locations – for example, the apostrophe may be to the right of the semicolon, but also is often found as the shift of "6" or "7."

Even though the letter keys are in the standard arrangement, it may be difficult for the student to be certain she is on the right keys, because of various additional specialized keys which may surround them. Many computer keyboards have built-in tactual markings on two keys of the "home row;" if yours does not, it may be helpful to apply them. Blind people often find it helpful to make a Braille chart when dealing with a new computer keyboard.

Sighted children experiment with computers from a very early age, long before they have formal typing instruction. Unfortunately, this encourages strong habits of hunt-and-peck. This same problem occurs with partially-sighted children. Totally blind children may be less likely to use hunt-and-peck, but it is possible with Braille labels or speech output.

Because of this problem, more and more schools are now teaching standard touch-typing to all students in the elementary grades (often calling it "keyboarding," presumably to emphasize the computer aspect). If a computer is to be used extensively, then regular touch-typing instruction should be provided – individually, if necessary – and children should not be allowed to revert to hunt-and-peck. See the chapter on "Keyboarding" for more detailed discussion.

Some keyboards also include a separate pad of number keys which allow one-handed entry of strictly numeric information. A tactual mark usually is built-in on the "5" key, and should be sufficient labeling.

Various specialized keys, such as those which move the cursor, will be in different places on different models. Often it is desirable to label some of these in Braille. Alternatively, a Brailled template or chart may be placed near the keyboard.

For a very young child who cannot type, it may be desirable to place Braille labels on certain letters used in specific exercises – for example, *y* and *n* commonly indicate *yes* and *no*.

Unfortunately, some of the least expensive keyboards do not have true keys, but instead simply have "keys" painted on a flexible plastic surface with little bubbles underneath. (This is often called a "membrane keyboard.") If there are raised squares around the letters, the blind student may be able to proceed with normal touch-typing, although the "flat" arrangement may feel strange. Also, it is sometimes possible to feel the little bubbles underneath, but this is usually quite slow and inefficient. It is possible to apply Braille to everything, but this is difficult and may be only marginally successful. If at all possible, provide a keyboard with real keys. (Note: It is *not* desirable to label all the letter keys in Braille. It interferes with normal stroking, and discourages the thorough memorizing which makes fast typing possible.)

Look at All the Choices

If a specialized device is being considered, one possibility is to borrow or share. Even a completely separate district may be willing to lend something. Among other things, a brief loan can let you try out a device before purchase.

However, avoid assuming that a technical device (which tends to be glamorous and attractive) is the only solution, or even the best solution. Consider all of the following possibilities, each of which is discussed in detail later in this chapter.

(1) Speech output.

(2) Braille output ("paperless" or on paper).

(3) A live reader (that is, a person reading the display aloud). This is one solution which is always possible, and should always be considered. There are many ways to

provide a reader, often without any additional expense. (See the chapters on "Placement Options and Decisions" and "Other Modes of Reading," as well as elsewhere in this book.) For younger students and relatively short courses, using a reader is almost always preferable to purchasing special devices.

(4) Enlargement or enhancement of the visual display, if the student has considerable useful sight.

(5) An electronic device for reading the visual display – e.g., the Optacon.

(6) A combination of these approaches. For example, suppose that a speech output device is available to a high school student, but it is only compatible with some of the programs being studied. The student could use a live reader for the programs which have no speech.

Always consider the proportionate weight of various factors: available finances and other resources; the age and experience of the student; the length of the course; and the goal of the instruction.

Even when a speech or Braille output device is readily available, avoid the blanket assumption that it should be used. Always ask:

(1) Does the device do the job well enough to justify its use at this time? (Example: If the speech is difficult to understand, the student may finish the course before he is comfortable with the device. Other common difficulties are described later in this chapter.)

(2) Does the student have the maturity and skill to use the device independently? If someone must help him constantly, it might be more efficient for that person simply to read the display.

(3) Will use of the device change or restrict the student's work? (e.g., the second grade is using computers in math; a talking program is available, but the examples are different from those used by other students.)

(4) Is there a temptation to substitute computer use for important basic skills? Suppose, for example, that a first grader with low vision has difficulty reading math problems. "Talking problems" on the computer should not be substituted for learning to read Braille.

Speech Output

Computer output through a speech synthesizer is increasingly common. Some devices are designed especially for the blind, and some are for the general public. They can be used by anyone with adequate hearing, and generally are less expensive than Braille devices. Quality and versatility, however, vary greatly.

CHARACTERISTICS OF THE SPEECH ITSELF

(1) How natural is the sound?

(2) To what degree can the user alter the speed of speech? Does pitch vary when speed is changed?

(3) Can speech easily be turned on and off?

(4) How long is the delay after new lines, new input, etc.?

(5) How sophisticated is the speech logic? For example, does it pronounce "boathouse" with a "th" sound, or is it programmed to recognize the exception? Can you "teach" the machine correct pronunciation?

(6) Can the speech spell out words? Can it be made to pronounce individual letters of the alphabet as full words (e.g., Alpha for the letter A, Bravo for the letter B, etc.)? How easily can these be changed back to normal pronunciation? Will strings of capitals (e.g., KISU) ordinarily be spelled out, and if so, can this be stopped if the entire display is in capitals?

(7) Can the speech indicate punctuation, and upper and lower case? How easily can these provisions be turned on and off?

(8) How are strings of numerals pronounced? (For example, will "158" be called "one hundred fifty-eight" or "one-five-eight"?)

How will commas and decimal points affect this?

TOTAL PACKAGE

In total, what all is needed to provide the desired speech?

(1) Hardware. What computer will be used? Are extra serial or parallel boards required? Is the speech synthesizer separate? Are connecting cables required? Power converters? Good quality speakers or earphones? (Good reproduction of high-pitched sounds can be especially important for intelligibility, especially for synthesizers which increase the pitch along with the speed. Use of high fidelity earphones or speaker, and pointing the speaker directly at the user, can be important.) Have all of these been made entirely compatible with one another, and with the power source (e.g., electrical outlet in wall)?

(2) What software (programming) is required? (Caution: If you are planning to copy a program onto a blank disk, check the copyright provisions.) Is the software compatible with your hardware? Note that slightly different models of the same computer may not accommodate the same software. Will the software which you are considering actually permit the student to do what is desired? If a package will work with one computer program, how widely applicable is it? One must not assume that it will work equally well with all the software which the school may be using.

(3) What keys on the keyboard are needed for controlling the speech output? Will use of these keys interfere with the normal operation of the application programs (i.e., the programs that the class is learning to run)?

(4) If terminal emulation software (a program used in a small computer to make it act like the terminal of a large computer) is to be used, will the package work with it?

TOTAL COST

Consider the total cost in finances, time, and other resources.

(1) Be sure to consider *all* parts of the total package, as discussed above – even desk space and wall outlets. Can everything be assembled in time? Will the attachment of specialized devices make it hard for sighted students to use the computer?

(2) Monetary cost is not only a matter of the original package. How much does it cost to receive future releases of the product, to keep everything up to date? Is there a maintenance fee that must be paid so that you can receive help from the vendor? How will repairs be financed?

(3) How reliable are the software and hardware? What warranties are provided by the manufacturer?

CONTROL AND INTERACTION WITH THE DISPLAY

Most computers employ a "cursor" (defined above) to tell where the next character will be placed. Sighted people often manipulate the cursor with a set of buttons, a joystick (like the control stick in an airplane), a "mouse" (a remote control which is moved around on an open area of the desk), or some other gimmick. If the location of the cursor itself is anything other than obvious (i.e., anything other than right after the last location), then the blind person needs to be able to find out where it is. If screen reviewability is provided, the blind person needs to be able to manipulate something like a second cursor, for screen review with speech, without affecting the location of the visual cursor.

The type of adaptation for speech depends heavily upon the way the computer program interacts with sighted users. In fact, some programs are virtually impossible to use with speech output.

Programs, regardless of the computer they run on, handle the screen in one or more of several ways:

(1) The simplest programs just feed their output, a line or portion of a line at a time, onto the bottom of the screen. At the end of each line everything on the screen moves up a line and the top line goes off the screen. This is called "scrolling." Relatively simple speech devices often get along pretty well with this system; the tendency is for programs not to put out very much at once, so that information does not scroll off the screen before the sighted person reads it. Nevertheless, programs do sometimes put out a whole screenful of information, and this usually takes too long to listen to with speech. When this happens, some kind of screen review capability is needed, or a feature allowing program output to be saved in the file and later reviewed at leisure.

(2) Some other programs put out one screenful of information each time they put out anything. This eliminates the problem of data scrolling off the screen. However, large amounts of data are sent to the screen, and can overwhelm a speech device. Screen review capability is almost always called for when this type of program must be used by a blind person.

(3) Still other programs keep the data in a stationary position on the screen, and just change the characters in specific locations as new data is to be displayed. For example, the word NAME might be permanently displayed whenever the program is running, but the entry (e.g., John W. Smith) would frequently be changed.

This approach is used by many large business computers, as it minimizes the amount of information sent to the screen. Information to be displayed on the screen, however, may be accompanied by a great deal of other information such as where to put it, how bright to make it, whether it should flash, etc. This extra information confuses speech devices.

Also, the usual practice is to send only the data being changed (John W. Smith) and not the title or description of the data (NAME), since NAME is already displayed on the screen and need not be changed. Very sophisticated speech devices are needed for coping with this method of screen handling. Such devices have only recently become available, and are still relatively primitive in their capabilities. We can expect to see tremendous refinement and improvement in these devices in the next few years, since they are the ones in greatest demand by blind people for employment situations.

(4) The last of the common methods used by programs to communicate with the screen involves use of the "graphics" feature to "paint on" characters in various sizes, colors, and locations – sometimes intermixed with lines, shapes, and pictures. To our knowledge, no one has yet attempted to devise a widely applicable method of connecting speech equipment to screens handled in this way. The only methods blind people have used successfully with this type of screen handling, to our knowledge, are the Optacon and live readers.

Games are popular for recreation and for instruction. Unfortunately, most of them involve complicated graphics (pictures), and are especially hard to adapt to synthetic speech format. Some cannot be adapted at all with present technology, although the student might play with sighted assistance. Others may be read aloud only in part. Software designed especially for the blind may have games that have been adapted appropriately.

In addition to actual "games," many other programs for younger children make extensive use of graphics. A math problem may be shown in pictures. Sometimes large letters or numerals are made by graphics – that is, drawn rather than typed. If there are no regular numbers or letters, probably the speech synthesizer cannot read the display meaningfully.

Computer programs are notorious for their use of complicated text formats–tables within tables within tables; mixtures of labeled data, some of which may be labeled above, some below, and some beside; and portions of the screen whose purpose and format change in midstream. So-called "pull-downs" and "windows" are examples of this last category: they are methods of breaking into existing text to insert temporary information, or to allow interruption of one task to perform another. Most speech equipment is quite difficult to use with complicated screen formats. Even speech equipment which has screen review usually does not provide much help with complicated formats.

A "spreadsheet," such as a budget form, cannot be used at all unless the entire display is under control at once. If the speech arrangement cannot deal with the spreadsheet as a unit, or cannot move the cursor around at will, probably the spreadsheet cannot be used with the device.

Braille Output

For the student who reads Braille comfortably, Braille output is even more desirable than speech output, other things being equal. Braille also eliminates sound distractions for classmates.

Unfortunately, however, Braille computer output devices are generally less available and more expensive than speech devices. Furthermore, a particular Braille device may or may not be superior to a particular speech device. Good speech is better than bad Braille.

Following is a discussion of considerations in evaluating Braille output devices.

QUALITY AND SUITABILITY OF THE BRAILLE DISPLAY

(1) Is the Braille embossed on paper? Or is it formed by tiny pegs which rise to form the dot patterns? Computer devices most commonly have the latter, called "paperless Braille." It is not difficult to read, but may require some practice.

(2) How many Braille cells are displayed at one time? The fewer there are, the slower it is to read.

(3) How quickly and easily is the display "refreshed"–i.e., replaced by a new set of symbols?

(4) What is the quality of the Braille itself? Is each dot either clearly present or clearly absent, or is there a problem with weak dots? Are the dots properly aligned? If you do not read Braille well by touch, ask the opinion of experienced blind persons.

(5) Braille displays generally include the standard Braille letters of the alphabet. However, this is not the same thing as standard Grade I Braille which merely spells out every word. Computer Braille is a code that has more or less been agreed upon by manufacturers of Braille output devices in this country–one Braille symbol for each character that the computer can generate. Furthermore, even the letters of the alphabet are sometimes altered by adding an extra "dots 7 and 8" below dots 3 and 6, respectively. Dots 7 and 8 indicate upper case, lower case, or control characters.

(6) It is very unlikely that you will find an output device which transcribes into Grade II Braille. If you should find a device which claims to do so, check its accuracy and consistency for literary applications. Also note that for the writing and modification of actual computer programs, it would probably be inappropriate. Check to see that such a translator can be disabled.

(7) How is capitalization indicated?

(8) How is punctuation displayed? Most devices use computer Braille punctuation, which is not standard English Braille. Computer Braille is preferred for programming, while a translator is preferred for literary applications.

(9) Are special computer symbols such as "Control-D" shown? If so, how are they displayed, and can this feature be turned on and off at will?

(10) For mathematical expressions, how similar is the computer's Braille to regular Nemeth code? Two-celled signs (such as "equals"), especially, are likely to be different.

(11) How are new lines, paragraphs, etc., indicated?

(12) Does the Braille display indicate video attributes from the screen – e.g., highlighting, reverse video, blinking text, etc.?

Note: The discussion below is abbreviated, since the following questions are somewhat similar to those for speech output devices. See also the detailed discussion above under "Speech Output."

TOTAL PACKAGE

What is the total package needed? This may include:

- Continuous-feed Braille paper
- Braille embosser or paperless Braille display
- Special cassettes for storing digital data
- Grade I or Grade II Braille translation software
- Screen review Braille software or hardware
- Maintenance fees

CONTROL AND INTERACTION WITH THE DISPLAY

How well can the display be controlled and correlated with the video display? How are special formats such as "spreadsheets" and games handled? Braille devices may work better than speech devices for some complicated formats, because the amount of information displayed at one time in Braille is so small. However, often it is best to use a sighted reader.

Live Readers

A reader (that is, a person reading aloud) is universally possible. If the blind student is quite young and/or taking a very short course, usually this is the best solution. Depending on circumstances, it may be best for a very long time.

Remember that the use of a reader does not preclude some use of other methods. For example, a serious student of computer science might borrow and try out various devices, while continuing to rely mainly on readers.

The chief problem in the use of a reader usually is the old bugaboo: the tendency of the sighted to do too much for the blind. The reader should not make the decisions. The reader should not do the keyboarding (except perhaps for a very young child).

Another problem is the intermittent nature of the reading required. The reader may become bored and inattentive.

Seek agreement on terminology between the student and the reader. Format and symbol usage tend to be much more complex than with a typical book or magazine. Are special symbols described in a consistent manner? For example:

- Does everyone understand the distinctions among parentheses () and brackets [] and braces{}?
- The symbol ^ may be called "circumflex," "caret," and "arrow up" by three different people. (And someone from a sorority or fraternity might call it the Greek letter lambda.)
- Are the terms "rows" and "columns" used consistently?

Acquiring proficiency in the use of live readers will prove extremely valuable: it will teach the blind student how to deal with the computer on the same basis as everyone else. Live readers enable the blind student to use computers in any physical location, and with *no* special modifications.

The chapter on "Other Modes of Reading" has further discussion about readers.

Use of Partial Sight

When a student has useful sight, it may or may not be wise for him to rely on it to read a computer screen. Even those who ordinarily read regular print may experience headaches and fatigue, and make many errors. On the other hand, some students find that the lighted screen is actually easier to read than a printed book.

Often a combination approach is good. The student might use his sight for short exercises but have someone read aloud during long sessions. Or, he might use a speech or Braille output device whenever the program is compatible, and read visually at other times.

When a partially-sighted student plans to read computer output visually, there are two general approaches–(1) enhancing the regular display, and (2) actually changing the size of the characters on the screen.

ENHANCING THE REGULAR VISUAL DISPLAY

Most screens have contrast and/or brightness controls. In addition, some systems allow separate control of character, background, and border color. Experiment. The student may be much more comfortable with the background and/or the characters brighter or dimmer. If a "reverse of contrast" (e.g., black on white *vs.* white on black) is available, try it also.

Consider the room lighting, as it may cause glare or affect the apparent brightness on the screen. Consider placing a hood over the screen.

Various overlays or special screens are available, to be placed between the regular screen and the user. These may maximize contrast, cut glare, and/or magnify.

Usually regular magnifiers are not practical with a video screen. However, a large magnifier can sometimes be turned sideways (with its light off) in front of a screen. If the screen is small, the lens may cover all or most of it.

It is often possible to direct the camera of a Closed Circuit Television (CCTV) magnifier toward a regular video screen.

Printers are commonly provided with computers. Some students can read printed matter more easily than the screen. (This usually is not, however, satisfactory as a complete substitute for reading the screen.)

SOFTWARE AND/OR HARDWARE TO ENLARGE CHARACTERS

Many computers can be equipped with special enlarging systems. Such a system actually changes the size of the characters on the computer screen.

However, there are disadvantages and problems similar to those with speech or Braille output. In fact, problems may be especially insidious because the large-print output *seems* so similar to the regular output.

Carefully examine the aspects described below. (Note: Because many considerations have already been discussed for other kinds of output, less detail will be given here.)

(1) Is the system compatible with the regular hardware?

(2) Is the system compatible with the regular software?

(3) What extra equipment, adapters, space, power, etc., is required?

(4) What keys on the keyboard are needed for controlling the enlarged output? Will use of these keys interfere with the normal operation of the programs that the class is using?

(5) How easily is the size of the characters controlled? Does the size increase or decrease in large increments, or is fine adjustment possible?

(6) Is clarity and contrast at least as good as that of the regular display?

(7) Is the appearance of any characters (e.g., mathematical symbols) changed in comparison to the regular display?

(8) The larger the characters, the less can be displayed at one time. If an entire line of the regular display cannot be shown, how is this handled? If a word is continued onto the next line, is it broken between syllables? Are parts of several lines displayed simultaneously, in the manner of a CCTV?

(9) To what extent is screen review capability provided? That is, can the student readily view a particular portion of the screen? How quickly and easily can the viewing be moved to another portion of the screen?

(10) Are graphics (pictures) enlarged in their original form? If so, will the entire picture fit on the screen?

THINK IT THROUGH

As discussed previously, look at all the choices. Consider speech output, Braille output, other special devices, live readers, and a combination of approaches. Do not assume that an enlarged display is always the best for a student with useful sight.

Other Methods

Other specialized devices are useful for some users. Probably the best known is the Optacon, which is described in "Other Modes of Reading." If a person has an Optacon and knows how to use it, it may be the best method for certain programs which do not lend themselves to Braille or speech output. However, the Optacon does not permit fast reading.

Conclusion

All aspects of computers can be handled by a blind person with appropriate skill–routine use, programming, design, maintenance, repair, and use of auxiliary devices such as modems and printers. A printer can be set up and the paper aligned by techniques described in the "Keyboarding" chapter. Blind students should choose computer courses on the same basis as other students, and should have the same assignments.

If your student is having trouble, or if there is difficulty in finding appropriate equipment, seek further help. The National Federation of the Blind has technically-oriented groups and committees which would be glad to assist you.

Technology, in and of itself, is neither good nor bad. To the extent that sighted people are becoming involved with computers and computer technology, so should the blind. However, technology is not going to end problems of employment discrimination, lack of opportunity, insufficient reading materials, etc. These can only improve through public education, positive attitudes, and a greater acceptance of the blind as equals in our society.

Technology *misused* can actually decrease opportunities for blind people. A good example is overemphasis on computers for routine classroom assignments in various subjects. It should not be assumed that the blind student needs to use a computer for composition. This is true even if other students do so, *unless it is computer use which is being studied.* Unfortunately, today some blind students are tied down to *one* location for writing because of misguided overemphasis on computer use and computerized Braille translation. With a portable typewriter, a Braille slate, and a Perkins Brailler, the blind student can write his/her assignments in any room and in any location (especially if a manual typewriter or a battery-operated machine is available, so that electrical outlets are not required).

Technology, if properly used and understood, can do much to help our progress. Misused, it can be a hindrance instead.

Additional Sources of Information

Portions of this chapter have been adapted from the following articles:

"Speech Output for the IBM Personal Computer," by Curtis Chong, in the *Braille Monitor,* January, 1986.

"Some Comments on Technology–Print-Reading Devices and Braille," by Curtis Chong, in *Future Reflections,* January-February 1984.

See the "References" section at the end of this *Handbook* for sources of computer-related devices and publications. See the chapter on "Keyboarding" for discussion of typing skills.

CHAPTER 34

HANDWRITING

My student was ecstatic. "Now I can write checks!" she exclaimed. "My dad won't have to sign for me. And now I can sign letters...and Christmas cards...yearbooks...." She excitedly named off more and more ways to use her new ability.

I too was excited, but I also felt regret that this had taken so long. Why hadn't her previous teacher started to work on this, before the youngster came to me in high school? It was hard to spend much time on handwriting; and since the skill was not easy for this student, it took until her senior year. In the meantime, she felt acute embarrassment every time there was need for a signature.

It is far better to start earlier. The kindergartner can mark with a crayon. The first grader can mark a Braille answer sheet with a pencil. This early practice builds proper habits of holding and manipulating the writing implement. A logical time to begin the actual signature is when all students learn cursive (script) writing – typically early third grade.

The Concept of Handwriting

"But is it *legible?*" my high school student kept asking. Again I explained that her emerging signature was reasonably legible and quite satisfactory, but that one couldn't necessarily recognize each and every letter perfectly. I repeated various jokes about doctors' handwriting, as I tried to get this concept across. It is *not* essential that *anyone* have a perfectly legible signature. It is customary to type the name under the signature, to take care of any ambiguity. It *is,* however, essential to have a signature that is distinctive and consistent. Banks generally will not accept printed "signatures," since they are too easily forged. Also, it is hard to rely on a signature that is immature and still changing. If we teach the student each letter, show how to link them together, and spend a reasonable amount of time working toward legibility, a usable signature will emerge.

The Braille student is accustomed to perfectly consistent size, spacing, and quality of characters. (This, by the way, is one of the advantages of Braille. It helps to show that Braille is not categorically harder to learn than inkprint.) Explain that print may vary in size and proportion; that capital letters may be shaped differently from lower case; that some letters have alternative shapes. Discuss the idea of critical features *vs.* individual variations (e.g., a cursive *e* must be a loop, but individuals may make them fatter or thinner, etc.)

When to Use Handwriting

Usually it is not worthwhile for a Braille student to try to do general writing in cursive. Typing is much more efficient for most purposes. Even when signing something, it usually is unwise to rely *solely* on handwriting. For example, the name should always be typed under the signature in a letter. Depending on the legibility of the signature, there may be other situations when it would be wise to ask someone else to write the name – for example, signing a list to request activity tickets.

Techniques for Learning

Consult any good handwriting instruction book to check posture and hand position, noting both right- and left-handed versions. Begin with simple marking, being sure that the pen moves smoothly. Illustrate upstrokes, downstrokes, etc. A regular ballpoint pen should be used.

Start with the easiest letters, not necessarily those that come first in the name. I find the cursive *e, l, i, r, m,* and *n* to be easiest. Omit "curlicues" and other embellishments that are not essential. Consider whether a square corner might be substituted for a curve and be easier for the student.

Learning the first few letters may take a long time, but it is worth the effort. After a few letters have been learned, others will be learned faster: some strokes will be similar, and more and more comparison becomes possible. Work to make each letter as standard as possible, but do not spend vast amounts of time striving for perfect legibility. The important thing is to have a unique, consistent legal signature.

Emphasize how letters are connected. The student will need to judge how far to stroke horizontally between letters. With a letter such as lower-case *o,* the connection to the next letter is different than for letters which end at the baseline. Help the student realize where each letter begins and ends. It may be interesting to practice connecting letters in a different sequence.

How about dotting i's and j's, and crossing t's? It is easier to do this when the letter is initially made, rather than going back as sighted writers do. At the top of the *i* or *j,* a slight motion of the pen can easily approximate a dot. On the *t,* a four-way motion can form a cross. This avoids the problem of losing one's place. Alternatively, one might put a finger of the non-dominant hand on a place to dot or cross, and come back to that place when the word is completed.

What about *g, j, p, q, y,* and *z,* which reach below the baseline? With a rigid signature guide this is a problem. One solution is a guide with an elastic line, such as the one from the American Printing House for the Blind (APH). (Note that it is possible to use either the larger or the smaller space, by turning the guide over.) Other possibilities are to regard the baseline as being slightly ***above*** the bottom (thus leaving room to go down); to move the guide slightly for the downward-reaching letter; or simply to squeeze in the extra portion. If a horizontal fold in the paper is used as a guide, there is no problem.

Materials

Many different teaching aids can be used for variety and clarity. Letters (singly or in groups) are available in raised form and in recessed form, from the American Printing House for the Blind (APH) and elsewhere. Letters may be traced with a pen or pencil, or with the fingertip. There are many kinds of raised-line drawing kits. Experiment with writing in sand, clay, etc., and in the air. Various helpful materials are available commercially, such as "string" which will hold a shape and adhere to a surface.

A system using Braille cells to teach script writing is described in an article by Johnette Weiss and Jeff Weiss (see "References"). The dots of the Braille cell serve as a guide for the script letter formations.

Practicing part of a letter, or a single stroke, is often helpful.

Help the student learn to retract and extend a ballpoint pen, and to be sure the ink really is flowing. (Testing the pen on scratch paper is a good idea.)

If the student has some sight, experiment with various implements while practicing: china markers, extra-heavy pencils, crayons, etc. However, for the signature as finally developed, a ballpoint pen should be used even if the student cannot see his own writing.

Size

I often start with letters up to one inch high, to make it easy to demonstrate shapes and motions. Then when the student can write several letters, we work on reducing the size.

APH offers paper with raised lines spaced approximately like ordinary wide-line notebook paper; writing between two lines is a good way to begin. Various line guides, to be placed under or over regular paper, are also available.

There are many kinds of signature guides to frame an individual signature. It is important to reduce the signature to appropriate size before the student becomes too accustomed to writing large.

Some students can write with appropriate size from the beginning.

One student commented, "I'm trying to make each letter fit into an imaginary Braille cell." You and your students will think of other ideas.

Defining the size is related to *where* the signature is to be placed. Your student should be able to help a stranger direct him/her where to sign. A signature guide works well. So does a request to fold the paper horizontally and then unfold it, producing a raised line which can serve as a guide. However, it is not wise to say merely, "Place my finger where I should start." Unless the student has enough sight to see the line, this often results in writing at an angle.

Students with Considerable Useful Sight

If you are helping a kindergartner or first grader learn manuscript writing (printing), use strictly the alphabet which is taught in that particular school. If the classroom teacher says the *q* should have a curved "tail," and you write it with an angle, your young student will be confused.

Various kinds of bold-line writing paper are available from APH and elsewhere. However, many students prefer the regular paper. Some students have difficulty even with mass-produced bold-line paper, and seem to need custom-made paper with very dark lines. Braille should be considered for such a student, since it is unlikely that she will read her own handwriting well.

Avoid using darker lines than necessary. Students with some eye conditions, such as nystagmus, report that a series of very heavy lines can be extremely uncomfortable visually. ("They jiggle and make me dizzy.") Also, if beginners' paper has guidelines for the height of lower-case letters, very dark guidelines will make the letters hard to see.

IEP DECISIONS

How Much Cursive Writing Is Practical?

When a visually impaired student can easily use manuscript writing, should he also learn cursive? If he does, he will be following the regular curriculum more closely; he will be able to write in all the ways that others customarily use; and he will easily and naturally learn to read others' handwriting. On the other hand, some visually impaired students have much more difficulty seeing the connected and less precise letters of cursive. If they continue to use manuscript lettering, they will write more legibly and read their own writing more easily.

Visual acuity alone may not indicate how easily a partially-sighted student will use cursive. It seems to be an individual matter. For a young student who is able to read and write manuscript lettering well, it is often best to begin by assuming that he will learn cursive along with his classmates. Provide good, clear models of the cursive letters at close range–he probably cannot see wall cards well. Have him use an extra-dark pen or pencil, and possibly paper with bold lines. Try the new erasable pens.

With a beginner, teach the exact alphabet used by all students at the particular school. (An exception occurs if the student is learning only his signature and will not be doing general writing in cursive.) However, after students have been using handwriting for some time, classroom teachers no longer insist on a particular model.

Be Specific

If learning cursive writing appears to be a problem, decisions should be consciously made by the IEP team. Too often everyone drifts into assuming that the student cannot learn cursive, and alternatives are not really discussed. Just why is he not learning? Is it his sight, or something else? Does he have trouble following the class presentation, but do well when instructed individually? Does he have materials he can see well? Is his physical coordination normal? If not, has the problem been diagnosed medically and then analyzed educationally by an expert in physical disabilities?

If the student is not to rely on cursive for general writing, the IEP should provide for:

- Learning and maintaining the cursive *signature,* which is very important for legal purposes.
- Learning to read the cursive writing of others, when it is large and plain enough. High-interest material might be presented in large, plain cursive.
- Using effective means for general writing–probably manuscript writing (printing) and typewriting. (If the student cannot read his own *printing* easily, then he should be learning Braille.)

Maintaining and Extending Skills

When the signature is learned, develop a plan for maintenance. Could the student sign each class paper, or certain selected papers? Might the older student open a checking account and use it regularly? Some concrete plan must be followed, or you will be starting over again in a year or two.

CHAPTER 35

HOME ECONOMICS and DAILY LIVING SKILLS

A young blind woman stated confidently that she knew how to make doughnuts. It soon became apparent, however, that she had only been allowed to *sugar* them.

A blind eighth-grader wanted to learn to cook. Her parents rearranged their kitchen extensively, even relocating electrical outlets.

Opposite Extremes

These examples illustrate two opposite problems: complete omission of certain activities (or parts of them), *vs.* fancy and unnecessary arrangements.

Complete lack of experience is obviously harmful, but it occurs for a number of reasons. Parents and classroom teachers may not know effective alternative techniques and lack the experience to invent them. Resource/itinerant teachers may not know techniques for a particular activity, may believe that those techniques are too cumbersome, or may explain them poorly. It is especially unfortunate when, as with the doughnuts, the student does only part of the job but is encouraged to believe she has done it all.

Home/School Coordination

Since daily living skills are rather personal, and some of them are not usually done at school, encouraging good techniques can be touchy. Parents may feel that the resource/itinerant teacher is intruding into their personal family life. Encourage parents to study checklists of daily living skills, meet various blind people, read articles such as those in *Future Reflections,* etc. Cultivate tactful approaches such as:

- "That can be a good way to begin. Now could we try..."
- "Yes, some blind people do it that way. Here are some other ways..."
- "Here is an idea that works well ..."
- "Now that Jimmy is older, let's see if we can teach him to ..."

Continual vague remarks about "giving him more responsibility at home" are only vaguely helpful. Concrete suggestions, such as "Let's teach him to make a peanut butter sandwich without any help at all," are more effective. Moreover, the definition of "independence" should be frequently discussed. For making a sandwich, this should include getting everything out of the cupboard or drawer (peanut butter, bread, knife, plate) and putting things away.

Similarly, avoid making assumptions based on mere discussion. Suppose, for example, that you inquire, "Do you have some money of your own, and do you buy things by yourself?" and the student answers "Yes." Exactly what does this mean? It could mean that the *parent* sometimes gives the child some money at the store and helps him to buy something. Ask more detailed questions and do some spot-checking. ("Tell me about the last time you bought something. Was anyone from your family with you?

...Here's a billfold and some play money. I'll give you some bills and tell you what they are, and you show me how you would sort them in your billfold."

Lists Can Be Helpful

Below is an informal checklist. It may be desirable to have two or more checkoff squares beside each item, with headings such as "With Family," "With Teacher," and "Other." Items can easily be listed in the IEP.

Many other lists of daily living skills have been compiled. Often they are age-graded and otherwise categorized, and contain much detail. For most purposes, however, simplicity promotes efficiency and prevents certain problems. If a list is too detailed (e.g., showing several steps in learning to lock and unlock a door), it encourages the incorrect assumption that blind children cannot grasp the whole task easily. Age-grading can be helpful; however, it may be discouraging if the student appears too old or too young to be learning the task. Also, learning is often dependent on circumstances such as apartment living *vs.* one-family home.

Other categories may make it easy for students or parents to omit a group of tasks due to stereotyping. Common examples include "Boys don't need to cook" and "Gardening is very hard for a blind person." Also, many people assume that a person who does not drive has no need to learn any tasks associated with a car. On the contrary, it is important for the blind passenger to do his/her share of routine tasks and to help in case of emergency.

Here is a useful list:

- Use screwdriver
- Climb ladder
- Lock and unlock door with key
- Mow lawn
- Shovel snow
- Rake leaves
- Work in garden (outdoors)
- Raise plants (indoors)
- Assist in caring for young child
- Care for young child when no one else is in the same room
- Care for young child when no one else is present in the home
- Use vacuum cleaner
- Make bed (not changing linen)
- Change bed linen
- Tidy up own bedroom
- Empty wastebaskets
- Insert or replace batteries (in small appliance, flashlight, etc.)
- Sweep with broom
- Scrub floor
- Wash dishes by hand
- Load and run dishwasher
- Select clothing for the day
- Shop for minor items of clothing
- Shop for major items of clothing
- Hand wash article of clothing
- Use washing machine
- Use drier
- Fold and sort clean laundry
- Change light bulb
- Plug in and unplug electrical device
- Play Monopoly
- Play checkers
- Play chess
- Play Scrabble
- Play card game (not standard four suits)
- Play card game with standard four suits
- Practice social dancing
- Participate in a school (or other) dance
- Turn on lights for others' convenience
- Buy a ticket to stage performance or movie
- Use coin phone
- Use Directory Assistance ("Information")
- Wash car
- Feed parking meter
- Check oil in car
- Pump gasoline at service station
- Change tire on car
- Sort bills in billfold
- Identify coins
- Make change up to $5.00
- Use school library (in person)
- Use public library (in person)
- Use state library for the blind (by telephone)
- Use state library for the blind (in person)
- Shop for incidentals (e.g., toothpaste)

Use vending machine
Cut meat on dinner plate
Serve self from serving bowl
Serve others from serving bowl
Make cold sandwich
Cook with microwave oven
Cook with conventional oven
Heat saucepan on burner
Make grocery list
Shop for groceries
Prepare light meal for self
Prepare light meal for at least two people
Eat at fast-food restaurant
Eat at restaurant with table service
Eat at cafeteria (other than school)
Pay bill at restaurant or cafeteria (other than at school)
Leave tip for waiter/waitress

Avoid Gimmicks

Unnecessary gadgets and fancy arrangements often create more problems than they solve. Unfortunately, it is usually people who call themselves "professionals" who are responsible for this kind of thing. It may be due to ignorance of better techniques, rigidity in using methods previously learned, or even a desire to justify one's existence through impressive-appearing procedures. We owe it to our students to learn the simplest and most effective techniques possible, and to teach flexibility.

Following are just a few examples of unnecessary gadgetry or artificially complicated arrangements:

- Special coffee mugs for the blind
- Button-on neckties for the blind
- Especially constructed electrical outlets
- Traffic lights which make special sounds

Blindness – The Myth and the Image, by Kenneth Jernigan, deals with this problem in depth. Occasionally a device is so unnecessary and inappropriate as to be ludicrous. More often, however, the problem is more subtle: although the device might be helpful to some blind people under some circumstances, it is bad to assume that it is always needed.

Brailled labels for clothing are an example. Many competent blind people use them, especially for articles of clothing which are similar to the touch but differ in color. However, there are many other good techniques, even for articles identical to the touch. And it is usually rather silly to sew a color label into the one and only mohair sweater which a person owns.

Worst of all, dependence on gadgets fosters the belief that one cannot get along without them.

Organizing Belongings

[Note: Much of the material under this heading and under the heading "Clothing Management" has been adapted from the book, *A Resource Guide for Parents and Educators of Blind Children,* also by Doris M. Willoughby.]

The blind child, as any child, must learn to organize her belongings and keep track of where they are. If others always find things for her, she will learn organization slowly if at all.

Help her to follow an orderly system for putting things away. If other people must move her things, they should inform her of the change. At the same time, the youngster should not become so rigidly organized that she is immobilized when an article is misplaced. If she drops something, teach her to hunt around on the floor with her hands in an organized pattern of search. If the family has left the shampoo in the wrong place in the bathroom, the blind youngster can look around by touch.

If every child in the family assembles his or her books, clothes, etc., for each school day the night before, morning crises will be minimized.

With forethought, the child can learn to distinguish items which a sighted person would tell apart by color, pattern, or label. Often the object itself will have other characteristics which distinguish it – weight, size, odor, shape of bottle, etc. With clothing, one can feel the texture, seams, pockets, buttons, shape of sleeves or neck, etc. If two or more items really are alike to the touch, such as three shades of the same brand of lipstick, consider these ideas:

- Keep each item in a separate place.
- For clothing, sew a few stitches in a hidden place.
- Put a different number of rubber bands, bits of tape, or safety pins on each item.
- Apply a Braille label. For the young child who cannot read, "labels" can be made from different textures, or with simple arrangements of Braille-like dots.
- File one or more small notches in an inconspicuous place.
- Pay particular attention to clothing which will be mixed in with that of others. To aid in finding one's coat, for example, one might add a distinctive belt or pin. If one's coat already possesses a fairly distinctive feature such as a furry collar, it is still wise to consider other characteristics such as the contents of the pockets. When hanging up a coat, the blind person should pay attention to where it is hung, and also should realize that hangers may move when other coats are added.

Clothing Management

Rob and Bart were among the blind teenagers at a young people's seminar. As the speaker discussed how to manage one's wardrobe, each reflected upon his problems with matching clothing. Rob had two suits which felt almost alike to the touch; discouraged at trying to keep track of them, he usually asked his mother which was which. Bart had four pairs of pants which felt exactly alike; he had worked out a rather time-consuming system of pinning them to the sport shirts with which they looked best.

"There are many ways to keep track of your clothing efficiently," said the speaker. "Usually, different garments will feel quite different. But if you really have two or more garments that are just alike except for the color, try putting some stitches in a place where they won't show. You can make a pattern of stitches – bunched together so that they feel almost like Braille dots – and work out a simple system for remembering what's what."

"Now, why didn't *I* think of that?" reflected Rob.

"Why did I go to all that bother?" thought Bart.

That evening, Rob sewed several stitches together in a hidden place on the pants, the coat, and the matching tie for his first suit. He did nothing to the second suit. When he bought a third suit a few weeks later, he sewed two "dots" in each part of it. Bart worked out a similar system.

The most important thing which Rob and Bart learned at the seminar was not this specific technique, or any particular technique, but rather the attitude of believing that an efficient method can be found. Previously, Rob had given up on finding an independent technique for color matching. Bart had found a solution, but a cumbersome one. Both had already become more independent than some of the other teenagers at the seminar; some had hardly learned to manage their own clothing at all.

Some schools of thought tend to rely on rigid, complicated formulas for the exact "best" way to do each task without sight. If such an approach is used, the blind person tends to be defeated if circumstances prevent use of a particular technique, and tends to be at a loss when suddenly faced with an unfamiliar task. For almost any activity, there are several reasonably good techniques, each of which has some advantages. The methods given in this chapter are examples only, and should not be taken as formulas. It is far more important to realize that one *can* figure out effective methods for any necessary tasks, and to make a habit of doing so, than it is to have a "specific technique" for each particular task.

When a young child is first beginning to dress himself, show him how to feel the different parts of each garment. He will find some kinds of clothing easier than other kinds, and gradually work up to handling the harder ones. At first you may decide to hand the clothes to him right-side up, or to lay them out carefully in a certain position. Get away from this help soon, however, and teach him to orient the garment himself. He can learn to take hold of the waist correctly as he puts on his pants, to keep the jacket buttons in front, to feel for the opening in the mitten, etc. He can feel the arches of his shoes to tell the left from the right. (You might say, "The arch curve goes to the inside, toward the other foot.")

Whenever a child has learned a small part of a larger task, be sure to maintain and reward that knowledge without overwhelming him. Suppose that a child has finally (after much struggle) learned to button a button–and refuses to button more than one. Also, he cannot figure out which button goes with which hole. If you start the job by buttoning the top button (usually the hardest one) and then expect him to do one button before you will finish, and if you praise him for doing his part, soon he will probably be willing to fasten two buttons and more.

While a child is learning a task, you will probably simplify it for him. You may do part of it yourself, as above. Or, you may give him a particularly simple version of the task, as in starting with large buttons and loose buttonholes. This is necessary and helpful, but again be careful that the child does not rely on such things indefinitely.

SHOPPING FOR CLOTHING

Urge parents to include blind children on shopping trips. Many people assume the blind child will not understand or care about appearance (especially color) and/or would make unwise decisions. Urge them to involve the child through feeling and examining the cut and style of the fabric, and through a description of the visual appearance. Remind the parent that *all* youngsters will make some unwise purchases, and should be guided through increasing responsibility. The five-year-old can choose between two garments which the parent is already considering. The seventh grader can select some of his or her own clothing. The college student should take complete responsibility for budgeting and purchase.

As a teacher, you can help the teenager learn to elicit information from a sighted person. The blind customer may shop with a friend or relative, or may get information from a salesperson. If possible, accompany your student to a clothing store to practice this, even if you cannot have the student actually purchase a garment. Emphasize that the blind customer–not the clerk or other sighted assistant–makes the actual decision.

As with every young person, the blind student must learn what styles and colors are most becoming. General rules (such as avoiding vertical stripes on a very thin person) should be learned. However, it is important to keep up with changing styles, through discussion, observation, and reading current publications.

Give attention to concepts and definitions. Does your student understand the meaning of *plaid, polka dots, stripes, pin stripes, pastels,* etc.?

TYING KNOTS

Ideas for this skill include:

- Use a heavy string or rope at first. Experiment with different textures of string or rope.
- If the child has partial sight, make the two ends different colors.
- Make the two ends different tactually, as by putting a rubber band on one end.
- Get two strings with very different textures, and cut each in half. Take one half from each string and sew them together in the center. Then the two ends will feel entirely different.
- Have the child grasp the string or rope while you move his hands and explain.
- At first, tie part of the knot for the child, thus asking him to perform only part of the task.

LAUNDRY

Even young children can place dirty clothes in the hamper and assist a parent in doing laundry. The older child can sort his/her clothes and organize drawers and closets. Plastic holders can keep socks paired in the washer.

Offer to go to the home and Braille the dials on appliances. In time the family should develop enough experience and creativity to make their own markings; but at first it is usually necessary for someone to do it for them.

If the blind person keeps track of how often each garment has been worn, recognizes its characteristics (light or dark color, likelihood of wrinkling, etc.), and notes circumstances which soil clothing faster, then he/she will only rarely need sighted advice about the need for laundering. An appropriate schedule should be set up for each category–e.g., white blouses washed after one wearing, brown jacket dry-cleaned once a month, etc.

Most modern fabrics wrinkle very little, and with others the "crushed look" is fashionable. Nevertheless, pressing is still a necessary skill. The beginner may practice with a cold iron. Soon he/she will learn to smooth a portion of material by touch and then carefully go over it with a heated iron.

General Appearance

Combing hair, applying makeup, and other aspects of general grooming can be done by touch. Again the key is to learn good techniques and to recognize situations which are likely to muss hair or smear makeup. Perhaps you can arrange a demonstration on grooming and/or makeup, with the adult rehabilitation agency or the National Federation of the Blind. If a cosmetics dealer is willing to give a demonstration but has no knowledge of blind techniques, invite a well-groomed blind woman to join in and offer suggestions.

Again, give attention to definitions and concepts. One of my students thought the term "redhead" referred to skin color as well as hair color.

Eating Skills

The article, "Blind Pre-Schoolers ... Some Personal Experiences," by Susan Ford (in *Future Reflections,* October-November, 1982), includes a dramatic account of one mother's efforts to teach her blind foster son eating skills *after* he had passed the normal age for learning them. Work closely with parents and preschool specialists to keep blind children out of such situations. Using alternative techniques as necessary, blind children should learn the same skills that others their age are learning.

Learning table manners takes time and effort for anyone, sighted or blind. This effort leads to being accepted as a mature person. The blind boy or girl can reach this goal as well as anyone else, but he or she will use some different methods at times. No one idea is best for everyone.

Avoid unnecessary gimmicks and gadgets. A baby will probably learn to feed himself more easily from a baby's bowl than from a flat plate, but the older child who becomes blind should not return to baby dishes. It is not necessary or desirable to buy special eating utensils designed for the handicapped. Look for a method that is easy to use, making use of whatever is on hand.

If you work directly with preschoolers, especially in the home, you will probably have ample opportunities to work on eating skills. With older children it may be harder to arrange but it can be done. Plan to join your student for lunch sometimes–in private, so that you need not discuss personal matters in front of peers. Encourage the family to meet a competent blind adult and eat with him or her occasionally.

Below are more selections from *A Resource Guide for Parents and Educators of Blind Children,* by Doris M. Willoughby. Also note that the chapter on "Early Childhood" discusses how babies first learn to feed themselves.

MATURE TABLE ETIQUETTE

The following selection speaks to blind young people with practical advice:

- Avoid depending on someone else's telling you where the food is on your plate. If food has been dished out by someone else, it may be convenient to have him or her tell you what the courses are; but it should not be necessary to have someone explain exactly where each item is on the plate.

- If food is passed around family style, you will learn what each one is as you help yourself. (If the person passing a dish does not tell you what it is, ask her.) Helping oneself from a serving dish is not difficult after some practice.
- Asking to have food passed is no different for the blind person than for anyone else. If you ask about a nearby dish for which a sighted person would have reached, someone else should either hand it to you or reply in a matter-of-fact tone with information such as "It's behind your glass of water."
- When there is quite a bit of food remaining on your plate, it can be easily found by checking with the fork or spoon, and a bite can easily be taken onto the utensil. If not much of the food is left, it may be possible to push it against the side of the plate or bowl. Also, a spoon may be used to help collect the food onto a fork (or vice versa). Another approach is to use a piece of bread, celery, etc., as a "pusher." Avoid messiness. It is well not to expect to find every last bit of food.
- A competent blind person will occasionally touch some part of her food with her fingertips, but she does it quickly and deftly so that little or no food sticks to her fingers, and immediately wipes her fingers on the napkin when necessary.
- Sometimes you may lift the utensil to your mouth and find that there is no food on it after all. This is really no problem at all, and should be given no attention or concern. Just try again.
- Soft meat can be cut with a fork. To use a knife, the following is helpful: Feel with your fork for the near edge of the meat, and insert your fork into the meat just behind the front edge. With a knife in the other hand, cut around behind the fork. A small morsel is then on the fork and ready to be lifted to the mouth.
- With the butter dish resting on the table near your own plate, hold onto the butter dish with one hand. Use a knife in the other hand to feel for the butter itself. Cut carefully and turn the knife to support the piece as you bring it to your plate. Remember that etiquette requires you to place butter or jam on your plate first, rather than directly onto the bread.
- Pouring ketchup, salt, etc., takes experience. At first someone else might help decide when enough has been poured. With practice you can use clues such as the angle of the container, size of the opening(s), sound of the ketchup as it comes out, etc. Using a squeeze bottle or spooning from a wide-mouthed jar may be easier ways of dispensing ketchup, and at home you may choose to use these containers.
- If you have some sight, be careful not to form the habit of leaning down close to your food. Learn alternative techniques such as those above, and use them when you cannot see the food clearly while sitting with good posture.

Money Management

Dimes, quarters, and half dollars have ridged edges, while pennies and nickels have smooth edges. The fingernail can distinguish this easily. The dime, quarter, and half dollar can then be told apart by size. Although the nickel is slightly larger and thicker than the penny, if a person has just one of these it may be hard to tell which one; therefore the student may wish to keep a "sample" penny on hand for comparison.

United States bills cannot be distinguished by touch. Therefore, the blind person should determine what each bill is when she receives it, and file it in the billfold in a distinctive way. Most blind people fold each kind of bill differently (usually not folding one-dollar bills at all), but it is also possible to place each kind in a different location.

The signature, as on a check, is one place where typing is not suitable. This is why a blind youngster should learn to sign her name in handwriting, even if she uses handwriting for no other purpose, and even if her signature is not very legible. She can locate the place for a signature by using a signature-guide frame, by having a sighted person crease the paper, etc. The other portions of the check may be typed at home (after determining the layout of the particular check), or dictated to a reliable person. Raised-line checks are sometimes available.

A blind person going into business should talk with other blind business people, to learn "tricks of the trade" for handling the few customers who are dishonest.

The Telephone

A blind person is obviously at no disadvantage in a telephone conversation – no one, blind or sighted, can see through a telephone line.

Dialing by touch can easily be done. There are many ways to dial quickly and effectively. (Great speed, however, is not really essential.) A partially-sighted person often can dial much faster by touch than by sight.

The pushbutton dial can easily be memorized, and three fingers can be placed on a row rather than counting buttons one at a time. On a rotary dial, the finger stop serves as a reference point, and holes may be located in both directions – forward from "1" and backward from "0." Resting several fingers in a group of holes can save time.

Shopping

The competent blind adult, selecting from many alternative methods, chooses the way of shopping which works best for her under a particular set of circumstances. It is the blind customer herself (not the sighted assistant if there is one, and not the salesperson) who makes all purchasing decisions.

Store employees are often willing to describe items and assemble an order as directed, especially during the less busy hours. Shopping with a friend or relative is sometimes helpful. Telephone ordering for home delivery is a good method at times, but should be only one of many alternatives. If a reader or driver is employed, he or she may be hired as a shopping assistant also.

The mature blind customer has her plans clearly in mind, asks appropriate questions, and makes her own decisions. Competent blind people usually shop alone for most things because of the convenience of arranging one's own schedule.

Due to public misconceptions, the blind customer sometimes must remind salespeople to speak to her directly rather than ignoring her or speaking to someone who is with her. It is also necessary to insist on the salesperson's giving all the information which is wanted, rather than making unwanted omissions or additions. For example, an appliance salesman may assume that a blind customer would only be interested in automatic controls rather than manual ones.

BEGINNING TO LEARN

Urge parents to allow younger children to make purchases involving very little money and no major decisions – an ice cream cone, toothpaste, etc. During travel lessons, have the youngster make such purchases as you gradually stay farther and farther away. Explain the importance of having the child actually carry out the entire transaction, including locating the cash register and talking with the clerk.

Use a vending machine, even if it is only the soda pop machine in the teachers' lounge. When a particular machine is used frequently, it is almost always possible to memorize the prices and levers for the desired merchandise. At an unfamiliar vending machine, or one in which merchandise rotates behind a window, the experienced blind person can quickly gain information from a sighted person and then operate the machine independently.

Housecleaning

It is important to anticipate the need for cleaning, and to follow an organized pattern in cleaning a given surface.

In vacuuming the living room, for example, the student might keep checking that she is gradually moving farther from the north wall as she walks across parallel to it. (From time to time she can pace off the distance from a wall, note what furniture she is passing, etc. With practice one can remain aware of position without much effort.) In wiping off the kitchen counter, the student may need to be reminded to move her hand gradually toward her body as she wipes back and forth.

Sometimes it is advisable to go over the same surface twice–first across the length and then across the width.

Child Care

The chapter, "Dating, Marriage, and the Family," contains suggestions about child care. However, these are brief and oriented toward babysitting. The best preparation for parenthood is to get to know blind parents and their families.

See also the references listed at the end of this chapter and at the end of this *Handbook*.

Thinking It Through

Think through–on a broad general basis–the day's routine, the week's activities, and special occasions. Ask your student about various tasks, and from time to time actually practice a given activity. Anticipate future needs. Examples include:

- Telling time with a Braille watch (Talking clocks are convenient, but often silence is golden)
- Public rest rooms: towels, liquid soap dispensers, napkin/tampon dispensers, urinals, etc.
- Procedures for voting

Cooking

The paper, *Suggestions for the Blind Cook*, is reprinted as an Appendix of this *Handbook*. Written by Ruth Schroeder (a retired home economics teacher who is herself blind and who taught blind students for many years) and Doris M. Willoughby, it offers detailed information on valuable techniques. It is also available from the National Federation of the Blind as a separate publication. Detailed suggestions are given about equipment and labeling, as well as methods in general.

See also the references listed at the end of this chapter and at the end of this *Handbook*.

A SENSE OF PERSPECTIVE

Even though we as teachers may know many good techniques, it may be hard to get them across to others. Emphasize the fine line between too much adaptation (e.g., "special kitchens for the blind") and not enough (e.g., failing to mark dials). If you are not permitted to make permanent marks on someone else's property, make temporary markings. Also, point out that clean hands touching the food will not bring disaster (in a non-commercial setting), and that the blind person learning to cook really needs to use the sense of touch. Different techniques can be used by the experienced cook who is in a commercial setting.

READING RECIPES

Your young student may need coaching in some of the Braille conventions that are slightly different from ordinary literary Braille, as shown on this chart:

(Inkprint) = (Braille)
400 degrees = dg#400
2 1/2 oz. = oz#2-1/2
2 tsp. = tsp#2
2 tbsp. = tbsp#2
1 can = #1 c
1 cup = c#1

For the student who usually reads regular print but cannot easily read a recipe lying on the counter, provide large print. Also, be creative about where to place the recipe. A recipe in either print or Braille, for example, might be taped to the cupboard door.

HIGH EXPECTATIONS

Remember the young woman who said blithely, "Yes, I know how to make doughnuts–I've done it many times," and then came to realize that she only knew how to sugar them. Any student can make comparable errors if she has had no exposure to the *complete* procedure. Prepare your student as much as possible beforehand. Help him/her be included in the regular class activities. Follow up afterward to maintain skills.

Sewing

The article, "The Blind Can Sew–Some How-To Ideas," by Ramona Walhof (reprinted from the *Braille Monitor*), appears as an Appendix of this *Handbook*. Added remarks by Doris M. Willoughby are also included in the Appendix.

See also the references listed at the end of this chapter and at the end of this *Handbook*.

Pacing

With appropriate training and opportunity, the average blind student can proceed at the same general pace as other students, in the sewing or cooking class as well as in personal skills outside of class.

In the classroom, the question sometimes arises: If a particular student does take longer to learn and/or perform certain tasks, must he/she become permanently "out of phase" with the class? Generally students are required, for instance, to thread the entire machine independently before they go on to sew. A student having great difficulty with threading could easily still be working on that when the others have finished the first project.

After several trials, we should help the student if necessary (e.g., thread the needle for her), and go on to the next activity–*but* keep track of the unlearned task and work on it at another time. This way, the student is able to benefit from class presentations about the other tasks and not appear hopelessly behind. At the same time, she is not simply excused from portions of the work.

Quite a bit of individual attention is usually needed for beginning sewing. Some assistance from an aide or volunteer is highly desirable. An advanced student, however, should know the basic techniques and not need much help.

In cooking class, students customarily work in groups. If one student has difficulty with a given task, other members of the team can help. This advantage brings the threat, however, of *too much* help. Emphasize the importance of rotating tasks. Don't let the blind student be continually relegated to doing the stirring after others have put the ingredients together.

Ask, "What is expected of other students at this level?" and guide the blind boy or girl to the same achievement.

Other Sources

The 4-H Clubs (under the Extension service of the state university) are not only for farm children. Projects include sewing, food preparation, home improvement, home furnishings, electronics, and computer work, as well as farm-related activities. Scouting and Camp Fire also have activities related to daily living skills.

The following chapters in this *Handbook* also particularly address the topic of daily living skills:

"Early Childhood"
"Fitting In Socially"
"Dating, Marriage, and the Family"
"Suggestions for the Blind Cook" (Appendix)
"Sewing" (Appendix)

Additional sources are listed in "References" at the end of this *Handbook*. Particularly note:

Lifeskills: A Can-Do Program for Living With Blindness (tips on daily living skills), by Janiece Betker

Parent Tips: A Guide for Blind and Visually-Impaired Parents, by Janiece Betker

Parent Tips: The Challenge Years, by Janiece Betker

So What About Sewing, by Adelle Brown

CHAPTER 36

INDUSTRIAL ARTS AND RELATED SKILLS

By John Cheadle
and
Doris M. Willoughby

Many men and women today (blind or sighted) earn their living as auto mechanics, cabinet makers, tool die makers, electricians, etc. Others enjoy hobbies in industrial arts fields. Everyone, to one degree or another, works on home repair, maintenance, and remodeling. Every person should learn basic mechanical skills so that he/she will not be helpless when faced with hanging a picture or sawing a board. Some will choose to learn advanced skills. It is a matter of individual ability, interest, and initiative – not sight.

Furthermore, the knowledge that one *can* make repairs and operate power tools is a very important confidence builder.

"But what about safety?" is a question often asked.

If a blind person turns on the power when his hand is touching the saw blade, he will be injured. But so will a sighted person. Problems arise from carelessness, lack of knowledge, or attempting a task beyond one's skill – not from lack of sight. A blind person using appropriate techniques and proper care is just as safe as anyone else. This chapter will describe some techniques in detail, and indicate sources of further information.

If a person with partial sight leans closer and closer to the blade of the power saw, straining to see, this is indeed dangerous. He may cut his hand. He may even cut his nose. But the problem is not the lack of visual acuity. The problem is lack of appropriate techniques and practices, compounded by the incorrect belief that poor sight is more helpful than good alternative techniques which do not use sight.

The methods described in this chapter are safe and efficient. They can be used by the totally blind. They are much superior to attempts to rely on inadequate sight, and hence also are the best method for the partially sighted. However, these techniques will not be learned while the eyes are uncovered and the student keeps trying to rely on vision. While learning, the student should wear sleepshades in order to learn the alternative techniques thoroughly and efficiently. At the same time, she will really become convinced that the techniques work (whereas, if she used her sight at the same time, she would believe that the sight was helping even when it was not). After training is completed, the blind person with some sight can then make an intelligent, informed decision as to whether she will sometimes choose to rely on sight. This matter is discussed at length in the chapter called "Sleepshades".

Overcoming Misconceptions

"In what sequence will Alyssa be taking the Introductory courses?" asked Ms. Cramer as she checked a blind eighth grader's schedule.

"Let's see–first Typing, then Home Ec, then Computers, then...a study hall."

"A study hall?" repeated the itinerant teacher in surprise. "What happened to 'Introduction to Woods'?"

"Well, I think I heard Mr. Kovaks say that Alyssa couldn't really take that," replied the secretary.

Alyssa's IEP clearly called for her to take all regular classes; and all four Introductory courses were required of eighth graders. Ms. Cramer had already provided a booklet of methods for industrial arts, and thought that the classroom teacher was ready. Yet as she unraveled this situation, Ms. Cramer found several layers of problems:

- The wood shop teacher believed that a blind person could not possibly work safely with power tools.
- The principal was sure that insurance rates would go up if Alyssa were in the class.
- Alyssa herself was nervous about Industrial Arts, and so were her parents.
- An unwritten policy excluded all mentally and physically handicapped students from Industrial Arts. Alyssa was the first blind student.
- The shop teacher and the principal were both older men who felt that a young woman teacher could not possibly give good advice about power tools. They also felt that industrial arts was less important for girls than for boys.
- Other than Alyssa herself, the only blind person whom the family and the classroom teachers knew was an elderly man who always clung to his wife's arm.

Ms. Cramer decided, correctly, that this was a critical point in Alyssa's growth as a competent person. Fortunately she had several weeks to work on the problem, since the course was offered during all four quarters.

Ms. Cramer arranged for Alyssa and her family to meet Ben Wilken, a blind man whose hobby was woodworking. They visited his basement workshop, and Alyssa drilled several holes with a drill press. Also, Mr. Wilken was able to take time off from his job as an estate analyst and visit the school to demonstrate and advise.

Ms. Cramer explained that insurance is based on group rates and is not affected by an individual. Furthermore, a blind person is *not* a greater-than-average risk, assuming that proper procedures are followed.

Ms. Cramer's supervisor talked with the superintendent, who had not been aware of the situation.

The IEP team was convened in December instead of the usual March date. They wrote, "Alyssa will attend all regular classes, including Industrial Arts, for which consultation will be obtained from a skilled blind adult."

Some of the parents of students with other disabilities heard about this. They began insisting that all classes be scheduled on the basis of actual individual abilities, rather than on stereotypes of a particular disability.

Alyssa did indeed participate in Introduction to Woods. She, the teacher, and her parents were pleased with her achievement. However, Ms. Cramer learned afterward that while the others had all made a modest project from "scratch," Alyssa had used a prepared kit of materials, and that the teacher had applied most of the finish. Next time, she resolved, she or Mr. Wilken would discuss each step beforehand, and keep in close touch with the class throughout the term.

Unfortunately, Industrial Arts is an area where fear, misunderstanding, and lack of knowledge may be extreme. A live demonstration and discussion by a competent blind person is a tremendous help, and worth a lot of effort to arrange. A film or videotape, such as that available from the Iowa Commission (Department) for the Blind, is very good also. Lay this groundwork with all parties–parents, student, classroom teacher, and the school administration. If you cannot give sufficiently detailed explanation yourself, get someone to help you.

Learning the Basics

EARLY BACKGROUND

Children ordinarily learn to change a light bulb, place a battery in a toy, etc., at a young age. Preteens can saw, hammer, and use a screwdriver or wrench. The blind youngster, too, needs to get a good start in these simple matters, to avoid a pattern of believing that such things are difficult. Urge parents to include the blind child in such activities; seek out opportunities at school. Following are a few examples which, though they may often be considered in another category such as "daily living skills," also fit the discussion here:

- Using "play tools," such as a wrench-and-bolt set or a hammering bench
- Using Erector Sets and other construction toy sets
- Identifying real tools and getting them for an adult
- Assembling a toy or other item from a kit
- Changing light bulbs
- Inserting or changing batteries in toys, flashlights, etc.
- Tightening screws (regular and Phillips)
- Using various keys and locks
- Operating record player, Talking Book Machine, tape recorder (various models with differing features)
- Driving nails or tacks (The very young beginner might hammer nails or tacks into Styrofoam.)
- Plugging in appliances (various locations, various plugs)
- Operating appliances (using dials, pushbuttons, etc.)
- Recognizing dangers with appliances and taking safety measures
- Adjusting the thermostat for the heating or cooling system
- Operating vending machines
- Hand sanding
- Painting or finishing
- Noticing a leak, placing a pail under it, and deciding what to do about it
- Resetting a circuit breaker or changing a fuse
- Making simple repairs
- Taking a toaster, can opener, etc., apart for cleaning, and then reassembling

All of this lays the groundwork for advanced skills to be learned in junior high and high school. There is enough to learn in Industrial Arts class without having to begin with "how to hold a hammer."

GETTING STARTED

Remind parents that often it is beneficial for a child to do only part of a job, or to assist. This step is important in developing readiness for the whole task. The child might assemble part of the new toy, or finish driving a nail which someone else has started. At the same time, it is vital that the older boy or girl *does* complete the whole job independently. For painting a fence, for example, she should: get out all the materials; prepare the paint; prepare the brushes or rollers; protect nearby surfaces if necessary; paint the fence; clean the brushes or rollers; put everything away. If someone else consistently does any particular part of the job, everyone tends to assume "a blind person can't do that very well."

If there are printed directions, a sighted person could read them aloud without actually helping. If the same task is to be done again (e.g., inserting batteries), the blind youngster should remember the directions or take Braille notes.

Many devices, such as screw starters, are not designed especially for the blind but may be especially helpful. A board can be squared with a hand saw by using a regular Try Square–keep the saw against the square while cutting (see below, in John Cheadle's article and elsewhere, for further suggestions). Other devices, such as the Rotomatic measuring device, are designed specifically for the blind. The key, however, is not a device or method, but the *attitude* which presumes success.

Hitting the Mark with Attitudes

Below is an adaptation of an article by John Cheadle in the March/April, 1983, issue of *Future Reflections*. Copies may be obtained from the National Federation of the Blind.

–John Cheadle is employed at the National Center for the Blind in Baltimore, Maryland.

He began his career as a cane travel instructor with the Nebraska Services for the Visually Impaired. Shortly thereafter, he was asked to begin a woodshop class in the Orientation Center for the Blind in Nebraska. Mr. Cheadle explains that the most important purpose of the woodshop class, like all other classes at the Center, was to provide the opportunity for blind persons to develop confidence in themselves.

Later Mr. Cheadle worked for the Missouri Bureau for the Blind and for the Idaho Commission for the Blind, before coming to his present position at the National Center.

Mr. Cheadle is also the father of three children, one of whom is blind.

Home repairs, lawn work, woodworking and automobile maintenance and repair have long been considered the domain of men. It was expected that fathers would teach their sons how to hammer a nail, fix the sink, change a tire and mow the lawn. Mothers would teach their daughters how to cook, sew, do the laundry, clean house and perhaps some gardening.

Those expectations have changed and I believe that is a good thing by and large. Now, boys and girls are both encouraged to take home economics and woodshop in high school. Mothers insist on their sons learning to cook, and fathers are showing daughters how to use power tools.

Expectations are also changing for our blind youngsters. In the December, 1982, issue of *Future Reflections,* we had an article entitled, "Let Your Blind Child in the Kitchen, Mom." The point was made that blind children (especially boys) are often short-changed in culinary experiences. The article encouraged parents (especially moms) to give their blind children more experience in the kitchen.

The same can be said of some areas typically associated with fathers, namely home repairs, woodshop, lawn work and automobile maintenance and repair. It is often erroneously assumed that blind persons are necessarily limited in these areas. If we believe that, it is only natural that fathers will *not* take the time to teach their blind son or daughter how to change a tire, use a power saw, or mow the lawn. And such has too often been the case. The purpose of this article is to (1) dispel the myth that blind people are less safe or capable at these tasks than others and (2) provide some ideas about alternative techniques that blind people can use to perform these tasks safely and efficiently.

First, the myth that blind persons are necessarily limited in these areas. The best response to that is to point to the thousands of blind men and women who routinely mow their own lawn, fix the kitchen sink and plant a flower or vegetable garden. Jim Walker (in an article in the March-April, 1983, issue of *Future Reflections*) is but one example of a blind youngster, now grown up, who learned these things from his father or on his own. There are others: a pig farmer in Nebraska who fixes the roof on his barn; a teacher in Idaho who changes the oil in his van; a federal employee from Virginia who fixes his kitchen sink; a housewife in Missouri who cans vegetables and fruits from the huge garden she plants yearly; and a radio announcer who designs and makes a combination desk/bookshelf for his study.

These people are *not* amazing or exceptional. They are simply ordinary people going about ordinary tasks. Most of the techniques and tools they use are the same as sighted people use. Sometimes, alternative techniques and adapted equipment are necessary, but there is nothing mysterious or difficult about them.

Thomas Edison once said, "Genius is 1% inspiration and 99% perspiration." Neither you nor your blind child have to be "geniuses" or "professionals" or even very creative to be successful in teaching and learning the common skills associated with home, shop and auto. Belief and persistence are the keys. Following are some specific suggestions:

Automobiles:
When you are working on your auto, encourage your child to observe and help. Show him or her what and where the different parts are. Have them learn about the tools you use and ask them to help you by finding a particular tool. As they become older or more experienced, begin to show them how to do some of the tasks and then let them do it. Changing a tire, checking and adding oil, changing the oil and changing filters are some common things you may want to teach them.

Your youngster also needs to learn from you how much vehicles and their parts can differ. For example, jacks are made differently and some cars will have a certain, special kind of notch or fitting for the jack, and others will not. Some may use a scissors jack, some may need a bumper jack and some may use a screw jack. And there are many varieties within these three types. In some cars, the gas tank will be in the back under the license plate, in others it will be in the front, or on the driver's side to the back or on the passenger's side to the front. It will help if your child becomes aware of these kinds of differences.

For most of the basic tasks, nothing special is needed. The jobs can be done by sound and touch with few if any modifications. Most dipsticks, for example, have "full" and "add" markings which are easily felt. If yours is not, just file a notch or scratch a mark where needed. I would also suggest that you *not* slide your finger down the dipstick when locating the oil. It is best to lightly tap the index finger up and down, beginning at or above the full mark and working your way down. This way you can feel the "tug" or adhesion of the oil as the finger pulls away from the stick. When you have located the oil, leave the finger there and locate the "full" and "add" marks with your thumb or thumbnail.

Sounds are helpful, too. If you are working on the engine and drop a part down through it, stop and listen. With experience, you can tell by sound what part or parts of the engine the item hits. Knowing that, you can track the item to its probable location. For example, a generator makes a dull-hollow sound and the engine block has a distinctive sound. Since no one, sighted or blind, can see down through an engine, you may find yourself adopting this technique.

Most of us and most of our blind children will only learn enough about automobiles to serve our own personal purposes or interests. Some of our blind youngsters, however, may become interested in related vocations. There are blind people who are auto mechanics, engineers, machinists, small engine repairmen and machine operators in industry.

For the more technical and sophisticated levels of work, some adapted equipment may be necessary. Items such as Braille micrometers and Brailled meter-readers and torque wrenches are available. Other tools, including regular modern torque wrenches, are easily adapted.

Home Repairs and Woodshop:

[*Note: The original article includes descriptions of several specific methods and tools, one of which is reprinted as follows.*]

Hand Saw (Cross-Cut):
After measuring and marking, put your wood in a vise or secure with clamps. Find the mark, place your index fingernail on one side of the board where the mark begins, and your thumbnail in the mark on the other side. Bring your saw-blade over

till it touches your thumbnail and fingernail (it should then be right on your cutting mark). Draw the saw back once to start the cut. Leave the saw in place, move your hand away from the blade, slide a square up to the saw blade (this acts as a guide to keep your saw in the proper place) and make your cut.

Partial Vision:
We use the term "alternative techniques" instead of "substitute techniques" because "substitute" connotes inferiority while "alternative" implies equality. It is accurate to say that some blind techniques are just as good as sighted techniques, some are superior to sighted methods, and a few are inferior.

I currently employ many of the alternative techniques of blindness in my own work [as a fully sighted person]. My experiences demonstrate that these techniques are often safer, more efficient and more accurate than the "sighted" methods I had been taught. For example, the use of templates and edge-guides provide a safer cut (there is less chance of binding the saw blade), are more efficient (it takes less time to set up templates and a straight-edge than it does to measure and mark), and more accurate (templates are consistent, pencil marks aren't, and the straight-edge reduces the chances of straying off the cutting line).

In regards to teaching alternative techniques to partially-sighted kids, I am a strong advocate of sleep shades (blindfolds). First of all, it makes learning the alternative techniques faster and easier. Secondly, it builds confidence to know that sight is *not* required to do the task. Finally and most importantly, your youngster will be able to make informed decisions about when his sight can be used safely and efficiently and when an alternative technique is better. That kind of decision cannot be made unless one has the appropriate alternative skills.

Lawn Work:
Again, most lawn and gardening work needs no special comment. Touch, sound, memory, special markings or systems are utilized here the same as in any other area. Each person should work out his/her own methods and systems according to personal preference and specific circumstances.

Many blind people do mow their own lawns and perhaps a comment or two would be helpful. The technique used will vary according to personal preferences, type of equipment used and the size and shape of the lawn. Guides or straight edges, such as a moveable rope between poles, or a cyclone [chain link] fence rail laid out on the ground, might be helpful. [Editor's note: a tactual border around gardens, etc.–such as the cut-up rubber tires often used for this purpose–can also be helpful, especially for beginners. The person should slow down somewhat in anticipation when he/she is near such a barrier, and will easily perceive when the machine actually encounters the barrier.]

Whether your child ever mows a lawn regularly or not, it would be good for them to know about the equipment used. They could learn where the blades are, how to start it and how to fill it with fuel. As with the automobile, they should be aware of the different kinds of mowers. In fact, it is always a good practice to let your child know and experience the variety of shapes, sizes and brands modern-day equipment and products can come in.

Electrical Work and Electronics

How can a blind person work with "hot" electrical wires? The answer lies in common sense and an appropriate level of skill, and is really the same as for anyone else.

First, no person should attempt something beyond his skill. A three-year-old is very carefully watched in relationship to anything electrical. A teenager learning to repair appliances should work under careful supervision.

Second, everyone should learn and obey safety rules –e.g., knowing where the "hot" wires are, and turning off the power when necessary. Instructors who teach this kind of work know the normal safety precautions against shock and injury, as well as the conditions under which shocks are likely to be dangerous. In the absence of unusual health problems such as heart conditions, blind students should not be assumed to be more delicate than others.

Simple techniques make electrical and electronic work possible for the blind as well as the sighted. A number of blind persons are qualified electricians, technicians, or electrical engineers.

Most household wiring employs sheathed or jacketed cable which consists of three wires side by side in an outer jacket, and which is much wider than it is thick. The uninsulated wire is the ground wire and easily distinguished by touch. The problem is to determine which is the white wire (usually used for "neutral") and which is the other color (usually red or black, and used for the "hot" wire).

Usually the most convenient method is for the student to ask someone which color is which. After the wire is once identified, usually all that is needed is to make that wire identifiable to the touch. One wire might be cut, stripped, connected, or bent; or a splicer (such as a wire nut or Scotch Lock) might be screwed onto the end. This identification can be applied either to the wire being worked on or to the one *not* being worked on, whichever is more convenient. Often it is best to bend one wire out of the way while the other wire is being worked on.

In more complex situations, labels or markers can be attached – simple markings such as bits of tape, or Braille labels if needed. It is also possible to use an audible continuity tester.

Buzzers, or other readily available auditory or tactual testers, may be used in place of light bulbs for testing circuits. More sophisticated auditory test equipment can be obtained if needed. However, live readers usually are more available and more economical in educational settings. (In this context, "reader" is used in a very broad sense, to include anyone who might tell the blind student the color of a wire, read a few printed labels, etc. This includes lab partners, classmates, the instructor, etc. See also the chapter on "Other Modes of Reading."

In some parts of the electronics industry today, most electrical connections are "crimp" or "wire-wrap" and do not require soldering. However, many blind people have developed methods for soldering. The Smith-Kettlewell Institute (see "References") has extensive information on soldering and other techniques in electronics.

The serious student may wish to purchase special adapted devices such as audible voltmeters.

Diagrams

Various options exist for producing raised diagrams, as described in the chapters on "Maps" and "Mathematics." Often, however, the best option is to describe a diagram aloud, and/or to show the student the actual arrangement with real tools and materials.

In mechanical and technical drawing classes, the blind student does not expect to produce a perfect product with his/her own hand. However, it is important for the blind student to (1) learn the concepts involved, and (2) learn the standard appearance and form of the symbols. Understanding how the drawings are made will allow him/her to work with a sighted reader (who may have no technical knowledge) and interpret or produce diagrams.

Power Tools

Many persons will readily grant that blind students can use hand tools, but nevertheless feel panic about power tools. Despite P.L. 94-142, vociferous objections are sometimes encountered from teachers and administrators, as in Ms. Cramer's experience.

This problem often includes resistance to the use of sleepshades, as persons illogically assume that attempting to rely on partial sight must be better than using alternative techniques. Explain why and how alternative techniques are safer and more efficient. Note that standard safety goggles can have dark cloth or paper inserted to make "safety sleepshades."

Before a problem arises, help parents become aware of their rights, and of the normality of blind students' taking Industrial Arts. Enlist the help of school administrators who have a positive attitude. Provide demonstrations, discussions, written suggestions, and films. Plan well ahead, so that staff can consider ideas without immediate urgency.

To do accurate work, blind persons often find it helpful to use more guides, jigs, templates, clamps, etc., than a sighted person might. This does not mean, however, that special safety guards must be used. The competent blind worker uses the ordinary guards and safety procedures which are important for anyone.

HAND-HELD POWER SAW (CROSS CUT)

(*Note: This description of the hand-held power saw is adapted from the article, "For Fathers (And Others): Some Tips On Alternative Techniques," by John Cheadle.*

> You will need an edge-guide for this cut. Protractor-style edge-guides are available from most stores that carry a good selection of tools or you may build your own. A template cut from hardboard would also be helpful but not necessary (see description below for explanation of its use).
>
> Measure, mark (using tactual marking), and secure your wood. Then, take your saw and measure the distance between the tool's blade and the outside of the saw's guiding-edge. (Let us call this the saw plate width.) Then use either of the following approaches: (1) starting at your cutting mark, measure back as far as the saw plate width, and secure your edge-guide at that point; or (2) beside your cutting mark, place a template which has been cut to the dimension of the saw plate width. Secure the edge-guide next to the template on the side opposite the cutting mark, then remove the template.
>
> Finally, bring your saw into position by lining up the guiding-edge of the saw with the edge-guide. Place the teeth of the blade against the piece to be cut and draw it back an inch or so. Turn the saw on and let it come to full speed. Move the saw forward along the edge-guide until contact with the wood is made. Make your cut. (See Figure 36-1.)

DRILL PRESS

Follow this procedure:

(1) Hand-punch a small hole at each point to be drilled. (A grid of tactual lines is sometimes used, with the intersections locating the places for the holes.)

(2) Consider the depth of hole desired. If drilling entirely though the wood, it is possible merely to listen for the bit to come through

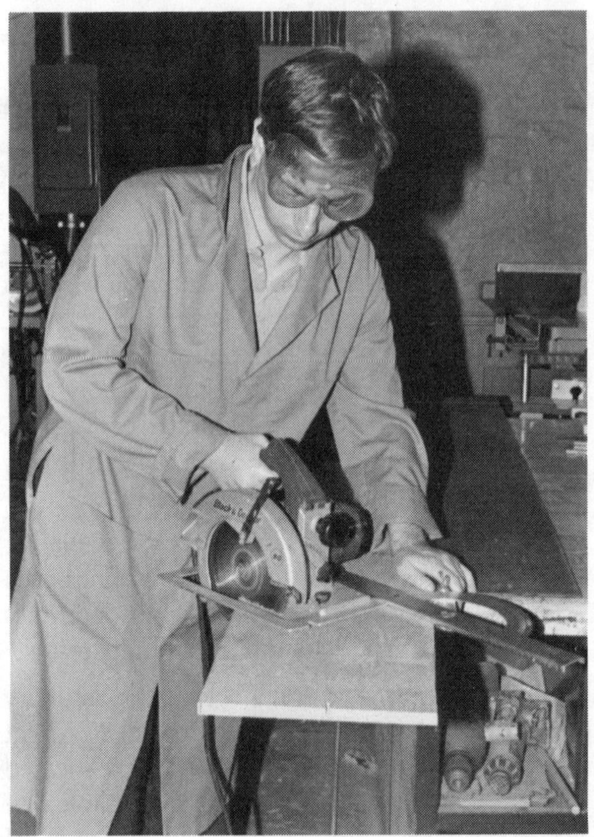

Figure 36-1
Hand-Held Power Saw

the underside. Usually, however, it is preferable to use the depth gauge, which is a threaded rod easily set by touch.

(3) Place the bit (drill point) in the chuck (the holder for the drill point). With the machine still off, bring down the bit and align it with a hole. Lock it into alignment.

(4) Raise the drill.

(5) Turn on the power and lower the drill.

(6) Listen as the drill engages the wood and proceeds through.

(7) When the drill reaches the desired depth, raise the drill and turn off the power.

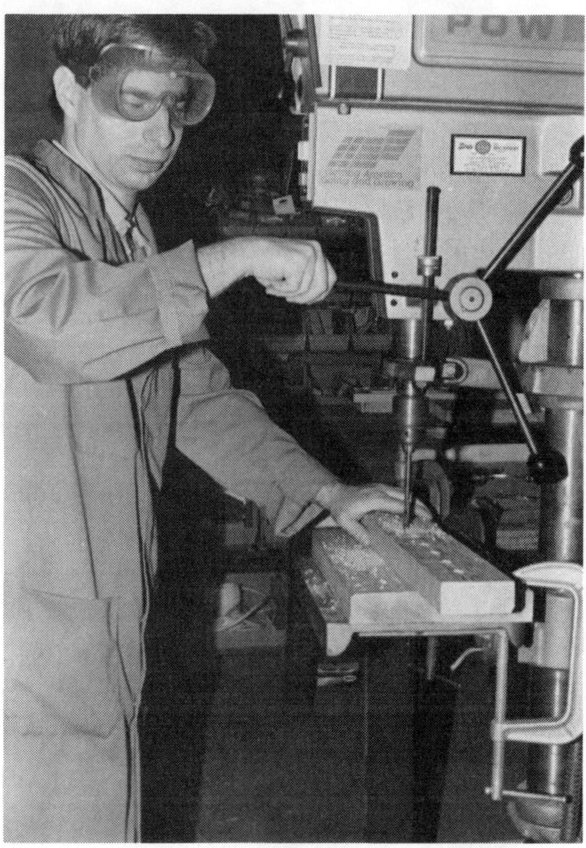

Figure 36-2
Drill Press

FURTHER INFORMATION IN APPENDIX

This chapter, "Industrial Arts and Related Skills," is intended as general background for anyone working with blind students. A detailed description of the use of two power tools is included here as part of this background.

The Appendix, "Alternative Techniques with Power Tools," gives detailed technical descriptions of high-accuracy measurement devices, and of techniques for additional power tools. The Appendix assumes that the reader has considerable background in industrial arts. Tools and devices discussed there include:

Rotomatic (measuring device)
Braille Micrometer (measuring device)
Band Saw
Scroll Saw
Radial Arm Saw
Router
Power Sander
Push Stick
Feather Board

Finishing

Hand sanding is easily done by touch.

The beginner should choose a finish which can be touched without spoiling it. It is often helpful to touch the surface deftly with the fingertips. (Keep a can of appropriate solvent close by for cleaning the fingers to avoid obscuring the sense of touch.) With practice, however, it is possible to tell whether the brush or roller is being applied to a dry surface or to one which is already wet. An experienced blind worker can use any finish desired.

"Feathering" the surface (that is, making long strokes over the whole area after applying the finish) is often helpful. Strokes may be made across the grain as well as with the grain. This evens out the finish, and also is one way of being sure that no surface has been missed. Not all finishes can be "worked" in this way, however.

Every worker, blind or sighted, should observe standard procedures which keep the proper amount of finish on the brush or roller.

Conclusion

Industrial arts classes (especially introductory classes) are not necessarily vocational training. *Everyone* should have some background in this area. Girls were once excluded, but now participate routinely. For blind students it should be the same. With the proper approach, the average blind student can succeed as well as his/her sighted classmate.

Appropriate techniques sometimes involve added guides or adapted devices, but they do not involve added safety guards. Blind students use the same safety procedures and guards as anyone else.

Remember the teacher who limited Alyssa to a prepared kit instead of an original project. Other teachers may incorrectly assume that blind students cannot find their own tools, cannot put them away, cannot walk around alone, need constant individual help, must work very slowly, etc., etc. Keep in close touch as the class proceeds. Do not merely ask, "Is everything OK?" Ask probing yet tactful questions such as, "What machine is she using now?" "How much of that job is she doing all alone?" and "What is the rest of the class doing now?" Visit the classroom if possible (or if you have a consultant helping you, ask him or her to do so).

If a particular tool or procedure is not discussed here or in the Appendix, this does *not* mean it is inappropriate or difficult. Space has limited this discussion to a few representative procedures. Often the ideas here will directly apply to a similar situation.

Ingenuity, plus the knowledge of several techniques, permits figuring out a different procedure. Basic principles apply in various areas – plastics, metalwork, lathes, machine tools, etc.

For example, Small Engine work is taught in many high schools. Techniques in this area are easily figured out by emphasizing the sense of touch and making use of hints found throughout this book.

There are many helpful tools and devices which were not mentioned here; but often a little ingenuity will do as well as expensive special equipment. For example, in place of a carpenter's level, a ball bearing in an angle iron serves well. Furthermore, in evaluating an entire flat surface, a marble may simply be placed in the center to check all directions at once.

If you need information on a procedure not covered here (such as welding), or would like further detail on the material which is included here, consult other sources such as the following. See "References" for complete bibliographical information.

Industrial Arts – Methods for Blind Students (videotape)
Techniques for the Blind Student in Industrial Arts, by David Hauge
"On Driving Nails and Hitting the Mark with Attitudes," by John Cheadle
"For Fathers (and Others): Some Tips on Alternative Techniques," by John Cheadle
"Growing Up: Some Reflections of a Blind Father," by James D. Walker

See also the Appendix, "Alternative Techniques with Power Tools," in this *Handbook.*

CHAPTER 37

MATHEMATICS

"Girls' math anxiety" has received a lot of attention recently. The stereotyped image, formerly accepted by girls as well as boys, is now rapidly disappearing: the fluffy-headed woman who can't balance a checkbook, let alone comprehend geometry or algebra.

"Blind students' math anxiety," based on an equivalent stereotype, should be similarly banished. There is no reason why, with proper teaching and a positive attitude, blind students as a group need have special trouble with math.

The Nemeth Code

Before the invention of the Nemeth Code by Dr. Abraham Nemeth in approximately 1965, there was much difficulty and inconsistency in representing scientific and mathematical symbols. With the Nemeth Code, there is a one-to-one precise correspondence between each ink-print symbol and its Braille equivalent.

Many elements are the same as in literary Braille. Letters and words are the same, with a few differences in the rules about use of contractions. Numerals are the same shape, but appear in the lower portion of the cell instead of at the top. Punctuation which appears immediately after a numeric symbol must have a special "punctuation indicator."

All Braille materials prepared today for math or science, from kindergarten through advanced college level, use the Nemeth Code.

It is appalling, however, how poorly some university programs prepare future teachers of blind students. Recently I asked a colleague, who seemed to have difficulty with math materials, whether her college program had taught the Nemeth code. "Oh, yes," she replied, "but I was sick and missed most of that week." A complex code – the basis of math instruction for all blind students today – to be learned in ONE WEEK??? If your college has left you with this incredible gap, seek out an additional source of instruction. Formats and symbols common in elementary school should be memorized. (Many expressions once considered "advanced" are now used in the early grades.) If you have to look everything up, you will work slowly and make mistakes. For less common signs which it may not seem necessary to memorize, it is essential to know where to find them and how to use them.

Even kindergarten materials use the Nemeth code. It is not recommended that students begin math instruction with some other notation and then learn Nemeth later. However, of course, a particular format or symbol might be simplified in a particular situation. For example, if a first-grade text has circles, squares, triangles, etc., as spaces in which to write answers, the young Braille student might be given the same "blank" symbol each time.

The Braille teacher should have a thorough understanding of the Nemeth Code overall. However, it may be possible for someone else to prepare certain materials despite a limited background. Simple problems drilling on the four operations are good examples. Someone who does know Braille well must monitor this carefully, watching for difficulties and exceptions to rules.

A student who uses Nemeth code from kindergarten will learn it naturally and easily.

Even such a student, however, can be careless or vague in the use of technical symbols. Check this carefully, and be especially vigilant when starting a new area such as algebra. Does your student really understand the notation for superscripts, subscripts, complex fractions, etc.?

REFERENCES ON THE NEMETH CODE

A helpful summary of the most common symbols, by Sharon L. M. Duffy, appears in the Appendix section of this *Handbook*. However, a complete description of the Nemeth Code is beyond the scope of this book. For the complete code, refer to *The Nemeth Braille Code for Mathematics and Science Notation* from the American Printing House for the Blind, or *An Introduction to Braille Mathematics* from the National Library Service for the Blind and Physically Handicapped.

Improved Skill Through the Use of Braille

Delaying the use of Braille often causes difficulty in math. In general reading, a student who can barely see the print may just barely get along with liberal use of context clues. But the context won't help him read the numbers in a math problem! Also, even if he can read ordinary numbers, he may have difficulty seeing fractions, decimal points, etc.

Following are some suggestions to aid in the transition to Braille for a student who formerly used print:

- Consider giving non-competitive grades (e.g., pass/fail) during a transition period.
- Note that the numerals may require almost no teaching if the student already knows literary Braille. The four common signs of operation (+ - x ÷) and the "equals" sign can be learned very quickly. Much work can be done by using these symbols only.
- At first it may be helpful for an adult to read each problem aloud while the student examines the Braille copy.
- As another transitional step, the student's "reading" might be separated from his "working the problems." He might practice reading problems without actually working them (meanwhile doing math assignments orally or in some other way). Alternatively, he might read each problem aloud before working it, with an adult available to correct misreading. (Caution: Do not continue this help too long, or the student will fail to take responsibility for correct reading.)
- At first have the student do only part of his work by using Braille, while the rest is done orally or with large print. Gradually increase the use of Braille.
- Anticipate unfamiliar formats.

Math Workbooks for Young Children

What about all those rows of bunnies or bears to be counted; all those bees that are supposed to have lines drawn to the flowers? Must we make realistic raised pictures for all of those?

PICTURES AND DIAGRAMS

Raised pictures, and especially raised diagrams, have their place. Several suggestions are described here in this section, and also under "Maps." But don't wear out your transcribers in attempting to convert every picture into tactual form "as is." There are many alternatives. A raised-line picture is *not* necessarily the best alternative – it may be much slower and more confusing for the student.

First, those groups of bunnies to count. Instead of a shape resembling a rabbit, it is customary to provide a row of simple raised shapes – perhaps little squares – or a series of Braille r's (the same number as there are rabbits). Line them up in straight rows, even if the printed pictures are not. Hunting around in a jumbled arrangement is a difficult and irrelevant task.

How will the bees get to the flowers? The same system can be used to represent the pictures themselves, of course, using two different symbols. However, whereas with the bunnies the child was simply asked to indicate the quantity, here we have a matching task. The child could draw a line from each bee to a flower, preferably using a waxy crayon that can be felt. But often another method is better. One idea is to pin or otherwise mark each flower which has a bee (without necessarily drawing a line *from* the bee *to* the flower). Or, two sets of small objects can be used to represent bees and flowers (e.g., marbles and cups), so that the child can physically place each "bee" into or onto a "flower."

You may want to consult in person with transcribers preparing workbooks for young children, as they often appreciate suggestions on format.

WHAT IS THE PURPOSE OF THE LESSON?

Always consider the *purpose,* and select priorities and methods accordingly. The purpose of matching bees and flowers, most likely, is readiness for the problem: "There are six flowers. There are four bees. If each bee visits one flower, how many flowers are left without bees?" With this in mind, you may be able to move a bright student on to this step quickly. Soon he will be able to examine the picture and simply say, "Four flowers match the bees, so two are left over." For independent work, he could write the Braille number to show "how many left over."

Coloring, cutting, and pasting may be called for in the printed workbook. Again, consider the purpose. The blind child might manipulate real objects. Or, he might place pins on the objects to be "colored." Unless art or handwork is the real purpose of the activity, it is usually best to seek a faster alternative.

Sometimes a lesson can be done entirely orally, although for a young child it is usually best to have some concrete objects or symbols.

When the purpose is learning the actual symbols for numbers, or simply counting items, a ready-made game may supplement the printed page. Various games such as Rack-O have Braille numbers on cards; the student might read the cards, place them in sequence, or actually play the game. Games using dice and dominoes require the counting of dots.

Methods and Equipment

Collect simple and practical items and ideas.

Large primary *clock faces* may be adapted by adding Braille markings, or obtained ready-made from the American Printing House for the Blind (APH). Regular clocks, without glass and with suitable tactual markings, may be used. Collect old Braille watches for practice purposes. Enlist the help of the Lions Clubs or others to see that every blind student beyond grade school has his/her own watch.

Provide Braille *rulers,* yard sticks, and meter sticks.

Work with *real money* at every opportunity. (It is unfair to ask a blind child to identify coins that are glued or reproduced flat on a page. It is important to be able to feel the thickness of the coin and the texture of its edge.)

United States bills cannot be distinguished by touch. Therefore, the blind person should determine what each bill is when he receives it, and file it in the billfold in a distinctive way. It is possible to place each denomination in a different location. However, a more flexible method (usable with any billfold) is to fold each bill in a distinctive way. For example, ones might not be folded at all; fives might be folded the long way; tens folded the short way; and twenties folded twice. Practice making change and sorting money in a real billfold.

Fraction "pies" and other concrete aids are available from APH and commercial sources.

Number lines are frequently used in today's classrooms, and may be constructed in Braille or large print. It can save time to draw several number lines on one page, (without numerals) and make copies. Thermoform can be used to copy such a Braille page, and large print can be photocopied. At times a Braille student may dictate directions to a sighted reader who draws answers on printed number lines. The "APH Number Line Device" provides a ready-made choice of ranges in which pegs may be moved.

The *Cubarithm Slate,* very popular in the past, is still helpful today. Small cubes, which can be turned to depict the various Braille numerals, can be arranged and moved about in a plastic grid. Possible uses include displaying spatially-arranged problems, and providing variety to any lesson.

The *"talking calculator":* What is its role? The best plan here is also the simplest: follow the regular policy of the school district for the use of calculators by sighted students. Usually calculators are forbidden in certain situations (notably where mathematical processes are being initially learned); optional in others; and expected in still others. Provide an earphone for classroom use.

An exception may be made for any student–sighted or blind–who has tremendous difficulty in math. Such a student may be permitted to use a calculator more than usual, in order to move on to other important skills rather than working on the same things indefinitely.

The Cranmer Abacus

The Cranmer Abacus, available from APH, is in very wide use. Its role is comparable to that of paper and pencil rather than a calculator, and it should be an option at any time. Even in kindergarten or first grade the child can begin. The older student can save a great deal of time by doing all calculating on the abacus, and writing down only the problem number and the answer. Also, sometimes the abacus can be used to "note down" an answer which was figured in some other way, and to "hold" it temporarily. This might occur with mental arithmetic, or when a student looks at a Brailled problem and does not write the answer directly under it.

A wide variety of computation is possible on the Cranmer Abacus–fractions, decimals, etc., as well as the four basic operations. A coupler (also from APH) can join two abacuses together for large problems.

TEACHING THE PAPER-COMPATIBLE ABACUS METHOD

Many teachers of the blind in this country have avoided the abacus because the calculation system was so different from traditional Western on-paper methods. If a blind child learned the traditional Western methods of calculation (in print or Braille), then it was difficult to devote time to developing skill on the abacus. If, on the other hand, much time and attention was devoted to learning abacus skills, the student would not understand the on-paper computation used by her classmates.

In consultation with Tim Cranmer, the inventor of the Cranmer Abacus for the blind, a completely new system of instruction has been worked out which *is* compatible with traditional Western methods of computation. A complete description appears in the Appendix, "The Paper-Compatible Abacus." This exciting new method overcomes the difficulties arising from differences between Western and Oriental modes of computation, while retaining the great value of the abacus as an efficient and speedy tool for blind students.

TEACHING THE ORIENTAL METHOD

Many students today have already learned the Oriental method and should not be asked to change. Others may prefer that method. The instruction book I have found most helpful in teaching the Japanese method is *Detailed Instruction on the Use of the Cranmer Abacus,* by Nancy Jacquat Foster. It proceeds in logical sequence, with clear explanation and many examples.

Teachers will find the Appendix on "The Paper-Compatible Abacus" (in this *Handbook*) useful even if they are using the Oriental method; many aspects of instruction and calculation are the same.

PARTIALLY-SIGHTED STUDENTS

Abacus methods should not be restricted to students who use Braille. However, partially-sighted students should use touch rather than sight, because they are likely to see two beads as one. Sleepshades should be worn during practice, to promote accuracy and consistency.

General Speed and Efficiency

HOW CAN THEY FINISH ALL THOSE PROBLEMS?

Speed, flexibility, and accuracy are good weapons against "blind students' math anxiety." Guide your students, from the very start, to assume they can accomplish the same quality and quantity of work as others. Although any individual might need adapted or shortened assignments at a particular time, there should not be a regular policy of shortened assignments.

"Why must the blind student learn the longhand method of division, etc., when he will just be using an abacus or talking calculator anyway?" This dilemma has no pat solution. In general, it is desirable to do some work on the longhand method (with Braille problems written out in full, and with answers written in the conventional way) until the child gets the general idea. A well-informed blind person avoids unnecessary gaps of knowledge, and finds it useful to know the conventional method of computation. However, once the student has the idea, it is usually best to rely mainly on the abacus. (Note that if the Paper-Compatible method is used, as described in the Appendix of this *Handbook*, calculation on the abacus is very similar to calculation on paper.)

SUGGESTIONS

Following are some general hints to maximize speed, flexibility, and accuracy in mathematics:

(1) Practice the basic number facts with flashcards, just as sighted children do. The answer can appear on the back of a Braille flashcard if plastic is used to counteract wear.

(2) Make a tape recording of basic math facts, with a pause before the answer. There are commercial recordings, sometimes with humorous sound effects.

(3) Keep speed charts.

(4) Teach the abacus early and well.

(5) Emphasize mental arithmetic whenever practical.

(6) It is possible for the student to roll a sheet of Braille problems into the Perkins, and write the answers in the conventional locations. However, this is possible only if the paper is aligned carefully in a machine that does not slip–otherwise dots will be destroyed. For best results, use the same machine that was used in preparing the sheet, and be sure the screw which maintains the left margin does not move. Always roll the paper all the way in, start the linespacing, and *then* roll the paper down to the desired spot.

When writing the digits of the answer to an addition problem, it is not difficult to proceed from right to left. Simply write the digit; backspace twice; add the next column and write its answer; backspace twice; etc.

The Nemeth Braille Code for Mathematics and Science Notation explains the official way to write a subtraction problem and allow room for a two-digit number at the top (e.g., when a "1" is borrowed and a "4" is converted to "14.") Since Braille numerals are always the same physical size, an extra space is needed for a two-digit number written above a single digit. Note, however, that many students will be able to do the borrowing or carrying mentally, and may not need to write in the extra numbers.

Multiplication and division problems, too, can be lined up in a manner similar to print. *The Nemeth Braille Code for Mathematics and Science Notation* describes "spatial arrangements" for each process. If a problem is written horizontally in a book, the student can learn to recopy it vertically when desired.

(7) Answers can be written with the slate as follows: Do not try to write the answer in the conventional place. Write it on a separate paper or on the reverse side of the same paper. In this way you can examine the problem continuously while the answer is being written. For conventional addition or subtraction, remember it is necessary to write the last numeral first and proceed in the reverse of the usual direction on the slate; this need be no problem after a little practice. When finished, recopy the answer onto an answer sheet if necessary.

(8) The Appendix, "The Paper-Compatible Abacus," describes a complete system of abacus usage and also offers a number of general suggestions for mathematics. The Oriental method (also mentioned in the Appendix) is another approach to abacus usage. Furthermore, the abacus can be used to note down answers when doing problems in longhand format. Any answer or number can be set on an abacus for convenience, to "hold" it until it is used in another process or written down.

(9) Usually only the problem number and the answer must be turned in; this saves a great deal of time. When there is a real need to see the student's computation, however, this should be shown in whatever detail is necessary.

(10) Anticipate various Braille formats, and try to introduce them before they appear in the textbook. The first grader can be stymied by horizontal problems if he has only seen vertical notation. The middle school student will need practice with exponents and other more advanced symbols.

(11) If your school uses an innovative method for math computation, such as "Fingermath," or if you yourself like such a method, consider it for the blind student as well. However, whereas the abacus is in general use for the blind in this country, methods such as "Fingermath" are not widely used. Consider whether the methods you teach would be continued if the student moved away.

Advanced Work

Your advanced student may get ahead of you, unless you have an especially strong background in math. The itinerant or resource teacher need not apologize for this, as we cannot be experts in everything. But it is our obligation to find additional sources of information if necessary, and to see that proper materials are available. A blind adult in an engineering or scientific field should be glad to meet with you and your student. The National Federation of the Blind in Computer Science is always interested in helping students.

Braille protractors and other specialized devices may be obtained from Howe Press. Logarithm tables and other charts are available from the National Braille Association. (Note that such tables are sometimes omitted in a Brailled textbook. It may be assumed that the tables will be obtained separately.)

All Those Diagrams, Tables, Graphs, Etc.

IS IT APPROPRIATE?

A tiny or very cluttered diagram may as well be no diagram at all. Most tactual diagrams should be to a larger scale than for the sighted, regardless of the size of the original. To be meaningful to a blind student, any diagram (however simple) should be at least two inches in each dimension. If there are labels, the diagram should be at least four inches each way.

If many different characteristics are shown on the same diagram, it is usually best to make two or more Braille diagrams, each with certain items shown.

Often there are alternatives to reproducing the whole thing, and sometimes the alternatives are more effective. You might reproduce a curve or figure in simple raised outline, and then take the student's hand to show him where various things appear in the print, while describing or naming them verbally. When concepts are well understood, often the written caption or the teacher's description are quite sufficient without any tactual version.

On the other hand, sometimes you will want to bring in extra materials – more than a mere reproduction of the printed diagram – to show important concepts. For example, the Mitchell Forms kit from the American Printing House for the Blind (APH) contains solid mathematical shapes (sphere, cone, etc.) as well as equivalent two-dimensional flat shapes and wire outlines. This is very good for showing relationships of various kinds, such as a cross-section. The Geometric Area and Volume Aid, also from APH, contains units to be assembled in various structured ways. Many aids, from APH and elsewhere, demonstrate fractional parts. Sometimes a regular object, such as a ball, will demonstrate concepts well.

MAKE IT MEANINGFUL

These ideas are helpful in making tactual diagrams:

(1) The single most useful tool is probably a tracing wheel. Common ones may be purchased from a sewing store; special ones are available from art stores, craft stores, and agencies for the blind. Braille paper must be placed face down on a fairly soft surface – a rubber pad is ideal, but a large blotter, several newspapers, etc., will do.

Unfortunately, the tracing wheel must be applied to the back of the paper – that is, the side opposite from where the final drawing will appear. An easy drawing may simply be copied (in reverse if not symmetrical) on the back, and then gone over with the wheel. Otherwise, follow this procedure: Place carbon paper under the Braille paper, facing upward toward the back of the Braille paper. Place the original diagram, face up, on top of the Braille paper. Hold everything together with paper clips. Place the materials on a solid surface, and trace the original diagram firmly with a pen or pencil. The drawing will appear, in reverse, on the back of the Braille paper – ready for the tracing wheel.

(2) Often a regular ruler may be used to guide the wheel while making straight lines. The "glue-down ruler" (from the American Printing House for the Blind), which is very thin, is helpful for complex drawings.

(3) Ways to make contrasting lines, various sizes of dots, different symbols, etc., are described under "Maps."

(4) A "Proportional Divider" is useful in enlarging complex diagrams exactly to scale. It is available at college bookstores and drafting supply stores, and works best with straight lines. This device does not actually do any drawing; rather, it automatically shows the length of the line to be drawn, at up to four times the original size.

(5) With a "Pantograph," used by draftsmen, you trace an original diagram while the device actually draws the same diagram to a larger scale, a few inches away. The larger diagram will be in pencil and will still need to be transcribed into tactual form.

(6) A compass with a spur wheel is available from Howe Press.

(7) The Sewell Raised Line Drawing Kit, from the American Foundation for the Blind, can be useful for spur-of-the-moment drawings. Its stylus is applied to the same surface where the drawing appears, and thus no reversal is necessary. However, the drawings are on flimsy plastic, and are not high-quality or long-lasting.

(8) The Thermoform machine uses plastic sheets for copying Braille or other tactual materials. A plastic sheet is heated until it takes the shape of the Braille page under it. Clever materials can be constructed very simply. It is not even necessary to fasten items onto paper; it is only necessary that they be thin enough not to interfere with the vacuum. A great time-saver is the use of pennies for simple counting

exercises for young children, or arrays to teach multiplication and division. (Caution: It is *not* recommended that students attempt to *identify* coins on a Thermoform copy. Real coins should be used for that purpose.) Simply place a piece of regular Braille paper on the machine (do not place the pennies directly on the machine surface.) Arrange the pennies or other objects as desired. Place the Thermoform paper above as usual, taking care not to disarrange the objects. Proceed in the normal manner to make a copy. Several copies can be made of the same arrangement, or a new configuration can be arranged in an instant. For delicate arrangements, fasten the objects to the paper.

(9) The American Printing House for the Blind offers various kits and aids.

LEARNING TO USE TABLES AND GRAPHS

Using tables and graphs is an important skill for all students, but all too often neglected with Braille students. Spend time with the beginning student, and with the older student having difficulty, to be sure he understands *how* to read and interpret the materials. Ask questions such as, "Read the vertical scale aloud," and "What is the highest point reached, on the vertical scale, by the curve representing Problem A?" Ask the student to move his finger along a particular line while you ask questions about it. Provide enough basic drill and practice so that the student really can *read* tables and graphs before he is expected to make advanced interpretations.

It is especially helpful for the student himself to construct graphs and tables from time to time.

Although these skills are important and relevant, often the time involved in preparing exactly the same materials that classmates use would be prohibitive. Imagination and resourcefulness may be needed. Look at various alternatives and ideas:

(1) For a lengthy unit, consider using a ready-made package which is equivalent. Perhaps your library for the blind has a mathematics text or a "Tables and Graphs" series already in Braille, or perhaps you have prepared similar materials for another student. This approach has the disadvantage that the work requires individual attention and is not exactly the same. Also, the sighted teacher will probably want a printed copy of the material. However, with limited resources this sometimes is the best approach.

(2) Braille graph paper is available, with various sized squares, from the American Printing House for the Blind (APH). Almost any method for making raised markings can be used in conjunction with it. However, be especially careful that lines are suitably contrasting and that clutter is minimized.

(3) The "Graphic Aid for Mathematics," from APH, is very versatile. This is a hard rubber board, 18" x 19", with built-in coordinate lines, and with a supply of rubber bands, pushpins, and flat spring wires. Other items, such as Braille labels, can easily be stuck on. Graphs can be constructed easily and quickly. Moreover, sometimes this can make it unnecessary to use paper at all. Instead, the teacher can quickly construct one graph, go over it with the student, and then construct the next one. The Graphic Aid is also an especially good way for the student himself to construct graphs.

(4) Bar graphs can easily be constructed on graph paper or the Graphic Aid. There are many ways to fill in the appropriate squares – hatch the paper with a tracing wheel, use strips of tape, etc. Bar graphs can also be made on plain paper with the Perkins Brailler, especially if bars are made horizontally.

(5) Especially on a cluttered graph, it may be best not to use graph paper, and best not to show the coordinate lines in their

entirety. Instead show each coordinate line at the edges only, and have the student use rulers to follow them in.

(6) Bold-line graph paper is available from APH. Even students with slight visual impairments may find this helpful, since standard graph paper is often quite faint.

(7) The beginner must have tangible aids in order to understand what a graph is. For the advanced student, however, it is not practical to try to provide all graphs and tables in Braille. Working with a reader is a necessary alternative and valuable experience. Furthermore, there are situations where working with a reader (using regular inkprint materials) is faster and more practical even if a Braille version could be prepared. For example, suppose the student is asked to draw a series of graphs. He might prepare one with his own hand, using tactual aids (to be sure he understands the idea), and then dictate the rest to a reader who draws them in inkprint.

Additional Information

The chapter on "Maps" discusses the preparation and use of tables, and contains other suggestions which are useful in preparing math materials.

CHAPTER 38

MUSIC

Regular Classes

The blind boy or girl should expect to take all required music courses, and decide individually about elective courses and/or private lessons.

Often it is not necessary to transcribe vocal music into Braille. The entire song may be learned by rote, or just the words may be Brailled.

Since musical instruments are generally designed to be played by touch (probably on the assumption that the musician will be using his eyes to see the printed music), the actual playing of an instrument generally presents few technical problems. Tactual labels can be used where necessary, as for organ stops.

Braille Music

One cannot, however, play an instrument with both hands while at the same time actually reading Braille music. Generally it is necessary to memorize. A suggested method is to read a short passage (the length depending upon one's skill), play that passage, read another passage, play it, and then at some point review the entire piece as far as it has been studied.

On the piano it may be best to play each hand separately first; in this case it is possible to read with one hand while playing with the other. There are a few instruments which are played chiefly with one hand, and with these it may be possible to read Braille while playing. The trumpet is one example. The French horn can also be played with one hand if a mute is used during practice.

With vocal music, the hands are free to read Braille. However, the words and music do not have the same relationship as they do in ink-print. To read the music, read the words, and sing–all at the same time–is a difficult task. Usually it is best to learn the tune either by listening or by studying the music separately. The words themselves, however, can easily be read while singing.

Although Braille music uses the usual six dots, its code is entirely different from literary Braille and from Nemeth Code. Furthermore, although any musical score can be written in Braille, the *system* of representation is very different from that of print music. For example, the notes *A, B, C,* etc., are not represented by the same letters in Braille. For example, the note which is read as *C* is represented by dots 1, 4, and 5, which represent *D* in English (literary) Braille. (When Louis Braille introduced raised-dot notation in France, musicians in that country used syllables rather than letters to refer to notes. A movable "Do" was not used.) Also, some of the pitches in a chord are indicated by their interval rather than by lettered notation.

You may need to search to find someone who can produce materials in Braille music for you. It may be difficult to find someone to teach Braille music to your student or to you. The state library for the blind, the residential school, or a special day school may be able to help you locate someone. A blind student or adult who knows Braille music may be very helpful even if he or she is not a "serious musician." If sources are hard to find locally, the Music Department of the National Library Service for the Blind and

Physically Handicapped may be consulted. Also, the Hadley School (see "References") offers correspondence courses for the older student.

Sometimes a combination approach is necessary. For example, a transcriber may assist the student and the band leader in interpreting the score. As another approach, the student who knows Braille music might transcribe it himself: the score could be described by a sighted person who can read the inkprint but knows no Braille.

Large Print Music

Many persons who generally use print efficiently find that some alternative techniques are needed for music. Large print music or memorization may be necessary to avoid "singing into the book."

A special adjustable music stand may help to position instrumental music. To evaluate the practicality of reading music while playing or singing, the student should try reading a selection with many especially small symbols–e.g., sixteenth notes and dotted notes–at the required distance. If this is not easily done, the student is well advised to use memorization.

The Value of Written Music

All of this sometimes raises the question, "Why bother to get the musical score at all if he cannot watch it while he is playing?" The serious student needs the experience of reading the actual score and understanding written music, be it in print or Braille, regardless of whether he/she finds it necessary to memorize before actually playing the piece.

The easiest time to introduce Braille music is when other students begin actually studying notation in regular school classes–usually around third grade. In many schools the "recorder" (a very simple wind instrument) is used to introduce music theory in an enjoyable way. The blind student can easily learn the basic symbols at the same time as others, and then extend his knowledge as he grows older. If it is difficult to get all the music transcribed, produce certain selected pieces. Also, flashcards for the basic symbols are a good way for a beginner to drill.

It is also helpful for the Braille student to have some knowledge of inkprint music notation. This can be done through raised symbols and oral discussion.

Private Music Lessons

The library for the blind and other teachers of the blind may suggest a piano teacher who knows Braille music. Usually, however, it will be a matter of public relations in helping private teachers realize that they can include a blind or visually impaired student by using suitable methods. A teacher may be willing to learn Braille music along with a beginning student. An advanced student may not need a teacher who knows any Braille.

Playing by Ear

Many persons prefer to play by ear. This, of course, presents no technical problems to the blind individual. Playing by ear is a skill which can be developed, and many blind musicians choose to do so. Chord structure and other basic elements of music theory may be studied. It is also possible to learn a selection from a recording. However, blind students, like sighted students, vary in their ability to learn by ear.

It should not be assumed that a person who plays well by ear has no need to learn written music.

Performing with a Group

What about watching the director's baton or hand? During practice it may be helpful if occasionally the director taps the rhythm audibly. But usually–at practices as well as performances–the blind member should become especially sensitive to listening for changes in interpretation as reflected by the members around him/her, in addition to knowing the music thoroughly.

It is also possible for the person behind or next to the blind singer to give unobtrusive touch signals. For example, to prevent the blind student's singing a note too long, the student beside her might squeeze her hand when the director signals a cutoff. As another example, if the blind student is not sure in what direction to face during a concert, the student behind her might gently turn the blind student's head in exactly the right direction.

Many blind students march with regular marching bands. The blind student can listen carefully to surrounding players and thus keep track of his/her own position. Another student can give cues if necessary, especially for turns. Partial sight can be helpful also (however, as always, remember that alternative techniques may be more reliable.) Keeping in step, of course, is done by listening anyway.

Keep Music in Perspective

There is a fine line involved in encouraging blind youngsters to develop all their potential skills, including music, while on the other hand avoiding the stereotype that "the blind are especially musical." We have all seen blind youngsters who are continually hailed as "marvelous" musicians, when actually their musical talent is only moderate, and mobility and other skills are being neglected. Even worse, some blind children seem to withdraw into a world of music - sometimes only passive listening accompanied by rocking or other mannerisms.

Help your student, however gifted, to regard music as one and only one aspect of a normal, balanced life.

References

The following provide further information. See "References," at the end of this *Handbook*, for complete bibliographical information.

Introduction to Braille Music Transcription, by Mary Turner De Garmo

"Experiences of a Music Enthusiast," by Deborah Caldbeck

How to Read Braille Music, by Bettye Krolick.

CHAPTER 39

PHYSICAL EDUCATION AND RECREATION

Very Young Children

If a baby is always held in someone's lap or kept in a playpen, and if people believe that everything is hard for her because she is blind–then her physical development will indeed be slow. If she is placed in a variety of interesting places and positions, and if everyone continually thinks, "How can we best help her learn to do this?" –then she will have equal opportunity with other babies.

Does a child need to be taught to play? Yes. But with sighted children this learning is taken for granted, whereas with a blind child the parents usually need some guidance. Help them meet older blind children and blind adults, to see how they carry on normal activities. Help the parents select toys. Demonstrate how to give physical guidance to *show* the child (many times if necessary) how to ride on a rocking horse, put a doll to bed, build with blocks, swing, etc. Help them avoid toys which really are particularly difficult for blind children, such as especially tiny and flimsy items.

Find constructive ways to discourage stereotyped behavior or mannerisms–especially by keeping the child busy with desirable activities. The book, *A Resource Guide for Parents and Educators of Blind Children,* contains many suggestions for guiding a young child's play and self-help.

You may be especially helpful with the child who is learning to walk. Urge everyone to assume he will soon learn, and to use the methods that are customary with other babies–supporting him in various ways, calling to him from nearby, helping him walk along the sofa, etc. Pushing a large object (a chair, baby buggy, toy lawn mower, etc.) is helpful in building confidence and readiness for cane travel. Explain the value of cane travel itself, and see that it is begun before bad habits are built up. The videotape, *Kids With Canes* (see "References"), shows how cane travel is begun successfully with very young children.

Kids With Canes also shows the use of the cane at a playground. Although the child does not take the cane up a ladder or on a swing, he can place it nearby where he can retrieve it himself. Other children can be taught to leave the cane alone. Thus the blind child can find his way to and among pieces of playground equipment with safety and independence.

Other chapters in this book deal in depth with cane travel and with the general development of very young children.

Physical Education Classes

Is Adaptive Physical Education desirable for a blind student? Sometimes it is, but it should be oriented toward keeping the child in regular P.E. as much as possible. The Individualized Educational Plan (IEP) should spell out how much (if any) P.E. is to be separate from that of the group. Only rarely is it best to make all P.E. separate.

REGULAR CLASSES

Discuss various methods for including the child in regular classes. For example:

(1) *Teaching a specific body motion* (as in calisthenics, swimming, etc.): Give clear verbal directions. Supplement as needed by taking hold of the student and showing her the position, and/or letting her examine someone else's posture. It may be desirable to teach some of the motions before the class meets.

(2) *Ball games and races:*

- Pair the blind student with a partner for running.
- Provide a sound at the goal or base. This may be a mechanical noisemaker or a person's voice. The student can then run without a partner.
- The blind batter may use a batting tee, or may throw the ball straight up for himself and then bat it as it comes down. A kickball pitch may be rolled slowly, or the ball may be placed stationary in front of the batter.
- A ball containing a noisemaker may be used.
- Consider modifying the rules slightly to give the blind player a fair chance. Example: She need not catch a fly ball to put a batter out, but need only touch it before it hits the ground.
- Assign the blind player to a particularly appropriate position and allow her to stay there longer than usual.
- Provide tactual indications (or bright, clear markings for those with useful sight) for sidelines, tracks, etc.

(3) *Tag:* "It" may be provided with a bell and be required to make a continuous sound.

(4) *Trampoline:* The "spotters" around the trampoline may call out directions if the blind jumper moves off center. Also, a small bell may be attached beneath the center of the canvas.

(5) *Bowling:*

- Use a bowling rail (available from the American Foundation for the Blind), the side wall, or some similar guide. The blind player lightly follows this guide with her free hand while walking forward. This is one of the very few situations where counting steps is desirable.
- Some people prefer to walk forward (using the guide rail) all the way to the foul line, then walk backward the appropriate number of steps, and then go forward again to release the ball.
- After the first ball, someone informs the player which pins are still standing.

Individual Assistance In Class

If sighted assistance is to be provided on a regular basis, it is often desirable that the helper *not* be a member of the same physical education class. Despite the teacher's best efforts, classmates tend to feel that they have less fun and achievement if they must help the blind student continually. Using student volunteers from outside the class often solves this, as such helpers will tend to feel they are getting *added* fun and achievement.

Sometimes it is best to provide individual adult assistance in the regular class. However, you will face serious and well-justified resentment if you suggest that the regular P.E. teacher should do very much of this (with the possible exception of a class where two or more adults are present anyway). If the teacher is guiding the blind student, who will supervise the other students? If they see the teacher's attention taken up, they will soon be roughhousing and misusing the equipment.

ALTERNATIVE ACTIVITIES

There may be times when it is best for the blind student to work on something entirely different. Fast ball games are the most typical example: tennis, ping pong, basketball, racquet ball, etc. However, do not assume that all ball games are inappropriate. Use ideas such as those listed above to provide assistance or adaptation as needed.

Avoid substituting an activity which is sedentary for one which is strenuous. Following are examples of appropriate alternative activities:

rope jumping
weight lifting
running or jogging
riding an exercise bicycle
calisthenics
trampoline or Rebounder
martial arts
wrestling
swimming
track
archery

At the secondary level, there is usually a choice of units or sections. Often a student can, by using the regular arrangements, select swimming or tumbling instead of badminton or baseball. Even if most students are not given a choice, it may be easy to arrange it for the blind student.

Arrange individual sessions only when it is really the best alternative; include the blind student in a class for as many sessions as possible.

Where can we find someone to provide individual attention when needed? Consider teacher aides, student teachers, adult volunteers, and older student volunteers. For the child to work alone (without an adult close by) would be inappropriate and possibly dangerous.

If the Adaptive Physical Education (A.P.E.) teacher works with the student, the A.P.E. teacher will take care of some of the individual attention and provide guidance for everyone. He or she should provide a detailed sequence of skills, with activities designed to achieve them. This is especially useful if the youngster needs help with things that have already been mastered by other students.

Work closely with the A.P.E. teacher for mutual benefit. Probably you do not have as much detailed knowledge of P.E. programming as he or she does. At the same time, the A.P.E. teacher may have very little knowledge about blindness. I once talked about a "bowling rail" (meaning the type for the blind, which is merely for orientation), and the A.P.E. teacher thought I meant the kind for the physically handicapped, where the ball goes down a chute. Another time, an A.P.E. teacher asked a blind boy to "step on the footprints" to pattern his foot movements-but the child couldn't see the footprints, and couldn't feel them through his shoes. (She soon thought to have him take off his shoes. But that still didn't help much, since the texture contrast was very slight, and since he had to reach out tentatively to feel for each footprint. After talking to me, she decided to use verbal description and physical prompting instead.)

Learning ABOUT a Game

If the student does not take part in a given game, he nevertheless should learn how the game is played. He might examine a Braille diagram of the field, learn the terminology and rules, practice individual skills such as dribbling, etc.

THE PARTIALLY-SIGHTED STUDENT

The youngster with a relatively slight loss of vision may need fewer adaptations, but it should not be assumed that he needs no attention. Even a student who reads small print easily, sees traffic lights, and has a relatively high visual acuity may have great difficulty following fast-moving balls. Talk with him and his teacher about using bright-colored balls, avoiding unnecessary glare, judiciously planning which positions he should play, etc. If a partially-sighted student has difficulty even when visual arrangements are maximized, he/she should have the opportunity to use alternative methods which do not require sight.

Informal Settings

THE SCHOOL PLAYGROUND

A blind boy or girl with a well-rounded background can fit in and have fun at recess, but it may take planning and guidance. Without guidance, the child (especially a boy) may be left out while the others chase each other across the playground; may be constantly shepherded by a couple of "mother hens;" or may always play with a very sedentary group (usually girls). Think of ways to provide guidance. Often considerable help is needed when the child is getting acquainted with a new playground, and much less help is suitable later. Ideas include: intermittent assistance by an adult aide; a rotation system of child "buddies;" reminders or suggestions by the playground supervisor (Caution: Most playground supervisors are much too busy to give detailed assistance); reserving certain equipment for the blind child part of the time; and showing the child how to do various activities.

Following are some activities with which I have had particular success on playgrounds:

- swings, climbing equipment, etc.
- jumping rope
- beeping balls or beeping Frisbees (if playing alone, the child may throw it, retrieve it, and throw it again)
- playing with suitable toys brought from home (trucks on the sidewalk; toy parachutists; toy animals; etc.)
- walking around and exploring unfamiliar portions of the playground
- building snowmen, sand castles, roads for toy cars, etc.
- sliding or climbing on hills or snow piles
- apparatus such as tin-can stilts

EXTRACURRICULAR ACTIVITIES

Extracurricular activities are important opportunities for recreation and general development. According to Section 504 of the *Rehabilitation Act,* a handicapped student enrolled under an IEP must not be excluded from extra-curricular activities solely on the basis of handicap.

Encourage individual interests, rather than permitting a stereotype of "activities suitable for blind students." Like others, blind students must recognize the dangers of over-commitment *vs.* the benefits of activities. They may also need guidance in understanding just what is involved. One very non-athletic girl insisted she would try out for cheerleading – until her parents realized that she thought a cheerleader simply led vocally, as one might lead a choir! When this student learned about the physical contortions of cheerleaders, she joined the Pops Chorus instead.

ORGANIZED ACTIVITIES OUTSIDE OF SCHOOL

Overcoming Discrimination

[The following is reprinted from *A Resource Guide For Parents and Educators of Blind Children,* by Doris M. Willoughby.]

> At the close of the year-end conference with Mrs. Wathan, the Braille teacher asked, "And what will Billy be doing this summer?"
>
> "Well, he'll be playing around the neighborhood," answered Mrs. Wathan. "But I was sorry to find that there are no organized playground activities for eight-year-olds here in town."
>
> "Oh, I think there are," commented the teacher. "I'm sure I saw a group that age in Westview Park last summer."
>
> "No," replied Mrs. Wathan, "Billy and I went and asked at the Parks Department last week, and they said they had nothing."
>
> "Hmm," replied the teacher thoughtfully. "I'm afraid I suspect that what they meant was, 'We don't have any special programs for *blind* eight-year-olds, and we assume that blind children couldn't fit into our regular programs.'... I'd suggest you call them up, without mentioning blindness, and just ask about programs for eight-year-olds. Then after you learn what the programs

> are, take Billy to the park and enroll him, with advice to the leaders as to how to handle blindness. I'll give you some pamphlets you can offer them; in fact, I'll join you in talking with them if you like. I'm sure they'll include him after they have more information."
>
> Mrs. Wathan did as the teacher suggested, and found that there were indeed several suitable groups. Soon Billy was happily participating every morning.

This is one of the few situations where it may be wise to purposely avoid mentioning blindness for a time. In gaining information, one must somehow get the basic facts without their being distorted by misunderstandings and misconceptions. Discuss this with parents along with the other extreme: it would be most unwise to have Billy actually start out in the play group without anyone's having mentioned blindness.

Tell parents that you would be glad to help and that you would talk directly with the leaders if they wish. Look for others who could help also – especially blind adults with experience in the matter at hand. If transcribed religious materials are requested and you cannot provide them because of legal limitations, locate volunteers without these limitations.

Unless firm guidance is given, it is likely that the blind youngster will often be excluded or that too little will be expected of him/her. Even written manuals on "Including the Handicapped" often sell the blind short. Leaders are likely to excuse the blind youngster from hikes; assume that reading cannot possibly be done if the book is not immediately available in Braille; assign a "buddy" even when one is not needed; etc. Of course, a public-school teacher cannot insist on becoming involved in private activities, but most parents welcome advice.

Regular Or Special Activities?

Especially with summer camps, a thorny question is whether a regular setting or a special group is preferable. This should be an individual matter and not based on anyone's personal prejudices. Usually it is possible to include a blind child in a regular camp or club. On the other hand, sometimes a special group will be better for a particular child. Note the possibility of first attending a special group for one or more sessions, and then later a regular one.

Help teachers of music or dance to realize that they can include a blind or visually impaired student by using suitable methods. It is helpful to keep track of teachers who have had a blind student before.

Participation in community ball teams and other sports is another thorny question. Since organized sports are often competitive and based on tryouts, it may be reasonable for them to exclude a youngster who cannot follow and catch a fast ball. At the same time, exclusion should not be automatically assumed. Be sure the blind youngster really is given equal opportunity at tryouts – a given individual may indeed be able to excel. Playing a particular position may be a solution. Furthermore, there are many sports in which blindness need be no disadvantage at all – swimming, wrestling, and gymnastics are just a few.

See also the chapters on specific topics such as social adjustment, music, etc.

UNSTRUCTURED RECREATION

In some ways this is the hardest situation for teachers and parents to help with, since youngsters choose their own activities and companions outside of class.

Build a Background of Experience

Help the blind youngster to develop the skills needed – both social skills and activity skills – and help peers to develop favorable attitudes. Every activity which the blind child learns will come in handy in joining his/her peers. Can she join in easily to play checkers? To roller skate? To sit around and talk? To go to the park? To go to the movies? Whenever we get a chance to guide relatively informal activities, as at recess or a class party, we should look for opportunities to guide the blind youngster in taking part assertively and appropriately. Encourage parents to invite other youngsters to the home to socialize. Encourage membership in Scouts, religious groups, etc.

Watch For Gaps In Experience

There are some skills which most children learn from each other and which are rarely taught by parents or teachers, but which you may need to teach a blind child. The grade-school child may need to be shown how to hang upside down on the bars. The older child may not have learned "Chopsticks" and the other informal piano "duets" enjoyed by preteens and teens.

Personal Independence

Social and personal skills become vitally important in the teenager's leisure-time activities. Can the young person select food, eat neatly, and handle money efficiently in a restaurant or cafeteria? Can he/she join peers on a shopping trip without being a burden? Does he/she pay for part of the gas when others drive? Again, the more experiences and skills the teenager has, the more easily he or she will fit into varying situations.

A common and tragically unnecessary problem is that of independent travel. Many youngsters reach their teens still very fearful of shopping alone, traveling on a bus, walking on the street outside of familiar areas, and even going into a rest room alone. Do not let this happen to your students because of a rigid school of thought which may have told you that a cane travel teacher must have years of very specialized training and a total absence of personal disabilities. See other parts of this book, and contact the National Federation of the Blind for further information about cane travel.

CHAPTER 40

SCIENCE

Building Equal Opportunity

When Curtis Willoughby first thought about becoming an electrical engineer, most people were skeptical; in fact, he himself thought he might be aiming too high. He knew of an electrical engineer who had become blind in later life and continued in the profession, but in 1961 he knew no one who had gone through engineering school using alternative techniques. Nevertheless, with encouragement from the National Federation of the Blind, he graduated from Iowa State University with a BSEE degree and secured a good job.

Four years later, Lloyd Rasmussen wondered whether electrical engineering was too difficult a course for a blind person. He decided it wasn't, since Curtis Willoughby had succeeded. Today these are only two of many blind engineers in good jobs throughout the country. Once again we observe that the real barrier was attitudes. New methods and equipment have come into use, but there was no sudden revolution in 1961. What was needed was for someone to say firmly, "Yes, I can do this."

Unfortunately, science is still a subject where blind students sometimes are left out partially or completely. The principal of a grade school with several blind students was recently heard to say, "Science is so highly visual–there are a lot of things they can't do." This chapter offers suggestions on overcoming this misconception.

Techniques and Adaptations

Sometimes a modification does need to be made in assignments such as using a microscope. But any modification should provide a logical *equivalent,* rather than a substitute which is easier and/or irrelevant.

The blind student can learn to operate the microscope itself, and set it up for someone else to look into (with the sighted person guiding the fine adjustments). The blind student should be able to make a verbal description of the typical appearance of each item studied, and learn all the concepts which the others learn. If a test requires students to look into a microscope and name the specimen, the blind student can instead be provided with a written description of the characteristics of the specimen. (Sometimes a student with considerable sight will be able to use pictures satisfactorily but not see into the microscope. He could use pictures for study and on a test.)

Generally, the blind student will examine things tactually, and should listen carefully to all descriptions. Sometimes he/she may need an individual oral description. Real specimens or models should be provided when reasonably possible, and a field trip may facilitate this. Be aware of resources in the community such as a taxidermist, a private collection, a museum (especially one with a "hands on" exhibit), a petting zoo, a college science department, or a private laboratory. For anatomy, get a skeleton and/or a life-sized model with removable layers.

DIAGRAMS

There are numerous ways to make two-dimensional diagrams. Many ideas are described in the chapters on "Mathematics" and "Maps."

Be creative. Good representations of living cells can be constructed by making a raised outline and then gluing in various beans and peas for the parts of the cells. In tactual representations of such things as electrical circuits, it is not necessary to make each symbol look just like the print; simple Braille symbols can be used with a key to their meaning.

For the student with some sight, large-scale diagrams made with a very soft lead pencil, with a heavy feltpen, or on a blackboard may be helpful.

Remember that some verbal description is appropriate and is better than a frantic effort to secure every single thing in tactual form. Also, often one diagram can be used to explain several variations. If the student has one or two diagrams of living cells, other cells can be explained verbally by comparison. When a few electrical circuits have been shown in tactual form, others can be described aloud.

Suggestions about class presentations on the chalkboard are included in the chapter, "General Classroom Arrangements and Study Skills."

In a technical drawing class, the goal should *not* be for the blind student to make perfect drawings with his or her own hand, but rather to understand the concepts, comprehend a drawing when it is described aloud, and direct someone else how to make a drawing.

The blind student should study how each symbol appears visually. One reason for this is answering questions on tests. Another reason is that it is often necessary to use a reader who does not know the symbols. The knowledgeable blind student may explain a symbol and ask the reader to name it correctly; alternatively, the knowledgeable student can understand that the "zigzag" described by the reader is an electrical resistor.

LABORATORY WORK

Laboratory work is usually done with a partner, and often the work can easily be divided equitably with very little special planning. When reading a printed dial or judging colors is done by the sighted partner, the blind partner might make the computations or type up the results. Most activities can be done by either partner.

Because of the specialized vocabulary and concepts, it is especially important for the blind student to read the related chapter or workbook pages before class. This will minimize misunderstanding and reduce the need for individual attention. It may also have the pleasant result that the blind student understands the experiment better than his sighted lab partner.

If there is uncertainty about handling equipment that could be dangerous, practice beforehand is desirable. Using Braille labels on dangerous chemicals is just as safe as using printed labels. If the blind student is able to carry out a particular activity, but simply takes longer, additional time can be provided during a study hall or before or after school.

Dissecting may pose special problems. If the student has considerable sight, extra lighting and magnification may help. Organs can also be found by touch; it may be necessary for someone to take the student's hand and show him. In some delicate tasks, it may be best for the student to observe tactually the dissecting which is being done by others, in a manner comparable to that suggested for microscope work, rather than doing the cutting himself. When a test is given, the student's hand might be placed on each organ (with the opportunity to examine its surroundings), or a pin might be placed in the organ to be identified.

Regardless of the exact methods used, the blind student can learn the concepts involved, and learn them with real meaning rather than just verbalization.

If a student partner would have an undue burden because of the nature of the work or the blind student's experience level, it may be best to have an aide or volunteer come in for certain activities. Assistance should always be directed toward increasing the student's knowledge, understanding, and independence.

SPECIAL DEVICES

A program for blind students should provide Braille measuring devices. The serious advanced student may want to purchase other aids. However, for courses below the college level, regular equipment is generally appropriate, with the use of ideas such as those described above.

What Is the Real Problem?

Terry was a good student, but he was failing seventh grade science. When the itinerant teacher analyzed the problem (finding, unfortunately, that no one had told her about it until two tests had been failed), she found a cluster of causes which all made one another worse:

- Many activities depended on pictures or chalkboard presentations, and Terry had had very little experience with this.
- The textbook was on tape, while Terry felt most comfortable reading Braille.
- The tapes of two important chapters were defective.
- Terry did not take notes when using a tape or listening to a live reader, and he read each chapter only once.
- The teacher did not insist that all students read the textbook assignment before class, and Terry did not do so.
- Tests were administered in Braille, using several Nemeth Code symbols that were new to Terry. When he had listened to the material spoken aloud, he had not realized there were any special Braille symbols.
- Since Terry was intelligent and very verbal, he usually could give an adequate oral explanation when asked. However, there were several important concepts which he merely "verbalized" and did not really understand.
- He had no idea that he was having serious trouble until he failed the first test. Even then he thought it must have been just that particular test, or the fact that he was tired that day. He expected to do much better on the second test, but did not change any of his methods.
- Although Terry's parents were well educated, they were not personally interested in scientific matters. Terry's personal background in science was rather weak and did not help him compensate for the above problems.

Terry's parents were very upset after the second test, and asked for a conference. The itinerant teacher analyzed the above causes, and made several recommendations:

- In seventh grade, Terry was old enough to take some responsibility for his own needs. He should speak up and look for alternative arrangements if chalkboard presentations or demonstrations are not made clear.
- Using the tape of a science text is not like listening to a recorded novel. It is usually desirable to go over the material more than once (a general overview and then detailed study). Taking notes is essential. The same is true if it is read aloud "live."
- Science material often has special symbols in Braille and/or inkprint. The student should learn what they are, even if the text is on tape. The specialized teacher or the Braillist should teach these to the younger student; an experienced student should anticipate this and ask about possible special symbols.
- It is especially important for a blind student to read the assignment before the material is discussed in class.
- It is desirable to have someone ask probing questions to be sure that new concepts are really understood.
- A student should be alert to signs that he is not doing well: the feeling of not quite grasping things; uncertainty during class discussions; any low grade; the realization that there are many new and difficult ideas and terms involved. If danger signs continue, he should get help at once.

The itinerant teacher made these recommendations and presented a plan to help Terry catch up. She explained that she would provide certain parts of the textbook in Braille–especially passages with new symbols–but that because of availability it was necessary to use tape for most of the text.

Unfortunately, however, Terry's parents had already concluded that the problems were entirely due to the textbook's being on tape rather than in Braille. They discounted the other causes, and complained that tapes were difficult to use.

The teacher described ways to make effective use of tapes, and again explained that it was impossible to obtain all secondary-school and college materials in Braille. However, several similar situations occurred before Terry's parents really joined in to help him change his approach to "heavy" subjects.

Role Models

Dr. Geerat J. Vermeij is a noted biologist who is blind. The Spring-Summer, 1989, *Future Reflections* includes a reprint of his address, "To Sea With a Blind Scientist." It is vital for blind youngsters–especially those who are particularly interested in scientific fields–to read about and meet successful scientists such as Dr. Vermeij.

CHAPTER 41

TESTING AND EVALUATION

Can a blind student be tested fairly? Generally, yes. But it is important to examine the arrangements for each test to be sure it is appropriately given and non-discriminatory.

Classroom Tests

GIVE SUGGESTIONS

Most classroom teachers give short quizzes and/or lengthy tests on their particular subject matter. The resource or itinerant teacher should offer suggestions and help such as the following:

(1) Transcribe tests into Braille or large print. If the student uses regular print, be sure that the test is a clear, readable copy. Some students who usually read regular print prefer large print on tests.

(2) Despite the advantages of having a test on paper, every blind student should have experience with oral tests. There will be times when Braille or large print will be unavailable. Even if currently it is possible to provide everything in the ideal mode, at some later date the student will encounter the "real world" and need to take a test orally.

(3) Often it is best for the student to give answers aloud for someone else to write down (usually directly onto the test paper).

(4) At other times the student may write down her answers in Braille and then read them aloud.

(5) The student may type her answers, either directly or after making a Braille draft.

(6) Some students with partial sight use handwriting on tests; however the option of typing should be encouraged.

(7) For multiple-choice and true-false, it is often helpful to provide a Braille answer sheet. The Braille letter symbolizing the answer choice can be marked with a pencil even by someone who does not ordinarily use handwriting. An answer sheet helps to ensure that the student works independently without receiving inadvertent hints.

(8) Many tests involve "matching." A typical example would be matching a list of ten characters in Roman history with descriptions of their roles. Unless one set of choices is very short and easy to memorize, this task is extremely difficult to do orally. If there is no time to provide the entire test in Braille or large print, the teacher should nevertheless provide at least one set of choices in written form, so that the student can examine it while the other set of choices is read aloud. (In this example, the names of the characters should be written down.) If even this cannot be provided, the *student* should write down one list of choices (possibly in abbreviated form) as it is read aloud. Also, a way should be provided for "checking off" the choices on each side as they are used.

(9) When questions and/or answers are given orally, it may be hard to avoid giving extra help unconsciously. Offer tips such as the following.

- Be aware that during ordinary class discussion, when a teacher presents two choices he often indicates the correct one by vocal tone. When reading a test aloud, one must make a conscious effort to avoid this. It may be helpful to adopt an arbitrary vocal tone or stress, such as always reading the last choice with finality.

- If some wrong answers are amusing, the reader should not acknowledge the humor until the test is over – not even if the student laughs. Otherwise, the reader is agreeing that the student is interpreting the matter correctly.
- Consider carefully how to elicit the student's answers accurately without actually giving hints. The reader should ask the student to repeat if necessary. The reader may need to say, "That's not one of the choices. I'll read the answers again."
- If the student seems uncertain of an answer, the reader should wait for a decision. He should make sure the student knows about available resources. (For example, a younger student may need to be reminded that she may reread the paragraph even if it is on a different page. Also, any written directions for the test always should be read aloud, even if they seem obvious.) However, these kinds of things can very easily shade into giving extra help (e.g., whenever the reader notices a wrong answer, he suggests rereading the paragraph). Avoid superfluous chatter.
- The student should have as much as possible of the same freedoms that others have. Encourage the student to decide how fast the reader should read, how many times a difficult question should be repeated, etc.
- The reader should steel himself to say calmly, "I'm sorry, I can't tell you," if the student asks for too much help.
- Note that these procedures are also good for reading daily worksheets or handouts, even though they may not be considered "tests," if the other students are expected to fill in the answers independently.

(10) A reader must read *well.* Asking a student to take a test which is read aloud poorly is manifestly unfair. A blind college student recalls, "I have blown tests because the wrong person gave me the test, either someone I was afraid of or unable to direct adequately, or who insisted on working out the answers for themselves, slowing me down." The reader should take direction from the student (to read faster or slower, skip, repeat, etc).

(11) The blind student should be given the very same test as others. This may seem obvious; but especially with an oral test, there is a temptation to simplify or shorten. Suggestions for special formats, such as map skills or microscope work, are given in other chapters of this book.

A blind adult recalls: "My speech teacher wanted to skip the quizzes. She said it was not that important since I was doing well anyway. I disagreed. If she was right, then every good student should have been excluded from taking them. The fact was that she was too lazy to give them to me. Because of that, I, English major that I am, did not take senior English in order to avoid this teacher and her degrading notions about blindness."

(12) For an oral test it is usually necessary to work in a separate room.

VERY YOUNG STUDENTS

Note that the *Patterns* Braille instruction series (as any good reading curriculum) has tests correlated with the various levels. They are "diagnostic" tests, which indicate not only overall success, but also the nature of any difficulties (e.g., Inflectional Endings, Reading Comprehension, etc.) With a good student, these are reassuring. For a student having trouble, they are invaluable in analyzing problems.

Very young children sometimes are frightened or confused by a testing situation. They may balk when the teacher cannot tell them an unknown word; they may fear punishment; they may be intimidated by a difficult page or unfamiliar format. One cannot, of course, give actual help. However, there are many things that can improve the atmosphere. Explain carefully beforehand, and do some "practice test pages." Make sessions relatively brief, early in the day, with frequent breaks. Be relaxed and reassuring. Frequently make remarks which are encouraging yet do not give actual hints: e.g., "You're doing a nice job" or "You're really reading carefully." (Note: This should *not* be continued beyond the earliest grades. For an older student such comments tend to be interruptions and may seem condescending.) For an especially nervous child, consider giving a scented sticker each time she completes a page (explain that you cannot tell her whether or not there were errors, but that the sticker will be for "trying hard and not giving up.")

With a young beginner it is sometimes necessary to give considerable guidance in *how* to take a test. In the earliest grades it may be appropriate to direct the child, during the test, that he must do certain things–e.g., read every example, or use the abacus on every problem. (Note again, however, that this is *not* appropriate beyond the beginning stage. The older student should develop her own style of test-taking, including such things as not reading every answer choice.) Even when the older student is clearly doing poorly, she should not be coached *during* the test itself–after all, this is not done for other students.)

In kindergarten and first grade, tests may consist of pictures or other format difficult to transcribe or read aloud. The chapter on Braille for younger students has suggestions relevant to this chapter.

WHAT ABOUT TIME LIMITS?

Many people routinely assume that a blind student should be given extended time for tests. They note that if he must flip back and forth between a chart and the questions about it, while the others can see everything on one page, the same time limit seems unfair. If the test has not been Brailled, and the student is unaccustomed to working with a live reader, it will take more time to work through the material.

Other people point out that if a blind student expects to compete in the real world, she should not expect to "play by different rules." If alternative techniques really work efficiently, why should there be any need for extended time?

A simple answer to this dilemma is not yet possible. Some analysis of individual circumstances is necessary.

Regular Time Limits Are Often Appropriate

For many reasons, usually the blind student *should* be expected to complete tests during the usual time limit. The chapter on "General Classroom Arrangements and Study Skills" explains ways that appropriate techniques should enable routine assignments to be completed within the usual time. If the student reads print slowly, she should learn Braille and work up speed. If handwriting is laborious, typing should be used, along with oral dictation when appropriate.

Sighted students are forced to learn many ways to speed up on a timed test; blind students can learn them too. Moreover, studies show that in case of indecision, the first impression of an answer is usually correct. Agonizing in a perfectionistic way is likely to produce a *lower* score.

And remember, "Work expands to fill the time allowed."

Exceptional Situations

With the present state-of-the-art in education, there are some situations in which a rigid time limit would indeed be unfair. Tactile maps and graphs may be more time-consuming to interpret, even with the best transcribing and a skilled student; it is not possible to glance over the entire field instantly, and the student must study it somewhat before getting the whole picture. As another example, if the student must copy math problems into Braille (perhaps from oral dictation because a Braille copy is not available), work each problem, and then write or dictate the answer–all while the sighted students merely read each problem, work it, and write the answer, all on the same page–it will take more time.

Avoid, however, the blanket assumption that *every* test or assignment involving mathematics or graphs will be slow. If the test is multiple choice, true-false, short answer, or essay, it may be entirely possible to work within the time limit. It depends on whether a graph must actually be read, problems actually copied, etc. It also depends on how similar the blind student's task is to that of sighted classmates.

A different exceptional situation occurs when a student is just learning to use a particular mode of reading or writing. There will be an adjustment period of relatively slow work.

If every test were given in an optimum manner, with optimum materials, and if each student already had adequate experience in using the chosen mode of reading and writing, there would be no need for time extensions. Even with only a reasonable degree of opportunity, most students can meet time limits most of the time. Since tests are so crucial, however, and since there are situations where the time limit would be truly unfair, we cannot now say flatly that tests *always* should be taken in exactly the standard time limit. We *can* say, however, that ordinarily the blind student should work within the time limits, and should continually strive for greater efficiency. Note that this applies also when tests are not formally timed; if the blind student regularly takes longer than the others, something is wrong, even if there is no "official" time limit.

Building Speed

Following are suggestions for increased speed:

(1) Every student should have at least one mode of reading in which she can read with excellent speed. Too often, plowing through inkprint with poor vision slows a person down. Obtain the most efficient mode whenever possible.

(2) Many things, such as maps, diagrams, and tables, can be hard to work with orally. Every student should be skilled with reading from paper (i.e., either print or Braille).

(3) Despite the importance of learning good Braille skills, each student should become skilled in working with a live reader. It will not always be possible to obtain a test in Braille, and the same is true for large print.

(4) A reader should read quickly and clearly. The reader should also *take direction from the student* (with the possible exception of very young children). Many blind adults recall doing poorly on tests because the reader read poorly or did not read the way the student wanted. Sighted students taking tests may skip around; answer easier questions first; reread a hard question six times; stop reading the choices when the answer has clearly been found; go back to a related question; etc. Blind students should learn to do the same, but too often the reader resists such things as annoying or odd. By the middle grades the blind student should be building experience with the use of a reader in many different situations (not just tests), with the student controlling the manner of reading. If the student really needs guidance in test-taking skills, it should *not* be done *during* a test. The student should take the test in her own way, and at another time discuss and/or practice how it might be done better.

(5) Consider the optimum method for reporting answers in each particular test. For essay tests it is probably typing, although some prefer oral dictation. For a multiple-choice or even a short-answer test it is usually best to dictate answers aloud for the reader to mark them on the printed sheet.

(6) Work to improve test format. For example, it is unfair to expect a blind student to flip bound pages back and forth, within the same time limit, if others have it all on one page. But if a table or chart is removable so that it can be placed beside each set of questions, and if each set of questions is on a separate page to prevent the need for hunting around, the format *is* competitive.

(7) Work on skimming and scanning to seek out the needed information quickly. This can be done in Braille, and it can be done with a reader. However, it may be virtually impossible to do in print with limited vision – another reason to learn alternative modes of reading.

(8) Develop a mind-set toward working within the usual time limits. Remember that unlimited time implies that a person is unable to work normally. It also encourages laziness.

(9) If the student reads well in the chosen mode, and seems to have adequate test-taking skills, yet still does poorly, probably she is not well prepared in terms of content. When sighted students do not know the material, we do not alter the test or its conditions. It should be the same for the blind.

Formal, Standardized Tests

Following are definitions of a few common terms: *Reliability* ensures that the same test will keep giving essentially the same results. *Validity* ensures that the test actually measures what it purports to measure. A *norm-referenced* test compares an individual's performance to that of his peers, while a *criterion-referenced* test measures against an absolute standard.

Often the question is raised, "Since this test was standardized on a non-disabled population, how can it be either reliable or valid for a blind child?" Some may carry this farther and lament, "Why bother to give the test at all?"

In a strictly technical sense, a test given in Braille (or large print or oral form) is not the precise equivalent of the regular print version. Nevertheless, the results are useful in the same general way as for a sighted student. Strengths and weaknesses are brought out. In most cases, scores can be meaningfully computed, and achievement can be meaningfully compared with various standards.

ACHIEVEMENT TESTS

An achievement test is designed to measure specific skills or concepts which the child has learned (as distinguished from a test which claims to measure general ability).

Most schools give a major standardized achievement test at least every two or three years. Examples include the *Iowa Tests of Basic Skills,* the *Iowa Tests of Educational Development,* and the *Stanford Achievement Test.*

Although these are considered group tests, often the blind student should work individually for reasons such as the need to read aloud. It may be appropriate to be flexible with time limits (see above discussion).

PLAN AHEAD

Arrange for a suitable mode of reading. Keep in mind the format to which the student is accustomed; an important test is not the place to practice with a new mode of reading. Plan ahead carefully – these are very long tests, resulting in major scheduling problems if plans go awry. Make direct contact with the publisher if necessary, being sure that the correct Level and Form are transcribed. Find out exactly when the test will be given, since your local textbook service may pass copies around.

Short sample tests or practice tests are sometimes available beforehand. These are just as important for the blind student as the sighted – possibly more so, if unfamiliar formats are involved.

Plan carefully for the actual administration of the test–when, where, and by whom. It should be given at the usual times (several sessions are normally necessary for everyone), with a plan for extra time if needed. Note that it may take extra time to assemble the materials, even if extra time is not needed for the test itself. You may be the logical one to give the test, even if you do not ordinarily work directly with the student. In a metropolitan area, consider transporting all visually impaired students to one location for the test.

Often the test is administered by a counselor, principal, or multi-categorical resource teacher. A paraprofessional may administer the test under proper supervision.

WORK CLOSELY WITH THE TEST-GIVER

Work closely with the person who gives the test, helping him to anticipate needs and to work efficiently. The test-giver must have a Teacher's Guide as well as a copy of the student's pages. Look through everything beforehand, and consider using paper clips and other markers to aid in keeping the place in a multi-level test. Consider some pencil marking of Braille pages, to help a test-giver who does not know Braille. Discuss ways to give the student every advantage to which she is entitled, while at the same time avoiding inadvertent hints.

Give very specific suggestions, especially for complex format. Sometimes it is best for the student to read certain things in Braille while other things are read aloud to her. For example, the student might examine a table while the aide reads the questions about it, to avoid constantly flipping pages. As another example, the student might read math problems in Braille but prefer that another section of the test be read aloud.

SPECIAL FORMATS

Certain formats may present a dilemma. You may find that maps, for instance, have been completely omitted from the Braille copy. For a student in the primary grades, try to transcribe the missing material yourself. In the higher grades, it may be necessary to omit that particular section; there may be no way to produce a real equivalent in Braille. Usually the rest of the test can still be scored meaningfully.

Even though all Braille material for math and science should be transcribed in Nemeth Code, I have seen standardized tests in which this was not done. Arithmetic problems look very peculiar when written in literary Braille. When a student is accustomed to doing all math in Nemeth, it is unfair to present a math test in literary Braille format. Try to get the material redone. Alternatively, go over the material with the student, explaining the situation and being sure she can read everything. Another possibility is to read the test orally, with the student writing down as much Braille as necessary and/or making some use of the poorly-transcribed material.

The chapter on "Maps" contains suggestions on handling pictures. Consider preparing a written description of each picture, for the examiner to read aloud.

Usually the principal and others will readily agree to appropriate arrangements. Be firm, however, in case of misunderstanding. Do not give in to a blanket statement such as "None of our special-education students take these tests." Instead assume the student will take them unless *individual* needs (not just the fact of blindness) compel otherwise. Note that partially-sighted students using print may need accommodations as well as Braille students–for example, the use of a typewriter or other alternative arrangements for answers.

STANDARDIZED ANSWER SHEETS

Standardized answer sheets are easily handled, but somehow seem to worry people. Explain that the student should give her answers in some alternative format, and then they should be transferred onto the standard sheet by someone else. The student might:

- Use a large-print or Braille answer sheet which has been prepared for the occasion, and underline choices with a pencil. (Caution: Do *not* use a "generic" answer sheet with an arbitrary number of items and answer choices. The regular answer sheet is carefully customized to the test. If no appropriate answer sheet is available, use one of the methods below.)

- Indicate the answer choices on a blank piece of paper, using Braille, typing, or handwriting. (For example, if answer choice "c" is the correct response for Question #2, the student would write "2 c.")
- Give answers orally.
- Mark directly in the test booklet, if a consumable copy can be made available.

Note that many students who use regular print have difficulty with computer-scannable answer sheets. Don't let them struggle with all those little ovals.

The IEP

See that the IEP states (or clearly implies) that the student shall take all the regular classroom tests and standardized tests, in appropriate form.

IS THERE A GOOD REASON FOR AN EXCEPTION?

Should it seem that exceptions are warranted, examine them in detail. Often someone is merely assuming the test is inappropriate, or there is concern about how to administer it. Tactful inquiries and discussion of arrangements will usually overcome these problems. The chapter on "Your Professional Role" contains suggestions on how to deal with persistent problems. Excluding blind students from tests is a serious omission.

Occasionally a student (sighted or blind) really does have great difficulty with tests *per se.* This should be dealt with immediately and assertively.

The psychologist or counselor can help if extreme fear seems to be the problem.

Some students need help in "test-taking skills" (e.g., viewing a multiple-choice question as a series of true-false questions). A counselor or a specialist in Learning Disabilities can offer suggestions.

If problems really seem severe enough that a student should be excused from certain tests, help the IEP team analyze the situation carefully. Make it clear that blindness in itself is not the reason. Be specific. Shall we work on test-taking skills and set a schedule for resuming regular testing? Does the student have an additional disability which in itself makes the testing inappropriate? Will we omit certain tests until the student learns Braille (again, setting a definite timetable)? *Which* tests, exactly, are to be modified or omitted?

Beginning Braille Students

A special, temporary problem arises with young students who do not yet know all the Grade II Braille signs. For example, the prefix *dis* is not used until Volume II of the third-grade *Patterns* book, yet often appears in standardized tests at lower levels. An oral test is generally not suitable when evaluating reading skill. One solution is to delay regular standardized achievement tests until the end of second grade, by which time the student should know all the common signs of Grade II Braille. (If *Patterns* is still being used for the reading curriculum at this point, provide supplementary work to see that the most common signs have all been introduced.) This approach also avoids the problem of test pages which consist solely of pictures – a common situation at the earliest levels. Write up the plan precisely, lest it be assumed that standardized tests will never be given. Provide alternative means of objective evaluation – e.g., the tests which accompany *Patterns.*

NORMAL EXPECTATIONS

Most boys and girls are nervous about tests. They are not excused. Blindness is no excuse either.

Tests of "Aptitude" and Vocational Interest

I put "aptitude" in quotation marks because of the shakiness of assuming that pure "aptitude" is measurable in isolation from experience, and of assuming there is one certain way to measure ability. If a child cannot see the marks he makes, will a pencil-and-paper test really measure his hand coordination? If a high school student cannot write numbers rapidly into tiny squares, should we conclude that Accounting is impossible for her?

IS THE TEST APPROPRIATE?

The question of experience *vs.* "pure ability" extends into cultural background. A youngster transplanted from an isolated region of Brazil might fail all our "aptitude tests," yet be highly skilled in his family's traditional activities and fluent in his native language. An American inner-city youth whose family has no books or pencils, and does not speak Standard English, has a comparable situation.

Aptitude should be evaluated in an appropriate manner. Unfortunately, traditional "school readiness" tests for young children emphasize drawing, printing, and cutting–skills which the young blind child usually cannot do in the conventional manner. Too often, evaluators assume the child "is not ready for first grade," when actually the child lacks alternative techniques or was not given a chance to use them.

Ideas for adapting materials for young children appear under "Intelligence Tests" in this chapter, and in the chapter on "Early Childhood." Verbal skills can be evaluated orally, or through suitable tactual tasks, including Braille itself. Coordination can be observed in fastening clothing, playing, and other activities not based on vision. If the child does poorly even on appropriate tasks, consider whether he needs better instruction and practice in alternative techniques, instead of flatly assuming "poor ability for schoolwork."

This problem is particularly insidious with partially-sighted students. It is very hard for adults to realize that the child's vision is very different from normal vision. (See the chapters, "The Partially-Sighted Child" and "Explaining the Idea of Sight and Partial Sight.") For a young child, all evaluations should avoid relying on vision. With older partially-sighted students who read print and write with a pencil, be wary of tests which use faint and crowded print or diagrams.

SCHOLASTIC "APTITUDE"

"Aptitude" tests in high school usually purport to give vocational advice and/or show readiness for college.

The *Pre-Scholastic Aptitude Test* (PSAT), *Scholastic Aptitude Test* (SAT), and *American College Test* (ACT) are commonly given in high school. College admission often requires one or more of these, with preference varying in different parts of the country. This kind of test is given only by specifically designated persons, and sometimes a particular educator specializes in giving them to blind students. It is customary to administer these without a time limit for blind students.

To some extent these important tests are available in Braille, large print, and recorded modes. They may also be used with a live reader. Unfortunately, however, there are many problems. The desired mode is not always available, and usually blind students are given a different (older) Form of the test. If it is to be read aloud, the student may have no choice of reader, and may be given one who reads poorly.

After sighted students take the PSAT, they are given the correct answers and shown which of theirs were wrong. Unfortunately, this important preparation for the SAT is often unavailable to blind students. Producers of the tests assert that because they have very few Forms in transcribed modes, they cannot afford to give out the correct answers.

The producers are also rigid in defining what they consider "standard conditions." When the Educational Testing Service (ETS), which provides the PSAT and SAT, sends a blind student's score to a college, the score may be accompanied by a most unfortunate letter. It states that the test was given under nonstandard conditions, and that the ETS cannot really validate the score. This makes the college wonder about the student's ability. It also deprives the student of the opportunity to decide when and how to inform the college about his/her blindness. The National Federation of the Blind is working to eliminate this and other problems. Various laws prohibit discrimination due to a non-validated test.

TESTS TO GUIDE VOCATIONAL CHOICE

Another type of testing is the vocational *interest* test or checklist. It is intended to indicate what jobs the student would enjoy or find interesting. A vocational *aptitude* test or checklist is intended to show where the individual would be most likely to succeed.

Blind students should have the same opportunities for vocational guidance which counselors typically offer sighted students. For example, there are a number of easily-administered inventories, such as the *Strong Vocational Interest Blank.* Too often, it is incorrectly assumed that this would be irrelevant for the blind student. Job exploration is a vital area in education, and these tests can help a student think about areas to which he has never given thought. Appropriate testing can help develop an IEP that will aid the student in making vocational decisions. Again, remember that all of this applies to the partially sighted as well as the totally blind. It also applies to those who are college-bound as well as those who are not.

AVOID UNWARRANTED CONCLUSIONS

Such tests can be helpful, but should be used with caution. If such a test shows a blind student to have high interest and/or aptitude for a given job, this is probably accurate. But indications *against* a job may be very misleading. Assumptions are often built in, making it appear that excellent vision is a prerequisite for Accounting work, or that a driver's license is required for a traveling job. In actuality, a Certified Public Accountant can use a computer, or direct another person, to "place the little numbers in the little squares;" the key factor is understanding and applying the principles of accounting. A blind salesperson can walk, use public transportation, or hire a driver.

Job Opportunities for the Blind (JOB) is a program administered jointly by the U.S. Department of Labor and the National Federation of the Blind. Applicants throughout the country are matched with jobs throughout the country. JOB can help a student to plan ahead for employment, and to meet blind people who are already working in a field which the student is considering.

Intelligence Tests (IQ Tests)

Tests can provide important information for planning a student's program. However, the results of a test must be used appropriately. Good educational practice requires, and P.L. 94-142 provides, that no single test shall be used as the sole criterion for placement of a student. If general achievement and adjustment are normal, but the child scores very low on an intelligence test, then probably something was wrong with the testing situation. It is not appropriate to conclude flatly that she is mentally retarded.

It is generally accepted that the odds are against a student scoring above his/her actual ability. Most inaccuracies underestimate the intelligence of the individual.

Intelligence tests, sometimes regarded as measuring innate ability, involve the same controversies described for other "aptitude" tests, above. Accomplishment of the tasks is actually based on a background of experience. This re-emphasizes why no single test should ever be used as the sole basis for program planning.

Nevertheless, intelligence tests are a part of the educational scene. If all students are tested except the blind child, this in itself sets her apart. And usually a meaningful score (as meaningful as for any student) can indeed be obtained.

Today most psychologists do not view IQ tests as iron-clad decrees of "innate intelligence," but simply as indicators of current intellectual functioning. That is, the test measures how the child is *currently functioning* in certain sample tasks which are school-oriented. It does *not* necessarily indicate how the child will perform later under different circumstances, or how the child now functions in other life skills which are not measured by this test. Even the score itself is not an absolute figure, but an indication within a range of figures. There are many causes for possible error, including fatigue and nervousness. There is only a moderate relationship between scores on intelligence tests and actual success in life.

INDIVIDUAL INTELLIGENCE TESTS

Regular individual intelligence tests can be used from approximately age four. Examples include the *Wechsler Intelligence Scales for Children, Revised* (WISC-R), the *Wechsler Preschool and Primary Scale of Intelligence* (WPPSI), and the *Stanford-Binet Intelligence Scale.* These generally contain a *Verbal* scale (oral questions) and a *Performance* scale (involving eye-hand coordination). For the general population, both portions are given. However, most of the Performance scale is unsuitable for a blind youngster. A common solution is to give the verbal portion only – it can be scored independently, and generally is regarded as giving a reasonably good indication of the level of intellectual functioning. This often is the best solution for visually impaired students who read print as well as those who use Braille. (Note that no reading is required by the test itself.) A student may appear able to take the Performance test, yet score artificially low because of seeing poorly.

There are some tests which claim to be especially adapted for measuring the intelligence of blind persons. Many examiners feel, however, that such tests tend to feature tactual tasks which have been awkwardly contrived to appear to resemble the visual tasks on the original test, without really being equivalent.

GROUP TESTS

Group tests such as the *Otis-Lennon Mental Ability Test* may not be appropriate for blind students. Often, the time limits are an integral part of the scoring; and if these are changed because of an alternative reading medium, the score may appear meaningless. Individual intelligence tests are generally regarded as much more reliable than group tests. Ask the psychologist or counselor to analyze the nature of the test *vs.* the needs of the student and the direction of the IEP. Sometimes a test is partially "intelligence" and partially "achievement," and this may or may not be reflected in the title of the test.

TESTING THE VERY YOUNG

Below the age of four, estimates of intelligence are particularly indefinite and subject to change. Infant scales of intelligence, such as the *Cattell Infant Intelligence Scale,* may be used from the age of one month; however they tend to be based on assumptions which may be inappropriate for blind babies. Social maturity scales also are often regarded as indicators. However, in interpreting such scales, even more caution should be applied than was described for older children. A very young child has an extremely restricted background of experience. Often a child will miss an item on the test simply because she has had no experience with it. The overprotective attitudes of society and of the parents frequently deprive a blind child of experiences which others routinely enjoy. Information about the child's background is very important in interpreting the meaning of any weaknesses.

Furthermore, small children are easily fatigued or frightened to the point of being unable to function.

Usually the best indicators of a child's intellectual functioning are careful observations of the child's behavior and general development. Interviews with parents, babysitters, and preschool teachers are valuable. Speech and language patterns are particularly good evidence of intellectual development.

See the chapter on "Early Childhood" for additional suggestions.

LOOK AT THE WHOLE PICTURE

Even for older students, other indications of ability should always be used in conjunction with intelligence tests. Much can be inferred from classroom performance, achievement tests, and general behavior.

If there is more than one disability, finding an appropriate way to test may be a challenge. Consult the residential school for the blind, and others accustomed to testing multiply handicapped blind children.

Psychological Tests of Personality

Tests of emotional balance or personality are a touchy subject. Various controversies exist as to whether schools and employers should be able to require such tests at all. For a blind student the problem is compounded by the common misconception that blindness itself causes emotional disturbance.

If a personality test is given to all students, then the blind student would participate on the same basis as others.

When a student is first being evaluated for special services such as Braille, it is appropriate to "screen" for problems other than blindness – that is, to give brief tests checking for difficulties with hearing, speech, etc. It is appropriate to check, in a relatively brief and generalized manner, for the presence of substantial psychological problems. Furthermore, at any time the school counselor may talk with any student about personal problems. However, to go beyond behavioral observation and probe deeply into the student's personal feelings, or to give lengthy personal counseling, should be done only for good reason and with parental consent. The chapter on "Multiple Handicaps" comments on distinguishing between genuine psychological problems, and problems which are really due to mistakes in handling blindness.

Screening for Other Disabilities

During a general check of the school population, or a special-education evaluation, you may be asked to advise about testing the blind student.

Speech tests often consist solely of pictures, since the therapist wants to observe pronunciation without the child's simply repeating what someone else has said. For a partially-sighted child, make sure the pictures are large and plain, and consider supplementing them with some description.

If the child cannot see pictures, the therapist might describe them, being careful not to use the word she wants to elicit. ("The baby drinks milk from a – –.") Real objects can sometimes be used. Some tests rely less on pictures than others, and by a combination of methods an adequate evaluation can be accomplished. If no problems are reported by parents and teachers, the therapist may simply converse with the child to obtain a representative sample of speech.

Hearing tests require no adaptation, since the student simply listens and responds. It is, however, important that the examiner knows the child is blind, and does not expect her to follow hand signals or other visual cues.

Vision screening may seem superfluous if the child is already known to be visually impaired. For a child beyond second grade, it may be best to omit screening by the school nurse, since it may be embarrassing and confusing. However, a very young child may be upset if the class lines up to see the nurse and she is left out. In this case the nurse may contrive a "test" for purposes of getting acquainted and helping the child feel included. A student with some sight could stand close to the chart or count fingers, even if the nurse does not really wish to record an acuity figure. A totally blind child might read some Braille letters or words, to "show the nurse that she can read."

Regular medical testing of the eyes is discussed in the chapter on "Dealing With Medical Matters," in this *Handbook*. The chapter on "Assessment of Functional Vision for Reading" deals with the educational analysis of visual functioning in daily life.

Tests of *Motor Functioning* evaluate the ability to use large and small muscles. The examiner should be aware of the child's visual status, to avoid asking a child to imitate motions at a distance, or to "walk on the green squares." Plan alternative modes of giving directions – e.g., verbal description instead of visual demonstration. Help everyone distinguish actual physical problems from those related to blindness. A first grader who uses Braille should not be expected to write and draw fluently with a pencil, but this does not mean "poor hand coordination." Unsteady walking may simply indicate the need for a white cane, not a balance problem.

Individualized Academic Evaluation: As a part of a general evaluation, it is customary for someone to give a brief individual test of the student's functioning level for academic skills. Usually the test is partly oral and partly written. The *Woodcock-Johnson Psycho-Educational Battery* is an example.

Transcribing such a test into an appropriate medium, and administering it, is very similar to giving a classroom test or an achievement test. If you are not giving the test yourself, work closely with the test-giver. If the student reads print, be sure that suitable copy is provided, with appropriate lighting and positioning.

If Braille is used, be sure that the test-giver knows where to find the various examples (especially if it is necessary to skip around), and that a means for handling pictures is planned. It may be desirable for you to accompany the test-giver and assist if needed. For example, if the child is examining a symbol and asks "What is this?" you could determine whether or not the question should be answered.

Related Chapters

The following chapters, particularly, contain additional suggestions about testing:

"Early Childhood"
"Dealing With Medical Matters"
"Assessment of Functional Vision for Reading"

CHAPTER 42

FITTING IN SOCIALLY

Ann is painfully shy. She has hardly any friends, and has never been asked for a date.

Louise has many friends, and is always elected as a class officer. However, she looks down on everyone who is not "popular." Gradually, even her friends are beginning to feel that Louise is aloof and bossy.

Tom has a pleasing personality and tries hard to make friends. Most of his classmates, however, are repelled by his dirty clothes and unpleasant odor.

All three of these teenagers are sighted. None has any disability, visual or otherwise. These instances show that all youngsters have problems, sometimes serious ones. Had these teenagers been blind, many people would have assumed their social problems were due to blindness:

"Poor Ann – it must be very frightening not to be able to see."

"Louise can't see how people frown when she acts bossy."

"It must be hard to keep clean if you are blind."

Development of social skills is the same for the blind as for the sighted. The blind person will use different *methods* on occasion, such as making more use of the sense of touch in applying makeup; but the young blind person needs to learn the same things as the young sighted person.

Attitudes Are the Key

It is unfortunately true, however, that the blind person is sometimes behind in social skills – due not to inability to learn, but due to the belief that he/she cannot learn, or to mistaken sheltering from social experience. Individual help should be provided if a specific technique is lacking; in general the blind youngster who is behind in social skills will be helped by the same general approach as any other youngster with such a problem.

One young woman said, "When I was in high school I never mentioned my blindness. My friends never mentioned it either. When I joined the NFB, I learned to be frank and positive about blindness. Several of my friends said to me later, 'You know, in high school we were always afraid we would offend you by saying something about your vision. We were always nervous about it. We feel so much more comfortable now that *you* are comfortable.'"

The Preschool Child

The social development of a preschool child is a part of his general development and maturity level. Learning to talk, feed oneself, and use the toilet are skills that come with physical maturation and proper guidance. The chapters on "Early Childhood" and "Home Economics and Daily Living Skills" include practical suggestions for this age group. It is vital that (a) blind children are not deprived of regular guidance, and (b) when the blind child really does need some different or additional help, he gets it.

All children need to be taught how to play, but with sighted children this often occurs without much thought. While encouraging children to think up ways to use play equipment, we also should demonstrate the standard use. For example, a child may enjoy pushing an empty tricycle, but he should also be taught how to get on and ride it.

When a child plays with other children, he learns many things besides the obvious matter of sharing toys. He learns to enjoy other children's company, and how to participate in structured games and unstructured play. He learns how to react when another child annoys him, and what to expect if he does the annoying. He even learns how other children talk–some blind youngsters sound quite stilted in their speech because they have talked mostly with adults.

Very young children usually need little guidance in accepting a blind playmate. They quickly learn to take his hand to show him a toy, for example. The preschool teachers may, however, need considerable support. Also, parents often find that playmates never seem to be available in the neighborhood. Suggest to parents that they specifically invite other children over to play, perhaps sharing some especially interesting toys, and perhaps inviting the mother over as well. This usually results in return invitations to play elsewhere. Avoid the extremes of pushing too hard, on the one hand, and passively letting the blind child be left out, on the other hand.

Preventing Undesirable Habits

Teaching standard play is a vital part of minimizing mannerisms. The child who has a suitable construction set (one which will stay together when he examines the construction by touch), and is taught how to use it, is unlikely to simply tap the pieces on the floor. Watch for overly repetitive or stereotyped motions, even when the motion would be acceptable or desirable in moderation. If a child spends great amounts of time on a rocking horse, climbing up and down the same jungle gym, etc., insist that he vary his activity. Remind parents that it is especially important to provide something to do if the child must sit still for a long time; examples include playing with a toy while waiting for the doctor, and reading or conversing in the car or bus.

Some blind children tend to poke or press the eyes–a very undesirable habit. As with other habits, physically move the child into better positions with something else for the hands to do. Nip this habit early before it becomes ingrained.

A few children develop a very unfortunate way of showing excitement: they clasp their hands together, tense all their muscles, tremble, and make squeaking noises. One father said, "Son, when you feel excited, show it! Put your arms up over your head and jump up and down! Yell 'Yea' or 'Wahoo!'" He was helping his son to substitute a more socially acceptable way of expressing emotion. He was also encouraging more physical movement. Increased physical activity makes this kind of mannerism less likely. When this boy complained that he could not jump up and shout in school, his father said, "Well, at school you might just raise your arms a little bit and *whisper* 'Yea! Wahoo!'"

PERSISTENT MANNERISMS

However, as with sighted children, undesirable habits sometimes persist in spite of our best efforts. Gentle reminders are usually more effective than scoldings, since the latter tend to make the child still more tense and prone to mannerisms. Vary verbal reminders with physical ones–as, simply move the child's hand out of his mouth and onto a toy. Another idea is to replace an objectionable habit with a more socially acceptable one. A child who continually twists her hair might carry a plush toy and stroke that instead. One three-year-old always picked up toy cars and dangled them by the wheels, jiggling them instead of really playing. His parents phased out this habit by saying, "You may twiddle only the little wooden cement mixer. All other cars and trucks must be played with in the regular way or not at all." Then they gradually reduced the time he was permitted to have the cement mixer.

Blind children (even those with useful sight) often do not realize exactly what others are doing. They hear adults say, "Quit scratching your head!" and "Quit fiddling with your shoe!" and so on, and may not realize that these positions are inappropriate only *in excess.* The child may think he or she is expected to keep the hands rigidly in place on top of the desk, never moving or stretching at all; but to attempt this causes great strain. Recently I asked a girl to show me ten different positions in which it would be OK to place her hands for a short while. I had to help her after the third one. "I'm teaching her to fidget in class," I said jokingly as I told the classroom teacher about my efforts to help the child relax normally and keep her fingers out of her eye. Later I sat beside this child in class for a few minutes, and quietly described how other children stretched slightly, jiggled their feet, placed their hands on their knees, etc.

As another idea, eyeglasses (with plain glass if no correction is possible – even if the youngster is totally blind) may serve as a physical reminder to prevent eye-poking.

Keeping the child busy and happy, with plenty of appropriate physical activity, is the best way to prevent and counteract mannerisms.

An older child may respond well to rewards for avoiding the habit. If the habit is well-established, start by working on it only part of the time. Avoid making the child extremely nervous by expecting perfect control immediately.

All youngsters chafe at repeated verbal reminders. Older youngsters, in addition, often are very sensitive about personal corrections in front of their peers. A "secret signal," therefore, is often the best approach to an undesirable habit. Talk privately and agree that, for example, the teacher will touch the youngster's shoulder if she is twisting her hair or rocking. The adult agrees not to mention this aloud, and the youngster in turn agrees to respond to the "secret signal." A euphemism can work in a similar way – instead of "Ellen, don't rock back and forth," we can say, "Ellen, please sit up straight," and thus make a more socially-acceptable comment.

A speech therapist once told me that when a child first began to use a new speech sound, it was unwise to say, "Now use your good *s* sound all the time." The child would continually forget, feel overwhelmed, and give up. Instead, she explained, the child might first be told, "Be sure to use your good *s* sound when you read aloud in class." Gradually more and more time spans would be included, until eventually the child was expected to remember "all the time."

Gina, in fourth grade, was not conquering her habit of eye-poking, despite all the conventional approaches. Indeed, it was growing worse. Suddenly remembering the speech therapist's advice, we instituted the "limited-time" approach. During a 30-minute reading group (a good choice because her hands were especially busy) we made it clear that Gina *would* remember to keep her hands away from her eyes. (A small reward was given each day, and a negative consequence was available if needed.) At other times we reminded her frequently but did not expect perfection. One month later (having had good success) a 30-minute period in the afternoon was added. Gradually (reminding ourselves not to botch things by moving too fast) we expanded the time.

Informal Play

"But the others all just run around and play ball."

Sometimes it seems that way. How do we integrate a blind grade-school child (especially a boy) into play groups?

In the first place, let's not assume he couldn't possibly play ball. He certainly can in a supervised situation with appropriate adaptations; and his friends may be willing to include those adaptations during informal play. He can bat a ball from a tee which holds it stationary at the right height, or use a beeper ball. "Batting" in a kickball game can be even easier, especially if the pitcher stands close in, rolls the ball carefully, and calls out when he releases the ball. The blind player can run to a voice calling him on each base, or run with a friend.

Let's not assume, either, that the blind child cannot "just run around" during very informal play. He can be flexible, take someone's arm when they are actually running, ask questions, and figure out what is being played. Sometimes it does seem, however, that informal play is the hardest to join, and it may take some time and guidance before he is able to do so. Watch the other children awhile and see what different things they actually do. Do they stop to play in a sandbox? Play catch? Jump rope? Swing? If the youngster participates in some specific informal activities at first, he can gradually come to be included in more and more.

Actually, of course, other children do many other things besides "run around and play ball." Swimming, skating, and other non-team sports are popular. Playground equipment usually presents no real problems. As with preschoolers, the blind elementary student needs to know the standard uses of playground equipment and other devices. Provide table games which are suitably adapted, and be sure he knows how to play. Offer to attach Braille labels to games.

Sometimes it is desirable to structure an otherwise informal situation. A "buddy" might accompany the blind child at recess–with the responsibility rotated among various willing children, and perhaps only part of the time. During an indoor playtime, all children might be assigned to specific activities for the first few minutes, thus inconspicuously assuring the blind child an appropriate place. Sometimes an aide might accompany the child at play. Usually a combination approach of various types of guidance is best. Avoid the extremes of constantly hovering, *vs.* always letting the child fend for himself.

Show parents how informal play is handled at school, and encourage them to give some similar guidance at home.

See also the chapter on "Physical Education and Recreation."

Conventional Behavior

School-aged children notice when others ignore social conventions, even if they themselves rebel at society's standards. A child who always eats with a spoon, sits in strange positions, and constantly speaks out of turn will be viewed as quite "different."

Since a blind child will not see a frown, and since many people will think he cannot learn social conventions, it is necessary to give specific attention to matters such as this. Take the child's hand and show her how to hold her fork. Teach her conventional posture. If she speaks out of turn, belches audibly, etc., correct her tactfully. Show her various gestures and motions such as raising her hand or waving, and be sure she understands when and how they are used. A blind kindergartner may not understand just when to raise her hand and when to take it down, and that if one arm gets tired she can use the other one. Show the child where the movie screen is, and see that she faces it.

Talk with the student about what looks good or bad visually. Describe other people's appearance. Include descriptions of other people's errors and problems, whenever it can be done tactfully and appropriately. (Encourage parents to do this too, since they are particularly in a position where they can talk confidentially about other people's personal appearance.) Often a blind child feels that he/she is the only one who makes mistakes. Suggest to aides, parents, and others that they look for chances to mention (quietly and appropriately, of course) various things which a sighted child would notice about others' problems: "Billy dropped his pencil." "Annette has her head on her desk." "Mark is crying because he skinned his knee." With a teenager we might mention: "Josh forgot the answer, and looks really upset." "Two girls over there haven't ever been asked to dance, and look like they're about to leave."

Because blind children are often singled out–partly to meet their special needs and partly because other people feel sorry for them–often they are allowed to get away with unacceptable behavior at home and elsewhere. For example, a bus driver said that a blind student was rude and disruptive on his bus, but that he didn't want to discipline him as he would any other child who did the same thing. When this kind of thing occurs, the child does not learn what is acceptable.

General Appearance

With proper guidance, blind students can achieve good grooming and normal appearance as part of their peer group.

Sue, age 15, had never carried a purse. At school she kept things in her notebook or her pockets; but her teachers observed that personal items were often visible to others. A sensitive inquiry revealed that Sue did not own a purse of any kind. "What do you do at church?" asked the homeroom teacher. "Some clothes don't have pockets. Suppose you need a Kleenex?"

"I borrow one from my father," replied Sue.

Sue had no idea what to keep in a purse, or how to carry one. At the age of 15, she was dependent on others to manage her personal items when she had no notebook or pocket.

Watch for things like this, and seek the parents' help. Another example is a girl who never wore a skirt (not even to church, where her peers often wore them), and had no idea how to put on a dress. Even if the student and her family say they have personal preferences against something such as skirts, explain that you are trying to make the normal choices *available* to the blind student. If a sighted girl grows up wearing jeans and then decides to include dresses in her wardrobe, she simply does so immediately. If the blind girl has never worn skirts, she may have a major hurdle to overcome in knowing how to put them on, and also how to walk and sit appropriately.

Matt's schoolbooks were in an old, tattered bag which looked vaguely feminine and was often slung carelessly about his neck. "But how am I going to carry stuff?" he protested when the counselor talked with him about personal appearance. "I need one hand free for my cane!" The counselor helped Matt get a backpack like many other boys used. He also advised, "When you're grown and working in an office, you'll want a briefcase."

Guiding Acceptance by Peers

Classroom teachers often ask how to help sighted youngsters accept a blind classmate. It is best to speak openly about the disability (without dwelling on it unduly), and to encourage the student to do the same. The new student can introduce herself to the class in the normal manner, including other characteristics as well as blindness, and explain study methods. It is usually better not to discuss blindness with the class before the student arrives. Unless the subject comes up naturally (as when Braille materials arrive before the student does), a preparatory discussion seems to say that blindness is such a special situation as to require a great deal of preparation, and that we should avoid discussing it in front of the blind person. It is better to be open and matter-of-fact.

You and the classroom teachers will, however, need to guide classmates in including the blind student as an equal. Often this can be done publicly, as when a new student is introduced, or when someone speaks to the class about blindness in general. When specific problems arise, it is sometimes best to talk to the individuals privately.

Emphasize to teachers that, while overt rejection is usually easy to recognize, it may be harder to note and deal with the opposite problem – namely, overprotection. The latter is, in my experience, the more common problem and the harder to solve. Do little girls "mother-hen" the blind child's play at recess? Does someone always carry his tray even though he could do it? Do classmates jump to pick up dropped objects? Deal directly and tactfully with things like this, and be firm. To allow overprotection is to interfere with education.

Joining Others

CONVERSATIONAL SKILLS

Teach children to face the other person during a conversation. Urge sighted people to say things like "Please reach over here," rather than moving to accommodate the blind child. Help the blind youngster to be flexible and attentive, noting other people's needs and actions. See that voice volume is appropriate to the situation. If a child consistently talks too loudly or too softly, despite reminders, have his hearing checked. If he talks too much or too little, give him feedback and guidance.

Some children need extra guidance in what to say during conversations. The younger child may remain in a stage of self-centered questions, constantly asking "Who is he talking about?" or "What do you mean?" The child needs to learn to listen awhile and see what can be learned without asking questions. Textbooks sometimes have exercises on "Making Inferences." Besides reducing annoying questions, such exercises should improve general "incidental learning"–that is, learning things without their being formally taught. Too many blind children wait passively for someone to *teach* them the names of their classmates, for example, rather than listening attentively to conversation.

Many young people converse in a very self-centered way. For example, one boy always expounds about his own musical interests, without ever encouraging a friend to describe *his* interests. The student may need to practice thinking of open-ended questions to draw people out, and consciously using them. He may also need to broaden his own interests and experience.

Another type of self-centered conversation is the self-putdown. No one enjoys talking with a constant complainer. The counselor may be able to help direct thoughts and speech in a more positive, outward direction.

Teach alternative techniques for personal contact, and the confidence and assertiveness to use them. If Alicia finds the counselor's office open but silent, she can ask, "Mr. Brown, are you there?" or simply, "Mr. Brown?" If she is waiting to buy tickets and is uncertain whether she is being spoken to, she can ask, "Did you mean me?" or "Am I next?"

Encourage the blind youngster to be good-natured to people who say, "Do you know who this is?" but, if necessary, to refuse a guessing game politely but firmly. At the same time, you as a teacher can discourage others (including adults) from this practice which is really annoying and unnecessary.

PARTICIPATION

All young people need guidance–some more than others–in making and keeping friends. A school counselor should be able to provide suggestions appropriate for all children, including books for teachers and for students.

When various students are standing around, the blind student can orient herself by the voices and join a group as anyone else would do. See that your students learn how to join a group in a conversation or activity: look for a natural pause in the conversation, and say something to indicate interest. Join into what is already being said or done. Avoid changing the subject abruptly or for no reason.

Some youngsters may need coaching on what to say during informal chatting. ("What's for lunch?.... What did you think of that assembly?.... That test sure was hard.... Only three days till vacation....")

All children need to learn how to take turns, and how to be good losers/winners. Overt crying is not the only way to be a "bad loser"–it is also bad for the older youngster to stalk away in silent gloom.

It is important to look attentive when others are talking, even when not saying anything oneself. A person should be sensitive to others' moods–i.e., judging whether or not a friend wishes to talk about something bothering her.

Giving compliments is an important part of relationships. The blind girl or boy cannot easily use one of the most common, namely, complimenting a person on what he/she is wearing. Nevertheless, there are many kinds of compliments that can easily be used–about athletic or personal achievements, about clever ideas, etc. Also, sometimes an article can be examined by touch and admired (if, and only if, the social situation makes this appropriate.)

Jon depended heavily on Ken, his close friend. When Ken had the flu, Jon asked the counselor about finding a place at lunch, carrying books, etc. The counselor helped Jon get better acquainted with Brad, another friendly and compatible boy, and also took the opportunity to help in developing friendships.

"You're making a new friend here," she said. "I can see you're really enjoying Brad's company, and he likes you. It's good for a person to have more than one friend, for lots of reasons. When Ken gets back you'll want to socialize with him again, but I do hope you don't just drop Brad cold. Keep both of them as friends – you can spend some time with each, and maybe some with both together. And also – I think we all have realized that you were awfully dependent on Ken. Let's work on how you can find a seat yourself when you want to, and how to organize your things so that nobody needs to carry your books."

Remember that many well-adjusted youngsters (disabled or not) have only one or two best friends, and that recreational interests vary greatly. Look for many different types of activities as you help your student select those which he or she enjoys most – chess, swimming, bowling, ham radio, etc. Joining structured groups such as Scouts, religious organizations, etc., can be very helpful. Offer to help parents confer with leaders of such groups. Although laws covering private groups may not be the same as for public-school activities, often there will be a legal or organizational requirement for equal opportunity. Even if there is not, you can help the parent use persuasion and education (possibly with help from others such as the National Federation of the Blind) to build equal opportunity.

Protecting Oneself

Unfortunately, today it is also necessary to coach youngsters about when they should *not* be friendly. On a city street, it is usually unwise to converse at length with a stranger; invitations to ride in a car are totally unacceptable.

Parents may fear that blind youngsters cannot handle such problems. Talk about ways to identify persons reliably without using sight. A student old enough to walk alone on the street should be able to prevent most problems, and also to shout and go for help in case of emergency.

Learning to avoid harmful strangers is sometimes undermined by a seemingly innocent practice – the tendency for people to *give* blind youngsters things. This practice is undesirable enough because of its implications of pity, but it can confuse the child's safety training as well. Recently I have observed:

- a cab driver deliberately leaving change on the seat so that a young blind passenger will find it
- a high school principal giving a Homecoming corsage to the blind girl
- a sixth grader bringing several art projects to a blind first-grader

Examine situations like this, and apply a test recommended by booklets on child molestation: Does the role of this person make the action appropriate? Ask also, "Would it be considered appropriate if the child were not blind?" and note that blindness should not change one's general role in life.

A different dilemma about "friendliness" may occur in a play situation. The child who has been coached to cooperate may not realize that she too has rights.

Denise found herself being chased by several boys and girls at recess. It was not even a real game of tag, but a form of unkind teasing. Wanting to be friendly, Denise ran here and there for ten minutes; when the bell rescued her, she was near tears.

The playground supervisor, who had sympathized but hesitated to intervene, described this to Denise's resource teacher, who then coached her about ways to leave a really undesirable situation. "You can say, 'I'm tired – I don't want to play this any more,'" he counseled. "Just go and do what you want. Now, they might call you a 'chicken' or something, but just ignore them. And remember, if they really scare you, you should get help from the playground supervisor."

The Teen Years

New to the public Middle School, Paula very much wanted to be part of "Charlene's crowd." However, Paula's mother became very concerned about the way these girls seemed to treat Paula when they came home with her. They played Paula's records and ate the food she offered, but they talked to one another instead of with her. Never did they invite Paula to join them elsewhere.

Finally Paula's mother decided that the arrangement was harmful. She insisted that her daughter invite only one or two girls at a time. Although some girls declined the individual invitations, eventually two girls (one who was part of "Charlene's crowd" and one who was not) became Paula's close friends.

As this example illustrates, it is usually easier to get acquainted in a smaller group than in a large one. Informality is usually better than fancy entertaining. It is helpful to have equipment or skills which are valued by the other young people–cooking skill, a guitar, an interesting collection, a tandem bike, etc. However, the youngster must not let others lose respect for her and treat her like a "doormat."

DEVELOPING ONE'S OWN RESOURCES

As we consider the free-time activities popular with teenagers, we see all the more the importance of good travel and other skills of independence. Can the young woman shop independently, or must she constantly cling to a friend? Does the young man use various alternative methods of transportation, or does he feel helpless if his parents cannot take him? Are skills like table manners, dialing a telephone, etc., routine matters or causes of embarrassment?

Often a teenage brother, sister, or friend can provide transportation or reader service. Avoid, however, a situation where the blind teenager is smothered by too much help and attention, or the sighted teenager resents constant duties. Encourage reciprocal arrangements. Perhaps the blind brother or sister can do an extra stint of dishwashing in return for articles read aloud. A friend who provides transportation might be invited for dinner. As the student gets older, it is more and more desirable that readers and drivers be paid on a businesslike basis.

A great many teenagers have part-time jobs, with benefit both financially and socially. Blind teenagers, too, need to have this opportunity.

ADULTS SHOULD BE SENSITIVE AND CONSIDERATE

Teachers and parents should watch what they say to teenagers in front of peers. Be discreet about mentioning personal mannerisms, clothing, etc. Work on eating skills in privacy.

Always phrase remarks in a careful and dignified way, such as, "Parking meters are next to the street rather than close to the building. Consciously think about where the parking meters are, and use that as a clue to where you are." Matter-of-fact words and tone are important even if no one overhears, as it helps the student not to feel belittled. It is especially important if you are teaching something which peers have learned at an earlier age.

The chapter on "Dating, Marriage, and the Family" is actually an extension of this chapter. It contains many things which might otherwise have been said here.

As always, the teenager's problems in regard to blindness boil down to a matter of attitudes. The article, "I Remember," reprinted at the end of this chapter, shows this especially well.

Dealing with Problems of Acceptance

Generally, when their natural curiosity has been satisfied, youngsters respect the blind student's methods and accept them as a matter of course. If anything, young people accept a disability better than adults do. To prevent or minimize those problems which do occur, the following ideas are helpful:

(1) Help the blind student to improve his/her own individual skills and general self-confidence, and to contribute to the group.

(2) Help him/her to determine when help is needed, and to accept or refuse help pleasantly.

(3) Help all youngsters understand that we are all different, and that it is rude to overemphasize *any* characteristic (such as freckles, height, etc.) School counselors should be able to suggest many structured and unstructured ways to help students realize the universality of "differences" and the hurt caused by misplaced emphasis.

(4) Explain the physical cause of the disability in appropriate terms, and help the blind child do so also.

(5) Emphasize that blindness is a physical limitation and nothing more.

(6) Encourage other students' interest in such aids as Braille, and point out their value. A few students may be seriously interested in learning Braille.

(7) Help the blind youngster not to be oversensitive. He/she should be willing to answer friendly questions, and to be objective about tactless questions. He/she should also realize that some teasing and arguing are unavoidable, and learn to ignore it in most cases.

(8) Teach the blind youngster to be reasonably assertive rather than passive. He/she can speak up and say, "How about my turn next?"

(9) Look for possible problems apart from blindness. Is the group a tight clique, rejecting all outsiders? Do health problems seriously curtail the blind child's energy?

(10) Insist that the disability never be "used" to escape work or responsibility.

SPECIAL PROBLEMS

Conspicuous physical characteristics tend to magnify problems of acceptance, but the same principles apply nevertheless. Stress that we all have our own individual strengths and make our own particular contributions. The child may also want to meet others, if possible, with his particular physical characteristics.

When a child has extremely short stature, consult an expert on physical disabilities and architectural barriers. Get desks the right size, and a step-stool for reaching. Especially in junior high and high school, make sure the student can reach things like drinking fountains, sinks, and shelves.

Albinism also involves physical characteristics which may bring misunderstanding. One boy was teased as a "little old man with white hair." A kindergartner became furious at the many adults who gushed, "What beau-ti-ful hair you have!"

Albino Black youngsters face prejudice from both races. A Black adult may be especially helpful in discouraging prejudice by Black youngsters. I discussed this recently with an albino Black man who recalled that his Black playmates sometimes teased him and called him White. He advises emphasizing that all characteristics differ among people, and explaining albinism in a scientific way. He noted that prejudice decreased as he and his classmates grew older. And, of course, improving the general climate of race relations helps minimize any problem related to racial identity.

A Personal Description

The following is reprinted from *Future Reflections,* January, 1982.

I REMEMBER

By Mary Ellen Halverson

[*Editor's Note: Mrs. Halverson graduated from the University of Iowa with a major in Spanish. She has taught Spanish in the elementary schools and is now a full-time wife and mother and an active volunteer in the NFB and in her children's school.*]

When I look back on my high school years and consider all of the negative ideas I absorbed about blindness, I really wonder how I survived with any self respect left at all. I'm sure one reason I did is that I had a very positive, supportive family who believed in me and expected me to do well in school and other activities....

I began losing my sight in junior high due to a disease in the retina. When I had long reading assignments, my parents would read them to me in the evening. Many times I had difficulty in reading the blackboard or tests, but I struggled along. I can remember worrying about tests–not about the subject matter to be tested, but about the quality of the mimeographed pages of the test. I knew that frequently the print was faded or blurry and I was reluctant to use a magnifying glass in front of my fellow junior high students.... Neither my parents nor I realized that by eighth or ninth grade I was definitely legally blind. We told ourselves and others that I just had a "sight problem."

By the time I entered high school, I had lost a little more sight and was enrolled in the Sight Saving program in our school district. My parents and I were quite relieved since this program provided books on tape for me, and a lot of material in large print. There were different types of magnifiers available, and such things as large print dictionaries. However, the only skill I was actually taught by one of the sight saving teachers was typing, which is a valuable skill to have. I attended my regular high school classes in the morning and then went to a resource room for the afternoon. At first, this room was in an elementary school which I found rather embarrassing. I traveled there every day with several other students by cab. Eventually the resource room was moved into the high school, which was an improvement.

I remember the first day I met the sight saving teacher, who was a very kind, well-meaning person. Right away she told my family and me that "we never use the word 'blind,' we say, 'partially sighted.'" This suited us quite well since the word "blind" conjured up terrible and frightening visions in our minds. She further reassured us that I would not have to learn Braille, but could use large print books. I should tell you right here that in order for me to read even the large print, I had to put my face right down on the page and even then, I could only read several letters at a time. I can remember spending three hours trying to read a chemistry chapter in a large print book one evening. I imagine my fellow students read and studied the chapter in thirty minutes. Although we didn't realize it at the time, Braille would have been much more efficient and faster for me to use. Braille is not an inferior reading system, and can be easily learned.

Another area which caused me some anguish was traveling about both in the school building and outside. It was especially hard to see the down stairs, and I could not read the room numbers. When I approached the stairs I just slowed down and probably looked rather awkward. I developed my own techniques for finding the right room, such as the second room past the drinking fountain or the room next to the main front door. I did not attend many school or social activities at night because I could not see after dark. My excuse to people was usually that I had to study. Therefore, I missed out on dances, dates, and sports events, all of which are an important part of high school life. Now I know that this area of travel could have been solved so easily with some training in the use of the long white cane....

I am now convinced that the key to being an independent, successful, and happy blind person is your attitude about yourself. Along with attitude, but secondary, you must also learn some skills like typing, Braille, cane travel and other techniques that will work for you. During my high school years I had neither the positive attitude about myself nor the skills. I suppose the sad part is that there was no one to teach them to me. My classroom teachers were sympathetic for the most part, but they could offer no real encouragement or worthwhile advice concerning blindness. In some of my classes I felt that I was a nuisance to the teacher. I was very apologetic when I had to ask to have something read from the blackboard or from a test....

By now I'm sure you can understand how all of these experiences can cause a young person to feel very inferior to her peers. Even though my grades were high my self-respect was low. Of course, I did not realize this at the time. I should add here that my high school experience was not totally gloomy. I did have a good group of friends, some very cooperative teachers, and a terrific family. I graduated high in my class of 528 classmates and went on to the University. I entered college prepared to struggle on as before, but the unexpected happened.

I met several well-adjusted, confident blind students who had received training in the skills of blindness and had acquired that all-important attitude I mentioned earlier. They knew without a doubt that they were equal to anyone and they were willing to take on their share of responsibilities both in school and any other area of life. They also had another thing in common – they were members of the National Federation of the Blind and met for monthly meetings. At first I tried to avoid these meetings since I did not wish to admit that I was blind. But on the other hand, I liked these friends personally, and I wanted the same confidence and freedom they possessed.

After a couple years of college I attended an Orientation and Adjustment Center which taught skills and began the long process of improving my attitude toward myself and my blindness. It was, beyond a doubt, the most valuable year of my life. Very few places and very few people can restore a person's self-dignity and respect so effectively.

[*Editor's Note: Unfortunately, many orientation and adjustment centers have low expectations and are not very helpful. This student was fortunate.*]

Sometimes I think about how those teenage years might have been. I also think about the young people who are living my experiences right now, and about their parents who are worried and don't know what to do. If this article reaches you and helps any of you in one small way, those years of worry and embarrassment will have all been worth it! Parents, your children who are partially or totally blind, do have the opportunity to become independent, happy and successful individuals. It is respectable to be blind.

CHAPTER 43

DATING
MARRIAGE
AND THE FAMILY

The blind youngster needs to learn the same things about sex and family life that any child does. The things which are not said are just as significant as the things which are said. For example, if a father often says to his sighted son, "When you have children of your own, you will ...." but never says such things to his blind son, he is telling the second boy by implication that he probably will never have a family.

Learning physical facts about the human body should begin in early childhood, and be refined as years go by. One of the best ways to learn, with a minimum of self-consciousness, is to help care for babies, including changing diapers. Models and raised diagrams of the human anatomy are available also. (One good source is a Rape Crisis Center. Anatomically correct models help abused children explain their experiences, but can also be helpful to blind children for a very different reason.)

Preteen girls should examine tampons, sanitary napkins, and rest-room vending machines. (Blind boys should have an opportunity to examine tampons and pads also. These things should not be a mystery.)

Who Should Teach?

Personal subjects must be handled with great tact and discretion, especially where touching something might seem even more personal than merely discussing it or looking at a picture. Many things are discussed most comfortably at home. However, many parents find it hard to discuss anything related to sex. Help parents find appropriate books on dating, marriage, and the family. Try to provide anatomical models and raised diagrams.

Any teacher should be very careful about personal matters, especially with a student of the opposite sex. It is easy to cause great embarrassment unintentionally. Nevertheless, often someone at the school can be very helpful. Nurses, physical education teachers, and counselors commonly discuss personal health and development. In sixth or seventh grade, units in Health or physical education typically cover the changes of puberty. Furthermore, any sensitive teacher may happen to gain the personal confidence of a student.

It is important for a teenager to have someone to confide in *at any time.* If you are itinerant or working with a student of the opposite sex, be sure that there is someone other than yourself who can help meet this need.

Teenagers' typical self-consciousness about the body can involve major misunderstandings. One girl, already nervous about public rest rooms, steadfastly refused to use one particular rest room. Tactful discussion revealed that she thought everyone could see in. She knew the windows had no drapes, and she had never heard of translucent glass (that is, glass which lets light pass but cannot be seen through). She also was uncertain about how much could be seen over and under the doors of the stalls.

Another student was laughed at because she never closed the toilet stall door. She needed to understand why it was important to close the door, and also needed practice in handling various locks.

In each of these cases, the woman itinerant teacher was able to work on the problem during cane travel and general orientation. Had the teacher been a man, help would have been obtained from an appropriate female staff member.

A third student refused ever to kiss her boyfriend; she felt she never knew when they had enough privacy. A sensitive counselor talked with her about social conventions and degrees of privacy. She discussed various ways to determine whether other people are likely to be watching, and if so how much they could see. She also encouraged the girl to talk more freely with her parents.

Dating

The boy or girl approaching dating age will begin to wonder, "Will the other kids want to go on dates with me?" and "Should I marry a blind person?" Various suggestions about dating and marriage appear below and in the chapter on "Fitting In Socially." See also *A Resource Guide for Parents and Educators of Blind Children,* also by Doris M. Willoughby.

When one blind girl lamented a lack of dates, her resource teacher said, "Those boys are only hurting themselves when they don't ask you out! They're missing a *beautiful* experience!"

This remark came across as condescending rather than helpful. *"I'm* the one sitting at home and not having a good time!" protested the girl to her mother later. "That teacher just doesn't understand!"

It would have been better to say, "I'm sorry you are unhappy," and "I'm sure you will have more dates as time goes on." It would also have been valuable to provide constructive help in developing social skills and good grooming.

On the question of whether to marry (or date) a sighted or blind partner, we suggest this advice: Blindness is merely one of many characteristics, and not the most important one. It is wise to select partners on the broad basis of general compatibility. Personality, religion, education, etc., are far more important than sight. It would be foolish to restrict one's choices by ruling out *all* blind people or *all* sighted people. However, the partner's *attitude* toward blindness *is* a crucial factor. For example, if a fully- or partially-sighted boyfriend or girlfriend persists in being overprotective, he or she is a very poor prospect for marriage to a self-reliant individual who is totally blind.

The article, "Dating and Marriage," also by Doris M. Willoughby (*Future Reflections,* January, 1982), extends many of the ideas introduced in this chapter. Part of this article follows:

A young blind woman once told me of a teacher's saying to her, "You are an exceptional blind person. You are attractive enough to marry a sighted man." She and I analyzed that comment and thought of several implied statements within it:

- Most blind people aren't attractive.
- Marrying a sighted person is categorically much better than marrying a blind person.
- This young blind woman would be still more attractive if she were sighted.

The National Federation of the Blind emphatically disagrees with all these implied statements, briefly commenting as follows:

- Individual blind people are attractive or unattractive according to their individual characteristics and one's personal opinions.
- Since the majority of the population is sighted, it is to be expected that frequently a blind person will marry someone who is sighted. However, although sight is a helpful thing to have, it does not make a person "better," either in intrinsic value as a person, or as a partner in marriage. The blind

individual is wisest to date a variety of people, and to choose the marriage partner (sighted or blind) who is best suited for him or her based on *all* characteristics. Also, the *attitude* of each partner toward blindness is far more important than the mere fact of being blind or sighted.

- We don't compete in life with what we might have been under other circumstances; we compete with others as they *are.* A blind person with a reasonable degree of poise and competence can fit in socially on the same basis as others.

Having dealt with the statements implied by the teacher's remark, let us consider her original remark itself. No doubt you have heard many variations of the comment, "She does so well, we would never know she is blind." Although often one must accept such remarks in the spirit intended, it is well for you and your growing youngster to recognize the problem of the implied statements. (Compare the remark sometimes made to a sighted person, "You drive so well I almost forget you are a woman!") This type of remark is a symptom of the unfortunate social attitudes which still expect the blind to be inferior and incompetent. Try to avoid statements such as the above, and say instead,

"My, you are getting to be an attractive young woman!"...
"That new hairdo looks great!"...
"I'm glad you had so much fun at the party"...
"You and Bob seem to be really hitting it off well"...
"I think you showed a lot of social poise in that situation."

SUGGESTIONS TO YOUNG PEOPLE WHO ARE BLIND

[The following is adapted from *A Resource Guide for Parents and Educators of Blind Children,* also by Doris M. Willoughby.]

Remember that all teenagers have a great many adjustments to make in growing up, and all feel nervous and confused at times. Time and experience will help you feel much more confident.

When it is appropriate to shake hands, hold out your hand and the other person will probably grasp it. If the other person does not grasp it soon, simply put your hand back down. No embarrassment is necessary.

In a cafeteria, it may be convenient to go with a sighted person and have him or her tell you the choices. However, it also works well to ask the people behind the counter, or any employee of the cafeteria, to explain the choices and hand you what you want. As you move your tray along, feel the rail ahead to be sure it is there. At many cafeterias, an employee will carry your tray and find you a table if you so request.

Salespeople and others will sometimes ignore you or talk to someone who is with you, instead of talking directly to you. Be assertive. If you are not sure whether the question really is for you or for someone else, say something such as "Am I next?"

If you are a girl, you may feel that it is hard to get acquainted with boys because you cannot take the initiative in dating. Society is changing in this respect, and there are more and more situations where it is proper for a girl to ask a boy. Among other ideas, you might help arrange a girl-ask-boy party, or you might invite the boy over to sample your cooking.

If you are a girl, do not assume that being feminine allows you to depend on others.

If you are a boy, remember that being blind does

not make you less of a man. Do not hesitate to ask a girl for a date because you fear she may not accept your blindness. Every boy is turned down for dates at times. If she refuses, ask someone else.

If you are a boy escorting a girl for the first time, it may be helpful to go to a place where you have been before. Later, with experience, you will have the confidence to go to unfamiliar places on dates.

Anticipate that a waiter is likely to give the check to a sighted person, even if that person is the girl you are escorting. You may want to say, "May I have the check now, please," to prevent this. You may also wish to warn your date about this, and gain her cooperation in getting the check to you.

There are many ways to find transportation. Double dating, group activities, and car pools offer alternatives to driving one's own car. (Be sure to help pay for the gas.) Perhaps you can take the bus or a taxi, or walk. Perhaps a friend or relative will drive you; again, be sure to pay your share of expenses. A sighted girl dating a blind boy may be quite willing to drive if her date buys gas and provides a pleasant evening.

Individual dating is not the only way to get acquainted. Informal clubs and other group activities provide excellent opportunities for meeting people.

If a new friend says nothing at all about blindness, bring up the subject before too much time goes by. He or she probably has several questions but is afraid to ask. You might include some humor to help put your friends at ease.

Be alert to the likelihood that people will try to help you unnecessarily. Sometimes this can be anticipated and prevented. Sometimes you will guide the sighted person in giving you the right kind of help – as, "Let me take hold of your arm, instead of the other way around." At other times you will say, "Thank you, but I'd rather do that myself." If you cannot avoid unwanted help, be polite and try to think of a way to handle a future encounter differently.

The creative individual who is blind can find a way to take part actively in any activity, including dancing, skating, etc. Think how to apply methods and ideas you have already learned. Be creative and figure out new ideas. Talk with an experienced blind person who is older than you are. Believe that you can do it, and then go ahead.

Marriage and Family Responsibilities

Boys and girls also wonder whether they can manage the responsibilities of married life, particularly raising children. A number of suggestions for child care appear below; however, these are brief and oriented toward babysitting. The best resource is continual contact with successful blind parents.

Answering questions about hereditary conditions is a touchy matter. Encourage parents to get accurate medical facts, preferably from a clinic specializing in genetics, and to be frank with their children. The question of whether to have children is a personal one, regardless of whether the eye condition is hereditary. Many people, learning that their eye condition is indeed hereditary, have children and resolve that they will provide the very best education and training if a child is blind. Other people make other decisions. Many types of blindness are not passed on to children at all. Of course, blindness or the possibility of passing blindness on to children are only two of the many factors that people must consider as they approach marriage and raising a family. As a group, blind parents are as successful at raising children as are sighted parents. Blindness need not prevent successful parenthood.

Learning to Care for Children

The following is adapted from *A Resource Guide for Parents and Educators of Blind Children*. These suggestions are oriented toward babysitting in a home situation, and are written in a style directed toward parents; but they will be useful to teachers also.

> Can a young person who is blind stay alone in the house, deal with the possibility of unwanted callers, and care for young children? Certainly, if he or she has the necessary training and uses alternative techniques.
>
> The blind person alone in the house will deal with visitors in the same way that others do, but will use voice. If the visitor cannot suitably identify himself by calling through the door, then the youngster should not let him in. Teach your child security cautions which are suitable for your locality.
>
> Under supervision, a young child can learn to hold and amuse a baby, and can fetch things needed for the baby. By the teen years, he or she can be a responsible babysitter.
>
> In most respects, a blind youngster learns child-care skills in the same way as anyone else. First, he or she helps an adult to care for brothers and sisters, cousins, or other younger children. Formal or informal classes in child care are often available.
>
> Sighted young people, prepared in this manner, often simply begin to babysit on their own when they reach their teens. Blind young people may do the same. Often, however, the blind boy or girl faces two types of problems at this point. First, the adults who are teaching may not know how certain tasks could be done without sight. Secondly, potential customers may assume that a blind teenager could not really be responsible.
>
> Throughout this book are many suggestions which will help in solving both of these problems. It is a good idea to increase the level of responsibility rather gradually, so that the final step is a relatively small one.
>
> The first step (beyond merely assisting) could be to become a "Mother's helper"–that is, to be responsible for the baby while a parent is nearby but busy. Peggy began by taking care of her two young cousins while her aunt caught up on housework. As Peggy became more and more able, her aunt began to pay her a small wage–less than for regular babysitting, but enough to reflect some responsibility. Peggy's aunt told friends and neighbors about this arrangement, and soon Peggy had two more such jobs: the mother of infant twins took much-needed naps while Peggy amused the babies, and a teacher graded papers while Peggy watched her three-year-old. Thus, over several months Peggy built up an employment record showing her capability. One day the teacher made a quick trip to the grocery store, leaving Peggy alone with the child. Seeing that there were no particular problems, she decided to begin hiring Peggy as a regular babysitter.
>
> Peggy might also have brought a child to her own home, to care for him under her own mother's supervision. If your teenager does this, form a plan to gradually give her less and less help. Later (with the approval of the child's parents, of course) give all the responsibility to her, and make a point of frequently leaving the house while she is babysitting. An older, capable blind babysitter may still prefer to bring a child in rather than going to a strange home, because of the effort involved in becoming acquainted with a strange house well enough to babysit safely.
>
> It was reasonable for Peggy to be paid less when she was taking only partial responsibility. However, it would have been a mistake for her to accept low wages for a regular job in an attempt to attract business. If she is ready to offer the same service as others, she should expect the same pay and the same respect.
>
> When a blind teenager plans to babysit in a strange home, she should take the time to be well prepared. She should know the general characteristics of children of various ages. She should go to the home beforehand, if possible, to get acquainted with the children and with the layout of the

home, and also to take Braille notes regarding emergency phone numbers.

Any teenager, blind or sighted, always should be aware of the option of declining a job which really appears too difficult, and should have ways to summon help in an emergency.

In caring for an infant, the sitter must remember that, if she is not holding onto the baby, he must be in a safely defined space from which escape is impossible. She must anticipate that the baby may suddenly learn something new – the young baby may roll over for the first time, or the older baby may suddenly stand up. If there are older children, the sitter must anticipate that they may try to move the baby or give him a forbidden object.

All necessary care – preparing bottles, changing diapers, etc. – can be done without sight. Some suggestions for spoon-feeding are as follows: Protect the baby's clothing and the surroundings to minimize the mess. Do not fill the spoon completely – offer just a little at a time. Expect to scoop food off the chin and the bib frequently. Sometimes a baby will cooperate and eagerly seek the spoon; however, some babies wave their heads around and expect the spoon to seek them. The blind person may place his/her free hand gently at the edge of the baby's mouth to aid in getting the spoon to the right place. Feeding a young baby is a job which should be practiced first with help from an adult.

A toddler must also be watched carefully and kept in a safe environment. It may be necessary to block off stairways, lock the basement door, etc. A babysitter is well advised to stay right with the child, and play with him quite a bit more than a parent would. This accomplishes two goals: it keeps the child happy and amused, and it enables the sitter to know exactly what the child is doing. The sitter should examine the environment by touch frequently to be sure she knows what is there. In checking the child's hands for forbidden objects, the sitter can make a game of it – perhaps counting the fingers humorously or reciting a rhyme.

Parents may worry that young children will hide or run away so that the blind sitter cannot find them. Tying bells firmly to the shoes of very small children may be a good idea. A harness or stroller may be used when walking outside. A child who deliberately hides can usually be enticed out if the sitter begins to read an interesting story aloud or prepare a snack. (The blind sitter can read from a Braille book which also has inkprint and pictures.) If necessary, a blind sitter can search by touch in likely places, while talking about a pleasant game, and while listening for telltale sounds.

School-age children can be controlled by reason and discipline, with very few things being different for the blind babysitter. Parents may fear that older children will deliberately take advantage of a blind sitter, but handling this potential problem is actually not very different from handling any attempt by a child to get away with something. The sitter must be alert to what the children are doing at all times, listen for suspicious sounds (or a suspicious lack of sound), and check on the children continually. Sometimes she may use techniques which were described above in connection with younger children.

If children ask a blind sitter to draw or print something for them, she might describe or spell the item or use lines that can be felt. Also, the children may greatly enjoy describing their own drawings to the sitter. They are likely to be fascinated by Braille and other alternative techniques, and may eagerly amuse themselves for quite awhile if allowed to try them out.

These suggestions are by no means comprehensive. It is most helpful for the blind teenager to talk with successful blind parents and blind teachers, or at least to correspond with them. The teenager should also realize that, even if circumstances should prevent any paid babysitting, learning to care for children is an essential part of becoming a responsible man or woman.

Two detailed and helpful books are *Parent Tips: A Guide for Blind and Visually Impaired Parents"* (information on baby and child care), and *Parent Tips: The Challenge Years* (for blind parents of school-age children). Both books are by Janiece Betker (see "References").

Facing the Attitudes of Others

The blind adult needs to be knowledgeable and assertive in order to stay out of an abyss – namely, the passive and helpless role which society presses upon him or her.

This book has many suggestions for facing this problem as it relates to a young person still in school. However, many aspects of facing the world as a blind *adult* are beyond the scope of this book.

Jobs are denied to capable workers just because someone *thinks* a blind person could not perform well. Teachers teach sighted children that their blind parents (however competent) are dependent on *them.* Social workers sometimes take children from their parents solely because the parents are blind.

The National Federation of the Blind deals with problems like these every day, with ever-increasing success. The "References" section of this book lists several especially relevant publications, and there are many others. Help your student maintain regular contact with the NFB, so that he/she will build a background of knowledge to resist prejudice, and know how to get help when it is needed.

Blind people today serve on juries (although sometimes judges still ask, "But how can he see the evidence?") Blind people today hold good jobs (though many are still unemployed or underemployed). Blind people today raise families (though some doctors and nurses still say, "How can *you* care for a child?")

Here is another short excerpt from the article, "Dating and Marriage":

During the months when Curt and I were dating, someone said to me, "I think it's simply wonderful of you to date him." I had a vague feeling at the time that there was something wrong with that remark, but I really didn't know what to say or think about it. Today I would say something such as, "It is not a matter of *my* doing something for *him.* He is a terrific guy and we *both* really enjoy each other's company." And I would realize the remark means that we have a lot of work to do in educating the public about blindness.

CHAPTER 44

STARTING ANEW EACH TIME

The New School Year

Susannah made excellent progress in second grade, reading Braille as well as the best of the print readers. However, when the itinerant teacher arrived after the first day of the following year, the third-grade teacher exclaimed, "This will never work out! Why on earth didn't her parents send her to the school for the blind? I don't have any special training for this!"

The truism about a "stitch in time" fits whenever a blind student starts a new year or a new course, with a new teacher, or in a new school. Susannah's itinerant teacher assumed that because second grade went well, everyone in the school would accept and include Susannah easily. She assumed that the second-grade teacher would explain things to the third-grade teacher. "Surely," she thought, "if I come on the first day of school I can head off any problems that might come up."

Not so. This classroom teacher has been building up worries and barriers all summer, and has had them confirmed by an all-important first day which evidently went very badly. For any possibility of a reasonably successful year now, tremendous effort will be required.

Never assume anything.

A successful transition to a new year for a Braille student generally requires more preparation than for a student who uses print. This is not because the student necessarily requires more attention, but because more attitudinal barriers must be overcome. (As discussed throughout this book, it is vital that we do indeed overcome these barriers, rather than letting them be an excuse for the student to attempt sighted techniques which are not really best in the long run.)

ADVANCE PREPARATION

If your student has already been attending this school building, the most important groundwork should already have been laid – namely, enlisting the informed support of the administration. Keep in touch with the building principal. Many districts also have a Director of Special Education. In a small district, try to meet the superintendent.

In the spring, talk with the administrator about ordering transcribed texts, and discuss your student's methods and abilities in general. Probably there will also be a formal Program Review or Staffing near the end of the year; be sure to include the appropriate administrator(s) and, if possible, classroom teachers.

Especially for the younger student, I try hard to find out who the classroom teacher(s) will be, in order to have some discussion in the spring. I offer a copy of *Your School Includes a Blind Student* and other materials, and discuss methods in a general way. This enables both of us to assess possible problems and plan ahead; it also lessens apprehension over the summer. If the teacher has not already met the blind student, I try to arrange this.

When there are several teachers, it saves time to have a group meeting. I use the following outline:

(1) A brief statement of general philosophy (the blind student as a regular student, the value of being in regular classes, etc.)

(2) My role, plus any other individual help available. I may say, "When there is a need for individual attention, I will help find a way to arrange it without an undue burden on the classroom teacher."

(3) Explanation of methods and materials.

(4) Description of any special needs or problems, including those not directly related to blindness.

(5) Answering questions as time permits (this tends to be continued into meetings with individual teachers).

(6) Determining which staff member will coordinate arrangements and materials.

(7) Explanation of how to reach me.

WHICH TEACHER

Asking that a student have one particular classroom teacher (or not have him/her) is a type of preplanning I try hard to *avoid*. Such requests tend to imply that only certain teachers can work effectively with blind students, an idea with which I thoroughly disagree.

Sometimes it is said that the student should have a particular teacher because of a smaller class, a better personality match, a particular need, etc. I usually say, "That problem should be carefully considered. But the class assignments are a complicated matter." I might say to the principal, "I feel that Jim has a strong need for ____, and I know you'll want to take that into account in selecting his teacher for next year." But if I, as the teacher of *blind* students, make a strong statement about the assignment of classroom teachers, somehow it comes across as meaning, "Only certain teachers can work effectively with blind students." It is a very small step from this to "No one in our school (grade, department, etc.) can work effectively with blind students." Next time there may be only *one* available teacher–with the very characteristics you considered so unsuitable!

If a student really does need a smaller class or special arrangements because of individual needs, this should be documented in the IEP. But "regular class placement" means "regular class placement."

Sometimes a student expresses strong preference for or against a given teacher. Especially in high school, there may be merit in such preferences; yet a student does need to learn to work with various personalities. In most instances I encourage a student to talk with his/her parents, or with the counselor, about this kind of thing. I also explore, however, whether there is any problem related to blindness which I might alleviate. One blind student avoided a particular English teacher who had embarrassed her by calling her "wonderful" and saying she need not take quizzes. This problem might have been easily solved by an alert resource or itinerant teacher.

If parents express preferences, I encourage them to talk with the principal or counselor.

I do sometimes make suggestions about class *groupings*, realizing that final decisions are the principal's prerogative. If a particular classmate persists in being a "mother hen" and overprotecting the blind student, separation may be helpful. Also, if another student is deaf, it may be hard for the classroom teacher to maximize the learning styles of both.

Sometimes two or more blind students are in the same grade at the same school. On the one hand, if they have needs in common it can be efficient to place them together. On the other hand–especially if their abilities differ considerably–it can be very important to separate them. Students and classroom teachers tend to believe that blind students' needs and abilities are similar, even when they are not. (All of this assumes that there is more than one section of each grade. In a small school where two students must be in the same room, make extra effort to emphasize individual needs.)

It is *not* necessary that blind students always be in the classes which have the fewest students.

ANTICIPATING NEW NEEDS

Look ahead for new situations. Perhaps the fourth graders must pass to several classrooms daily. Perhaps the sixth grade has many science field trips. Seventh or eighth grade will have home economics and industrial arts. Prepare carefully for such new situations, as by arranging for the sewing teacher to visit the adult Orientation Center or a blind homemaker. "Sell" your program and your student, just as though you were starting from scratch – because, in a sense, you are. Ideas described below for starting at a new school may, of course, apply to new situations in the same school.

In the fall, *before* school begins, recheck to be sure that plans are in place and there are no unpleasant surprises. You may find that the supportive principal suddenly retired due to poor health, and was replaced by one who believes residential schools solve all problems; or that the helpful science teacher left for a higher salary and was replaced by one who keeps talking about other handicaps; or that the history book was replaced last week by a brand-new edition. The sooner you learn of a change or problem, the more likely you are to minimize the difficulty. Even if there are no big surprises, you will find that the general discussions of the spring have been replaced by specific and urgent questions.

A WRITTEN SUMMARY

Especially at the secondary level where the student will have several teachers, hand out a summary of methods and materials. Teachers find it very helpful to be able to look up how to contact you, how to handle daily worksheets, where to get materials, what standards to apply to typewritten assignments, etc. Following are two examples of such summaries, which would be handled confidentially and given only to the teachers who work with the student in question.

The first, on the following page, describes a strong student.

SUMMARY – KAREN AINSWORTH'S METHODS AND MATERIALS

Karen very much appreciates the way she is being included as she starts high school. I hope that this written description of her methods and materials will be of further help in making things go smoothly.

Materials

Textbooks: These should all be here, either in Braille or on tape. If the book is arriving in installments and is not all here yet, keep Mr. Jones advised. It is not possible to get *all* books in Braille; let us know if you would like suggestions on the use of tapes.

Give Karen an inkprint copy of each book also. She will need it for reference.

Supplementary books, book reports, reference materials, etc.: If we have several days' notice, it is usually easy to get these kinds of things in Braille or on tape. We will help to order them, or you may contact the state Library for the Blind at ____.

Daily handouts, worksheets, etc.: If the item is available two weeks or more ahead of time, place a regular copy in Karen's box in the counseling office. Include your name and the date needed. If there are several items, indicate the sequence and approximate time schedule.

Delivery: Transcribed materials will be delivered via Mr. Jones.

In the case of items which are not transcribed before the class uses them, it is usually best to *read them aloud* "live." Sometimes a classmate can do this, or Karen can take the paper home to get it read. See Mr. Jones or Mrs. Willoughby if you have trouble finding someone to read aloud.

Equipment and Supplies

Karen has organized the materials she carries with her very well. Larger items, such as typewriters and tape machines, are readily available by arrangement. Please let us know if there are problems with equipment or materials, or if you have a need which might be met by a device of some kind.

Methods

Karen has an excellent attitude and is very conscientious. Usually she will know what method will work best for her in class. However, the following list may be helpful.

Written assignments: Karen should type all assignments unless there is a very unusual format. She can make corrections by using the correction key.

In case of an unusual format, such as diagraming sentences, she might dictate her answers aloud for someone to write down.

Note-taking: For most purposes Karen should now be using the Braille slate. For very lengthy notes she may use the larger Braillewriter. If material is to be *copied* verbatim from a visual arrangement (such as the chalkboard) provide a classmate with self-carboning paper, so that Karen can have a duplicate set of notes to be read aloud later. We do *not* recommend tape-recording lectures, because this is not notetaking: she would have no summary for review purposes. Karen should take notes on the same basis as others.

Tests: We will provide tests in Braille whenever possible. Otherwise a test may be given orally. Karen may give her answers by marking a Braille answer sheet, by dictating aloud, or by typing. She is expected to take the same tests as others, although extra time should be permitted if necessary. If you have a test for which it is not readily apparent how to administer it, please ask for advice.

Cane Travel

Karen is learning her way around Central High, and can travel to many locations independently. Where she is not yet independent, we have arranged for someone to accompany her until she has more experience. Karen should grasp the sighted person's arm, just above the elbow.

General Adjustment

Karen is eager to fit in and do what is expected. If she is doing something incorrect or not customary, she would very much like to know about it. (Examples: if she does not face the movie screen, or places the heading wrong on her papers.) Of course, anything of a personal nature would be discussed privately.

Contacts for Suggestions and Materials

Mrs. Willoughby, the itinerant teacher of blind students, is usually in the building on Tuesday and Thursday mornings. Her office telephone is ____ and home phone is ____. Mr. Jones and Mrs. Tauke are coordinating arrangements at Central.

Below is an example of a written summary for a student who has many problems.

To save space, the remarks about "Materials" are not reprinted here; they would be very similar to those in the summary for Karen, above.

SUMMARY–MATT BRIDGES' METHODS AND MATERIALS

Matt and his parents appreciate the personal interest shown by the Westlake staff in helping him to get started well in junior high. We hope that this summary will be helpful.

Materials

[Editor's Note: Comments on "Materials" are similar to those for Karen and are not reproduced here.]

Equipment and Supplies

We are helping Matt to organize the things he carries with him. He should have his loose-leaf notebook with a section for each class. He also has an organizer pouch for his Braille slate, pencil, and other small items. Please talk with Miss Curry if he has great difficulty finding things.

Larger items include typewriters, tape machines, Braillewriters, and talking book machines (record players with special features). These must be shared by arrangement among several classrooms. Matt should know how to operate all these machines. He also can carry any of them a short distance.

Methods

Note: Matt often needs guidance to avoid his assuming he cannot do something. Please ask Mrs. Willoughby or Miss Curry if you are not certain how he would participate in an activity.

For *written assignments,* the goal is for Matt to type them on a regular typewriter. We are phasing in this method, using it with short assignments at this time. He can cross out errors with x's.

If the assignment is too long or difficult for Matt to type, he may: (1) write it in Braille and then read it aloud to you; (2) write in Braille and then dictate it to someone (such as his parents or a teacher aide) who will write it out; (3) dictate it onto a tape; (4) dictate directly to you.

Note-Taking: If students are *writing their own notes* from an oral lecture, then Matt should learn to take his own. For lengthy note-taking, we can provide a Braillewriter, which he uses well. For short notes he can write on the Braille slate, which is quieter and much more portable. If you have not seen the slate used, please ask for a demonstration.

If material is to be *copied* from the board, etc., another student might use multicopy paper (which we can provide), and give a copy to Matt so that he can have it read aloud later. We do *not* recommend taping lectures, because this is not note-taking; no summary is provided for review purposes. Miss Curry is working intensively with Matt on note-taking skills.

Tests: Tests may be given orally or in Braille. Matt can give his answers orally, or mark with a pencil on a Braille answer sheet.

However, at this time he is having some special problems in taking tests. Miss Curry will administer most tests in the resource room individually. We will be in touch about your particular testing situation.

Daily Living Skills

Matt has difficulty with certain personal skills such as eating neatly, dialing the telephone, etc. Please advise if you notice problems. We are setting priorities as to what to work on first.

Mobility

Miss Curry will talk with you about just where Matt has already learned to go alone, and where he still needs help. If he cannot walk reliably from your class to the next, someone should accompany him or at least watch him. If he knows the way, he should not let other students help him.

Following are some suggestions for accompanying Matt when he does need assistance:

(1) If he is late or having great difficulty, it may be best for someone to walk right with him. He should take the arm of the sighted person just above the elbow; this works better than for the sighted person to push him ahead.

(2) On the stairs, Matt should walk by himself, with the guide ahead or behind. Go single file and let people pass. We are helping Matt to walk more normally and smoothly on stairs.

(3) If he knows the way fairly well but sometimes gets lost, the guide might follow and help only in case of difficulty.

When Matt walks alone, occasionally remind of these points:

(1) The hand which is holding the cane should be centered in front of the body at the waist. Except on stairs, the cane should be moved back and forth in front of the two feet, evenly on both sides.

(2) On stairs the cane tip should be about two steps ahead, and usually not moving back and forth.

(3) The cane should be used to find a doorway. If the door is closed, the cane makes a different sound when it strikes the door. If the door is open, the cane can easily find the opening. He should not hunt for doorways with his hand – this is slower, looks awkward, and makes it difficult to carry things.

(4) We keep encouraging Matt to walk faster. The Adaptive P.E. teacher will be helping us with this.

General Behavior

Matt is not disruptive. However, he needs considerable guidance as to what is expected, both academically and socially.

Mannerisms, or inappropriate motions, have been one area of concern. We suggest that if he makes any large motions (such as moving his hands in the air) he be firmly asked to stop. He seems well able to control any motions that are really distracting, and simply needs a reminder at times. With smaller motions, such as nodding his head, use your judgment – these are harder for him to avoid completely at this time.

In general we expect that Matt will meet the same behavioral standards as other students. For example, although he may be allowed to talk at certain times in order to gain visual information, he is not permitted to chat at will.

Health Concerns

Matt suffers from asthma which can be severe. Contact Mrs. White if she has not already briefed you about this.

Contacts for Suggestions and Materials

Mrs. Willoughby works with Matt during sixth period Monday, Wednesday, and Friday, in Room 310. She may also be contacted at ___ (office) or ___ (home), or by leaving a message with Miss Curry.

PREVENT PROBLEMS

Careful planning makes disasters far less likely. Suppose, for example, that a new student needing much attention appears just as school is starting. If your preparation has been done well, you will know just where the most urgent needs are for your other students, and can manage your limited time efficiently.

It is possible to give *too much* help to an experienced student who is not in a high-risk situation. The older student should gradually take on more responsibility for ordering books and materials, explaining his or her methods to teachers, etc.

The First Braille Student

Even if the student is coming along with his class from the same district, and even if there have been other visually-impaired students in this building, the arrival of the first Braille student will pose some hurdles. As always, the real problems are not the technical arrangements, but attitudes. Many people seem to feel that arrangements for a "partially-sighted" student are just an adaptation of "regular" methods, whereas the use of Braille seems somehow exotic. Your job is to show that Braille and all other alternative techniques are also merely variations of "regular" methods.

In a resource school with several blind students, of course, preparation for an individual will be less extensive.

Beware, however, of assuming that having had *one* (or even two or three) previous blind student(s) will make future arrangements easy. I once encountered a principal who told me over and over about the failures of their one previous blind student (evidently a very slow student who attempted to attend public school before P.L. 94-142, with no special help whatsoever) who finally "was sent to the Blind School, where she belonged." I also recall a high school where, despite explanations that Mark was a good student, a social studies teacher failed to mention the important supplementary text. She explained later that "we couldn't use that with Wayne" (a previous blind student with severe learning problems).

BUILD A POSITIVE IMAGE

As you keep in mind the *real* problems of blindness, you will emphasize meeting blind children and adults who are succeeding. Arrange for the teachers to visit a good adult Orientation Center, the home or office of a competent blind adult, and/or a school that already has one or more blind students. Go along yourself, to answer questions and compensate for possible misunderstandings. (With a trip to a special school, be prepared for the question, "Why aren't we sending our student there, too?") Arrange a visit to your prospective student at his current school. Show a *good* film or videotape (see "References"). Invite a speaker who is blind. Pay particular attention to classes needing specialized techniques, such as industrial arts.

It is important for the staff to meet teachers and administrators who have successfully included a blind student. If your student is simply moving up within the same district, this should be easy. For a kindergartner, help the teacher visit the preschool. It may be deflating to our egos as "specialized teachers," but when it comes to saying "This can work for you," the regular classroom teacher finds the greatest credibility in another classroom teacher. The administrator finds it in another administrator.

PLAN AHEAD

When a new student who uses Braille enters, do everything which is described above for helping an established student begin a new year, and then some. If you meet serious problems, get help. As always, it is especially important to have the support and understanding of the school administration.

A nightmarish vision of mine has fortunately never (to my knowledge) happened to any of my students: a substitute teacher says, "You can't see this?? What's the matter–are you blind?" I would hope that no teacher today would make such an insensitive comment, or that if it did happen, an experienced blind student could handle it. But for younger students who cannot yet express themselves well, an explanation should be included in the directions for substitutes.

A student coming along with a class to a new building will already know many classmates. For those not acquainted, there are many possible approaches. Generally I prefer *not* to talk to the other students ahead of time. While advance preparation for the *staff* is necessary for educational planning, there is no such practical need for the students. Indeed, prior explanation seems to emphasize differences, and to reinforce talking *about* the student rather than *with* him or her. After the student actually enters, we can then introduce him/her as we would any new student. The boy or girl can introduce himself/herself, and do at least part of the explanation of methods.

There are exceptions, of course, as with a very shy child or one with a great many special needs. Also, the matter of explanations to students in *other* classes points up the value of good preplanning with the *entire* staff. With suitable preparation, teachers will be more likely to say, "That's Mary Ireland, who just came into Mr. Pierson's class. She's blind and does her work in Braille," rather than, "That's the new blind girl, poor thing. We must all be very kind to her."

WATCH YOUR TIMING

One principal suggested I talk to all the parents in preparation for Shelley, a blind kindergartner. "This could promote better understanding," she suggested. "The speech therapist, the audiologist, and so on are all speaking at the Kindergarten Roundup, explaining the help they can offer. Why don't we include you?" As we talked over the advantages and disadvantages, I said I would speak *if* we could keep it on the same rather general basis of "help available," but that this would be hard to do since most people knew of the one particular blind child, and since I had never been to that district's Roundup before. Eventually the principal said, "No – I've decided we'd better not do it this time. I'm afraid Shelley's parents would complain that we were setting her apart too much – they've said they don't want that."

In a resource school where there would always be blind children, I would have been eager to speak to parents. It would have been easy to avoid discussing individuals; and "calling attention" to a program involving several children is justified. Even in Shelley's school, if the blind child had *already* been at the elementary school for several months, I would have felt comfortable in speaking to parents. But the danger of *creating* problems must always be considered. At that particular time (just *before* Shelley entered) it would have been awkward to deal with questions such as, "Why can't she go to a special school?"

A New Student Who Uses Print

With the new student who uses print, there is danger of two opposite errors: (1) giving too much help and special attention, or (2) assuming that because the student has some vision, he/she can do everything in the usual way. It is hard to tell which danger is the more likely, and it is common to have a mixture of both. The school might assume that the student could easily fill in tiny circles on a standardized answer sheet, and at the same time assume he could not possibly take industrial arts.

ANTICIPATE QUESTIONS

For the visually-impaired student using print, the same general approach described for Braille students is called for, although there may be fewer questions asked. A meeting with teachers is desirable, as is the follow-up written summary of arrangements. (We specialized teachers sometimes mistakenly assume that no explanation for the staff is needed unless Braille is involved.)

For a partially-sighted student the most common topics for planning are:

- Books and materials in large print or on tape
- Methods with the overhead projector and other visual aids
- Combination locks

- How to use a four-track, multiple-speed tape recorder, including finding the right place
- Arrangements for reading: magnification, lighting, etc.
- Specialized classes such as home economics and industrial arts
- Questions about eyestrain, headaches, and posture
- Methods for writing, including darker pencils, paper with extra-dark lines, etc.
- Typing
- Physical Education
- Deciding whether a problem is due to vision or to some other cause

MATERIALS

In my experience, the aids and materials most often used by partially-sighted students are: large print books, handouts, etc.; recorded books and the machines for them; magnifiers; paper with dark ruled lines; dark pencils and pens; a typewriter; alternative padlocks; a small rack to hold a book in reading position; and needle threaders. As new students arrive and others move up into secondary school, acquaint them with various aids and devices. Padlocks usually become necessary in junior high. Needle threaders promote independence in sewing class. Although teachers will bring up some of the discussion subjects, above, you will need to bring up others – especially the matter of carefully analyzing the real cause of any problems.

A short description enclosed with each cassette machine saves a number of frantic "trouble calls." The chapter on "Other Modes Of Reading" contains considerable material about the use of recordings.

When the Teacher Begins a New Territory

BUILDING A BACKGROUND

When you take over a new territory, try to talk with your predecessor in person as well as reading the required records. He/she may give many helpful insights, including tidbits of information that are not prudently written down. For example, he/she might say, "Billy's whole problem is his parents. They don't even let him take a bath by himself," or, "At South, don't worry if everyone seems chilly. It's not you, it's a carryover from the boundary dispute."

Such comments should be taken with a grain of salt. However, I disagree with those who say, "I don't want to know what the previous teacher thought. I want to form my own conclusions." I *would* like to know what my predecessor thought, but reserve the right to form my own opinion.

It is also helpful to talk with others who serve your same territory – speech therapists, psychologists, etc. Even if they know little about your particular students, they can advise you about agency relationships, authority lines, history, and general policies.

As you look over the records for your new students, give a high priority to (1) quickly getting acquainted with those in the greatest need of attention, and (2) taking advantage of the opportunity to make some changes as you begin.

Most of the ideas for starting with a new student, a new school, or a new year are also applicable when you are the one who is new. Meet the administrators at once and get off to a good start. Meet the parents and students, especially those with urgent needs, as soon as possible. It is well worth voluntarily taking some time during the summer, at least to telephone a few key people.

A GOLDEN OPPORTUNITY

Probably in most respects you will continue the work of the previous teacher. However, for a short time you will have a golden opportunity to make changes relatively easily, with people accepting them as the different approach used by the new teacher. Look for things which the previous teacher had tried to achieve without success – perhaps you, as new blood, can succeed. You may also find that you disagree with certain things and wish to make a major change. (Warning: try to learn the reasons for the previous arrangements before blithely assuming they were wrong. Perhaps the reason why Mai-Lan has no Physical Education is a serious medical problem you do not know about.)

The use of a particular alternative technique–especially the cane or Braille–can often be successfully started by a new teacher. Perhaps the former teacher has laid the groundwork by explaining the value, but did not quite convince the necessary people. Or perhaps he/she did not appreciate the value as well as you do. It is usually best to emphasize the idea of a "different approach" (even if you have a low opinion of the previous teacher's methods), rather than directly criticizing what was done before. It is, of course, always necessary to give good reasons for your recommendations.

Because fresh approaches are helpful, it is unfortunate that geography usually requires a resource/itinerant teacher to have the same students for many years. Trading students can be very beneficial. Visiting one another's students can provide some of the same advantages.

Starting a New Resource or Itinerant Program

Since even with P.L. 94-142 we still do not have all options everywhere, and since populations shift, new programs for the visually impaired are still being established.

Starting a "new program" today is usually much less of a pioneering effort than a few years ago. Probably there will already be one type of local service for blind students, as you branch out into another. Even if this is not the case, other services such as speech therapy can provide a helpful precedent. Probably several people have been aware of the vacuum which you are filling.

Nevertheless, starting an entirely new service offering is a weighty undertaking. Seek a middle ground between naively assuming that everyone will be immediately enthusiastic, *vs.* apologizing for your existence.

FINDING THE STUDENTS

An important but touchy matter is a search for prospective students. On the one hand, a survey is likely to turn up interested parties–for example, a new resource program may be welcomed by some who have found it a struggle to succeed with itinerant service, and by some who would like to leave the residential school. On the other hand, a new teacher who actively recruits students may incur resentment from other programs. Work with your supervisor to develop a suitable plan.

A comprehensive survey should include school nurses; all levels of school administrators; the library for the blind and other transcribers; the state residential school; all nearby special programs; the rehabilitation agency; organizations of blind adults; medical facilities; eye doctors; preschool specialists; etc. See if there is a school census with a question about disabilities. Survey as far ahead as possible.

MATCHING THE TEACHER WITH THE POSITION

If you are an administrator seeking a teacher, contact the colleges and universities which have courses in the education of the visually impaired. Also look for experienced teachers through the National Federation of the Blind (NFB), the Council for Exceptional Children (CEC), the Association for Education and Rehabilitation of the Blind and Visually Impaired (AER), and agencies you use in recruiting other teachers. Employment in this field is rather uneven, with an oversupply of teachers in certain geographical areas and a shortage in others.

If you are a teacher without full certification in this field, ask your state Education Department about a temporary certificate, conditioned upon further study.

Funding may be obtained from Federal sources such as Title VI; the state Education Department; county or multi-county school districts; and local school districts. A Quota allotment in the form of supplies from the American Printing House for the Blind (APH) is available for every legally blind child. (Note: schools usually do not deal directly with APH. Find out who administers the Quota funds in your state.) Service clubs such as the Lions often will donate equipment.

EQUIPMENT

The Basics

Following is a brief list of essentials. Quantities will vary according to student load, but these things should be available even if you know of no Braille students at first. Lack of Braille equipment will discourage introducing Braille to a student who is having trouble with print, and will cause a crisis if a new Braille student appears suddenly.

- Braille paper
- Perkins Braillers
- Slates and styluses
- Typewriters
- Paper with dark ruled lines
- Stencils for teaching the cursive alphabet
- Signature guides
- Long canes of various sizes
- Magnifiers
- Braille instruction books, including reading-readiness materials

The following items are also essential from the very beginning, but should be available from the library for the blind:

- Talking book machines
- Tape machines
- Earphones/headphones

In this computer age, devices for speech output or Braille output are highly desirable, especially for the older student. However, it is also possible for a a "live" reader to read the computer screen. See the chapter on "Computers" for further discussion.

The subject of transcribing textbooks, worksheets, etc., is covered elsewhere in this book.

Additional Helpful Equipment

Depending on the number, age, and characteristics of your students, you will expand your inventory to provide more variety and quantity, and to include the following:

Materials for Young Children:

- Simple wooden puzzles or form boards
- Modeling clay
- Soft bulletin board squares (on which the young child can place Braille worksheets or cards and indicate answers with pushpins)
- Models of animals, vehicles, etc.

Reading and Writing Aids:

- Peg sets to demonstrate Braille to beginners
- Braille alphabet blocks
- Reading stands (to hold an inkprint book in a comfortable position)
- Feltpens and extra-dark pencils
- Magnifiers
- Machines for reading practice (for example, a machine with which the student can read a word or phrase and then run a card through to hear the material spoken aloud)

Aids for Mathematics and Science:

- Braille rulers
- Brailled clock faces
- Tactile geometrical shapes
- Wooden or plastic fractional parts
- Raised-line graph paper
- Bold-line graph paper
- Cranmer Abacuses
- Braille thermometers
- Graphic Aid for Mathematics (available from the American Printing House for the Blind, this provides a rubber grid on which graphs may be built)
- Scientific models

Equipment for Physical Education and Recreation:

- Audible balls
- Audible goal locators
- Appropriate table games
- Sports Field Kit (available from APH, this

provides tactual maps of the playing field for various sports)

Other Aids:

- Loose-leaf notebooks for 11" x 11-1/2" Braille paper
- Transcribing-dictating machines with foot pedals (for typing from recorded copy)
- Plastic stick-on labels which can be Brailled
- Rotomatics (The Rotomatic, which is available from the National Federation of the Blind, is a tactual measuring device for industrial arts)
- Speech output devices for computers
- Braille maps
- Large print maps
- Braille globes

CHAPTER 45

SCHEDULING

When will we squeeze in time for the lessons? That is a continual dilemma never fully solved. Often it is necessary to juggle the schedules of several different people – the regular classroom teacher, the itinerant teacher, the local general resource or remedial teacher, and a reader or aide. Look at all of these *together,* enabling them to complement one another. For example, if an aide assists the child part time, it generally is best for the itinerant teacher to work at another time, so as to provide maximum total individual attention. (This, of course, brings the problem of lack of communication with the aide, so time for some contact should be arranged also.)

Priorities

Set priorities for a given student consciously, and get them into the IEP.

Try to avoid conflicts with regular class time, but recognize that sometimes the need for learning alternative techniques is so urgent that it temporarily takes precedence over some routine classwork. Cane travel might be appropriately substituted for Physical Education for a time. The need to learn Braille might be more urgent than Social Studies class at this moment. In setting priorities, however, remember that the child's morale is important. Although he/she may need to face facts and miss some enjoyable things, it is usually a mistake to let lessons eclipse a valued play period or an exciting assembly program.

PRIORITIES FOR THE SPECIALIZED TEACHER'S TIME

As a matter of policy, the specialized teacher of blind and visually impaired students should spend the majority of his/her time with those who most need his/her services. If a given need can appropriately be met by some other staff member, the specialized teacher's limited time should be saved for working elsewhere.

Following are the areas where the itinerant/resource teacher's skills are most specifically needed and where most of his/her time should be spent:

(1) Teaching Braille reading and writing

(2) Teaching cane travel

(3) Teaching keyboarding (typing) to students who cannot see the keyboard and cannot see the typed material

(4) Teaching the use of the Cranmer Abacus and other specific alternative techniques for use in the classroom

(5) Teaching alternative techniques for daily living skills

As discussed in the chapter on "Qualifications," misplaced priorities decrease a teacher's effectiveness. A prime example is overemphasis on "vision stimulation" in place of effective alternative techniques. (Refer to the chapter, "The Partially-Sighted Child.")

Another common problem occurs when the specialized teacher does work that could readily be done by others. Various educators can instruct the student in the regular curriculum, and provide academic tutoring if needed.

Various staff members can help the student practice techniques initially taught by the itinerant/resource teacher. A Braillist who is not a teacher can prepare materials.

When a partially-sighted student relies successfully on sight, regular teaching methods are appropriate on the whole. The itinerant or resource teacher should provide consultation and guidance, but not extensive direct teaching.

How Do We Find a Time and a Place?

When an aide or reader will be assisting part time, try to make his/her schedule flexible. Ideal situations occur when the aide is a homemaker willing to come at varying times, or when other assignments are general clerical work.

If the blind student's work takes the usual length of time, then the individual help is best provided at the same time as the regular lesson. The resource teacher should take the first grader out for individualized reading at the same time the class is reading; or an aide might join the student in the regular reading class. In the high school current events class, the reader might come in whenever students work on newspaper articles.

Often, however, individual help cannot all be scheduled in this manner. Especially in cases of occasional need, an aide may not be available at the ideal time. Sometimes the blind student may not finish during the regular class session. Specialized lessons such as cane travel have no counterpart in the general curriculum at all.

The experienced older student usually can absorb the responsibility for unfinished lessons, completing them during study hall or at home. When help is to be given at school, possibilities include working during study hall, during a long noon hour, or before or after school. Sometimes an alternative lesson may be substituted for the sighted student's equivalent. While the other fourth graders practice penmanship, the blind student could work on typing or the personal signature.

Often there seems to be no really convenient time. Perhaps you can use part of a long recess or play period, with a student who is not upset by this. If nothing else seems to work, a staggered-time arrangement, in which the student misses different classes on different days, may be possible.

Arrange schedules very carefully, both in terms of what the student misses and in terms of inconvenience to classroom teachers. Be careful also to stick to the time periods planned. If the student returns to class three minutes late, it might appear insignificant, but it may mean repetition of detailed explanations while other students wait.

SEEK OUT ALTERNATIVES

Sometimes you may give lessons at the student's home, your home, or some other location outside the school. This is often done when laws prevent working at a parochial school, but it can be useful for other reasons. With a kindergartner who attends mornings, you may go to the home in the afternoon. Cane travel lessons often are most relevant near home or elsewhere.

Be creative in looking around inside the school. Once when I was told there was no room at the hour I wanted, I walked up the stairs of the large old building and found a dusty, unused space more than big enough. It was beside the stairs, out of the way so that the fire marshal would not object. After a cleaning job, our only annoyance was a brief distraction when the third grade went by on the way to lunch.

In a large high school, there seemed to be no suitable location for Braille during first period. The library was crowded; the lunchroom converted to a gym; various remedial and special lessons took up every space. But the counselor solved the problem. He knew which teachers had a planning period, and arranged for us to use the Spanish room. (Note: Some classroom teachers would have found this an imposition. Having the counselor arrange it was important. And even with the unused space by the stairs, it was important to get permission from the administration.)

Which Days Each Week?

As I start in the fall, I talk to each school where I will be going regularly, and write down *all* the reasonable alternatives for scheduling. Often I note that a certain time would be "best," others "acceptable," and others not possible. When I have such a list for all my regular students, I work out the schedule which is the most practical total picture. Then I get back with each school to indicate when I will be coming. This approach prevents (well, usually prevents) my confirming a time at Westport and then having to change because that is the only time I can possibly go to Southview.

It may or may not be possible to have the luxury of regularly scheduled time in your office. You may need to work on records and phone calls in between lessons wherever and whenever possible. (But watch out for causing resentment through too much use of a school telephone.)

The bane of my existence is the "six-day cycle" favored by many secondary schools. Apparently this is designed to avoid the problem of having, say, Health on Tuesday-Thursday and Science on Monday-Wednesday-Friday, thus shorting Health. An arbitrary cycle of six school days makes the ordinary days of the week irrelevant. This is fine for the Health teacher. However, it is terrible for the itinerant teacher who wants to come every Tuesday and Thursday during study hall: the study hall may be Monday and Wednesday on alternate weeks. When I run into this, I try hard to schedule into a period where the student has the same class every day. Once, however, I had to tell a student that I would come "every Wednesday plus every other Monday."

Speech therapists gave me one good alternation idea. With some students they work intensively for six weeks, and then (while checking that the first student's skills are maintained) work intensively with different students for the next six weeks. By alternating, they can get in more intensive work than would otherwise be possible with their heavy load. This would not be acceptable for a beginning Braille student, of course, but is practical in some other situations.

Monitoring

Most itinerant teachers have many students who need only occasional service – advice, book orders, troubleshooting, etc. It is important to meet with them and their teachers in person at least two or three times a year. A personal visit usually turns up some problems and questions which no one has taken the time to telephone about. Also, if you will be ordering books and giving advice, you should keep abreast of the student's actual abilities yourself, not just second hand. If the student reads print, always have him read some selections aloud. Include the smallest print used, with some passages where context cannot help – math problems with fractions are good. You are responsible for justifying the medium provided. You also share the responsibility for keeping the total program appropriate.

Such occasional contacts usually can be fitted in throughout the year on an irregular schedule. It is helpful to keep a list of the "Monitored" students who should be visited soon, in order to fit one in quickly when a regular lesson is canceled. However, if you have a heavy load, it will sometimes be necessary to cancel a regular lesson in order to accommodate a "Monitored" student. To avoid procrastination, set a goal of seeing (for example) at least two of these students per month.

Flaws and Interruptions

What itinerant teacher has not had the experience of driving a considerable distance only to find that the student (a) has the flu, or (b) went to the museum?

Get a school calendar and keep track of scheduled holidays. Also, arrange for a reliable person to contact you if a lesson must be canceled. For appointments later in the day, this will probably be someone at the school. For the first appointment of the day, ask the student or parent to call you at home (if long distance, arrange to charge such calls to your employer). If the parent cannot or will not call you, perhaps he/she would be willing to call the local principal, who could in turn call you. Ask what radio station broadcasts weather-related cancellations. These arrangements pay for themselves if even one or two unnecessary trips are headed off.

Be conscientious about calling ahead when *you* cannot be there.

The life of an itinerant teacher is especially hard during the season for blizzards or sandstorms or whatever your local hazard happens to be. No one should expect you to travel under really dangerous conditions. Keep track, however, of how much time is lost with each student due to weather problems, your own illness, or other difficulties on your part. If you miss proportionately more for a particular student, arrange makeup time.

Especially if you work in more than one district, you may be summoned to two conflicting meetings. Sometimes this can be avoided by anticipating likely commitments, and by explaining your schedule. You may need to cancel a routine commitment for a vital conference. Sometimes you can send a written report. Another solution is to give your information to someone else from your agency, and have him/her represent you. If you are in the unfortunate position of having two equally vital conferences at the same time, go to the one that notified you first. This is a difficult problem.

Streamlining

Here are some thoughts on minimizing and streamlining the workload, and making a heavy schedule more manageable:

- Examine travel patterns critically. Can you rearrange your schedule to allow more compact routes? Could someone else look it over for new approaches? Would any exchanges with someone else's route be beneficial? Continually re-examine your procedures.

  Mrs. Ratcliffe taught in a resource school, and all transcribed textbooks were shipped to her. When she began to monitor a student elsewhere, she still had his books sent to the resource school first, so she could keep track of them. The list of outside students grew to twelve, and *still* Mrs. Ratcliffe received all the books. Each fall she delivered them in person, with frantic efforts and many delays. Finally her supervisor insisted that the books go directly to the students.
- Look for jobs that can be done by clerical personnel, and negotiate to get that help. Examples include typing up book orders; checking equipment in and out; typing reports; keeping records; etc.
- Minimize paperwork. Can you compose a form letter (for parent conferences, book requests, etc.) and just fill in the blanks? Can you put a notice in the school bulletin instead of writing individual notes to teachers?
- Distinguish between *wishes* and *needs* on the part of parents, students, and classroom teachers. Insist that no one take up large portions of your time just because they *feel* you should be there. Document needs through regular IEP procedures.
- If something is inconvenient it may not get done at all. Why make a trip to the home economics room to get a tracing wheel for diagrams? Why not buy a couple of extra tracing wheels? Emphasize convenience for yourself and others.
- Don't keep saying, "I'll get around to it." Make an appointment. If for two months you have been trying to catch the principal to ask about a conference–make an appointment through his secretary. If you have been meaning to enliven the Braille lessons with a note written to Grandpa, ask the child to remind you next time. He won't forget!
- Make your job description clear. Most itinerant teachers of the blind, for example, are *not* expected to do tutoring in academic skills as such.
- Don't fall into the trap of racing around to try to transcribe *everything* into Braille

or large print. As discussed elsewhere in this book, this policy is both unwise and unrealistic.

- If one particular child always seems to need more help, consider whether he/she should be restaffed for a different program.
- For streamlining of deliveries and messages, arrange for *one* person in each building to coordinate such things. This can be almost anyone (counselor, principal, secretary, librarian, etc.), but the time and confusion saved can be very great.

The Wide Open Spaces

Distances are relative. A city teacher may speak of a "distant school" four miles away, while in Wyoming forty miles might be considered a short distance. Also, traffic and quality of roads are important. Whatever your territory for itinerant work, get good maps, keep your vehicle in good condition, and consider joining an auto club.

Distance is relative in another sense also. I first taught blind children in a resource program; at that time it seemed hard to keep in touch with teachers at the far end of the building, especially if recess breaks did not coincide. Later in a County school district, I found that an appropriate program could be maintained with two or three visits a week. Today, traveling around several counties, I have found ways to handle extremely varying amounts of direct contact.

MANY POSSIBLE MODELS

The farther away you are and the less often you can reasonably go to a particular school, the more complicated it is to keep things going. More planning must be done for adequate help when you are not present, and sometimes problems will mushroom before you arrive.

However, this is only one side of the coin–continuous close contact brings its own problems and disadvantages. Southview School had a full-time resource teacher for the blind, plus a full-time Braille aide. Every book and every worksheet was provided in Braille, and students wrote assignments in Braille. When Don completed sixth grade, his parents transferred him to Westridge Middle School, near his home in another district. Although Don was a good student, the Southview staff insisted he could not possibly succeed without a Braillist at the school every day; this resulted in a frantic search by the middle school principal. The county itinerant teacher said that Don could learn to type his lessons, and that reader service could be provided when a Braillist was not present. But with everyone so accustomed to the special environment at the resource school, much unnecessary turmoil accompanied Don's transfer.

If Don had continued in such a sheltered situation throughout his school years, he would have faced a severe jolt upon graduation into the "real world."

Itinerant teachers must be familiar with many alternatives in placement and scheduling. Educators in special schools must realize that other models do work and do have advantages. Instruction should always work toward greater and greater independence.

Be Creative

For many students who have already learned alternative techniques, and for those using very few alternative techniques, infrequent visits by the specialized teacher are quite adequate. If more help is needed, aide service may be provided part time. Another form of individual help comes from the multi-categorical, or general, resource teacher, who can competently assist a blind student individually if proper support is provided by a specialist in work with the blind. Braille materials can be sent to the school, and sometimes a Braillist can come to the school part time. With these various types of help, properly arranged, even a small and isolated district can provide a suitable program.

Do not assume that the only possible help will be from local school staff. Other possibilities include: PTA volunteers; service organizations, especially those which emphasize helping the blind; volunteer Braillists and other library volunteers; blind adults in the community; the adult rehabilitation agency; field representatives from the residential school; and part-time contract work by a specialized teacher from another district. It is usually unwise for the student's own parent to work directly with him at school, since it is difficult for the parent to be objective, and since any home conflicts will be carried into school. However, the parent might prepare materials, or perhaps two parents could assist each other's children. Further ideas for finding and scheduling help appear elsewhere in this book.

When a beginner should have a lesson every day, and the specialized teacher cannot be there every day, arrangements can be made for someone else to work between times. The specialized teacher should introduce new skills and concepts, but someone else can carry on with more routine lessons or drill. The teacher's guide for the *Patterns* series is especially designed for use by someone who does not know Braille. In any Braille book, penciled helps can be written as needed. An Adaptive Physical Education teacher is a particularly logical person to learn to teach cane travel, but others could do it also, and everyone should reinforce good travel and correct poor habits.

EXTREME DISTANCES

When distances are great and the student is still learning basic alternative techniques, there may be a real dilemma as to which is better: to provide itinerant service on a less-than-ideal schedule, or to send the student away from home. Generally, the fewer problems the student has in addition to blindness the easier it is to arrange a good local program (although it does not follow that all multiply handicapped students should be sent away to school). Two factors which bode well for success are (a) school staff who seem optimistic and creative, and (b) parents who are assertive in insisting on appropriate service. However, these factors and others can be hard to assess and may keep changing. Examine all factors and be creative.

If you, as the specialized itinerant teacher, cannot be there as often as desired, spend more time when you do go there. If distances are extreme, consider spending an entire day – even staying overnight and remaining for more than one day. Spend part of your time observing the staff as they work with the child; then make suggestions. Leave plenty of directions and materials which are practical and easy to use. Provide a copy of this *Handbook*, as well as *Your School Includes a Blind Student* and *A Resource Guide for Parents and Educators of Blind Children*.

Australian children on remote ranches attend a "school of the air," with guidance from parents and only occasional in-person contact with a teacher. Sick children in the U.S. may attend class via speakerphone. Variations of these ideas can be used with blind students. Radio, speakerphone, picturephone, CCTV, etc., can enable a distant teacher to have a two-way "direct" lesson (with an aide present at the other end if the child is young). In combination with some actual personal visits, such an arrangement can permit a young student to remain in the local community when it might have seemed out of the question.

A SUCCESS STORY

In conclusion, consider the following selection from the article, "To Be the Best Person She Can Be," published in *Future Reflections,* December 1982 (see "References").

> Carol and Ed Syslo and their two children – Tara, nine, and Greg, four – live on a farm in central Nebraska. Tara, who is now a fourth grader, has always attended her local public school. That did not occur without a great deal of effort on the Syslos' part. Although they had the law, PL-94-142, to back them, they had to work hard to convince the local school board and officials that they should provide the necessary support services so Tara could stay in her local community. That is no small accomplishment for any parent in any school system that does not already have a vision program; but consider this: Tara attends a two-room school house with a

total of *20* students. Tara is the only fourth grader!

Carol Syslo speaks: She loves to read. She reads for hours at a time, and she's very good at reading. Last year when she was in third grade, they tested her and she had a 6.5 grade level on her reading....

A year ago she was in a track meet of all the rural schools in this area. And we had a little bit of trouble. A couple of the teachers from a different school thought maybe this would create quite a problem, having Tara in the track meet, [that] she would cause other kids to fall and this and that. And our teacher said if Tara wasn't going to be able to go, then the whole school wouldn't come. And the teacher we had before we had transferred school districts, said if Tara couldn't come, her school wouldn't come. So the other teachers said, "Okay, okay!" So the day came, and Tara was absolutely no problem. When she ran in the races, a real good friend of hers (Kathy) ran in front of her and talked the whole while, and Tara just followed the noise. There was nobody touching her or anything, and she won one race and came in second on another. And [in] the sack race, Kathy ran along side of her....

When we work with Tara, even in our school when we have to have our little battles with our school board, it isn't just for Tara. Because what we do... [is] going to affect all the kids. And I think in years to come, it's going to get easier. But the state is just within the last few years really supporting our kids staying at home and going to school.

And I hope we do a good job of it and prove to the state that it's a needed program....

But to me, well, I just can't imagine her not being here....

Related Chapters

The following chapters of this *Handbook* will be especially helpful in relation to scheduling:

"Qualifications for Itinerant and Resource Teachers"
"Early Childhood"
"The Partially-Sighted Child"
"Multiple Handicaps"
"The Law, the IEP, and the Blind Child's Education"
"Placement Options and Decisions"
"General Classroom Arrangements and Study Skills"
"Paraprofessionals and Volunteers"

CHAPTER 46

MOTIVATION

Molly spends half of every period bemoaning how difficult her lessons are. Shawn doesn't moan–he growls and slams books when he thinks the lesson is too hard, which is most of the time. Alice seems cooperative and pleasant, but somehow never seems to finish anything.

Problems like these are familiar to any teacher, including the specialized teacher of the blind.

Attitudes Toward Blindness

The greatest hurdle is building a positive attitude. Address this in the very beginning, and keep working on it–never assume the problem is solved for all time.

THE STUDENT'S ATTITUDES TOWARD BLINDNESS

One of the most important elements in helping a blind student build positive attitudes is often the most neglected–namely, meeting capable adults who are blind. Even if considerable effort is necessary because of geography, and even if student and parent resist the idea at first, do all you can to arrange this contact frequently. Just recently I asked a blind co-worker to talk with a high school student who was objecting to using a cane. My co-worker soon extracted a promise, backed up by a humorous bet with the principal–and the student has used the cane ever since. This contact was for a particular purpose, but ongoing contact is just as important.

See the chapter, "Learning About Blindness," for detailed discussion of the student's attitudes toward blindness.

THE TEACHER'S ATTITUDES

Examine your own attitudes and methods carefully for a "hidden curriculum." This means the attitudes and values which you teach without consciously doing so. If you really believe that Braille is a last resort and very hard to learn, your students will quickly figure that out. If you believe that cane travel is extremely difficult and of limited value, your students will pick that up and act accordingly. If you say such things as, "Ann can read print, but Mary has to read Braille," consider the ramifications to your hidden curriculum. You are saying that inkprint is innately more desirable than Braille, and that Braille is a last resort. Instead simply say, "Ann reads print, and Mary reads Braille."

Demonstrate the value of alternative techniques in ways that matter to the student. Show, for example, that reading Braille can be much faster than struggling with print; that Braille notes for a speech can enable one to look at the audience continuously; that typed papers are well received by teachers and easy to read. Try to incorporate other class assignments into your lessons on techniques, as by using the classroom spelling list for drill on the typewriter or slate.

Analyze your own attitudes carefully and continually. A common problem is avoiding teaching Braille or cane travel because the specialized teacher has little experience with it, has too little time, or views the technique as a last resort. Remember, both the law and common decency require providing what is best for the student, not what is most convenient for you.

Reasonable Expectations

PROVIDE VARIETY AND INTEREST

If a classroom teacher presents dull and repetitive lessons, he/she will soon be made aware of that by squirming, restless students. With a cooperative student in a one-to-one situation, however, it may be hard to judge whether the lessons are sufficiently challenging and interesting. The student may show boredom only by lessened enthusiasm. For maximum success, give continual attention to making lessons interesting and varied. (Sometimes it is helpful to make a written list of ideas.)

Jennifer, in tenth grade, gradually seemed less and less interested in her Braille lessons, although she agreed that they were desirable. The itinerant teacher suddenly realized that every lesson followed the same format: read for fifteen minutes from the Braille instruction book, then write the newest signs on the slate for fifteen minutes. She began varying the format, and asked Jennifer for ideas. Soon lessons included writing notes to a sighted friend who had learned a little Braille; exchanging riddles in Braille; reading short selections from Braille magazines, with a key to unfamiliar signs; and writing vocabulary words from the biology class. Enthusiasm returned immediately.

Timmy, in first grade, wanted to throw away his cane. "Why do I need it?" he complained. "I can find my way around the school. I can walk to the corner at home. And my mother won't let me go any farther!"

The travel teacher looked around the school for things that were especially interesting tactually, and checked on permission to enter any room where a class was not in session. Then, for a typical lesson at school, she would say, "Today I want to see you walk to the end of the north hall and back two times with your cane tapping in front of *each* foot. Remember that if you don't do that (or if you don't use your cane at all) you may trip over a bucket or run into an open locker. When you have walked back and forth twice, we will go into Mrs. Larch's room and look at her snails." The travel teacher also negotiated with Timmy's mother about beginning instruction beyond the end of the block. Timmy gradually ceased complaining.

MAKE LESSONS RELEVANT AND AGE-APPROPRIATE

Especially with an older student, make the lessons as relevant as possible. Try hard to incorporate assignments from other classes, as by practicing spelling words during your typing lessons.

Watch your tone of voice, especially when you work with various age groups – an older student may feel you are "talking down" to her, especially when she is working on a skill such as handwriting which her classmates have learned some time ago. Be matter-of-fact and complimentary, not "gushy."

ANALYZE THE REAL PROBLEM

Motivational problems in your students are deeply intertwined with everyone's attitudes toward blindness, a subject discussed throughout this book. At the same time, blind youngsters *are* youngsters, and are subject to the same foibles as any other group. While examining attitudes with a critical eye, we also must deal with the same problems faced by all teachers.

Especially if lessons are not going well, carefully consider their suitability in all respects. Are they too long for the student's attention span? Are they too hard or too easy?

Are the materials unsuited to the student in some way? Perhaps, for example, the student appears to have a problem with comprehension and attention span – when actually he is using up so much energy trying to see the print that he has no energy left for the content. (Such a problem is solved by using Braille and other alternative modes, not by trying to improve study habits.)

An extreme example of this problem is mistaken overemphasis on "vision stimulation" and/or on inappropriate visual aids. This is discussed in detail in the chapter, "The Partially-Sighted Child."

Just before a holiday, students become restless and achievement drops. The wise teacher anticipates this and tries to make lessons especially varied and interesting. Just before a holiday is *not* the time to press for the very best achievement, or to start something especially difficult.

Watch physical comfort. For various reasons students may not speak up, and instead will let the lesson suffer. The height of the table or desk, for example, is very important for Braille and typing lessons.

Be Calm but Firm

Shawn's teacher found it necessary to be "overprepared" for his lesson, with the most varied format possible and with everything ready to go. The slightest hesitation seemed a signal for more grumbling and slamming of books. Briskly proceeding through tightly-planned lessons was more helpful than anything else for Shawn.

Shawn's teacher needed to do more than is usually necessary, but a degree of her brisk and organized approach is a vital part of all good discipline. A vague approach, with frequent pauses to search for materials or decide what to do next, is an invitation to restlessness. Make your directions and remarks brief and to the point.

It is unfortunate that many specialized teachers have little or no experience with a full-sized class. Make the best use of such experience if you have it, and seek to get some if you have none. When you are familiar with methods for keeping a larger group organized and working, you will find it much easier to keep a small group or individual on the track. Never assume that a small group or a single individual could not present a discipline problem. In a resource room where you often work with one student while others are doing seatwork, keep checking on the others in some meaningful way, such as glancing at them frequently.

None of this, of course, needs to imply that you must be overly strict when it is not needed.

AVOIDING EXTRA CHATTER

In a group, if one student talks too much or in an irrelevant way, the teacher finds ways to curb this. In an individualized situation, extra chatter may be harder to recognize and harder to combat. Remarks may appear relevant, and there is no group to be considered. Moreover, the instructor may fall into the trap of following "social etiquette" rather than retaining the instructor's prerogatives. For example, the teacher may reply to everything the student says, instead of deciding how much and what kind of conversation there should be. Below are two versions of an illustrative exchange.

Version A

Teacher: All right, Matt, are you ready to go over your math homework?

Matt: Aw, I'm tired.

Teacher: Now, Matt, we've talked about this – we need to keep working even when we're tired.

Matt: [*Sigh*]

Teacher: What do you have for Problem 1?

Matt: Hmm, where did I put that?

Teacher: Matt, you *must* have things ready!

Matt: [*Hunting through papers in notebook*] Ah – er – 349.

Teacher: Right! What's Problem 2?

Matt: [*Sigh*] I'm so tired.

Teacher: You *must* get to bed earlier........

....

....

Version B

Teacher: [*Briskly*] Good morning, Matt! What do you have for Problem 1 in math?

Matt: Aw, I'm tired!

Teacher: [*Pleasantly but still briskly*] Problem 1, please.

Matt: [*Hunting through papers in notebook*] Hmm, where did I put that?

Teacher: [*Says nothing*]

Matt: Ah – er – 349.

Teacher: Great! A correct answer to a difficult first problem! You're off to a good start. What's Problem 2?

Matt: 406?

Teacher: Right again! Go on, please.

....

....

In the first version, the teacher nags Matt (obviously having done so before), and in the process takes up time. By responding to each complaint, she encourages him to complain more. Also note that her very first words invited the possibility of a negative response.

In the second version, the teacher proceeds very briskly, having consciously chosen this approach to help Matt keep on-task. She realizes she need not respond verbally *at all* to unnecessary remarks. She responds quite a bit, however, to the first correct answer – thus further encouraging appropriate, on-task behavior.

Imagine how each version continues, today and tomorrow and the day after....

Many students chat pleasantly, rather than complaining. Others ask questions – often good questions, related to the material at hand. But always the teacher should retain control of how much conversation there should be. Pleasant chatting can be restricted to times in between tasks. Good questions may need to be answered at another time, so that today's assignment can be completed today.

THE ENVIRONMENT

A major thorn-in-the-flesh for itinerant teachers is the need to scrounge places for lessons. Exchanging tales of out-of-the-way locations and various distractions is a wryly amusing activity for most itinerant teachers and some resource teachers. Up to a point this is a problem that must be lived with, and we try to be flexible. But sometimes the location and working conditions make the difference between success and failure. Creativity and negotiation are essential. I once found myself trying to instruct a particularly resentful and distractible teenager in one corner of a crowded resource room where his classmates (with a variety of disabilities) continually argued with one another and their resource teacher. I arranged to change my lessons to the counselors' conference room, even though this involved complicated scheduling and transporting of materials. It was well worth it.

Constructive Ideas

One of my Education professors often said, "Now, remember, don't nag!" By this she meant, "Don't just keep *telling* the child to behave; *do* something!" Below are several concrete ideas on how to take constructive action, rather than simply nagging a student to do better:

- Talk with the student and confront the problem directly, asking for suggestions in solving it. This can be very effective with older students.
- See the chapter on "Your Professional Role" for thoughts on building a businesslike atmosphere.
- Have the student reread or rewrite the unsatisfactory material.
- If the student continually interrupts with informal conversation, set a rule as to when such conversation may occur (as, only at the end of a page or the end of a lesson). Alternatively, have the student raise his hand, just as in a large class.
- Vary your own voice volume, which you may have gradually been raising unconsciously. Lowering it suddenly may increase attention.
- Use a stopwatch to time certain activities, such as words per minute on the slate. Keep a chart of progress, possibly with a small reward for a certain speed.
- Avoid making threats which you really would not carry out.

- Be sure your expectations are realistic for the age of the student.
- Give plenty of encouragement, and try to vary the exact words you use for praise. Also, according to noted author and psychologist Haim Ginott (see "References"), it is wise to praise *specifics* rather than giving a blanket compliment. Ginott feels that a comment such as "You finished the worksheet in just five minutes - that's great!" is better received than, "You are a very good worker!" With the latter, the young person may think about times when he was not a "good worker," and reject the compliment altogether.
- In case of serious problems, contact the parents. Do the same for substantial improvement.
- When working with more than one student at a time, make judicious use of the room arrangement. Moving someone away from another student and/or closer to you can make a big difference. Also, you can unobtrusively improve behavior by casually walking over near a student who is restless.
- Write a summary of your lessons on the regular report card - and make sure your student knows that you will. One sixth grade teacher used a letter grade from my individualized typing instruction in lieu of the regular handwriting grade (with explanation, of course).
- For serious problems, the principal's disciplinary assistance is available to you. But use this only sparingly and in careful consultation with the principal.
- Especially with a group, develop a hierarchy of consequences for breaking rules. Example: verbal reminder; change of seating arrangement; discussion after class; partial loss of recess time; note to parents; conference with principal.
- Even when expectations are age-appropriate, a given child may really be unable to meet them at first. Suppose, for example, a ten-year-old is exceptionally restless, both in your lessons and in the fourth grade. Expecting him to stay seated for an entire 40-minute Braille lesson is unrealistic. Begin instead with a lower standard (say, requiring him to remain seated for ten minutes at a time, and then providing a short break of some kind). Also provide plenty of variety within the lesson. Gradually work toward more age-appropriate behavior.
- With a young child, this idea may occasionally be helpful: have the child rest his head on his arms on the desk for a minute or two, with both student and teacher completely silent. This is a calming strategy sometimes used by teachers of younger children.
- The itinerant teacher who cannot easily keep a student after class faces a special problem. Make maximum use of methods which work during your lesson time. If staying after school really seems the most effective consequence for a behavior problem, you may be able to use it by saying, "I will mark one minute wasted each time you talk out of turn. If at the end of four lessons we have no more than fifteen minutes recorded, we will erase them. But if I mark down more than fifteen minutes in four lessons, then we will make up the time. I will arrange to come back after school." (Note: Strenuously avoid asking another teacher to discipline a student for you. The other teacher will probably resent dealing with a problem which he/she will regard as yours.)
- Counselors and psychologists can suggest many excellent ideas for keeping charts of work accomplished, with various kinds of motivational rewards.

"She Just Sits There"

What about the student who seems to accomplish nothing? She may appear to be working, but get very little done, like Alice. She may spend a great deal of time complaining or worrying.

Be sure to rule out medical causes–possibly the student really does not feel well. If there is a medical problem, try to find out exactly what the limitations really are, and not permit the student to "take advantage" by seeming even more limited.

Be creative in motivating a student who seems passively uninterested. Focus on what she *is* interested in. Would she enjoy a story about space travel? Can you use a game as a reward for accomplishment? Also focus on what she can do well, and if necessary reduce your standards for a time so that she can experience success.

Cross-age tutoring sometimes is helpful to unmotivated students. They may enjoy the attention if an older student helps them. They may like the prestige of helping a younger student, and at the same time reinforce their own skills.

The itinerant teacher felt that Alice was using passive resistance by appearing to work while actually doing almost nothing. The teacher began to keep a chart of pages finished. A simple reward system, involving an occasional game of checkers, helped a good deal.

How Much Time to Spend on Discussion

With a few students, the matter of counseling poses a problem of extremes: the student seems to need a great deal of advice and reassurance, to the extent that nothing else gets done. Every period could easily be taken up with discussing the student's problems, attitudes, and worries. The teacher must decide how much discussion time is reasonable, and take active steps to restrict it, probably by setting actual time limits. You might say, "For five minutes at the beginning of each period we will talk over any things that are bothering you that day, and then we will need to get on with the lesson. Each Friday we will talk about how the week has gone." Recognize that a student may deliberately talk on and on in order to avoid actual work.

Even when the student is not overly talkative, discussion time should be budgeted. Exact timing is an individual matter. Talking at the beginning of the lesson can set the tone and provide needed reminders. Part way through the lesson, it can be a helpful break. Postponing discussion to the last few minutes prevents endless chatter.

Often the problems being discussed will lessen or disappear as skills are learned. Pointing this out to the student is an important part of the teacher's guidance.

Another area where extremes are a dilemma is "how much special attention." Especially with a very self-conscious student, we don't want to call attention to his disability without good reason. On the other hand, it is undesirable to try to hide the disability; and if individual attention is needed, it should be provided. Use common sense and examine the importance of the matter at hand. Consider a high school student who usually uses regular print easily, but occasionally prefers large print, and who says, "I'd like to use those books just at home, and I'd like to talk about them only in the counselor's office." You would probably agree to these requests and hope to help the student gradually feel less self-conscious. Consider, in contrast, a sixth grader who is rapidly losing sight, has difficulty with all print, and makes the same requests. That situation merits careful planning *immediately* to help the student move *quickly* into working on alternative techniques and discussing blindness openly.

Occasionally a student may complain, "I can't," or "I'm so dumb," over and over despite every effort to reassure him. A last resort is to ignore these remarks, in order to get on with the lessons and to remove the possibility that the remarks are mainly for attention-getting. You might say, "Bill, we have talked many times about how you are *not* dumb, and about how most of your work is OK. But we are getting behind because of talking about this so much. Now, I am going to start ignoring you if you say 'I'm dumb,' and I want you to understand what that will mean. It will *not* mean that I agree you are dumb or lazy. It just means that we don't have time to talk about that right now, and you must get on with your work. Also, it means I've decided that Mrs. Johannes is the best one to talk with you about your feelings, not me."

Helping Others to Motivate a Student

It is even more difficult to help when you are not the one teaching the lesson. Often you will learn of problems in the regular classroom or problems while the student works with an aide, when you are not on the scene.

Frequent informal conferences, even if very brief, are important for this reason and others. Discuss what is reasonable to expect of the student, and offer concrete suggestions. (In talking with another professional, it is usually better to say, "I'd suggest..." or "Have you tried..." rather than "You ought to...") Frequent contact also makes it possible to be consistent and minimize possible attempts to play one adult against another. It is reasonable for you to expect the classroom teacher to follow through with skills you have taught, such as by having the student use the slate for note-taking. It is just as reasonable for the classroom teacher to expect you to be consistent with regular school rules such as no gum-chewing.

Helping an aide to motivate a student is sometimes easier because you can be more direct without offending. On the other hand, it may be harder because of the aide's lack of background in educational methods. Again, continual consultation is essential. Try to "back up" the aide in such a way that the student gains respect for both of you. Other suggestions are contained under the general subject of "Paraprofessionals and Volunteers."

Consider who is in the best position to talk with a teacher or aide who seems to be having difficulty. Enlist the help of someone else if appropriate – the counselor, the local resource or remedial teacher, etc. (Note, however, that asking the principal to talk to someone often implies that the problem is quite serious. Use this help with extra care.) In working with a paraprofessional, consider the lines of authority over him/her.

Contact parents about any substantial problems. Don't leave yourself open to the accusation, "You never told me about that!" Do all you can to keep your efforts and the parents' efforts on the same track.

Following Through

It is one thing for a student to perform well while you are watching, and quite another for him to do so at other times. This problem is discussed throughout this book. Following is a summary of ideas on follow-through:

(1) Demonstrate the value in ways that matter to the student.

(2) Ask a competent adult or older student to discuss his/her own use of the aid or method. A blind businessman could explain how he uses a cane for mobility and independence.

(3) Anyone whom the youngster particularly admires might mention the value. For example, the coach might say, "I hear you're learning to type! You'll be a whiz with computers."

(4) Encourage classmates' interest and acceptance. They might enjoy trying out the technique themselves. (Caution: Avoid taking the cane away from the blind student. Provide extra canes for practice. Also, be sure proper instruction is provided, to prevent floundering around.)

(5) In certain situations, other students should be told *not* to help the youngster who gets into difficulty due to non-use of a particular technique.

(6) Compromise at first, if necessary, by allowing the student to use the aid or method

only part of the time. Then increase use to full time.

(7) Watch for influences which might work at cross-purposes to your plans. For example, do parents or friends discourage use of the aid?

(8) Be sure that the aid or method is suitable, both generally and specifically. Is the child really mature enough to carry on without constant supervision? Have aids or materials been carefully chosen according to size, etc.? If a visual aid is used, is it really appropriate and helpful, or would a technique which does not require sight be more efficient?

(9) Calmly but firmly insist that he/she use the aid.

(10) Sometimes a student persists in misplacing a necessary aid, either carelessly or in an effort to avoid its use. Especially with a younger student, keep an extra one available.

(11) Emphasize "natural consequences." For example, if a first grader forgets his cane, he might not be permitted to walk to the bathroom alone. If an older student resists the cane, look for situations where he/she must walk slowly or depend on others. If poor techniques cause a student to be late, do not excuse him.

CHAPTER 47

WORKING IN PARTNERSHIP WITH PARENTS

The Rusts' first baby was blind from Retinopathy of Prematurity. Mrs. Rust was a devoted mother, and seemed to accept blindness calmly. When the home teacher for handicapped children suggested visiting the home of a blind three-year-old, she agreed but was not enthusiastic.

For several minutes Mrs. Rust stared at the active little girl in total silence. Then there were a flood of questions: Does she feed herself? Is she potty trained? When did she start to talk? How did you teach her to walk? Does she know everybody's voice?....... The home teacher suddenly realized that never before had Mrs. Rust asked any questions relating to her own baby's future. It became apparent that she had visualized her infant as growing into a helpless lump, for whom the normal stages of development would be irrelevant.

Such misconceptions are not restricted to first-time parents. The greatest problem for parents of blind children is the same as for the general public – attitudes toward blindness.

Practical and Positive Guidance

The magazine *Future Reflections,* published by the National Federation of the Blind, is a dramatically successful tool to help parents. (See "References.") All parents should be introduced to this magazine, offered back issues, and encouraged to subscribe. Should a particular parent not wish his/her name placed on a subscription list, you can lend your own copies to that family.

Future Reflections does an excellent job of giving really *practical* suggestions while at the same time developing the all-important positive attitudes. Too often we teachers overemphasize one aspect while neglecting the other: either we teach techniques and fail to see the total perspective, or else we preach good attitudes while failing to demonstrate how to put them into practice. Give detailed suggestions. If you say that a preschooler should have more experiences, provide a list of specific activities and keep adding to it. If you want a first grader to practice Braille reading at home, provide books that he can read, and inkprint copies for the parents. *Just Enough to Know Better: A Braille Primer* (see "References") teaches the basic Braille code to parents in an easy-to-read, enjoyable format.

The chapter, "Learning About Blindness, At School and At Home" (in this *Handbook*), describes other examples of good literature about blindness. It also gives examples of bad literature and how to deal with it.

It is important to demonstrate activities and techniques as well as to describe them. Ask the parent to visit class and see how well the child can read (and also to see how he holds the book and moves his hands, and how to prompt him when he has difficulty). Go to the home and help teach the child to make a sandwich.

A field trip to another school, to an agency for the blind, or to the workplace of a blind person can have many benefits besides the obvious ones. Recently I went to an agency for the blind with a third grader, her parents, and her classroom teacher. The main purpose was for all to see the services offered by the agency, and this was accomplished. However, this was also the first good chance for me to show the parents how the youngster could use her cane in an unfamiliar environment. Also, after the tour leader had shown the child several interesting objects, we observed her father guiding the child's hand to look at things–something we had never seen either parent do before. Their usual way of "showing" the child was simply to ask, "Do you see that?" And, having some sight, the child would usually answer "yes" but have little real grasp of what the object was like.

Discuss various aspects of daily living in enough detail to see where help is needed. Don't just ask, for example, "Does Billy dress himself?" Also inquire how he goes about it and what help he receives. You may find that he can dress himself only if the clothes are carefully laid out in a particular way, and he receives much coaching.

Blind People Are Regular, Normal People

Contact with real people who are blind is essential. Be creative in finding ways to make this happen. If geography is the problem, encourage telephone and written contacts; try to arrange at least one "field trip" a year; occasionally bring a blind student or adult with you when you travel to the school; look for special opportunities in the summer or during other vacations. If there are blind people nearby but the family never seems to meet them, try an informal get-together at someone's home or office; a discussion on a particular subject of interest; a seminar on blindness in general; etc.

Don't Give Parents the Wrong Idea

Mr. Savage was upset and discouraged. The itinerant teacher for young handicapped children had said that his daughter would reach developmental milestones more slowly than most children, because she was blind.

Mrs. Woods was upset and angry. As a blind parent, she knew that blind children and adults could learn normally, given the proper opportunities. She expected her blind daughter to learn normally at the regular pace. Yet both the itinerant teacher and the kindergarten teacher continually exclaimed, "She's so exceptional! Most blind children can't begin to keep up the way she does!" Mrs. Woods feared that this attitude would soon rub off on the child, causing her to achieve less.

Blind people as a group (including blind children and blind infants) are *not* categorically slower in development or achievement. Some statistics seem to show that they are slower; however, upon closer examination it is seen that the real causes are not blindness itself. The causes lie in lack of information, inappropriate techniques, negative attitudes, and lack of opportunity.

Blind children need to learn by using their other senses, which may mean that more time teaching certain things is required. However, this does not lead to the conclusion that blind children are slower in general. It may mean that the typical *sequence* of learning seems uneven–but this is a different thing altogether. For example, if a blind child has difficulty learning to use a spoon well, it may indeed be partly because she cannot see whether there is any food on it. But at the same time, she may (if given the opportunity) learn to use a fork at an age *earlier* than usual, because she appreciates the way that food can be firmly speared. And if she is taught to feel the food on the spoon (as a beginning method, to be phased out later), she can learn to use a spoon well also. This is one good example of where a wrong conclusion should not be drawn if she takes longer to learn something.

Another example is writing with a pencil or crayon. These skills figure prominently in evaluations of school readiness. A partially-sighted child may score low on tests because of difficulty seeing the materials, although actually she may be entirely ready for schoolwork if given proper alternatives. A totally blind child may score low because the "equivalent tests" given to her were not truly equivalent.

When proper training and opportunity are provided, blind people as a group do as well as any other group.

It is true, of course, that any individual blind person (as any individual sighted person) may have low ability. This, however, is strictly an individual matter and should not produce generalizations about blind people.

If you, as a teacher, lead parents to believe that children are slower *just because they are blind*, you do a grave disservice with far-reaching consequences. The result is lowered expectations, a self-fulfilling prophesy.

Putting Worry into Perspective

Sometimes it seems that feelings of guilt–perhaps the feeling that they are responsible for the blindness itself, or perhaps regret at the way things were handled in the past–cause a parent either to overprotect a child or to push him toward unreasonable perfection. Some schools of thought even allege that it is normal for a parent to feel rejection for a blind child, since blindness (supposedly) is such an overwhelming tragedy. I believe we should see guilt problems in perspective: *all* parents sometimes wish that circumstances had been different, sometimes blame themselves for things they could not have prevented, and sometimes feel negative toward their children. We should neither magnify this problem by dwelling upon it, nor naively assume it never exists. Be reassuring and remind everyone that we cannot control all circumstances. Help parents to obtain accurate information on medical matters and on child development. Continually work on general attitudes so that blindness is simply not viewed as an overwhelming tragedy.

Families with disabled children are not categorically different from other families. Dealing with blindness (or any other disability) is a stress; but all families face stress. When parents describe problems and worries, a teacher should not appear uncaring and hard-hearted. Show an understanding of the other person's feelings by saying such things as, "It's hard to know what to do," "You felt that he just couldn't learn," "That must have been embarrassing," etc. At the same time, help everyone avoid letting regret or sorrow lead to continual overprotection.

One experienced teacher who is herself blind says, "I generally tell parents that their feeling of guilt is probably an intense wish for everything to be better for their children than it was for them. Growing up as a blind child is sometimes painful, but growing up as a fat child can be just as painful. Then I say, 'But you can't do anything about having had a blind child. What you can do something about, is the kind of life your child will have.' And I go on to talk about the fact that blind people can lead normal lives with careers and families, etc. Parents need to admit and cope with their feelings of guilt, and get on with the business of raising their child."

A True Partnership

"But we *only* want what's *best* for your child!!" –This line brought down the house at a dramatization of an all-too-typical parent conference. A group of educators (played by amateur actors) pompously persuaded a parent that his child was not ready for a regular school, and instead needed a special school. They squashed the parent's feeble protests that his child was normal mentally and achieving well. As the informal "curtain" fell, the final line repeated: "But we *only* want what's *best* for your child!"

One parent in the audience quipped, "The next time they say that to me, I think I'll say, 'Are you implying that *I* do *not* want what's best for my child??'"

We educators may indeed get carried away with our own knowledge and prestige, and forget that parents are our equal partners. Recognize that parents may be right and you may be wrong–or, perhaps, a compromise or third solution may be best. Educators are not the "experts" on everything. Parents are the experts on their family's values, priorities, resources, and needs. Parents *can* teach skills. They *are* experts on their child's needs, although educators may (correctly) see some different needs from a different perspective.

One parent commented that a "staffing" conference was really a "stacking." The educators decided (together, beforehand) what plans they wanted to make, arrived with a "stacked deck," and treated the parent as an irrelevant afterthought. Although contrary to the intent of P.L. 94-142, this scenario is all too typical.

Build a relationship with parents, outside of formal IEP staffings. Often you will be able to come to informal agreement about such things as reading media and the general goals of your services. Then, in the formal meeting, you and the parents will be thinking along similar lines, and the specifics of the IEP can be worked out smoothly.

APPROPRIATE MEETINGS

Keep meetings as small and informal as possible. Frequently *ask* parents, "What do you think?" and "What goals or plans do you suggest?" rather than expecting them to break in on your monologue. *Listen* to their ideas, instead of concentrating on your planned report. Ask parents to describe what approaches they have tried, and what they might suggest for you. Arrange each conference at a time and place as convenient for the parent as possible. (Consider meeting at the home or at the parent's workplace, if that is desired.) Explain beforehand what the conference will cover and how it will proceed; provide written evaluations in advance. If, at the conference, parents find they need more time to study or think, recess the conference until a later date.

Even when serious, widespread problems must be faced, include some positive remarks and compliments.

Include older students in conferences. This involves the student in decision-making and sets a valuable precedent for adulthood. It also minimizes difficulties in putting plans into practice with the student.

FOLLOWING THROUGH

A common problem occurs when parents agree to carry out a plan at home, but never seem to follow through. Perhaps it has been agreed that the youngster should help with cooking and dishwashing, but it becomes clear that this is not happening. Avoid critical confrontation, but talk with the parent about what is going wrong. Was the plan too ambitious or too vague? Is more information needed (e.g., specific techniques for using the stove)? Often it is helpful for the student to practice while the parent watches, with the teacher assisting the student. One girl, who always planned to practice cooking at home but somehow never did, was delighted to be invited to dinner at the home of a blind lawyer. After several enjoyable sessions helping her new friend prepare dinner and clean up, the young girl (along with her mother) finally felt comfortable in sharing this work at home.

Avoid overdoing educational jargon, but do not "talk down" to the parent by using unduly simple words. Think about social backgrounds and local customs. Is it customary to use first names? How careful must you be about personal questions? Is there racial tension? Is there a sizable age difference between yourself and the parent? Would an attempt at humor be taken wrong? Are you being too formal or too informal? Consider each parent's background.

IF PARENTS SEEM BADLY MISGUIDED

During my first year with blind children, I was horrified when a parent said she planned (on her own) to patch the eye of her younger child. She said, "My older boy had the same thing, and that was what the doctor said to do for him." I felt like shouting, "No! No! You're practicing medicine without a license!" I realized I shouldn't quite say that, but was speechless trying to think of something better to say. Fortunately an older, experienced teacher was also present and responded with great tact. She said calmly, "I would *really not want* to patch an eye unless the doctor had directed it for that particular child at that particular time. It may be fine–I know they do both have the same eye condition. But, you know, Dr. Brown is so good–I'm sure you'll want to ask him about it right away. Sometimes there are differences that only the doctor can see." The parent agreed, and said she would make an appointment. I made a mental note to remember these words and others like them, to develop a stock of tactful comments for difficult situations:

"You'll want to consider ..."
"We suggest this approach ..."
"It seems that way, doesn't it? But most blind people have found ..."
"That is a very complicated subject. I'd like to talk with you about it when we aren't in such a rush. Could we plan a short conference tomorrow?"
"That's a good way to begin. And soon let's start ..." (Note: This is a useful phrase when the parent is helping the child too much.)
"I would really hesitate before I ..."

THE BLIND PARENT'S POINT OF VIEW

If a parent is blind and you are sighted, the parent will have a wealth of first-hand experience about blindness which you lack. Ask for suggestions. Blind children who have blind parents tend to be more independent than those with sighted parents. Should you feel disagreement with a blind parent's suggestions, consider them extra-carefully because of the parent's valuable personal experiences.

It is, of course, possible that a particular blind parent has not developed positive techniques and attitudes in regard to his/her own blindness. If the parent was blind in childhood, he or she may have grown up without many of the present-day methods and tools. Also, he/she may have attended a special school rather than being in the "mainstream." Try to separate the parent's personal methods from present educational issues–rather the way you might approach someone who says, "This crazy new math–I never did arithmetic that way!"

Suppose, for example, a blind parent says emphatically that he never used a cane and sees no reason for his child to use one. You can say (directly or indirectly), "I realize that you have developed other methods for your own personal use. But we do strongly recommend cane travel for your child at this time, because...."

Blind parents will have a great deal to teach *you*. Most blind parents complain of the problem opposite to the one above: they see that a child is ready to use a cane or read Braille, and it is the educators who hang back. Even if you disagree at times, be especially receptive to the ideas of blind parents. Blind children whose parents are also blind tend to be more independent, capable, and confident.

We each have our own ideas about "what is best for the child."

Finding Time to Communicate

Frequent face-to-face contact is the best way to build understanding. Try to attend all regular classroom conferences as well as all IEP meetings and staffings, and arrange as much additional contact as seems desirable. Often an informal conference before or after a formal one is important to full understanding. Accommodate to the parents' work schedules as much as possible.

One eighth grader became very agreeable to working on Braille after the teacher had a frank discussion with the parents about the benefits. For several months the student had resisted learning Braille; but after this discussion the teacher had no more difficulty.

When you acquire a new student, meet the parents as soon as possible–preferably before a major problem or decision must be faced. Avoid a pattern of meeting parents only when there are serious difficulties.

Short conversations between conferences often prevent problems. Call or send a note to keep the parent informed of your progress, problems, and new approaches. If your personal circumstances permit, allow parents to call you at home. Often both parents are employed, finding it difficult to telephone during the day.

Furthermore, most itinerant teachers are notoriously hard to find during the day.

RESPECT THROUGH COMMUNICATION

Recognize that parents have heavy responsibilities. Few mothers are full-time homemakers. Financial problems may weigh heavily. Non-blind siblings, elderly relatives, and others may have special needs and problems.

Never accept unthinkingly what a student says about his parents. He may be misinterpreting, either innocently or knowingly. One kindergartner convinced the lunchroom staff that he could not use a fork, despite having used one at home since he was three. Then, when the teachers taught him to zip his coat, he continued to be "unable" to zip it at home for several weeks. When his mother realized what was going on, she set up a regular system of messages about skills.

STARTING EARLY

Meet the parents of infants as soon as possible, and keep in contact. If a particular age group is not your responsibility, arrange at least occasional contact if at all possible. Accompany the preschool home teacher once in awhile and talk about the future. Attend program reviews for children who may soon transfer to your area. Work for cooperation between specialized schools and less restrictive settings, keeping parents well informed of their options.

WORKING THROUGH A PROBLEM

Mrs. TenHagen did not agree that her son should learn Braille. "He can see large print," she protested. "And they all read slowly in second grade anyway." The itinerant teacher urged Mrs. TenHagen to observe the second-grade class for a full morning. Al moved his entire body when looking from the top of the page to the bottom; he could not read his own handwriting; he finished every reading assignment several minutes late; and he never did finish his math. "I see what you mean," his mother finally said.

The school staff continued to confer frequently and thoroughly with Mrs. TenHagen. At first she only approved the use of Braille for a small part of the time. But gradually, through continued discussion and observation, she came to agree to the use of Braille as the main mode of reading, with large print as a supplementary method. Since a significant change was never made without at least a phone call, this matter was resolved with maximum mutual understanding.

KEEP IN TOUCH

A final caution: Don't assume that understanding and agreement, once built, will continue over time and into new situations. Keep showing the parent how eating skills, for example, can be refined and expanded as the child grows older. Keep checking tactfully on various self-help skills. Discuss how to apply skills to new situations such as gym locker rooms. Keep showing that you are well-informed, flexible, and genuinely interested.

A Parents' Group

Even if only one or two parents are interested, you can help to start a Support Group affiliated with the Parents Division of the National Federation of the Blind. Following are a few excerpts from a brochure describing this very effective organization:

> The NFB Parents of Blind Children Division (POBC) is working to achieve these goals:
>
> - To create a climate of opportunity for blind children in home and society.
> - To provide information and support to parents of blind children.
> - To facilitate the sharing of experience and concerns among parents of blind children.
> - To develop and expand resources available to parents and their children.
> - To help parents of blind children gain understanding and perspective through partnership and contact with blind adults.
> - To function as an integral part of the National Federation of the Blind in its

on-going effort to eliminate discrimination and prejudice against the blind, and to achieve for the blind security, equality, and opportunity.

In order to accomplish these goals, Parents of Blind Children has initiated many exciting programs and activities. Among them are:

- Seminars and workshops for parents and educators of blind children.
- An annual Braille Reading Contest for Blind Children.
- The "Slate-Mates" pen-pal program.
- Distribution of free literature about blindness.
- Circulation of videotapes about the education of blind children.
- A network which deals with the needs of blind children and blind parents in the adoptive process.
- Consultation about legislation.
- Assistance to parents and blind children whose rights have been denied.

DOs AND DON'Ts FOR PROGRAMS AND SEMINARS

- DO emphasize the positive, demonstrating that blind children can achieve as well as others.
- DO involve competent blind adults as role models and as speakers on the program.
- DO involve parents in planning.
- DO bring out the value of alternative methods such as Braille and cane travel.
- DO, when time permits, consciously plan to cover all major topics (reading, mobility, daily living skills, careers, etc.) and various age groups.
- DO anticipate the likelihood of wrong impressions and misunderstandings, and counteract them. (Example: If a program emphasizes certain job opportunities – such as those which do not require college – discuss other job categories also, and make it clear that they are open to the blind. As another example, if there is a program about children with academic difficulties, make it clear that many blind children are strong students.)

- DON'T use educational jargon without definitions.
- DON'T "talk down to" parents, using unnecessarily simple wording and making dogmatic statements.
- DON'T discuss the special needs of one group (e.g., mentally retarded blind children) at such length that other groups are slighted, or in such a way as to leave the impression that all blind children have such needs.
- DON'T portray alternative techniques as a last resort.

Related Chapters

The chapter on "Learning About Blindness" discusses relationships with parents of sighted classmates.

The following chapters discuss P.L. 94-142 and the IEP as such:

"The Law, the IEP, and the Blind Child's Education"
"Placement Options and Decisions"
"Paperwork, Ouch"

CHAPTER 48

YOUR PROFESSIONAL ROLE

"Hilary will be an asset to your class," said Ms. Fontana brightly. "The other children will have the advantage of knowing someone with a disability. And the new methods I'll show you will be good for everyone. I know you'll find it a very interesting challenge."

Ms. Fontana's enthusiasm was met with stony silence. Finally Mr. Conley replied, with icy self-control, "What kind of new methods? I have all I can do already! Why on earth isn't she in the School for the Blind?!"

Poor Ms. Fontana. This was the fourth school she had visited, in her new position after graduating from a highly-regarded university. She had been taught to demonstrate a "positive attitude," and she radiated enthusiasm. At the first three schools the staff seemed comfortable and accepting. What went wrong at the fourth?

Ms. Fontana's Mistakes

She was just lucky with the first three. Any teacher of blind students must realize that Mr. Conley's attitude is still not uncommon, and that Ms. Fontana's choice of initial remarks was poor. She made several errors:

She assumed that everyone shared her enthusiasm for integrating blind children into regular classrooms.

Although more and more people do feel this way, many still do not, and must be carefully guided toward acceptance.

Ms. Fontana assumed that the classroom teacher would regard her as an expert.

Actually, classroom teachers commonly maintain the opposite assumption: the various highly-touted consultants and "experts" have no idea what things are really like in the classroom. They come in with their marvelous-sounding ideas and lots of fanfare, and then they leave you to face a *real* class, where none of their fancy ideas work. The fact that Ms. Fontana was young, female, and just out of college added a few extra stereotypes.

She thought that the advantages of having a blind student would be easily seen.

She was right that there are advantages, and in time they are usually recognized. But the busy teacher with a large class may at first see nothing but an added burden. Gushing about advantages only makes things worse.

It might have been helpful to emphasize characteristics apart from blindness that are generally regarded as assets – pleasant personality, intelligence, accurate typing, etc.

She should have played down, rather than emphasizing, the idea of new or different methods.

Basic teaching methods and materials remain the same.

Ms. Fontana was naive in regard to understanding and dealing with Mr. Conley's attitudes toward blindness in general. Dr. Kenneth Jernigan states:

> From the beginnings of recorded history the blind have been the victims of unreasonable and detrimental classification. Today these discriminations are being recognized for what they are, and the blind and their friends are insisting with growing success upon justice and equal treatment. No matter how moderately it may be done this resistance to

discrimination will inevitably bring a certain amount of hostility.

–From *Blindness: Discrimination, Hostility, and Progress.*

As blind people come to expect equal opportunity, the traditional pity becomes intertwined with hostility. The effect is similar to that felt by Black people resisting "staying in their place." This book is dedicated to promoting genuine opportunities for blind students while anticipating and overcoming the pity, misunderstanding, and hostility which will inevitably be encountered from time to time.

Accurate Information and Positive Attitudes

The chapter on "Starting Anew Each Time" contains detailed suggestions on laying a positive groundwork. Just a few points will be emphasized here.

A positive attitude need not make you a Pollyanna. Recognize that there may be problems. "I am here to see that there is no undue burden on you," is a good phrase. Emphasize what the student is already able to do without any special help. After initial remarks, quickly settle down to a practical discussion of methods and arrangements, always talking *with* the classroom teacher rather than *to* him/her. Frequently ask, "Does that sound OK to you?" or "Do you see any problem with that?"

If possible, gain the support of the principal before you meet the classroom teacher, and have him/her introduce you. Speak to a faculty meeting. Provide names of other classroom teachers who have successfully included a blind student.

Tactfully counteract generalization. If another blind student's difficulties are mentioned by comparison, you can say, "Yes, he did have that problem. This student..." Help everyone distinguish among individual characteristics.

Tactfully dispel myths and misconceptions as soon as possible. (Sometimes, of course, it is best to ignore one problem in order to deal with something else more urgent.) If the "marvelously keen senses of the blind" are mentioned, you can say, "We will indeed want to teach Jimmy to develop his other senses to the fullest." If wrong conclusions are drawn about what a child can or cannot see, explain that this is often hard to judge; that small changes in contrast, etc., can make a great difference; and that we should seek a *reliable* technique for each task, rather than necessarily always trying to rely on sight.

Never assume you have convinced anyone of anything permanently and completely. Information can be forgotten. A new situation may be perceived as an exception. ("But surely you didn't mean that she could go with us to a *factory!*")

Many things which seem obvious to you will not be at all obvious to most educators. Explain, explain–tactfully.

PROVIDE RESOURCES AND REFERENCES

Provide some printed information for reference. A good initial selection for high school would be:

- –A folder describing your agency and its services to blind students, including your own name and telephone number
- –The book, *Your School Includes a Blind Student,* by Doris M. Willoughby
- –Any specialized references that might be needed immediately, such as *Suggestions for the Blind Cook* by Ruth Schroeder and Doris Willoughby
- –A brief paper about attitudes toward blindness in general, such as *Blindness–Handicap or Characteristic* by Kenneth Jernigan
- –Suggestions about the use of taped materials

For preschool or kindergarten, *A Resource Guide for Parents and Educators of Blind Children* (also by Doris Willoughby) may be the most helpful book initially. *Your School Includes a Blind Student* is also helpful even at this age level.

If too much is offered at once, it will probably not be read. On the other hand, some educators are eager to read everything they can find. Size up individuals, and try to provide the right materials at the right time.

When you begin something quite noticeable, such as the use of a cane, find a way to inform staff about it for better understanding and support. Often a brief general note or bulletin is a good idea. Check with the principal, since he/she probably wishes to approve anything sent to all staff. Following is an example:

TO: Central School staff and bus drivers
FROM: Doris Willoughby, County Schools

I am writing this memo to provide information about the use of a white cane by Tommy Barrett (second grade, Mrs. Smith).

Tommy does not see well and often runs into things, especially outdoors where there is glare. He cannot cross a street safely by using vision alone. The Barretts and I have agreed that Tommy should start using a cane. I have shown Mrs. Barrett how the cane should be used, and I will demonstrate for school staff as well.

Tommy will be using the cane at all times when he is moving around, except while engaging in a sport. When he is seated, the cane should be placed on the floor by his feet. I will have the main responsibility for teaching him to use the cane. However, if he should at any time really *misuse* it, please correct him.

Tommy will have the cane on the school bus. He could slip it under the seat, hold it beside him at an angle, or slip it between the seat and the wall. It should *not* be in the aisle, of course.

If children ask questions, a matter-of-fact explanation is generally best – comparable to explaining, say, leg braces. You might say, "Tommy doesn't see very well and sometimes bumps into things. The cane helps him to walk safely and easily."

Please let me know right away if there are any problems with the use of the cane.

Building Rapport with Classroom Teachers

Pity the poor classroom teacher who has to deal with various "experts" on her students' problems – learning disabilities, behavioral problems, speech impairments, and now blindness. These so-called experts appear as if by magic at exactly the wrong time. They distract the teacher while Marty and Jennie start another argument; they chatter on about nothing during a badly-needed break; they expect a complicated report during the five minutes while classes are passing (when the teacher would love to step out for a drink of water).

Keep out of this stereotype. Remind yourself how precious a five-minute break can be, and how difficult it is to talk when restless students are present. If you must come in unannounced, make only the briefest comments and seek a convenient time to talk longer. Use written notes and phone calls if necessary. Ask permission before staying to observe a class. Don't chatter endlessly to a captive audience.

In spite of these potential problems, it is essential to find a time to talk with classroom teachers. Begin with a conference before school starts in the fall. During the year, insist that a time be available on a schedule suitable to the situation. Otherwise problems will grow without your knowledge – even if you are in the building every day.

Make your suggestions practical, and seek plenty of feedback. If you have not taught a large class of students this age, it may be hard for you to foresee problems which are obvious to the classroom teacher. For example, it might appear that the P.E. teacher should be able to help a blind child through an obstacle course, if it is easy for the sighted students to handle. But who will *supervise* the sighted students? If they see the teacher's attention taken up, the class will degenerate into horseplay.

Schedule lessons as conveniently as possible for all concerned. Be scrupulous about following that schedule, and discuss any interruptions as far ahead as possible.

Often you will start something (such as the use of a new Braille symbol, a new cane travel skill, etc.) and ask others to help the student follow through. However, when you start something particularly difficult or unpleasant, be very careful about asking other adults to complete it for you. If a lot of individual attention will be needed, seek out someone other than the classroom teacher – even if this means calling a conference and arranging for an aide or volunteer. And if you discipline a child by taking away his recess, *do not* expect the classroom teacher to give up her recess break to watch him!

Conduct yourself as an equal co-worker, not a superior. Although you have more knowledge about blindness, the classroom teacher knows more about subject matter and general policies. Make a point of asking advice, giving sincere compliments, and otherwise showing regard for the other person.

If you have taught less than a year in a regular classroom, most teachers will regard you as having virtually no "real" experience. Even if you have taught for several years in a regular classroom, they may feel that you have left the ranks and no longer understand. Be judicious about mentioning how much or how little experience you have. Rather, emphasize that you each have certain types of knowledge and can work together.

Often a general resource or remedial teacher, who is not a specialist in work with the blind, will provide individual help to your student. The role of this person is midway between the classroom teacher's and yours. Although he/she is not a regular classroom teacher, the assignment is in one particular building and usually involves some groups of students. Daily work with the student and contact with classroom teachers is easily possible. The general resource teacher can be of great help in supplementing your work. However, your relationship is vulnerable to the same problems which can occur with classroom teachers. Find time for adequate communication and mutual understanding. Discuss the "division of labor" openly. Do not let yourself be excluded from talking directly with classroom teachers; even if the general resource teacher does a great deal of this, you should be free to do so also.

At IEP meetings and other conferences, try to include classroom teachers and others who work directly with the student. Excluding them leaves out a vital perspective, and strengthens the stereotype that "those so-called experts never pay any attention to my ideas."

The Delicate Art of Negotiation

Rarely will it be possible for you to *order* a staff member to do something. Almost always you will be attempting to reach a mutual agreement, or to persuade someone to your point of view. Develop the art of accepting a person's feelings or opinions without necessarily agreeing. Learn to negotiate without arguing.

Align yourself *with* the other individual. You might say, "We would get into trouble with the Department of Public Instruction if we..." or "The parents couldn't criticize us if we..."

Develop the art of quietly mentioning something without seeming to emphasize it. Contact the teacher about another matter, and then bring up the other (perhaps more touchy) subject casually.

At the other extreme, sometimes a *more* direct approach is what is needed. If for two years you have been nagging everyone to phase in the Braille slate, and the student still uses only the Perkins, call a conference. Get slate usage into the IEP, with a timetable.

If you wish to do a certain thing, but must check with someone else about it, be as definite as possible without being domineering. You might say, "If it's OK with you, I will..."

Much of this seems to go against the grain of modern thinking in public relations. Shouldn't one always ask for the other party's point of view and then talk it over? "Nondirective counseling" is advocated by many professionals.

For the itinerant or resource teacher of blind students, however, it is often very appropriate to be direct in making recommendations – regardless of the fact that other professionals may avoid that approach. The specialized teacher is usually the *only* person (other than the young student) with an in-depth knowledge of blindness and blind techniques. Thus it is quite proper to sell one's ideas assertively.

Size up individuals. Consider what approaches work best with whom.

When there is disagreement (overt or passive), try to find out where the real problem is. I recall expounding on the value of Braille for a low-visioned preschooler, and meeting a cool reception from Headstart teachers. Assuming they wished to emphasize his vision, I assured them that he could learn print also, and I described some blind students whose grades had improved when they began using Braille. Again there was a cool response. Later I realized that *none* of the Headstart children were working on formal reading readiness as yet, and that the teachers thought I was trying to push the blind child too fast. They had no objection to Braille as such.

Be specific. If you want the aide to complete about three lessons per week, say "three lessons per week," not "moving right along." Better still, leave daily written lesson plans. If you want the child to practice writing Braille in between your visits, provide word lists or other specific assignments.

USEFUL PHRASES

Following are some especially useful phrases. Having them in mind helps one be prepared for tactful negotiation:

"I strongly suggest..."
"I would vote against that."
"The State Department of Education insists..."
"Most blind people prefer..."
"There is a problem with..."
"I must disagree because ..."
"I'd suggest a somewhat bolder approach..."
"Have you tried...?"
"I'm sorry, but our Department policy..."
"We have generally found that..."
"What would you think of...?"
"At Southview High they really liked..."
"We tried that at Southview, and..."
"Yes, that is one way to get started. Soon let's try..."
"As you know..." (This is a tactful way of bringing in some information which you believe they may *not* know or fully appreciate.)

Avoid phrases such as:

"You should not..."
"I insist..."
"You will have to..."
"That is not a good idea."

Another type of useful phrase is pleasant but noncommittal. It may indicate understanding of the other party's point of view, or seek information, but does not necessarily indicate agreement.

"I see."
"You felt that she..."
"I hadn't realized..."
"It's hard to know what to do."
"Tell me more about what you mean."
"Thank you for calling it to my attention."
"That must have been very difficult for you."

Phrases like these can maintain rapport while you consider how to proceed.

Sometimes the best strategy is retreat – perhaps to try again at a better time, or perhaps to work on a higher priority. There will also be times to call on reinforcements. Is there someone else who could better deal with this problem?

Always keep an open mind. Often time will show the other party to be right, and you to be mistaken. Still more often, a "third alternative" or compromise will emerge as a solution.

Fitting In

We give much thought to helping the blind student relate well to others and "fit in." But how about ourselves? Partly because we deal with the stereotypes of blindness, and partly because we are not "regular" faculty members, we too face this problem.

Before starting a new assignment, resolve as closely as possible the scope of your responsibility. For example, will you or will you not routinely give remedial help with academic work (and under what circumstances)? Having determined this, you can be firm yet tactful. If you take on substantial work outside your job description, you are doing no one a favor; rather, you will probably neglect some aspect of the job you were hired to do. At the same time, don't become a spoiled "prima donna" unwilling to do anything tedious or unpleasant.

If you were planning a trip overseas, you would study the local customs and try not to offend. Crooking the finger to mean "come here," for example, is very offensive in Southeast Asia. There are analogous customs and traditions within school faculties, but if you have never taught in a classroom you may not have learned them. If you formerly taught in a classroom, realize that customs may vary from place to place, and that some things are different when you are not a classroom teacher yourself. Tune in to subtle hints. Be conservative in your behavior, at least until you are well acquainted. Ask advice about local customs.

Following are several suggestions.

(1) Take advantage of opportunities for informal, relaxed contact with teachers. Whenever possible, eat lunch at school, relax in the lounge at recess, etc. Also avoid "talking shop" so much that you keep others from relaxing.

(2) Ask about such things as coffee cups and snacks. In many schools, leaving food on the lounge table means "help yourself," but food elsewhere is personal property. Check on how to pay for coffee.

(3) The teachers' lounge is a refuge and an inner sanctum. Do not bring in a student or a parent, except for a good reason and by arrangement. Classroom teachers need a break from formality. They do not wish to be watched by students or parents when they take off their shoes, talk about their personal lives, or otherwise "let down their hair" in the lounge. If you want to show your student the vending machine in the lounge, choose a time when there are likely to be few people (or no one) in there; and ask if it is all right. Working regularly with a student in the lounge is not advisable.

(4) If you let a student (yours or someone else's) into an area where he would not otherwise be, you are responsible. If you are the last one out of the office at night, and a student persuades you to let him use the phone, you must stay until he leaves.

(5) If you work at just one school, take on the same "duties" as other teachers–playground supervisor, hall monitor, etc. This is usually not possible for itinerant teachers, however.

(6) Read the school rules, and see that your student follows them.

(7) If you see someone else's student misbehaving, consider carefully whether you should do anything. You may be judged as interfering. (Exceptions would be if there is a clearly dangerous situation, or if the student is directly bothering you.) If you are the only adult around, it is generally best to (a) ignore minor misbehavior; (b) correct major misbehavior if you can handle it; (c) get help immediately for situations you may not be able to handle. Report any substantial incident to the principal at once. Ask advice from a counselor or the principal in case of continuing annoyance–e.g., students disturbing your lesson.

(8) Be thoughtful about sharing resources. If telephones and rest room facilities are limited in number, do not monopolize them, especially during short periods when other

teachers are free.

(9) Often you will need to work within earshot of others–perhaps even in the same room. Keep noise down. If an activity is especially loud or attention-getting, go elsewhere temporarily.

(10) Although you may choose to give students your own home phone number, recognize that many classroom teachers do not want theirs given out.

(11) Consider local customs of the community at large, and watch for situations in which you may seem too formal or too familiar. For example, if you are from a large city and never speak to strangers in public, you may seem "uppity" in a small town.

Conducting Yourself as a Professional

PERSONAL APPEARANCE

Roy Brown strode up the hallway of the large city high school. Recognizing the principal, he called out, "Hi! I'm Roy. Could you..."

"Young man!" interrupted the principal. "What are you doing here? Class started five minutes ago!"

To the great embarrassment of both of them, Roy hastily explained that he was not a student, but the new itinerant teacher coming to give a Braille lesson. He was just out of college and looked even younger; wore jeans and a T-shirt; spoke very informally; and had not previously been introduced to the principal. Even if this spectacular misunderstanding had not occurred, the staff would still have regarded him as particularly "green," and would have been reluctant to accept suggestions from him.

Especially the first few times you go to a given school, dress and act rather formally and conservatively–particularly if you look young and if the location is a high school. If you are a man, wear a suit. If you are a woman, wear a skirt or a flattering pantsuit, and shoes that are not sporty. Consider wearing a nametag (with your title and last name, not your first name)–somehow this adds a great deal of authority. Conduct yourself in a mature and dignified manner. Rarely do staff members call the principal by his/her first name. Teachers typically address one another by first name, except when students are present.

If in time you find that more informality is justified, you can relax safely. Attune yourself to local customs. Be especially conservative in your manner if the other person is much older than you are.

PERSONAL CONDUCT

Keep other staff members informed about your work, and ask them to do the same for you. When many individuals advise a student, a situation of "too many cooks" can arise, with great confusion.

Be very careful about revealing personal information about students. If you can be overheard by other students, other parents, or the public, do not say anything about individual students. It is usually all right to discuss routine matters in front of teachers who do not have the student, but personal matters should be discussed in private.

When the student is present, avoid saying things that could be misinterpreted or which reveal information a young student should not have. If the industrial arts teacher is upset and nervous, do not let the student overhear your discussion about it (unless you have consciously decided that he/she is mature enough). If there is a possibility of repeating a grade, do not say, "We may not be using second grade books next year" if the student is listening. Instead say, "We are not sure what books will be used."

Do not reveal confidential information across district lines. This is especially tricky when you bring someone to observe a blind student. Be sure the parents approve of the idea, and do not reveal personal details. Be sure you *know* where district lines are.

BALANCING VARIOUS NEEDS

Often there is a delicate balance among different needs. For example, in general it is very desirable to involve blind students – even the very young – in explaining and demonstrating methods and techniques. This helps improve the general climate about blindness, educates adults and classmates, and helps the student himself to develop positive attitudes. At the same time, it would be unethical to push too much of this onto a particular student. If the youngster is very shy, speak for him at first, then gradually increase his ability. With a confident student, watch to see that too much time is not taken up with speeches. Avoid both extremes.

Another area of delicate balance is that of directing your own influence. A Spanish teacher can try to change the English curriculum, the school board's policies, student conduct rules, etc., etc., without diminishing his role as a Spanish teacher. This is not so true in our situation. We need all the margin we can get to influence attitudes about blindness. Someone who is tired of hearing you expound about the general English requirements will probably be less willing to listen to your suggestions about the blind student. Furthermore, if you are not directly employed by the school district, the staff may regard your comments as criticisms of their district. They also may conclude that your opinion is related to blindness – as, by assuming that you seek to reduce the English requirement because blind students cannot handle it. For all these reasons, I generally refrain from making much comment on educational issues apart from blindness.

Avoid the occupational hazard of possessiveness. I have seen this more in resource teachers, who tend to spend more time with a particular student, but it can occur with anyone. However hard you work to help the student, and however excellent your approach, no student is "yours" exclusively. If he/she "belongs" to anyone, it is the parents. Other staff members will work with the student; they may have different approaches; they may succeed where you have failed. Resist the feeling that you alone always know what is best for the blind student. Also avoid assuming that you are the *only* one who can possibly help the student with certain things.

Reject also the opposite extreme of disclaiming all responsibility when problems and handicaps are many. If some part of the responsibility is yours, keep plugging away at solutions.

YOU MAY FEEL ALONE

When you meet hostility and misunderstanding, you may be tempted to question your right to be there at all. On the other hand, when you help a student succeed in spite of serious problems, it may seem that you have tremendous power. The words of P.L. 94-142 are reassuring: "It is the purpose of this Act to assure that all handicapped children have available to them...a free, appropriate public education...."

Itinerant work, especially, is sometimes a lonely job. Often there is little time for socializing, and little identification with a group of teachers. Even where there is plenty of companionship, there may be no other teachers who are specialized in teaching the blind. In most fields, there are plenty of colleagues available for "comparing notes;" but a teacher of the blind may need to travel 200 miles to find another. Keep in touch with other teachers of the blind, and with blind adults, even if it must be mostly by mail and telephone. The National Federation of the Blind maintains a network among teachers with a positive philosophy. Do not sacrifice the valuable resource (both professional and personal) of exchanging experiences and ideas.

Rapport with Administrators

How much deference should one show toward a principal or other administrator? Somewhere between "obsequious" and "brash." The exact middle ground varies with local custom and individuals, but it is well to err on the side of conservatism.

Reporting to the office whenever you enter or leave a building is a good policy even if not required. At least whenever you enter a building for the first time, introduce yourself at once. If feasible, meet the superintendent and other administrators as well as the principal.

Do not address an administrator by his/her first name. (An exception occurs when you are well acquainted and observe that everyone uses first names. Even then, always use formal titles when students or parents are present.) Disagreement with an administrator requires a respectful demeanor–he/she is in a position of authority, however much you may dislike it, and mutual respect is a foundation for an improved relationship.

ASKING FOR HELP

When should you consult the principal about a problem? Always do so if (a) the problem has broad and important implications; (b) the problem is substantial and not getting solved; or (c) there is physical danger. Following are some typical situations in which you *should* consult an administrator. Note that in a secondary school, a counselor is often considered an administrator.

(1) You see a student flash a knife.

(2) A parent tells you that the classroom teacher is treating her blind child unfairly, causing an upset stomach. You yourself have great difficulty talking with that teacher.

(3) A parent is suing an eye doctor for malpractice, and asks you to testify about educational costs. (Note: In this case, consult an administrator in the agency which actually employs you. Consult *before* agreeing to do anything.)

(4) Three teachers give you three versions of an important school policy.

(5) The IEP calls for the student to take regular home economics. However, the sewing teacher says firmly, "I have arranged for the blind girl to do all her work in a separate room."

Asking for help too often, on the other hand, can annoy an administrator and weaken your position. Following are situations where another approach (given in parentheses) would probably be better than talking to the principal:

(1) A boy passing in the hallway calls your eighth-grade student "Four Eyes." (If this is an isolated incident, it may be best to ignore it. If it happens more than once, start by talking with classroom teachers and/or the counselor, as well as with your student himself/herself.)

(2) A parent tells you a sighted sibling is treated unfairly in English class. (This is not your student. Let the parent handle the matter. At most, you might help the parent contact the counselor or principal.)

(3) The new third grade teacher excludes your student from a science experiment. (Talk this over with the teacher yourself.)

Itinerant teachers often work under various administrators who may have conflicting ideas. Different policies in different buildings usually can be handled by a "when in Rome..." philosophy. But real conflicts can arise when the teacher travels to various local districts and is an employee of yet another jurisdiction. Usually through negotiation you can find a solution which satisfies both. In case of impasse, suggest various alternatives, being pleasant but firm. Have your supervisor talk with the principal if necessary.

Rapport with Other Professional Staff

The school psychologist commented that intelligence tests for blind students were irrelevant and invalid. I said, "Oh, no, it is very important, and it certainly can be done. Would you like me to show you some articles about it?" This conversation caused a permanently cold relationship with this psychologist, plus a lecture from the principal about not telling the psychologist how to do his job.

I am now careful never to give the appearance of *telling* someone in another profession what he should or should not do. Faced with this situation today, I would probably say something like, "Of course, I'm not a psychologist... but you might want to talk with Dr. Fontanelle, who has tested a good many blind students with the verbal portion of the usual test...." If the psychologist refused to consider the matter, I would ask someone else to help me negotiate.

Suggesting how to adapt tests given by other professionals is important but touchy. Try to hold strictly to your own specialty, as, "Jane can see large, plain pictures but not small or busy ones. Could I take a quick look at the speech test and talk over anything that might be a problem?"

Make a point of asking the school nurse's interpretation of medical matters. In fact, one of the best ways to build rapport with anyone is to ask advice. Could the nurse act as liaison with the doctor? Would the speech therapist have good advice about language development?

Remember that counselors are primary problem-solvers on almost anything, and usually have some administrative authority. If there is a problem with a classroom teacher, often the counselor can help without the escalation that occurs if the principal is brought in. When a math teacher continued making "humorous" remarks about the cane, upsetting the student and ignoring my protests, a visit by the counselor ended the problem.

Rapport with Other Staff

It may seem superfluous to remind ourselves of the social equality of those whose jobs do not require college. But some educators (probably without realizing it) coolly ignore a maintenance person in a conversation, or speak to the cooks condescendingly. We are all equal citizens. Moreover, the cook or custodian may be the one person who can help your student with a problem. Treat everyone with respect.

For minor requests, such as adjustment of furniture, normally you will deal directly with the staff person involved. For matters of policy or procedure, however, the non-professional staff are under a different line of authority. You are much less free to negotiate with them than with educators. Consult the principal before asking the custodian to build a new cabinet in your resource room; before asking the cooks to change the location of silverware containers; etc.

Get acquainted with the custodian. Remark that your blind student is learning to go around objects in the hallways. This helps prevent the custodian's rushing to move things when the student approaches.

Talk with the cooks about procedures in the lunch line. Can the student proceed independently if someone tells him what the choices are? Can he carry his tray?

When I was a resource teacher in a school where some children were brought by taxi, I had a most disconcerting experience. The driver dropped off a totally blind kindergartner, 50 feet from the building, and drove away. When I happened to look out, the child was wandering helplessly in circles in the broad driveway. At the opposite extreme, I have seen drivers literally carry children who had been walking independently for years.

Talk with transportation personnel about what should be expected. Especially with a young child, pin down who will be responsible for what at each point. Also discuss where to place the cane in a bus or cab – somehow this question causes a surprising amount of fuss.

Always consider whose scope of authority is most involved. If you set up an obstacle course for your cane travel student, judiciously placing chairs in the hall for a few minutes and then removing them, it is probably unreasonable for the custodian to object. But if you wish to give your student a tour of the boiler room, and the custodian says only maintenance staff are allowed in there, your protest would probably be unwise.

Your Professional Relationship with Students

Since working with students is discussed throughout this book, the topic here will deal with one's general professional image as it relates to students.

Classroom teachers quickly learn that being a warm and helpful teacher is not the same thing as being a "chum" on the student's own level. If this is not understood, the relationship degenerates and control is lost. Although this is just as true with individual students, it may not be so obvious, since overt misbehavior is less likely. Also, some of the conventions of formality are missing – e.g., standing before a large group. Furthermore, the itinerant/resource teacher may help with rather personal matters, and often is well acquainted with the entire family.

How can we exert direction and control, while keeping the informality which is desirable for personalized help?

If you and the family have personal friends in common, occasionally say, "Nothing we discuss will be mentioned to anyone outside of school unless you yourself want it to be. I am careful to keep my professional role separate from personal relationships."

What should your students call you? Note how classroom teachers are addressed by their students, and expect yours to speak to you the same way. If you are personally acquainted outside of school, you might say, "At church your family calls me Jan. But at school we teachers are called by our last names. At school I'd like you to remember to call me Miss Black." Even in a preschool where the staff may use first names, I prefer my title; otherwise the little child will have to relearn when I follow her into kindergarten.

Respect students' confidences whenever possible. If a ninth grader says, "The boys in P.E. pick on me because I can't hit the ball. But don't say anything – I'll work it out myself," you probably should let him solve the immediate problem himself. However, you can work on the background – i.e., redouble your efforts to arrange a suitable P.E. program and to build good social relationships. Retain your right to decide when, because of the seriousness of a problem, you should talk with someone else.

If you disapprove of behavior, try to determine the real reasons behind it. Recently I scolded a sixth-grade girl for repeated failure to comb her hair after outdoor cane travel practice. Finally she explained, "Everybody says we're not supposed to comb our hair in school." This student, with learning disabilities in addition to blindness, had taken the rule literally. She did not realize that others combed their hair in the rest room and discreetly elsewhere, and that the teachers meant, "Don't comb your hair in class."

When you maintain high standards of both achievement and conduct, you show confidence in your students, and they will tend to respond in kind.

THE STUDENT AS AN ADULT

Many students become 18 before they graduate, and this brings a change in role. No longer can parents and educators alone determine the IEP; the student must participate. Usually this transition is smooth, with the student gradually taking more and more responsibility. Although the student gains adult status, including the right to decline services, remember that you have not lost your role as a teacher. Continue to conduct yourself in a dignified manner; make your lessons relevant. Maintain the conventions that support your role. For instance, 18-year-old students still address classroom teachers formally, so there is no reason they should start using your first name at school. (If a student debated this, I would suggest we *both* use formal titles, as in many college classes.)

Defining your professional role toward students also helps gain the respect of school staff.

Selected Sticky Problems

PROBLEM: The third-grade teacher is doing an all-around bad job with the blind student. Johnny's work and adjustment are going downhill despite numerous discussions.

Poor approach: As soon as you realize this is happening, you insist that the principal switch Johnny to a different third grade class.

Better approach: Switching classes should be a very last resort, especially after the term has begun. It implies that many teachers cannot handle blind students. It brings the dilemma of what to do if the "poor" teacher is the only one for that grade or subject. It encourages teachers to do poorly in order to avoid having a blind student. Instead, "pull out all the stops" to improve the situation in the present classroom, using the suggestions throughout this book. Involve the parents. Enlist the help of the principal, but channel it toward insisting that the present teacher improve her methods. Consider increasing the individual help provided.

PROBLEM: The principal feels that all blind students belong in residential schools. He continually cites the case of one blind student who tried public school and failed miserably.

Poor approach: You tell the parent that the local school situation is impossible, and that placement elsewhere is necessary.

Poor approach: You confront the principal at every opportunity. You bring in vast quantities of literature about successful blind people.

Better approach: Realize that although the use of literature can be helpful, a very hostile person may reject all information at first. Discussion may always degenerate into argument.

If the classroom teacher is open-minded, this problem may be "worked around." But if hostile teachers are supervised by a hostile principal, you have a large problem indeed.

If the student's placement really is open to question, hostile staff may tip the scales toward a different placement. But if the student clearly belongs here, do not give in. This is what P.L. 94-142 is all about. Be sure the parents know their rights of Due Process. If you are employed by another agency, ask your supervisor's help. If you are employed by the same district, consider whether a higher administrator would be more supportive. Ask advice from the National Federation of the Blind and other advocacy groups. No child should be sent away to school just because a principal is still living in the Middle Ages.

PROBLEM: SueAnn has always done average or low-average work. But she is failing Mr. Pepper's math class. Two teachers comment that Mr. Pepper gives far too much homework, and that their own daughters nearly failed his class.

Poor approach: You get the parent to go with you to the principal and demand that SueAnn's homework be reduced.

Better approach: Look for solutions used with other low-average students. How did those two teachers help their own daughters?

Also consider what individual help is available for SueAnn. However, unless there are special circumstances (e.g., a late-blinded student just starting to learn Braille), reducing assignments is unnecessary and unwise.

CHAPTER 49

TWO REPRESENTATIVES OF MANY SUCCESSFUL BLIND TEACHERS

By Doris M. Willoughby

Since I am sighted, the following two chapters bring an important perspective which I cannot provide by myself.

The two chapters are quite different from each other, and these two teachers use different approaches to some situations. It is so with all teachers. Personalities and personal circumstances differ; job requirements differ. But both Sharon Duffy and Caroline Rasmussen, together with many other capable blind teachers in widely varying fields, emphasize the competent blind individual, with confidence in himself/herself, taking charge in a responsible manner. Caroline Rasmussen frequently uses her driver for duties other than driving; Sharon Duffy hardly ever does. Each teacher, however, directs the employee and maintains control, rather than turning over the job to him or her.

Note that classroom management and discipline is *not* an area where sighted assistance is needed. It is *not* necessary to use an aide to help control the students just because the teacher is blind, even if there are many students together and they may be difficult to manage. Blind teachers in regular elementary and secondary education teach regular-sized classes, and have no more difficulties than other teachers.

These brief chapters emphatically do *not* purport to be a complete description of methods for blind teachers. The best way to build solid knowledge of techniques and approaches is to meet a variety of capable blind teachers in both regular and special education fields.

All blind teachers, as well as future teachers, are cordially invited to join the National Association of Blind Educators (a Division of the National Federation of the Blind). This active group builds opportunities for blind teachers, facilitates sharing of ideas and methods, and defends teachers' rights in cases of discrimination. The National Association of Blind Educators produces a national newsletter and many other publications, and holds frequent conferences and seminars in various locations.

CHAPTER 50

THE TEACHER WHO IS BLIND

By Sharon L. M. Duffy

Many blind children today have relatively little contact with blind adults who may serve as role models. In some cases, being a role model can be the most important function a blind teacher can serve. This is not to say that the skills are not valuable; but the most important lesson to be taught is that it is okay to be blind. If this is achieved, resistance to the skills training will diminish, and the ultimate competence in a skill will be greater. It is hard for any of us to do well at anything we don't believe in, so this must be uppermost in the minds of teachers as they teach. Practice and achievement will help along the road to acceptance.

This means, of course, that a sighted teacher can compensate by introducing her students to competent blind people, but a blind teacher need only walk in and teach.

In addition, regular classroom teachers who get to know a capable blind teacher may undergo some attitude changes with regard to what they should expect of their blind students. Certainly, any teacher of blindness-related skills will routinely provide information about what can be expected of a blind student, but a classroom teacher who generally thinks of blind people as dependents of society will tend to expect less than is possible. If, through contact with a blind teacher, he comes to know that his students will someday earn a living, raise families, etc., he will probably expect more from his blind students and provide them a better education.

The other side of this coin is a very serious matter, however. Although it is true that a competent blind teacher can have a very positive effect on students and other teachers, an incompetent blind teacher can do more damage than an incompetent sighted teacher. It is critical that the blind teacher be proficient in the skills of blindness, and be a well-adjusted person–not someone who is in the field because of belief that he/she cannot do anything else. Unfortunately, there are a number of blind persons in the field of work with the blind for just this reason. The fact that a person is blind does not make him an expert on blindness. Proper educational preparation, the development of skills and positive attitudes about blindness, and a thorough study of organizations of and for the blind can achieve this.

In my work as a rehabilitation teacher and field representative, I have encountered many sighted itinerant teachers, most of whom know Braille, but few who teach it well. Most sighted people understandably do not use Braille as their primary means of written communication so they do not use it with ease or great confidence. This is transmitted to blind students despite the most dedicated efforts of the teacher.

A blind teacher who uses Braille daily knows exactly what can be expected of a Braille student. She will not be fooled into believing that Braille is difficult. Her proficiency in reading and writing Braille in the process of teaching will settle this question definitively.

We expect that our sighted children be taught by literate teachers who have been reading for a lifetime. Ideally, Braille should always be taught by a lifetime Braille reader of great competence. However, given the current teaching arrangements, this is not practical. Therefore, it is important that sighted teachers become as proficient as possible in the use of Braille–proficient enough to demonstrate its use to their students.

Lest I be accused of implying that, in all instances, it is better to be blind as an itinerant or resource teacher of blind children, I wish to focus on a few things which can be taught equally well by sighted or blind teachers. Teaching typing and cane travel fall into this category. I teach finger positions by putting my fingers on my student's fingers, and his or her fingers on mine, at different times. I rely on a teacher's aide, secretary, or my driver to do proofreading.

It is advisable for anyone teaching cane travel to have either driven a route or walked it in advance noting landmarks, etc. When I use a driver, I frequently have him drive a route with me, describing such things as location of parking lots and angled streets. In a large city, I walk the routes in advance if I am in an unfamiliar area, using public transportation instead of a driver.

In teaching a cane travel student, I observe how he/she holds the cane by placing my hand on my student's hand and having him/her demonstrate the wrist action. Also, by walking behind my student, I can hear the width of the arc. If a student is not arcing wide enough, the tapping will be muffled. If the student is arcing too wide, I can hear that, too. If indoors on a hard surface, I can also hear whether the student is in step or not.

With older students, junior high or older, it is necessary to assign a route and allow the student to carry it out without close supervision. Once the basic technique is mastered, the blind teacher need not be within arm's reach, but merely close enough to know where the student is. The teacher can choose to follow in the car or to observe directly.

The question as to whether it is safe for a blind person to teach cane travel has often arisen. If the blind person is a competent traveler and a competent teacher, it certainly is. The fact that many blind persons have been successfully teaching cane travel for many years bears this out. Those who question whether a blind person can teach cane travel are generally the same ones who do not really believe that a blind person can travel independently in general.

A young sighted woman, certified to teach mobility, questioned the advisability of my teaching cane travel. When I asked her if she believed blind people could travel safely and independently, she did not respond by saying "yes." Instead she said that she once knew one man who had better orientation than anyone else she knew. Clearly, she does not believe in what she purports to teach. Any teacher who can travel competently with a cane is definitely proving that it is safe to travel with a cane. This confidence will be observed by the student.

If the teacher is blind and travels competently with a cane, a blind student can begin to think it is okay to use a cane–a vital part of becoming a good cane traveler.

One other aspect of being a blind itinerant teacher bears mention. It is necessary to hire a driver to travel most efficiently in rural communities and towns lacking good public transportation. Occasionally, a driver can be used as a reader. However, I make minimal use of my driver as a reader, because it could easily interfere with my relationships with my students and with other professionals who may mistakenly assume that I could not function independently, undermining the image I wished to project. In contrast, my walking in with a cane and finding the means of doing my job is a positive statement about the competence of blind people–one not missed by the staff and others. They are watching.

Also, many drivers make poor readers and are even less likely to understand the subtleties related to blindness. The pay for this position is generally not high. The teacher's employer will usually provide payment for mileage, and the itinerant teacher must pay anything additional out-of-pocket. I have known some itinerant teachers who purchased cars in order to make use of drivers who did not have cars. I have never done this since it did not appear to be cost efficient for me.

The relationship between driver and teacher should always be a business one. I do these things to maintain the employer/employee relationship: I keep Braille records of the hours worked, the route traveled (such as Boise, Nampa, New Plymouth, Boise), the number of miles, the cost of meals and any other expenses. I ask my driver to keep track of mileage and hours also. In this way, I am able to monitor mileage reports and see that all reporting is done accurately. I always pay my driver at the end of each week. If I find that a driver will not perform as requested, is incapable of performing the job satisfactorily, or is consistently late or absent, I fire him. My job depends upon the reliability of my driver.

A driver can be used to perform such tasks as notewriting, proofreading, typing, and finding people, but I generally do not use him for these things since he rarely accompanies me inside. Sometimes, the contacts made in regard to minor tasks can be important in developing a good relationship with the school. The time I spend with teachers and their assistants pays off in the amount of cooperation attained with regard to my students, and can solve many attitudinal problems.

Clearly, the blind teacher must be aware not only that the fact of blindness can be of great benefit in projecting positive attitudes about blindness, but also that any negative characteristics a blind teacher displays can be doubly damaging since the behavior of the blind teacher will be taken as typical of the blind as a group. This must be kept in mind in every action, however trivial. This means that especial care about personal appearance and the way in which every task is performed is vital to maintain and encourage positive attitudes about blindness.

Please feel free to contact me, c/o the National Federation of the Blind, if you would like to ask me about my work as a blind teacher.

CHAPTER 51

A BLIND TEACHER'S METHODS

by Caroline Rasmussen

I am totally blind, and I have been an itinerant teacher for visually impaired children for several years. I would like to share with you in this article, how I handle my job as a blind person, and some of the many complexities involved.

First of all, you probably wonder how I get around in my capacity as an itinerant teacher. I use my cane everywhere I go. Of course, sometimes I may use a sighted guide but I still carry the cane for identification. I always explain to the child that there are two reasons for the cane: the identification to the general public that I am blind, and second, for my own direct use and benefit. I explain there's only one place I don't use my cane–and that's within my own home. Therefore, any student of mine in a cane travel program, is expected to carry out the same policy.

I hire a person to be my driver, since public transportation is not available where and when I need it. This person also does a fair amount of reading for me. There are many ways I have gone about finding drivers. They are hard to come by, no matter where you live. This is due to the fact that it is not a high-paying position, and I feel it is also partly due to the fact that the person must drive his/her own car. I have secured drivers in the following ways: ads in newspapers, ads in "Shopper" newspapers, write-ups in church bulletins, and word of mouth. My best results have come from ads in "Shoppers" and by word of mouth. Then, once several have responded, I interview them and select a person.

My driver and I must agree on certain things before starting:

- What wages will be paid? Are there provisions for a possible raise?
- Will there be any paid time off for illness or emergency?
- Often there is a time gap during which I do not need the driver (while I am teaching Braille, attending a meeting, etc.) Under what circumstances will this be considered "time off" so that the driver is not paid? Note that usually the driver could not go home because we would be too far away.
- Will the driver be paid mileage or be reimbursed for any other specific expenses? If so, does this include the distance from the driver's home? From the teacher's home to the first business stop?
- Will the driver be expected to perform any duties besides actual driving (e.g., reading)? If so, will there be additional pay?
- In case of illness or emergency, what responsibilities does the driver have for notifying me and/or contacting the substitute driver?
- When the driver does not join me in the schoolroom, where should he/she wait? If he/she enters the school (either to

wait or to accompany me), will a dress code be observed?

- Codes of conduct need to be outlined. (Do not use profanity or rough language; never touch students without specific direction; etc.) A very important rule is that *I* am in charge, and the driver is not to initiate anything without my instructions.
- How much notice must be given for ending the employment?

One driver went against some of the requirements, so I had to let him go. I made a few changes when I hired again in late September of last fall. The person had to commit himself to driving all year.

My driver receives an hourly wage from my personal funds, plus he receives the mileage payment from our agency. The mileage check is made out to me; I just sign it over to that person.

I have not really had any problems with my drivers taking over my responsibilities. I make sure that I make the decisions concerning the job. One driver got carried away with the thought that he could handle the time scheduling, and after several warnings I had to let him go. I do not mind their suggestions, but I want to have the final say.

At times other people have tried to give the responsibilities to my driver, but usually I just listen and step in and do it if that happens. Sometimes I might say, "I am the one who can handle that." People have talked to my drivers when they should have been talking to me. I warn my drivers of this in advance, and I ask them not to respond if I am present. People will also tend to look at my driver as they talk to me. Again, I simply ask my driver in advance not to respond to this. When things like this begin to happen, I just speak right up. If people talk to my driver about things when I am not present, the driver has been instructed to explain to the person that he/she will need to talk to me.

I have received several reactions from people about my being blind. They may be shocked when we first meet, but usually after a few minutes of talking they seem pretty relaxed. Sometimes it takes a few times of getting together, or my getting in there and proving to them I can handle things. One set of parents always come to mind when I think of this kind of thing. They were extremely shocked when I knocked at their door; but now they say that they are glad I'm blind and that I work with their child. I believe it is very helpful for parents and teachers to meet a blind adult, plus I feel it's very beneficial to my students. It shows these adults that these blind children will be able to function and carry on a normal life. It shows the children that they can and will be able to do things if they set their minds to it. I believe it's a source of encouragement to all, too. The children may become frustrated at times, but they cannot say to me, "Well, you do not understand how it is!" They have tried, but caught themselves in mid-sentence! At times I have my students meet other blind people also.

Some of the things I teach require seeing. I usually call on my driver to help out in these areas. My driver sometimes assists me during a cane travel lesson. He and I jointly plan the route, then I explain it to the child. I tell the driver what to watch for, and ask him not to help the child out unless I say so. I have demonstrated correct cane usage to my driver in advance.

Typing is another thing I teach that requires sight for certain things. My driver does most of the proofreading, and sometimes I have him sit in on a lesson to make sure the child is using correct fingering. I do not always do this, but I try to make a decision once I get to know the child. In the beginning, I always start out with the help of the driver.

Some people may wonder how I locate a teacher if I need him/her. I do it much the same way a sighted person in my capacity would do. I begin by looking in the obvious places. I enter the room where I think this teacher might be, and ask if so-and-so is in the room. If I'm unable to locate the person, I leave a written message.

In this situation and others, I do a lot of note-writing to teachers, aides, and parents.

Some of you may ask, "How on earth do you do that?" ... Very easily. If a typewriter is readily available, I may type the message myself. Alternatively, I may dictate my message to a secretary or to my driver to write.

Although in my job we do not do any medical eye testing or screening, we are expected to make educational evaluations of the student's functional vision. I have set procedures and questions I follow usually for evaluations, using pages with various print sizes and type fonts, various kinds of pictures, etc. I am familiar with what is on these pages, and each is labeled in Braille for my convenience. I take Braille notes during the evaluation, and explain to the child that I am writing things down so I won't forget them. I also say, "I want to see if I can be of any help to you." They are very accepting of this.

I may ask questions of my driver during the evaluation, but for certain things it is better to wait until the child leaves. A teacher has to decide this for him/herself. I am in total charge of what we do, but I may ask my driver how accurately the child has read or identified pictures if I use materials which are not yet familiar to me. I also ask my driver to make note of facial expressions, squinting of the eyes, etc.

I tell my driver/reader that any personal information which he/she may learn about a student is confidential.

Classroom observations are handled much the same way as my evaluations. I utilize my driver, and I have set procedures I follow. By now my driver knows pretty much how I handle these different activities, and what kinds of things I look for. I try to clue him in on as much as I deem necessary about the child and the school setting before we make each observation.

Teaching Braille is one of my favorite areas. I try to have a copy of the child's book as often as possible; then I follow along as the child reads. It is also possible for me to follow along in the same copy that the child is reading–like most sighted teachers, I have learned to read upside down for this purpose. As I face the child, my hands are reading a line or two behind his.

Unfortunately, I have never had a teacher's manual in Braille. I have received these manuals on tape on a loan basis, or I have had them read aloud to me, and then I have copied parts of them into Braille. Then this Braille copy I take with me as I teach the child. I find this much more effective than relying on the tapes alone.

When a classroom teacher hands me printed material and wants me to read it or transcribe it for the student, this is another area where I utilize my driver. Or, under certain circumstances I may call upon the school counselor to do some reading. Sometimes I will talk to the teacher who handed me the quiz, and we will work on the transcription together. I will get the teacher to do the describing of the diagrams as I write the descriptions in Braille.

On rare occasions I have been asked to transcribe a child's Braille assignments into print. The way in which I handle it might depend on the time element I'm given and the length of the assignment. I could type it out myself; or I could dictate it to someone to write down. Sometimes it works out for me to read the assignment onto a tape for the teacher to listen to. This may depend on what type of lesson it is.

Another favorite aspect of my job is giving talks on blindness. I usually encourage the teachers to group their classes together in large groups for me to talk to. The only time I really like to speak to one class separately is when this class includes one of my regular weekly students. This does not always hold true, however–it depends on that child's needs.

This job has much challenge and variety.

In closing, I want to emphasize that this is how *I* handle the job as a blind person, but it is not hard and fast. Another blind individual might go about it differently, and maybe in time I will do some things differently too.

Postscript

Since writing this article, I have decided to change my personal mode of travel. I now use a guide dog.

I continue to teach in the same general way, including teaching cane travel. I explain to my students that the choice of a travel aid is an individual matter. I also explain that children are not permitted to have guide dogs, and that guide dog schools generally require that candidates already know cane travel.

My use of a guide dog in no way hinders my teaching cane travel. I use my dog when following or watching a student. (I had to train him *not* to go around a student when the student is moving slowly!) If I wish to show a child, physically, how to do something, I place my dog in a "sit-stay" position.

CHAPTER 52

PARAPROFESSIONALS AND VOLUNTEERS

The IEP

The IEP should provide, if necessary, for a paraprofessional or aide (that is, someone who is not necessarily a certified teacher) to prepare materials and/or give individual attention. However, even for a newly-blinded student, it is unnecessary and overprotective to provide full-time individual attention – unless, of course, there are major problems apart from blindness. A description of the time allotment and duties should be written into the IEP.

Study the funding procedures in your state. Some states have "unit funding," based on the number of *classes* or the number of *certified special-education teachers*. Other states have "weighted" funding, based on the needs of *individual students*. Each system has its advantages and disadvantages.

In a resource room or a metropolitan district, you may be fortunate enough to have one or more full-time aides assigned to you permanently. In other areas, aide service may be arranged individually for each child. In any event, it is almost always practical to have someone at the central office to do such things as sending out materials and supplies; transcribing into Braille, large print, or recorded form; ordering materials from elsewhere; and keeping records.

The student's IEP should specify the kind and amount of aide service. Give careful attention to helping the student function without the aide.

Zach worked diligently and behaved well in first grade – until his aide was sick for two days. Then Zach began throwing erasers, talking out in class, pushing children on the playground, and accomplishing almost no work. His aide had always been nearby, nipping misbehavior before it came to the attention of the teachers. Zach needed to learn to be a normal student, *without* an extra person to supervise him. When the aide returned, she was asked to remain on the far side of the room unless specifically assisting with a given task. For certain periods she was to leave the room altogether. After consultation with all playground supervisors, she stopped going out at recess. This kind of problem is one reason to avoid full-time assistance to an individual student.

Hiring the Right Person

As the itinerant/resource teacher, try to discuss the matter of an aide before anyone is actually hired, to avoid misunderstandings over the time needed and the skills required.

Analyze just what the paraprofessional will be doing. Often the work can be done by a secretary or other non-professional staff member already employed by the district. If the student will be served by a multi-categorical resource room, there may be an aide already available from there.

Participate as much as possible in hiring procedures. Ask to take part in interviewing:

(1) Ask the applicant to read some materials

aloud for you. Observe fluency, accuracy, and diction.

(2) If the candidate claims to know Braille, give a test even if he/she has credentials. Allow the use of reference books, but observe how much is looked up, and note overall speed. If the aide is to learn Braille on the job, the best qualification is ability in writing, reading, spelling, and typing.

(3) For a job involving typing or hand-copying, give an actual test in both typing (or copying) and spelling.

(4) Talk with the candidate about attitudes toward blindness – explain that you expect blind students to achieve as well as others and to be independent. Note the candidate's reaction and comments. It is normal to need some educating about attitudes; but if the candidate gushes about the "poor little things" or shows great skepticism, it is a bad sign.

(5) If the aide will work directly with students, ask about previous experience with this. Patience and the ability to work with the age group are essential.

What Will the Paraprofessional Do?

Consider the skills and schedule of each professional person, *vs.* the skills and schedule of the aide. An especially competent aide may be given more responsibility. Be aware, however, of regulations governing what a non-professional person may appropriately be assigned. Aides generally may assist the child in carrying out an activity which has been planned and initiated by a professional, under the continued supervision of that professional. For example, an aide may:

(1) Read aloud from daily handouts and other material which is in regular print.

(2) Assist a young child with a lesson in the regular classroom. For example, the aide might help a beginning reader keep the place in the book; show tactual models or describe pictures during a science lesson; help the child construct a May Basket.

(3) Assist an older youngster in class when he/she is learning new practical skills, as in home economics or industrial arts.

(4) Continue Braille practice in between the itinerant teacher's lessons, using *Patterns* or another suitable book.

(5) Drill in typing or some other specific skill, in between lessons by the itinerant teacher.

(6) Provide extra help or drill in any skill (such as telling time), as directed by the professional staff, when the child is having difficulty.

(7) Prepare materials in large print, Braille, or recorded form.

When possible it is best to have the student follow the regular presentation and then receive extra help later if necessary. However, if the blind child's materials are very different, and attempting to reconcile them to the regular procedure is difficult (as may be the case with Braille maps), working elsewhere may be better.

Give strong guidance to all concerned. Worries over budgeting often lead to inadequate attention. On the other hand, misconceptions about blindness often lead to too much individual help. Also, remember that a child's needs can change greatly over time.

Should the paraprofessional know Braille? If there are several students in one location, or materials to be prepared for several students, it is reasonable to hire or train a Braillist. But when students are far apart geographically, it may not be possible to provide each location with a person who knows Braille *and* can be there every day for general assistance. Instead, it is satisfactory to provide an aide who does not know Braille, to work in cooperation with an itinerant teacher who does know Braille. The chapter on Braille for younger students explains how an aide can work with the *Patterns* reading texts. If the older student has trouble, he should be able to get help from a person using an ink-print copy. The student also should be able to use printed materials which are read aloud to him, rather than being dependent on receiving everything in Braille. He should be able to direct the reader, listen attentively, and take Braille notes.

Supervising the Paraprofessional

The first time I worked with a part-time aide, problems appeared immediately and grew ever larger. The aide was often late; she sometimes did not appear at all, without having notified us; she did not seem to accomplish much; the child said she was cross and unreasonable. The classroom teacher said that the aide was a busy college student with conflicting responsibilities. Problems dragged on until eventually the aide quit voluntarily.

In this case, the aide was already hired when I came into the picture, so I could not have influenced the original hiring. But I now realize that I could have:

- Talked with the principal immediately, and discussed the aide's responsibilities.
- Clarified how and by whom the aide would be supervised.
- Talked much more with the classroom teacher about how we would share the task of directing the aide.
- Talked with the aide herself, before serious problems arose.
- Reviewed the aide's work continually, through tactful discussions with all parties, trying to head off problems.
- If problems were not getting solved, I should have consulted the principal, since he alone had the power to discipline or fire the aide.

We teachers who work with paraprofessionals have a more difficult role, in some ways, than the administrator. Without formal training in staff supervision, we must guide an individual whom we have no power to discipline.

It can be done, however. Be tactful; work closely with other teachers who also work with the aide; and seek help from the principal when necessary.

Each time a new aide is hired, and each time there is a new classroom teacher with whom the aide will work, carefully discuss the aide's role. Be sure everyone understands how you and the classroom teacher will share the supervision, and what the aide will do. Spell out some things the aide should *not* do.

We teachers tread a fine line between (a) lording it over all non-professionals, talking down to them and acting superior, and (b) failing to supervise when it is our place to do so.

Make suggestions privately. Use matter-of-fact explanation rather than fault-finding. Seek opportunities for the aide to help *you* – as by explaining what happened when you were not there. All of this is especially important if the aide is older than you are.

Anticipate new situations, and avoid giving the aide too much responsibility. A teacher should be there the first time a high school student uses a sewing machine, and the first time a young child reads single-spaced Braille.

Consciously think over how to word your directions for the aide, trying to avoid seeming either too vague or too demanding. These phrases are helpful:

"Let's set a policy of ...."
"Please insist that Bill ...."
"I'd like to see you do this ...."
"Here are some things I'd like to see Bill do every day."
"I noticed a problem with ...."
"[A certain situation] doesn't seem to be working out well. I wonder what we should do differently."

Common Problems

OVERDEPENDENCE

Denise was in seventh grade and a good student, but Mrs. Ponce followed her around to every class. "I need to see that all her materials are ready," explained the aide. "I often sit at the back of the room and don't actually help – but I stay in case I'm needed." The classroom teachers seemed to like this arrangement. The itinerant teacher, however, set about to edit the IEP. Soon the IEP provided, "40% of the time, Denise will attend classes without the aide being physically present in the room." Denise learned to organize her own materials, and the classroom teachers learned to interact more directly with her instead of asking the aide to help.

ROLE CONFUSION

When a paraprofessional spends a great deal of time with a student, and the itinerant teacher is only present infrequently, a role-reversal problem may appear. The local staff may become accustomed to consulting the aide, rather than the itinerant teacher, for almost everything. Try to prevent this problem by keeping in touch regularly with all parties. The chapter on "Your Professional Role" contains suggestions which may be helpful with this problem.

STUDENT BEHAVIOR

Matt quickly perceived that the aide had less authority and experience than the teachers. He found innumerable excuses not to work – especially if he and the aide were alone in the room. He told the teachers that Mrs. Jackson (the aide) was cross. He told Mrs. Jackson that the teachers made him work too hard. He made many "mistakes" in delivering messages back and forth about assignments.

Finally the resource teacher set up an arrangement which brought rapid improvement. She asked the aide to write down each of Matt's excuses, and to time him on all assignments. Once a week Matt met with the teachers and Mrs. Jackson *together.* Any inconsistencies or "mistakes" were analyzed. Politeness was emphasized. The plan called for talking with the principal and the parents if the problems persisted, but this proved unnecessary.

Having the aide write down or count something can be very useful. It shows the extent of the problem objectively. It can be a basis for productive discussion. Sometimes the student will cease the behavior immediately upon learning it is to be recorded.

TIME MANAGEMENT

A busy aide may fall farther and farther behind in producing materials – missing deadlines or rushing to deliver materials at the last minute. Urge teachers to submit material as early as possible; look into all possible sources of materials production; strive for efficiency.

Also examine the possibility that students are being given *too much* transcribing service. If an all-out effort is devoted to having every daily handout in Braille or large print, and the student never has to use a reader or do the work at a different time, he or she will not develop the flexibility needed for college and vocational situations.

Be creative in scheduling everyone's time. For example, suppose that the social studies teacher did not get an article to you in time to have it Brailled, and there will be no one to read it aloud during the appropriate period. A solution would be for the aide to tape-record the article. Taping removes the need for the reader's schedule to match the student's. It also provides the student with valuable experience in the use of tapes.

LONG-DISTANCE SUPERVISION

If you are itinerant you may face a special problem: how to direct an aide when you are not even in the building! Let's say that a first grader has individualized reading instruction in *Patterns.* The reading lessons are taught by you three days a week, and on the other two days the aide helps the student continue in *Patterns.* The classroom teacher, while available for supervision, does not know Braille. Neither does the aide – she just uses the *Patterns* manual. How do you, as the only person who knows Braille, prevent problems arising in your absence – reading with one hand; incorrect fingering on the Perkins; describing the sign for "these" as *"b in front of the,"* etc.? How will each of you keep track of what was accomplished by the other? I have found these procedures important:

(1) Be very specific. I once was annoyed with an aide for proceeding slowly through a series of lessons despite my reminders to

speed up. Then I realized I had never explained just what I meant by "faster." When I said, "Let's take at least four pages a day," the problem disappeared.

Providing written, dated lesson plans is by far the best approach.

(2) Maintain a notebook with notes about daily progress. Keep it where you and the aide can get at it.

(3) Talk directly with the aide frequently, by telephone if necessary. Sometimes (especially at first) find a way for both of you to be there at the same time.

(4) Demonstrate your methods while the paraprofessional watches. Also ask the aide to proceed with a lesson while you watch.

(5) Be wary of accepting at face value what the student says the aide did, or even what other adults say the aide did. Ask the individual to explain for himself/herself.

(6) Ask very specific questions. Instead of "How is her arithmetic?" ask "How many problems does she usually do correctly alone?" Other examples might be,

> "Does he find his own locker and put on his coat by himself?"
>
> "When she types, how many errors does she make per page? Are they mostly typographical or spelling errors?"
>
> "When (if at all) do you assist her in going from class to class?"
>
> "I'd like to see samples of his written work – perhaps two or three a week."

(7) Provide written references and explanations. To prevent misunderstanding with the word "these," for example, provide a Braille manual for reference. Also provide an easy-to-read list of the new signs and their verbal descriptions – e.g., "Page 59, *these:* dots 4-5, *the.*

(8) Finally, involve the aide in planning and evaluating. If possible, include the aide in parent conferences. Remember that, although you are the one with professional training, *both* you and the aide are adults with good ideas.

Volunteers

ADVANTAGES AND DISADVANTAGES

Using a volunteer has obvious advantages moneywise. However, since a paid employee is generally more reliable and responsive to supervision, seek other alternatives before assuming that a volunteer is the only choice. If you do use a volunteer, follow the procedures above as much as possible. Interview carefully; work closely with the volunteer to assure that all tasks are being done acceptably; and look for someone else in case of persistent severe problems. The child's own parent is usually one of the worst choices for working directly with a child at school, since it is so hard to step into a different role.

The most common task for volunteers is preparing materials, especially Braille. There are far fewer chances for problems with this task, since the person does not work directly with the child – in fact, often there are no problems in having a family member do it. Note also that materials preparation need not be done at the school.

FINDING VOLUNTEERS

Occasionally a certified teacher who is not currently employed may be willing to volunteer.

College students studying education, or high school students interested in education, may be excellent volunteers.

The Jewish Temple Sisterhoods, Delta Gamma sorority, American Red Cross, and Lions International are examples of organizations especially helpful in volunteer work with the blind. The Library of Congress catalog *Volunteers Who Produce Books: Braille, Large Type, Tape* may help you find transcribers.

Sometimes a competent blind adult is willing to assist a student, thus providing a valuable role model as well as technical help.

The chapter on "Placement Options and Decisions" describes several possible sources of help which may be available without direct cost. In addition to volunteers, other agencies (such as the rehabilitation agency for adults) often can assist young students.

VOLUNTEERS SHOULD BE APPRECIATED

Since a volunteer is not compensated monetarily, give special attention to making him/her feel appreciated and successful. Explain exactly what is wanted, and head off problems quickly. Don't let the volunteer take on more than is reasonable. Provide a buffer to keep anxious persons from besieging a transcriber with last-minute demands: see that requests for Brailling are funneled through a third party. Remind everyone that some things will need to be read "live" instead of being transcribed.

Every volunteer should receive a thank-you note at least once a year, preferably from both the student and an adult. If the individual will be seeking paid employment soon, consider writing a formal letter suitable for use as a recommendation.

CHAPTER 53

WORKING WITH OTHER AGENCIES AND ORGANIZATIONS

Getting Acquainted

Whatever your position of employment, it is always important to be well informed about other agencies and organizations which deal with blindness. Ask around about local services, and read about nationwide services. Visit in person when possible. Learn what services can be expected according to law or custom, and what voluntary organizations may offer under various circumstances.

When there are services which your school or agency does not provide, you should refer families to them appropriately. Get your students in touch with adult services early, to arrange for possible services available for children, and to encourage a smooth transition in services later. If financial aid is needed, know where it may be found. Don't forget that sometimes a nationwide or out-of-state service may be the most logical source for certain things – for example, a specialized course of study from the Hadley correspondence school.

What If There Are Problems?

But what do we do when the other agency has a record of poor service? What if the adult agency tries to steer everyone into a few selected vocations? What if library service is slow and inefficient? What if the preschool counselor says blind children are typically a year behind developmentally? Judgment, tact, and strategy are required in such a situation, and the following ideas may help, alone or in combination:

APPROACHES TO PROBLEMS

(1) *Describe the problem frankly but tactfully,* avoiding a blanket condemnation of the agency. For example, you might say, "The preschool counselor will show you some specific games and activities for your child at home. She has a lot of good ideas I encourage you to use. I might mention, though, that I do not agree with her on one point: she seems to feel that blind children generally develop more slowly than others. In my experience it is an individual matter."

(2) *Emphasize how to get the best possible service:* "When you contact the library, I think you'll get the best service if you first call on the phone and then send a written note confirming what you want. Also, Ms. Wilder and Ms. Hancher are especially helpful – try to talk to one of them if possible. I think that this approach will get you the fastest service."

(3) *Bring in some others for advice:* "Hmm – you say that Mr. Smith from Adult Rehab thinks you'd be better off going to a junior college and taking computer programming, instead of going to a four-year school and taking engineering? Well...your grades are

very good, and it seems to me that you would do well in engineering. This is a big decision, and a person ought to get lots of information and several opinions. You remember the blind mechanical engineer and the two college students that we talked with last summer; I think they could give you some helpful insights. Let's call them and see if we could talk some more."

Bringing in someone else is helpful when you would endanger your job by taking too active a role. Suppose, for example, that your student will soon be graduating from high school, but cannot get the adult rehabilitation counselor to work with him in planning for college. The counselor is always "too busy," and has broken several appointments. Attempts to reach her supervisor have failed. Your student and his parents may need to lodge a formal complaint or appeal about the service (or lack of it) offered by the adult agency. However, you are aware that your employer (the public school) would frown upon your openly and actively working on such a complaint. You can, nevertheless, quietly steer the family toward those (such as the National Federation of the Blind) who can help directly.

You might say, "Well, you may have a major disagreement there. You recall that our school has always kept you informed of your rights in case you should disagree with what we are doing, or feel that we are not meeting our responsibilities. The adult agency must have a similar procedure, and I think you'll want to look into that if you haven't already. I myself would not be able to help you directly. But here are the names of a couple of individuals and organizations that could work with you and give you advice if you wish – they have helped others with similar problems. And of course you may know of someone else you'd like to consult. I do urge you to continue, just as you've done in the past, to really *participate* in educational planning, not just lie back and accept what someone else may say."

WORKING FOR GENERAL IMPROVEMENT

In addition to dealing with each specific problem, keep working for general improvements. Develop a friendship with the preschool counselor and compare notes on the real capabilities of blind children. Help recruit library volunteers, and offer constructive suggestions toward better service. Work with the National Federation of the Blind to bring about reforms of various agencies.

IN THE WORST CASE

A difficult problem occurs when weaknesses are so serious that a particular program does more harm than good, or simply wastes time. Perhaps there is a Christmas party, given by a civic group, where blind people are treated as charity cases and portrayed as such by media coverage. Perhaps an Orientation Center or summer school teaches techniques poorly or incorrectly, and encourages attitudes of inferiority. Usually you will not be able to prohibit anyone from attending such a program, but again you can tactfully comment while seeking to bring about reform. You can say, "We do not recommend that for our students because ...."

Stay Well-Informed and in Touch

The above problems are part of why an educator should be well-informed about other agencies and organizations. We hope to emphasize a more pleasant reason, however: keeping your students and their families in touch with additional services which complement and extend the services of your particular agency.

Keep up with changes in library policies. Be well-acquainted with educational options which are more and less restrictive than those you commonly work with. Are summer schools and other special programs available? Where may help and information be found in regard to special needs? What service organizations (e.g., Lions, Delta Gamma) are most likely to make funds available? What is available for college students, and how are arrangements made? How are blind adults helped to find employment?

The National Federation of the Blind, with its many members continually analyzing the characteristics of various public and private agencies, is the best single source of information.

Encourage Continuity

Often the services of another agency will overlap to some extent with what you offer. Particularly, you will be aware of alternative options in educational placement (residential school, special day school, resource program, itinerant service, etc.) Placement decisions are discussed elsewhere in this book; but it is well to note here the need to be tactful yet assertive. Make clear to parents the advantages and disadvantages of your particular program; work cooperatively when transfer elsewhere appears best for the child.

If staff from another school should try to misrepresent or disparage your program, be assertive in insisting on fairness and accuracy. Be careful about what you yourself say about others' programs. Unfortunately, despite P.L. 94-142, inappropriate pressures still can be found. Some residential schools still grab students without discussing other options. Some special-school personnel still say, "Oh, they don't have anything for blind students there," when they should have said, "They emphasize itinerant service there." Some itinerant teachers still exaggerate what can be done with a given amount of time and resources.

Maximize contact and continuity when a student does receive service from two or more agencies simultaneously or in sequence. When a student attends summer school elsewhere, send plenty of information and suggestions, and ask that they do the same for you. If someone from another agency comes into your school to teach a skill or describe her services, help that person to keep in touch with everyone. Consider whether you could visit a staff meeting of the other agency to describe your own agency, or vice versa. Unfortunate cases of "working at cross purposes" occur all too easily.

Arranging New Contacts

Arranging a new contact is usually most successful if you tell the family about the agency, and *also* tell the agency about the family. You may want to arrange a get-acquainted meeting with yourself included. Generally, if you share any personal information with an outside party, you will need the parent's express permission (or the student's permission, if he/she is of age). Keep well-informed about who is and is not part of the same agency you work for.

A Few Specific Agencies and Organizations

Following are brief descriptions of certain agencies and organizations (by no means a complete list). Your role as a specialist in blindness brings the responsibility to provide information about services such as these.

State Vocational Rehabilitation Agency

Each state has a department of Vocational Rehabilitation for the blind. There is much variation from state to state regarding the size and the administrative status of this agency, as well as the name by which it is commonly known. Its purpose is to provide services to help blind adults live independently and become employed. Various services to children may also be provided. Sometimes certain services are provided through other entities on a contractual basis–e.g., sending clients to a private agency for intensive instruction in daily living skills.

National Library Service (NLS) and Regional Libraries

The National Library Service for the Blind and Physically Handicapped (NLS) is a part of the Library of Congress. Most service is indirect, coming through the regional libraries. Each state (or group of states) offers a lending library of recorded materials, Braille, and large print. If you have not located this service in your area, the regular public library could help you find it.

Books are generally sent through the U.S. Mail (postage free) rather than being checked out in person. Annotated lists and catalogs are available. Tape players and Talking Book Machines–along with accessories and repair service–are available without cost, either through the library or through another state agency working in cooperation.

All regional libraries can offer books and periodicals from NLS. Often additional materials are produced locally. Textbooks are sometimes offered; however this is an additional service rather than being part of the NLS system. (Literature and many other materials, of course, which are important in education without being "textbooks" in the strict sense, are always included.)

The quantity and quality of materials which are readily available, however, varies immensely from state to state. If few materials are on hand, a lengthy interlibrary procedure must occur before a book is found. Service may vary from excellent to abysmal.

The NLS itself offers direct service and consultation on specialized subjects, particularly music and foreign languages.

American Printing House for the Blind (APH)

The American Printing House for the Blind is a major source of educational aids and textbooks. Many Braille and large print books are offered, plus a few recorded items. Educational aids include Braille writing equipment, preschool/kindergarten aids (including reading readiness), tape recorders, math and science aids, maps, games, and materials for the multiply handicapped.

Most items may be purchased by anyone. However, schools can also obtain materials through the "Quota," an annual allotment of Federal funds for every legally blind student enrolled in a formal educational program. The Department of Education in each state has a system of registration for Quota eligibility.

Recording for the Blind (RFB)

Recording for the Blind is a large private agency with an extensive library of elementary, secondary, and college textbooks on cassette tapes, which are loaned free of charge after payment of an initial registration fee. A catalog is provided. Any books not currently available from RFB can be recorded on request (within the limits of the agency's resources). Orders may be placed either directly or through a regional library, but an eligibility form must be filled out for each individual borrower.

National Braille Press, Inc. (NBP)

Children's books which have the text in both inkprint and Braille are offered by NBP. In contrast to most sources of Braille books, which will only lend for a limited time, NBP offers books for purchase at a nominal cost.

National Federation of the Blind (NFB)

The National Federation of the Blind has over 50,000 members, most of whom are blind. Its ultimate purpose is the complete integration of the blind into society on a basis of equality. The NFB works toward this objective through such means as public education programs; legislative changes; counseling the newly blinded; legal counsel for blind persons facing discrimination; Job Opportunities for the Blind (an employment service in cooperation with the U.S. Department of Labor); publications about blindness; scholarships for students; and sale of aids and appliances at nominal cost.

The Federation is a membership organization, supported through contributions from its members and the general public. The members of the Federation believe that, with proper training and opportunity, the average blind person can perform on an equal basis with the average sighted person.

Parents of Blind Children (POBC)

Parents of Blind Children is a national organization of parents, family members, friends, and educators of blind and visually impaired children. POBC offers information and support, and seeks to create a climate of opportunity for blind children in home and society. Literature and videotapes are distributed. Seminars and workshops are conducted around the country. The annual Braille Reading Contest for children has attracted international attention and grows more popular each year.

POBC is a special division of the National Federation of the Blind.

American Brotherhood for the Blind (ABB)

The American Brotherhood for the Blind offers a free, nationwide Braille lending library for blind children and blind parents of sighted children. The library features Twin Vision books–books which have inkprint text and pictures, and also Braille text. The ABB also distributes free Braille calendars each year.

Special services for the deaf-blind are available. For example, *Hot Line to Deaf-Blind* is a bi-weekly newsmagazine in Braille.

The ABB is a private foundation.

American Foundation for the Blind (AFB)

The American Foundation for the Blind offers aids and appliances for direct purchase, with listing in its catalog. Many publications are also available. The AFB is a private foundation.

Other Sources of Materials and Information

The "References" section of this *Handbook* lists complete addresses for all of the above agencies and organizations, as well as for a number of others not described in this chapter. Chapters on particular topics (e.g., computers) may list sources related to that topic. No part of this *Handbook*, however, is intended as an exhaustive list of agencies and organizations.

CHAPTER 54

POSTSECONDARY EDUCATION AND CAREER DEVELOPMENT

When an individual becomes blind, he or she faces two major problems. First, he or she must learn the skills and techniques which will enable him or her to carry on as a normal, productive citizen in the community; and second, he or she must become aware of and learn to cope with public attitudes and misconceptions about blindness–attitudes and misconceptions which go to the very roots of our culture and permeate every aspect of social behavior and thinking.

–From *Blindness: Concepts and Misconceptions,* by Kenneth Jernigan.

This final chapter has borrowed the main title of a publication which is really the "next volume" of this book: *Postsecondary Education and Career Development: A Resource Guide for the Blind, Visually Impaired, and Physically Handicapped.*

The scope of this *Handbook* cannot include a lengthy discussion of life after high school. It does not even do justice to the *preparation* of a young person for life after high school, because the best way to do that is to meet successful blind adults and to learn about many different problems and solutions. Preparation also involves actually practicing many different techniques, in various situations, in order to be thoroughly convinced of their effectiveness.

Therefore, you and your students will want continual contact with the National Federation of the Blind and its publications–particularly the one named above. Written from the perspective of blind and otherwise physically handicapped students themselves, it provides insight on the problems faced by blind individuals seeking higher education, and provides answers and solutions. Here is just a sampling of the many vital topics which are cogently analyzed in the book, *Postsecondary Education and Career Development:*

- Choice of a career
- Choice of a postsecondary school
- The role of the rehabilitation agency
- The role of the postsecondary school
- Tips on techniques
- Library/textbook services
- Employing a reader
- Organizations of the disabled
- "Section 504" and other legislation
- College admissions and recruitment
- Academic adjustments
- Housing
- Financial and employment assistance
- Nonacademic services
- Discussing blindness with college administrators, professors, employers, and others
- Resumes
- Interviews
- Getting a job and working toward promotions

Job Opportunities

Today blind persons are employed in most fields and most positions. Blind people are working as farmers, lawyers, doctors, teachers, assembly workers, secretaries, and janitors. Blind people are social workers, engineers, librarians, printers, sales people, machinists, dishwashers, managers, and writers. Blind people are a cross section of society; and, as such, they are doing the whole range of jobs.

Job Opportunities for the Blind (JOB) is a nationwide program operated by the National Federation of the Blind in partnership with the United States Department of Labor. A major factor in its success is a network of volunteer field service representatives, staff associates, and friends throughout the country. JOB conducts workshops for employers and seminars for applicants; collects job listings; consults about techniques and devices; offers information about services and materials available from various sources; educates employers, applicants, and the public about the capabilities of blind workers; provides general encouragement; and helps to solve problems and overcome barriers.

Adulthood Is a "New Ball Game"

Teachers can help the young person with social development in preparation for good citizenship and family life as an adult. However, this must be continued by contact with blind persons who are already successful citizens, spouses, and parents, and by publications such as those listed below.

With a schoolchild (even a high school student), teachers and parents can *require* that he or she use a given technique, and can authoritatively arrange opportunities for doing it. But after high school, all of that changes: if the individual is not really convinced of the value of a given method or technique, he/she will probably not use it. Furthermore, if the student has not learned resourcefulness and flexibility, he/she will simply give up if a "favorite" technique does not work in a particular situation.

As each student nears the end of high school, talk with him or her about life as a mature adult, and urge continued active contact with the National Federation of the Blind. But a quick talk in the spring of the senior year is not enough. Begin the transition early. In a sense it should begin in earliest childhood with the parents meeting blind adults as role models; the young child should gradually and naturally grow into the relationship of a mature colleague sharing ideas and methods with other blind people.

Discuss sources of services and materials – don't wait until the senior year. Talk about vocations in a general way in first grade, and in detail during high school – don't wait until graduation. Help your students seek out part-time jobs and volunteer work – don't wait until after college. Read through the book, *Post-secondary Education and Career Development,* with your older students.

A Tragic Case

When Pat finished high school, she attended college in her home town. After college she held a series of jobs, but never a permanent one – she continued to live with her parents, who assured her that it did not matter whether or not she contributed to the family budget. She was not idle, but spent her time playing the piano and reading Braille books.

When Pat was 40, her mother died. Suddenly Pat realized she did not know how to care for her clothing, go shopping, cook, or otherwise manage her daily life. She did not have a job. Pat's father, not feeling able to maintain a home for his daughter under these circumstances, placed Pat in a nursing home.

Avoid Dependency

Pat's case is tragic and totally unnecessary, but even this extreme example is not uncommon.

Even more frequent are the less extreme examples:

- A young man aspires to become a mechanical engineer, but is "guided into something more practical for the blind."
- A young woman learns to ride the city bus, but then decides that taxis and

rides with friends are "always so much easier." As time passes, she realizes that she often stays home because her friends are not available, taxis are so expensive, and she has become fearful of riding the bus alone.

- A university student had learned to take good Braille notes in high school. However, at the university he decided to use a tutor and a note-taking service. During his senior year, as he filled out job applications, he began to realize that he had no confidence in his ability to do things on his own.
- A young woman sought an apartment near her new job. Several apartment managers urged her to go to the special housing for the handicapped instead.

  "We don't have an elevator," said one.

  "You might start a fire in the kitchen," said another.

  Since the young woman had no experience in dealing directly with prejudice, and was uncertain where to go for help, she settled for a too-small apartment far from a bus line.
- Another young woman, experienced in the use of computers, located several job openings. In each case, however, she found a compatibility problem in regard to speech output from the computer–and she gave up. She never considered arranging for a person to read the material aloud, or using other alternatives.

Without regular contact with knowledgeable and experienced blind people, and without thoughtfully analyzing the big and little compromises which present themselves constantly, the relatively independent person slips deeper and deeper into the bog of dependency.

The National Federation of the Blind

The National Federation of the Blind has a truly positive philosophy. This is in contrast to many groups of and for the blind, who claim to believe in "independence" but really encourage helplessness in many subtle ways. One NFB member expressed it this way: "Federationists recognize that there is no such thing as a free lunch. Everything has its price, and we recognize that with every privilege comes a responsibility. Allowing others to help us do the things we can do for ourselves will make us seem more dependent and reduce our odds of competitive employment. The odds are enough of a problem as it is."

The National Federation of the Blind can help your student talk with college authorities and employers about blindness in a way that is tactful yet firm and effective. The National Federation of the Blind can help your student realize that if he/she does not know a technique for a given situation, or has forgotten it, a solution can be found through common sense.

References

Below are listed just a few of the publications which are especially relevant to the general transition to adulthood. See "References" for complete bibliographical information.

"Part-Time and Summer Jobs," from *Future Reflections,* April 1982

"Life After High School" articles in *Future Reflections,* July 1982 and May 1983

"About Dating, Blindness and the 'Little Things' of Life," from *Future Reflections,* January-February 1984

Movin' On Out (a general book for young adults who are starting out on their own)

Postsecondary Education and Career Development: A Resource Guide for the Blind, Visually Impaired, and Physically Handicapped

Blindness: New Insights on Old Outlooks

Blindness: The Myth and the Image

Blindness: That's How It Is at the Top of the Stairs

Blindness: The New Generation

Blindness: Concepts and Misconceptions

Blindness: Discrimination, Hostility and Progress

Blindness: Handicap or Characteristic

Have You Considered...? (a publication of Job Opportunities for the Blind)

Competing On Terms of Equality: The Goal and the Reality

Blindness: Of Visions and Vultures (A paper discussing public attitudes toward a blind person's dating and marriage)

I Am a Blind Mother Fighting to Keep My Children From Corruption

This is NOT the end......

APPENDICES

APPENDIX A

A DEFINITION OF BLINDNESS

By Kenneth Jernigan

Before we can talk intelligently about the problems of blindness or the potentialities of blind people, we must have a workable definition of blindness. Most of us are likely familiar with the generally accepted legal definition: visual acuity of not greater than 20/200 in the better eye with correction or a field not subtending an angle greater than 20 degrees. But this is not really a satisfactory definition. It is, rather, a way of recognizing in medical and measurable terms something which must be defined not medically or physically but functionally.

Putting to one side for a moment the medical terminology, what is blindness? Once I asked a group of high school students this question, and one of them replied – apparently believing that he was making a rather obvious statement – that a person is blind if he "can't see." When the laughter subsided, I asked the student if he really meant what he said. He replied that he did. I then asked him whether he would consider a person blind who could see light but who could not see objects – a person who would bump into things unless he used a cane, a dog, or some other travel aid and who would, if he depended solely on the use of his eyesight, walk directly into a telephone pole or fire plug. After some little hesitation the student said that he would consider such a person to be blind. I agreed with him and then went on to point out the obvious – that he literally did not mean that the definition of blindness was to be unable to see.

I next told this student of a man I had known who had "normal" (20/20) visual acuity in both eyes but who had such an extreme case of sensitivity to light that he literally could not keep his eyes open at all. The slightest amount of light caused such excruciating pain that the only way he could open his eyes was by prying them open with his fingers. Nevertheless, this person, despite the excruciating pain he felt while doing it, could read the eye chart without difficulty. The readings showed that he had "normal sight." This individual applied to the local Welfare Department for Public Assistance to the Blind and was duly examined by their ophthalmologist. The question I put to the student was this: "If you had been the ophthalmologist, would you have granted the aid or not?"

His answer was, "Yes."

"Remember," I told him, "under the law you are forbidden to give aid to any person who is not actually blind. Would you still have granted the assistance?" The student said that he would. Again, I agreed with him, but I pointed out that, far from his first facetious statement, what he was saying was this: It is possible for one to have "perfect sight" and still in the physical, literal sense of the word be blind.

I then put a final question to the student. I asked him whether if a sighted person were put into a vault which was absolutely dark so that he could see nothing whatever, it would be accurate to refer to that sighted person as a blind man. After some hesitation and equivocation the student said, "No." For a third time I agreed with him. Then I asked him to examine what we had established:

(1) To be blind does not mean that one cannot see. (Here again I must interrupt to say that I am not speaking in spiritual or figurative terms but in the most literal sense of the word.)

(2) It is possible for an individual to have "perfect sight" and yet be physically and literally blind.

(3) It is possible for an individual not to be able to see at all and still be a sighted person.

What, then, in light of these seeming contradictions is the definition of blindness? In my way of thinking it is this: One is blind to the extent that he must devise alternative techniques to do efficiently those things which he would do with sight if he had normal vision. An individual may properly be said to be "blind" or a "blind person" when he has to devise so many alternative techniques – that is, if he is to function efficiently – that his pattern of daily living is substantially altered. It will be observed that I say *alternative* not *substitute* techniques, for the word *substitute* connotes inferiority, and the alternative techniques employed by the blind person need not be inferior to visual techniques. In fact, some of them are superior. The usually accepted legal definition of blindness already given (that is, visual acuity of less than 20/200 with correction or a field of less than 20 degrees) is simply one medical way of measuring and recognizing that anyone with better vision than the amount mentioned in the definition will (although he may have to devise some alternative techniques) likely not have to devise so many such techniques as to alter substantially his patterns of daily living. On the other hand, anyone with less vision than that mentioned in the legal definition will usually (I emphasize the word *usually*, for such is not always the case) need to devise so many such alternative techniques as to alter quite substantially his patterns of daily living.

It may be of some interest to apply this standard to the three cases already discussed:

First, what of the person who has light perception but sees little or nothing else? In at least one situation he can function as a sighted person. If, before going to bed, he wishes to know whether the lights are out in his home, he can simply walk through the house and "see." If he did not have light perception, he would have to use some alternative technique – touch the bulb, tell by the position of the switch, have some sighted person give him the information, or devise some other method. However, this person is still quite properly referred to as a blind person. This one visual technique which he uses is such a small part of his overall pattern of daily living as to be negligible in the total picture. The patterns of his daily living are substantially altered. In the main he employs alternative techniques to do those things which he would do with sight if he had normal vision – that is, he does if he functions efficiently.

Next, let us consider the person who has normal visual acuity but cannot hold his eyes open because of his sensitivity to light. He must devise alternative techniques to do anything which he would do with sight if he had normal vision. He is quite properly considered to be a "blind person."

Finally, what of the sighted person who is put into a vault which has no light? Even though he can see nothing at all, he is still quite properly considered to be a "sighted person." He uses the same techniques that any other sighted person would use in a similar situation. There are no visual techniques which can be used in such circumstances. In fact, if a blind person found himself in such a situation, he might very well have a variety of techniques to use.

I repeat that, in my opinion, blindness can best be defined not physically or medically but functionally or sociologically. The alternative techniques which must be learned are the same for those born blind as for those who become blind as adults. They are quite similar (or should be) for those who are totally blind or nearly so and those who are "partially sighted" and yet are blind in the terms of the usually accepted legal definition. In other words, I believe that the complex distinctions which are often made between those who have partial sight and those who are totally blind, between those who have been blind from childhood and those who have become blind as adults are largely meaningless. In fact, they are often harmful since they place the wrong emphasis on blindness and its problems. Perhaps the greatest danger in the field of work for the blind today is the tendency to be hypnotized by jargon.

APPENDIX B

THE SEEING SUMMER

A Playlet in Three Short Acts
Adapted by Beth Couch from the novel

THE SEEING SUMMER
By JEANNETTE EYERLY

With Study Guide
By Doris M. Willoughby

This is a dramatization of certain scenes from *The Seeing Summer* by Jeannette Eyerly (Copyright Jeannette Eyerly, 1981. Published by J. B. Lippincott Company, Junior Books, a Division of Harper & Row, Publishers.)

CAST:

NARRATOR
TEACHER (MRS. COUCH)
STUDENTS WITH SPEAKING PARTS:
- LAURA
- MATTHEW
- MARTY
- MEGAN
- THANH
- SARAH
- TONY
- KATHY
- BECKY
- DAVID
- LINNETTA
- JOSH

OTHER STUDENTS
JENNY
CAREY
ICE CREAM LADY
OTHER CUSTOMER(S)
CASHIER
STAGE HANDS

There is a part in the play for every child in the group which is giving the performance. Those without speaking parts will play the other students in the classroom scenes. They may also double as stage hands, as "other customers" in the ice cream store, etc.

This adaptation of *The Seeing Summer* was the idea of Mrs. Beth Couch, the 4A teacher at Perkins Elementary School in Des Moines, Iowa. All the children in Mrs. Couch's class had previously read the book. The playlet was presented for the first time at the school on April 22, 1985, and has since been expanded by Jeannette Eyerly to include two more scenes.

ACT ONE

Scene 1

Scene: An elementary classroom. The teacher is sitting at her desk, correcting papers. Any number of children can be sitting on the floor or at their desks. They are reading or writing. There is an American flag on a standard in one corner of the room; perhaps there are some maps or a chalkboard on the wall. A narrator is standing at one side of the stage.

LAURA: [*looks up from her book and raises her hand*]

MRS. COUCH: Yes, Laura?

LAURA: What is it like to be blind?

MRS. COUCH: Class, Laura has asked a good question. Do any of you have any ideas to share on what being blind would be like?

MATTHEW: Well, I can answer that. I think it would be dark.

MARTY: Yeah. You'd bump into everything.

MEGAN: No, that's not right. People would have to lead you around so you wouldn't bump into things.

THANH: You would look funny when you got dressed. You can't see, so you would have on maybe one red sock and one pink one.

SARAH: You would lose all of your money because you couldn't tell a $20.00 bill from a $1.00 bill.

LAURA: Blind people are what you call handicapped people.

MARTY: Yeah! That's right. They can't learn things like we do because they can't see to read. If you can't read, you can't learn.

MRS. COUCH: You people have expressed a lot of ideas on what you think being blind is like. Does anyone have a suggestion on how we could go about learning more about being blind?

MATTHEW: Why don't we look in the card catalogue in our library. You said sometimes authors write about problems so we can have a better understanding of what the problem is really like.

MRS. COUCH: Good idea, Matthew! Why don't you go to the library and ask Mr. Knight if he could help you find a book about blindness.

[*As Matthew hurries off stage, the curtain falls.*]

Scene 2

Same as Scene 1

MRS. COUCH: That was a quick trip, Matthew! Did you have any luck?

MATTHEW: Yes! I found *The Seeing Summer* by Jeannette Eyerly. Mr. Knight said it was real good.

MRS. COUCH: Shall I read it to you?

CHILDREN: [*loudly*] Yay! Read it! Read it!

MRS. COUCH: [*reading from THE SEEING SUMMER*] 'Hopping on one foot, Carey glared at the chunk of cement that had worked its way up from a crack in the sidewalk. Tears came to her eyes–not because of pain, though her toe did hurt a lot, but from disappointment...'

Curtain

ACT TWO

Scene 1

Scene: Front steps of Jenny's house. Jenny is sitting there with her long white cane. Carey comes up the sidewalk, holding a plate of cookies.

NARRATOR: More than anything else, Carey wants a new ten-year-old playmate to replace the friend who has moved away. When she hears that the new family next door has a girl just her age, she straightens up her room and settles down to wait for the movers to arrive next door. But when they do, she is stunned to learn that her new young neighbor is blind and uses a white cane. Not fair! Surely, the new girl will not be able to do anything that Carey likes to do.

CAREY: [*loudly clearing her throat and yelling*] HELLO!

JENNY: [*in a cross voice*] I'm not deaf. You needn't YELL.

CAREY: [*in a squeaky voice*] I didn't yell.

JENNY: Yes, you did. When people first know you're blind, they always yell. They think because you can't see, you can't hear either.

CAREY: [*speaking in a low voice and staring fixedly at Jenny*] Well, if I yelled, I'm sorry. I came over to get acquainted. I live next door. My name is Carey Cramer.

JENNY: My name is Jenny Ann Lee, but I like to be called plain Jenny. I'm ten, just like you are. The real estate lady told me that. And you don't need to stare, either.

CAREY: [*loudly*] I'm not! [*She scrubs the toe of her sneaker over the sidewalk.*]

JENNY: Yes, you were. I can tell. I can feel you....You brought something over. Something to eat. What is it?

CAREY: [*stammering*] Coo-cookies. How did you know?

JENNY: Because I smelled them. Don't be stupid. Chocolate chip?

CAREY: [*admiringly*] That's *very* good! I was beginning to think... [*she pauses, then continues lamely*]... think that you weren't, well.....

JENNY: [*getting louder with each word*] Blind, blind, BLIND! So what?

CAREY: So...nothing....

JENNY: Why didn't you want to say blind, then?

CAREY: [*stepping backward*] I...I...don't know.

JENNY: [*scowling*] Yes, you do! You think blind is bad!

CAREY: [*winking back tears and starting to run back home*] Well, maybe I do, but I think mean is worse. [*She pauses, then looking confused, comes back to where Jenny is still sitting on the steps.*] Here are your old cookies. I forgot to give them to you.

JENNY: [*a little shyly*] I'm glad you came back. If you hadn't, I was going over to your house and say *I* was sorry. But sometimes, when people yell or stare or feel sorry for me, it makes me mad. Let's go in the house and you can meet my mom and my baby brother. [*She stands up*] You can carry the cookies, if you like.

Curtain

ACT TWO

Scene 2

Time: The next day.

Scene: The front porch of Carey's house. Jenny is knocking at the door; she is holding her long white cane.

CAREY: [*Coming to the door. She looks surprised.*] Oh! Hi! Did your mom bring you over?

JENNY: Nope. I came by myself. I knew you lived next door and that the first sidewalk I came to would lead to your house.

CAREY: *I* couldn't do it.

JENNY: You could if you had to. [*She shrugs.*] But right now, what do you want to do?

CAREY [*bewildered*] 'Do?'

JENNY: I don't care. Go for a walk. Swing. Climb that tree in my side yard. Anything that's fun. We could play cards. I brought mine, just in case.

CAREY: [*who obviously thinks Jenny can't do anything*] Play cards...I guess.... We can play here on the porch, if you want.... [*The girls sit down on the floor. Jenny takes a pack of cards from her pocket and then hands one to Carey*]

JENNY: Those little bumps on it tell you what card it is. If the card is the Jack of Hearts, there will be the letter 'j' and the letter 'h' in Braille. If it's the eight of hearts, it will have the letter 'h' and number '8' in Braille. Do you understand?

CAREY: [*dragging out the words*] I...guess....

JENNY: Now this – [*she hands Carey another card*] this is the king of diamonds. Right?

CAREY: [*inspecting it*] Right.

JENNY: Of course, *you* don't have to pay any attention to the bumps. I'm just explaining it to you. Now what shall we play? Fish? Go Dig? King's Corners? I don't care. [*She begins to shuffle the cards while the narrator speaks*]

NARRATOR: Carey knows how to play Fish, and Go Dig, but she does not know how to play King's Corners. So she says "King's Corners" because she thinks this will give Jenny an advantage. Bumps or no bumps, she does not know how Jenny can tell the cards apart. Of course, she plans to let Jenny win – though not by too much. Jenny would suspect something and that would make her mad.

JENNY: Now, this card [*she lays one down, face up*] is a clover. A ten.

CAREY: Club. A ten of clubs.

JENNY: I call them clovers, because that's what they look like. Mama showed me the shape.

CAREY: Well...O.K.

JENNY: You go first.

CAREY: No. You.

JENNY: Well, then, because this is a clover out here in the middle, if I have any clovers in my hand I can play them. Like this. [*She takes three cards from her hand – all clovers – and slaps them smartly down on the card in the middle.*] Now I draw one. And then, I have to throw one away, like this. Now it's your turn. [*She sits back on her heels.*] Just remember, whoever gets rid of all her cards first, wins.

[*Carey very slowly draws three cards from one of the piles in the middle, then plays just one. The game continues as the narrator speaks.*]

NARRATOR: [*in a rather conspiratorial voice*] Carey is being as careful as she knows how to be. But at times, it looks as if Jenny is helping *her.* She keeps getting more and more cards in her hand, and Jenny has fewer and fewer.

JENNY: [*kindly*] You shouldn't have thrown that card away. You have to remember which cards *I* played. You have to use your head. Now, it's my turn again. [*She plays two more cards in the middle and draws one from the pile.*] If you're not careful, I'm going to win. It's your turn again.

[*They play for a second or two longer, then Jenny lays down her last card.*]

JENNY: [*kindly*] I win. Do you want to play again?

CAREY: Not right now. I have kind of a headache. Why don't we go for a little walk?

Curtain

ACT TWO

Scene 3

Time: A short time later

Scene: Carey's bedroom. She may be seated at her desk, or lying on her stomach. She is busily writing in a small notebook. [*Carey's spelling is reproduced in this copy as shown in the novel; however the narrator will not call attention to the spelling.*]

NARRATOR: If we look over Carey's shoulder, we can see what she is writing in her diary:

BLIND PEEPLE

(1) Don't yell at them. They aren't deff.
(2) Don't stare at them. They can feel you doing it and they don't like it.
(3) Don't try to help them do anything if they think they can do it themselves. Sometimes they can.

Curtain

ACT TWO

Scene 4

Time: Several days later.

Curtain is closed as narrator begins.

NARRATOR: As Carey and Jenny get to know each other better, they start doing more and more fun things together. One day Jenny's mother suggests that they walk to a drug store in a nearby shopping center. She wants them to buy some ointment for Jenny's baby brother. Carey is surprised to see that Jenny pays for the ointment and gets back the correct change. She does not know how she does it! Jenny's mother has also given her some extra money to buy ice cream cones at Bobbitt's, a special shop that makes 50 different kinds. We see the girls now at the ice cream shop.

Curtain opens.

Scene: Interior of an ice cream store. The Ice Cream Lady is standing behind a counter. A big printed sign on the wall reads FIFTY DIFFERENT KINDS. The various kinds are listed but the letters may be too small for the audience to read. As the curtain opens, Carey is in the middle of reading the names of the 50 different kinds of ice cream. The Ice Cream Lady is waiting on another customer. The cashier sits at her desk at the other end of the stage.

CAREY: [*drawing a deep breath*] ...Karmel Krunch Pecan, Marshmallow Delight, Marshmallow Nut Fudge, *Nutty* Nut Fudge, Pecan Parfait, Strawberry Surprise, Wonderful Watermelon, and Youngberry Yummy Delight. So far, I've had 18 different kinds. So it's getting harder and harder to make up my mind. My ambition is to have all 50.

JENNY: My ambition is to have all 50, too. But it will take me longer to catch up.

The Ice Cream Lady has just finished waiting on another customer, who walks over to the cashier.

I.C. LADY: [*to Carey*] All right, my dear. And what will it be for you today?

CAREY: I'll have.....oh, let me see. Marshmallow Nut Fudge. A double-decker, please.

I.C. LADY: [*glancing at Jenny*] And your little friend, here? What will *she* have?

CAREY: [*in an exasperated voice*] Don't ask *me*. Ask *her*. She can talk.

I.C. LADY: [*embarrassed*] Oh...I didn't mean anything. It's just that...I thought....

JENNY: [*very politely*] I'll have a Karmel Krunch Pecan double-decker, please.

I.C. LADY: [*a little nervously*] A Karmel Krunch Pecan and a Marshmallow Nut Fudge. [*She hands Carey her cone. She fixes Jenny's cone but does not give it to her. She then speaks in a loud whisper.*] Will your little friend be able to handle the cone by herself?

JENNY: [*reaching for the cone, and laughing*] Try me and see. [*She starts gobbling down the ice cream. Carey and the Ice Cream Lady start laughing, too.*]

I.C. LADY: I *deserved* that. I'll know better next time. You can pay the cashier on the way out.

The girls walk toward the cashier's desk, Jenny swinging her long white cane before her.

JENNY: You'd better hold my cone while I pay her. But don't lick. [*Jenny takes two bills from her purse, hands one to the cashier and puts one back in her purse.*] Here's a five. And here's our check for two double-decker cones.

CASHIER: [*counting out three one-dollar bills and some change*] I've a nephew who is blind, and I've noticed he folds his five-dollar bills the long way, just as you do. The one-dollar bills he leaves just as they are. And the tens, he folds in half the short way.

JENNY: I haven't had any ten-dollar bills yet. But when I do, that's the way I'll fold mine.

CAREY: [*wonderingly*] I was wondering how you could tell the difference. But I guess anything is easy, once you know how.

[*Curtain falls as girls go off munching their cones.*]

ACT THREE

Scene 1

[*Curtain closed*]

NARRATOR: The summer moves happily along. Each day Carey and Jenny find some new things to do. Jenny teaches Carey to read and write Braille. They have what they call a "hot line" between their two houses – a coffee can, on a pulley, in which they write messages to each other in Braille. They also run races in the park. Then Jenny disappears! Two shady characters, who know Jenny's father is very rich, kidnap her and hold her for ransom. Carey, hoping to rescue her, gets kidnaped, too, and the two girls wind up together in a deserted warehouse in a run-down part of the city.

Curtain opens.

Scene: Inside the warehouse. Carey and Jenny are curled up side by side on a pile of old blankets. The whole room has been made as dark as practical. Carey, who has been crying rather loudly, sits up.

NARRATOR: [*in a spooky voice*] It is *very* dark in the warehouse. Though *you* can see what is happening on the stage, Carey cannot see a thing.

JENNY: While you've been crying, I've been thinking. I know something we can do to get out of here.

CAREY: [*sniffling*] What?

JENNY: Explore.

CAREY: You can't explore in the dark.

JENNY: I've told you about a million times that darkness isn't like being blind. Closing your eyes isn't like being blind either. When *you* close *your* eyes, your eyes are looking at the inside of your eyelids. And it's dark in there. I don't see 'black' and I don't see 'darkness' because I don't see anything at all – except with my mind.

CAREY: I still don't see how you can explore *this* place. It's big. Bigger than fifty houses. Besides, you don't know where anything is.

JENNY: [*sighing*] Listen. If you know where things are, you're not exploring. Come on. I'll show you the listening spot. I found that before you came.

[*Both girls get up and start off in the darkness. Carey is feeling ahead of her with arms outstretched. Jenny is moving briskly along using her long white cane.*]

Curtain

ACT FOUR

Scene 1

Scene: Same as Act I, Scene 1. Mrs. Couch is just finishing reading THE SEEING SUMMER aloud to the children.

NARRATOR: Will the girls escape from the kidnappers? You'll have to read *The Seeing Summer* to find out.

MRS. COUCH: '.....Carey dug her fists into her eyes until the darkness was sprinkled with tiny rainbow-colored dots and streamers. She was glad she wasn't blind.....yet seeing with one's eyes wasn't the only way of seeing. Jenny had taught her that.' [*Smiling, she closes the book and puts it down.*] Well, boys and girls. We've come to the end of *The Seeing Summer*. Have any of you changed your mind about blindness?

TONY: I have! They are people just like we are. They have feelings.

THANH: Yeah! When you learn how to do things, blindness is just an inconvenience....

KATHY: With a long white cane, a blind person can go anywhere!

BECKY: And in Braille they can read as well as we can.

DAVID: Yeah! They just use their fingers instead of their eyes.

LINNETTA: And they have neat ways to match colors, too.

JOSH: They can do the same things *we* do.

MATTHEW: *I* think we're lucky to have authors like Jeannette Eyerly who can write books like *The Seeing Summer* so we can understand what blindness is really like.

CHILDREN: Yay! Yay! [*All the children in the class shout and clap as the curtain falls.*]

Curtain

STUDY GUIDE
By Doris M. Willoughby

Credits and Honors

With the gracious permission of novelist Jeannette Eyerly and playlet originator Beth Couch, the National Federation of the Blind is distributing this dramatization as a public service. Royalties are waived, but credit should always be given to the authors. Additional copies of this playlet are available from the National Federation of the Blind.

The copyright to *The Seeing Summer* novel is held by Jeannette Eyerly.

The Seeing Summer has been nominated in a number of states as an outstanding book for children.

The Macmillan Co. reading textbook, *Winning Moments,* includes an illustrated excerpt from *The Seeing Summer. Winning Moments* is also being published in Spanish.

Suggestions and Remarks

This playlet is an ideal way to help children really internalize positive attitudes about blindness. Any class within a wide age range can use this play to build better understanding of blindness.

In a school where there is one blind child, or a small number of blind children, this playlet provides a way to dramatize and discuss day-to-day learning experiences.

A class of blind children in a special school can use this also; blind children may play the parts of sighted children. This can add to their understanding of sighted people and how to interact well with them.

Many classes do not have a blind student as a member or even an acquaintance. This playlet is an excellent introduction to the idea of blindness as a characteristic, not a tragic affliction.

A Scout group, religious instruction class, etc., may be especially interested because of the emphasis on understanding other people.

The beginning and ending scenes (where the class plays itself) provide added identification and involvement.

SUGGESTIONS FOR STAGING

Jenny's White Cane: It is best to obtain a real white cane of suitable size. One can be purchased from the National Federation of the Blind (1800 Johnson Street, Baltimore, MD 21230), or it may be possible to borrow one from an agency teaching blind children. A dowel rod or similar item can be used if necessary.

When held upright, a cane of appropriate length will reach approximately to the shoulder of the person using it. When the individual is standing still, as when Jenny arrives to play cards, she probably will hold the cane upright. It may be held loosely in the crook of the arm.

When Jenny is walking, she should hold the cane at an angle, so that the top of the handle is centered at waist height. (See Figure B-1.) She holds the handle in either hand, preferably with the forefinger extended slightly to direct the cane as it taps back and forth from side to side.

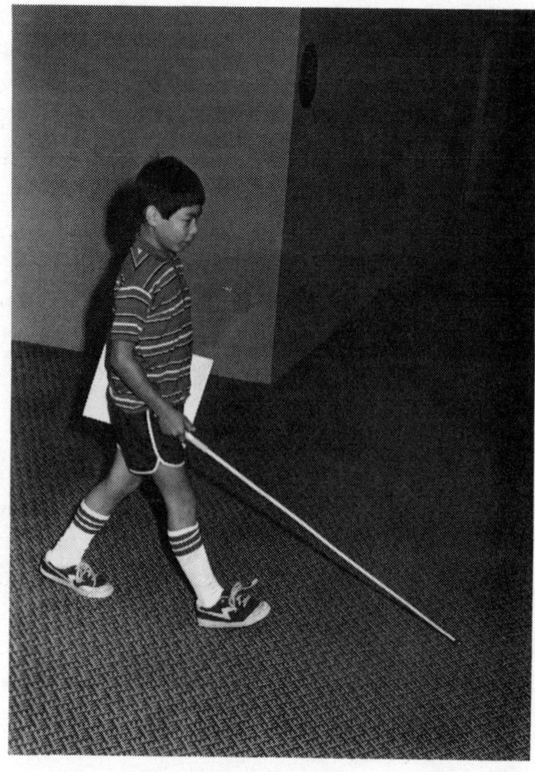

Figure B-1
Walking With Cane

If an object is in the way, the cane strikes it and Jenny then adjusts her direction to go around it.

When Jenny sits down, she should lay her cane on the floor beside her, in a position not likely to trip others.

Note that the cane goes along to the warehouse.

Brailled Playing Cards: Although the use of playing cards with real Braille is excellent, this is not essential. Brailled cards are regular playing cards with Braille added; an audience would probably not be able to see the difference. The girls could feel the cards and pretend that the Braille is there. As described in the text, the Braille marking consists of two symbols (e.g., 2h for Two of Hearts) at the top of the card. It is repeated in the opposite orientation at the other end, so that the card may be held either way.

Ice Cream: It is difficult to keep real ice cream from melting before it is used. A good substitute is pudding, which will look like ice cream to the audience.

Stage Setting: The setting can be extremely simple or rather elaborate, as desired. Note that if an actual curtain is used, some scenes can be performed in front of it while the set is changed behind the curtain.

Names: Except for Mrs. Couch, the originator of this playlet, the names of the school staff and students are arbitrary. The intent is that everyone in the class, as well as the teacher, play him/herself. The real names of the students, the teacher, and the librarian should be substituted for the names used here. (It need not be a fourth grade class.) All of this helps to make the dramatization a real life experience.

Portraying Blindness: Seek advice from a competent blind adult. Avoid two extremes in portraying Jenny: (a) exaggerated attempts to make her "look blind," and (b) inaccuracies which detract from her portraying a genuine blind person. A good example is the matter of how she reaches for the pile of cards. As an experienced blind player, she should not grope around with no idea where to reach. On the other hand, she would not always reach directly for the pile every time. Sometimes she would miss the pile slightly and then search gently to find it quickly.

As another example, Jenny *should* face toward the other person when she is conversing. A blind person listens to the voice and faces toward the sound.

It is *not* desirable for Jenny to wear dark glasses, which tend to encourage stereotyping.

FURTHER STUDY

The entire novel, *The Seeing Summer,* should be actually read. It is not long, and it is interesting and entertaining for all ages.

The playlet brings out a number of "study questions" which are answered by the end of the performance (e.g., "Can blind people get around by themselves?") Many other such questions will arise as the play is prepared and as the novel is read.

If at all possible, invite a competent blind adult to speak to the class and answer questions about methods and attitudes. While Jeannette Eyerly was writing the novel, she talked in depth with many blind adults and blind children. She also served for three years on the board of the Iowa Commission for the Blind.

All students will enjoy practicing using the cane and writing Braille.

In the *Handbook for Itinerant and Resource Teachers of Blind and Visually Impaired Students,* by Doris M. Willoughby and Sharon L. M. Duffy, the chapter on "Learning About Blindness" offers help in discussing literature. Also, the "Reference" section of the *Handbook* lists a number of publications which provide accurate information. *Questions Kids Ask About Blindness,* from the American Brotherhood for the Blind, is especially helpful.

Important Points to Emphasize

- Blind people are regular people, just like you and me.
- Blind people sometimes use different methods to do things, but accomplish the same tasks as other people.
- A blind person will not necessarily need or want more help than anyone else.
- Blind people are human; they are not perfect. Notice that Jenny overreacted to Carey's original hesitancy; later she insisted that Clubs were "Clovers;" etc.
- Sighted people usually have a lot of wrong ideas about blindness. These wrong ideas often bother blind people a lot.
- A white cane is an effective tool for getting around.
- Braille is another way to read. A blind child reads Braille just as others read inkprint.

A Safety Lesson Also

This dramatization can also be a springboard for discussion on a completely different topic: avoiding dangerous strangers.

Jenny and Carey were very fortunate: one of the kidnapers, at least, really did not want them to be harmed. Discuss the mistakes the girls made about protecting themselves against dangerous strangers. What could have happened if they had not been lucky?

How can a child (blind or sighted) protect himself or herself? Note that the mere fact of being blind does *not* need to make one extra-vulnerable to kidnaping or other dangers.

Jenny should remember rules such as the following:

Walk briskly and purposefully, thus showing that one is not helpless and vulnerable.

Pay attention to the general environment – e.g., high-crime area *vs.* serene rural community. (A youngster should be advised by parents. A more mature person can inquire about a new locale, and note clues such as rough speech and rundown buildings.)

It is *not* necessary or desirable to answer personal questions from strangers.

Avoid mentioning names and addresses in public.

Be wary of suspicious circumstances or conversations, and report them to parents as soon as possible.

Never get into a car with someone without being certain that it is someone approved by parents. The blind child can identify voices and think about what is said.

Do not believe stories of "emergencies" such as that told by the kidnaper. Many families have special code words to avoid this problem.

Never try to investigate a crime by yourself as Carey did.

Find a way to leave if a situation becomes unsafe. Learn to figure out how to get home on foot. When that is not possible or safe, locate a phone to call parents or a taxi. Carry a small amount of money for emergencies.

APPENDIX C

SUGGESTIONS FOR THE BLIND COOK

By Ruth Schroeder and Doris M. Willoughby

[*Note: This booklet is available separately from the National Federation of the Blind. The majority of the text is reprinted here.*]

The Regular Home Economics Class

Today more and more blind students are attending regular schools and colleges, thus taking their places in the mainstream of society. They participate in home economics classes as a normal part of their education. Recipes and other written material can be transcribed into Braille or large print. When a demonstration is given, the blind student listens to the verbal description, possibly with a classmate quietly narrating as needed, and examines equipment tactually. Using techniques such as those described in this paper, the blind student takes part fully in all class activities.

It is vital that the blind student actually *do* each kind of task, although he or she will often use alternative techniques. Other students may genuinely feel that they are helping the blind student by doing things for him; however, they must learn that unnecessary help is really a hindrance. If partners work together, they should keep track of how they divide the work (including clean-up duty) each time, and rotate this so that the blind student does each part of the work some of the time.

Cooking is one of the few situations where using a cane is not practical. Therefore, it is helpful to keep doors (including cupboard doors) either open flat or fully closed, and to inform the blind student about objects in the aisles.

The parents of a blind youngster should be careful not to exclude him from helping with cooking, dishwashing, etc., at home. A difficult time is in store for any student who enters a home economics course without having had any prior experience at home.

Equipment

In most situations no special equipment is necessary; all that is needed is to use the other senses well, as in listening for when the carrots begin to boil. Many items of equipment designed for the sighted are especially appropriate for the blind as well – pie-cutting guides, needle threaders, and metal measuring cups, for example. A kitchen timer which is sold on the regular market but happens to have well-placed raised markings is another example.

Plan the storage of your equipment and utensils so that you will not waste time unnecessarily in looking around for them. At the same time, however, you should realize that your plans will not always work perfectly in practice; you should be able to hunt around if necessary and find an item which someone else has put away in a different place.

Many helpful tools and appliances are available. However, in most situations it is a matter of personal choice as to whether to buy a special appliance or to use another approach (such as adapting a regular tool or appliance, or using a different method). Avoid overdependence on special tools or rigidly defined techniques.

Further discussion of specific types of equipment is included under many of the topics below.

What About Commercial Settings?

The blind person often uses the sense of touch to gain information that a sighted person would probably gain through sight. The beginning cook should keep his or her hands very clean and use them as necessary to gain information – touch rolls to see if they feel done, check the shape of a piecrust, etc.

The experienced blind cook can abide by any requirements of sanitation and formality as necessary. He/she is able to avoid directly touching any of the food with the fingers, by such means as wearing thin plastic gloves or using a utensil or appliance. Whenever this paper speaks of touching something, it should be assumed that the experienced cook can find a way to avoid using unprotected fingers if circumstances so require. Hundreds of blind men and women are successful managers or employees of commercial restaurants and snack bars. This paper, however, is *not* in any way a manual of methods for commercial operations. We invite you to write to the National Federation of the Blind and ask for information on commercial methods.

Recipes

Braille and large print cookbooks are available on loan from many libraries for the blind. A few cookbooks in recorded form also exist; these may be helpful to those who have severe circulatory problems or other special difficulties in learning Braille. If you do not know the location of your local library for the blind, you may inquire of your regular local public library; or contact the National Library Service for the Blind and Physically Handicapped, Library of Congress (see "References"). Also, cookbooks may be purchased from the American Printing House for the Blind and other sources.

Braille recipe files may also be made. Although the user of an inkprint recipe file prefers to have the front of each card facing toward him, with the title at the top, most Braille readers prefer a different arrangement. You will probably prefer to insert the Braille cards with the top down, with the Brailled side of each card away from you; this way your fingers will reach the Braille most comfortably. Because of this, the title of each recipe should be placed *below* the recipe as it is written on the card; the titles will then be easily accessible, as the bottoms of the cards appear at the top of the file box. Similarly, labels on file dividers should be placed upside down on the backs of the tabs.

A frequently-used recipe will last longer if a plastic page or card is used. It is also helpful, while using a particular recipe, to tape it to a cupboard door, or in some other way support it so that it is not lying on the mixing surface, and thus keep it as clean as possible.

Marketing

You will select, from many good alternatives, the method of marketing that works best for you in a particular set of circumstances. Most grocery stores, especially during the less busy hours, are willing to assign an employee to accompany you around the store and assemble your order as you direct. Alternatively, you may choose to shop with a friend or relative. If you hire a reader or a driver, you may decide to use him or her as a shopping assistant on occasion. You may wish to telephone a store that will deliver.

Be systematic as you place the groceries on your shelves at home. Plan where to keep each kind of item, and be consistent. If containers cannot easily be distinguished by touch, label them in Braille. (Store clerks and delivery people should be willing to read the inkprint labels for you as necessary.) One way of labeling is to write the name of the item on a 3" x 5" card, and then attach the card to the container with a rubber band. Reusable labels may also be purchased.

Measuring Ingredients

Metal measuring cups and spoons sold on the regular market are very convenient for the blind cook. Using measuring spoons with dry ingredients is no different for the blind cook than for the sighted. For liquids, however, we suggest that you bend the spoon so that the bowl is at right angles to the handle; keep each liquid ingredient in a wide-mouthed jar, so that the bent spoon may simply be lowered into it and then lifted out full. A popular convention is to bend the one-half teaspoon and one-tablespoon measures in each set, so that half of the spoons are adapted for liquids, and so that the spoons can be told apart by touch very quickly and easily. Steel spoons can be easily bent without damage.

It is very convenient to use nesting measuring cups, and fill the appropriate measure completely full in the usual manner. A one-cup measuring cup with raised fractional markings on the inside may also be used, however.

If a recipe calls for a measured amount of boiling water, we suggest that you measure the water *before* heating it. If you use the water immediately when it begins to boil, the evaporation loss will not be significant.

Cutting, Grating, and Peeling

The actual process of peeling, slicing, or grating is no different for the blind than for the sighted. As in all phases of cooking, safety depends upon competence and care rather than upon sight.

It is much easier and more satisfactory to grate or cut into a large bowl rather than onto a flat surface. The food is then automatically collected and easily manageable.

If you are a beginner who has had little or no experience in using a knife, you may find it easier and safer at first to cut downward toward a cutting board. The experienced cook uses a knife in various positions, however; and the newly blinded experienced cook will probably not change her ways of using a knife.

A suggested method for chopping vegetables into small pieces is as follows: Slice the vegetables into a large bowl. Then use a "Kwik-Kut Food Chopper," which resembles a round cookie or biscuit cutter but is very sharp on the bottom. (This cutter is available on the general market.) Chop the cutter up and down through the slices, moving around within the bowl and continuing until the pieces are the desired size and uniformity.

Pouring, Draining, and Mixing

If a tray or cookie sheet with raised edges is placed underneath the bowl while pouring and mixing, messiness and loss due to spillage can be minimized. A tray is also helpful for the same reason when carrying things which might spill–for example, a custard pie or gelatine dessert which has not yet set.

Place several small desserts or custards together on one tray in the oven or refrigerator.

Whenever possible, avoid unnecessary carrying: for example, measure ingredients immediately beside the mixing bowl, and prepare gelatine near the refrigerator. You may even wish to place a piecrust on the oven shelf before pouring in the liquid filling.

An "Oven Saver"–a round metal sheet with crimped edges and with a hole in the middle for heat circulation–is also good for prevention of spillage problems with pies both outside and inside the oven. This item is sold on the general market.

There are many methods for pouring and draining. For large quantities, a nervous beginner may wish to dip with a cup or ladle; however, pouring from one container to another in the regular manner may be accomplished with some practice. You may keep one hand on the receiving container to keep track of its location. With practice it is relatively easy to learn to judge the fullness of a container by sound and weight.

Depending on formality and other circumstances, you may determine when the desired level is reached by placing your finger over the lip of the container, counting the number of dips with your ladle, estimating, or using a liquid level indicator. With very thick mixtures such as cake batter, check that the level is even all across the pan. When filling an angel-food cake pan, cover the hole in the middle with a small plastic bag or a tiny jelly glass.

Using a screw-top jar or other shaker to mix the flour with the liquid is helpful in making white sauce and gravies.

Probably the easiest method of draining vegetables is to pour them into a colander or strainer: if the colander or strainer is placed over a bowl, any spilled vegetables will be retrievable. The experienced cook may prefer another method.

There are several good methods for separating eggs. One way is to break the shell into two unequal parts; lift off and discard the small end; then drain off the white. It is also possible to buy a special tool for separating eggs.

Stirring by hand usually presents no particular problem. Use a bowl that is large enough to minimize splashing, and be sure to scrape the sides of the bowl as necessary. If the bowl slides around annoyingly, set it on a damp cloth or some other non-slippery surface.

Although the beginner may feel nervous about an electric mixer, normal safety precautions make it as safe for the blind cook as for the sighted. The condition of the mixture may be observed and controlled by using a rubber spatula and/or by stopping the machine to check with the fingers.

For methods in pouring coffee or tea, see the paragraphs on "Serving the Food."

Plugging in an Appliance

If you are a beginner who has not yet learned how to plug in an appliance safely, the following suggestions may be helpful: First locate the outlet tactually and observe the orientation of the holes. With your right hand holding the plug by the insulated portion, bring the plug up to the outlet, but *do not* begin to push it in. Checking with your left hand to see that the prongs are oriented in the same direction as the holes, bring the plug up so that the prongs are over the holes, but *do not* yet push the prongs in, even part way. Remove your left hand, and be sure that your right hand is touching only the insulated portion of the plug. Now push the plug into the outlet.

Dials and controls

Dials and controls may easily be adapted to use without sight. With experience, you will be able to obtain the necessary information quickly from the appliance salesperson or some other sighted person, and arrange a plan to operate the dials easily and accurately.

For each dial or knob, you will need to define at least one reference point on the moving part and at least one reference point on the background behind it. You may have several reference points on the dial and just one on the background, or you may have several reference points on the background and just one on the dial.

Look first for already-existing features which you can use. Following are several examples of settings which can be used without any added markings:

(1) Turn the dial clockwise, or counterclockwise, as far as it will go.

(2) Move the dial to the next clearly-defined "click."

(3) Place the pointer straight up, straight down, etc.

(4) Place the dial halfway between two clearly-defined positions.

(5) Feel a screw, raised letter, or other tactual feature which happens to be on the dial already.

When the existing features are not sufficient for accurate use by the blind, you will need to add one or more tactual markings. Ideas include: filing small notches; applying actual Braille dots or letters, as with a special Dymotape set; placing drops of glue, paint, etc.; and etching glass. (Glass may be etched by using a portable high-speed grinder with a V-shaped silicon carbide stone, or a vibrating engraving tool with a silicon carbide or diamond point.)

Many knobs and dials can easily be removed to facilitate marking. Observe carefully before removing, however, so that you will be able to replace the dial correctly.

The tactile markings need not necessarily be the same as the inkprint markings, as long as they produce the desired results. If the dial is particularly hard to mark, for example, it may be possible to do most of the marking on the background instead of on the dial.

Use the minimum necessary marks, avoiding confusing clutter. Probably you will not mark nearly as many points as the inkprint dial has. On the heat control of a conventional oven, for example, marking every 100 degrees is entirely adequate. It is easy to set a dial one-fourth, one-half, or three-fourths of the way between two marks.

Microwave Ovens

On most traditional ovens, tactual labels can be placed in the obvious locations. On microwave ovens, however, sometimes there is a heat sensor behind the printed label. In this case, if Braille is placed in the same location as the print, the student searching for the correct control may inadvertently turn on several unwanted processes merely by gently touching certain spots. To deal with this problem, place Braille labels above, below, or beside the printed labels, in a strip or other consistent manner. The student can search for the correct label, and then move up or down to the actual control spot.

As a further challenge, sometimes controls are so close together that there is no room even for adjacent labels. Consider these ideas, alone or in combination:

- Use simple one- or two-symbol Braille labels.
- Experiment to see how large the heat-sensitive spot actually is. It may be much smaller than the printed label.
- Place double labels next to one row, indicating both that row and the next one.
- Label one row, and memorize the row next to it.
- If there is no room for regular Braille symbols, place simple tactual marks and memorize the meaning.
- "Braillabel" material (available from the American Thermoform Company), cut to size, often adheres better than Dymotape.
- File notches in the metal or plastic at the edge.

Using the Stove, Oven, or Electric Frying Pan

Food may be placed in a pan, and the pan on a burner, before the heat is turned on; this way, the pan and burner may be examined tactually with safety. However, with experience you will rarely if ever need to turn off the heat in order to replace a pan on the burner.

Similarly, if you are a beginner you may wish to examine a conventional oven carefully while it is cold. Once you are familiar with its arrangement, you will then be able to work confidently when the oven is hot, using a mitt or a potholder. It is usually better to pull out the oven shelf in order to insert or remove something; the danger of a hand burn is then minimized because you need not reach far inside the oven. Be sure that the shelves are properly attached so that they will not pull out too far or tip over.

Although the beginner may feel hesitant about lighting a gas stove or oven, the blind cook need only follow normal safety precautions and observe the operation of the stove by means other than sight. Listen for the sound of the flame lighting. If necessary hold your hand above the burner or pilot light, at a safe distance, to see whether it is still burning. With experience you will be able to set the flame to the desired level by observing the position of the control and the amount of heat generated. If matches are required, the beginner may prefer large wooden ones, and may need to practice lighting them; however the experienced cook uses any available match.

Usually you can tell when something starts to boil, by listening and/or by feeling the vibration of the pan handle. However, if the liquid is very thick, a Braille thermometer may be useful. A beginner may wish to have the mixture stop boiling temporarily before adding ingredients.

Monitoring the cooking of a confection by placing a sample in cold water and checking for the "soft ball stage," etc., is done by touch anyway, and should be no problem for the blind cook.

If you use a pressure cooker, select a type which makes use of sounds (as with a jiggling weight), rather than an inkprint dial. Notches may be filed in a weight which has multiple settings.

To turn meat which is frying, locate each piece by touch and flip it in the usual manner. If necessary, wad up a piece of paper toweling as a pad to protect your hand. (Especially at first, you may need to use your hand to find the piece of meat and/or to keep it in the right position while you are turning it over with a spatula.)

A suggested method for frying chicken is as follows: Tuck the ends of each wing together for greater compactness and ease in handling. Plan your arrangement of the pieces in the skillet so that you remember where each one is. Arrange the chicken in a relatively cool skillet (warmed only enough to melt the fat); turn up the heat appropriately until the meat is ready to turn; then turn the heat off again while you are turning the pieces. In turning large pieces, it may be convenient to exchange two of them with each other.

Since bacon is so thin and flimsy, a bacon decurler may be used to make turning unnecessary. This is a perforated metal plate with a small handle in the middle, available on the general market. The bacon cooks on both sides simultaneously when this device is placed on it. After the proper time has elapsed, touching the bacon with a spatula or lifting it up slightly will indicate its crispness. Scoop out the pieces with the spatula, pushing them against a paper towel to collect them.

In frying pancakes, the beginner will probably start with just one in the middle of the pan; however the experienced cook can fry several in the same skillet. Ladle in the appropriate amount of batter for the size of cake desired; for a thinner cake, shake or tip the skillet slightly. The appropriate time for turning may be judged by time and by the consistency of the cake as the spatula is slipped under it.

In preparing waffles, spread the batter around evenly as you dip it into the waffle iron. You will know when the waffle is done by observing such things as the amount of steam escaping, the odor, and whether the lid comes free easily.

The beginner frying an egg, and the experienced cook frying several eggs separately in one pan, may use an egg ring for each egg. Remove both the top and bottom of a small tuna or pineapple can, leaving a metal ring about one and one-half inches high and three inches in diameter. This ring is placed in the pan and the egg is broken into it. When the egg becomes firm enough to keep its shape, the ring is removed.

Time, touch, odor, taste, and/or sound will indicate when a product is done.

CHOICE OF COOKING METHOD

Many people today, sighted and blind, regard the microwave oven as extremely convenient and "the modern way to cook." Nevertheless, large numbers of people still prefer conventional stoves and ovens for many procedures, and/or cannot afford a microwave oven. Others use the "more traditional" methods when visiting friends or relatives, volunteering in the church kitchen, etc. Home economics classes teach various methods of cookery, not just the use of microwave ovens.

For all these reasons, the blind student needs to learn all the common means of cooking and baking. Do not permit the microwave oven to be the only method because "it is so much easier."

Serving the Food

Many aids are available for cutting cakes, pies, etc., into portions. From a restaurant supply house it is possible to buy a pie-cutting guide featuring slots for the knife. A different type of pie cutter, consisting of a wire frame with blades, is also available from restaurant supply houses. A hexagonal-shaped pie pan may be bought on the regular market, and a straightedge may be laid across between opposite corners to guide the knife. A straightedge may also be used in a similar manner with any metal pan if notches are filed at appropriate places along the edges of the pan; cakes, desserts, and gelatine may be cut evenly in this manner.

Setting the table usually presents no particular problem. If you have trouble spacing the place settings evenly, we suggest that you push each chair up close to the table in its proper place. Then you can center each place setting in front of the corresponding chair.

A tray or cookie sheet helps in serving soup or other liquids. A filled bowl may be carried on a tray to minimize the problem of spillage. Alternatively, the bowls may be filled at the table just before the diners arrive, with the tray being placed under each bowl in turn as a precaution.

Many blind hostesses prefer to serve food to their guests from a cart or sideboard. If each serving dish is passed around and then returned to this location, the hostess easily finds out when a dish becomes empty.

The popular custom of a self-service buffet style meal is particularly convenient for the blind hostess, as it is for the sighted. The hostess need only arrange all the necessary items appropriately, and then replenish empty serving dishes as necessary.

The beginner may experience difficulty in pouring from a coffeepot. We suggest the following: Set the cup near the edge of the table. Lift the coffeepot completely off the table, and lower it so that the bottom of the pot is lower than the surface of the table. Then place the spout so that it touches the lip of the cup and reaches inside. (With experience, you may or may not come to prefer some other method.)

To determine when the cup is full, you may place your finger over the lip of the cup; estimate the amount of liquid, according to sound, volume, time, etc.; or use a liquid level indicator.

Cleanup

Much of the need for cleaning up spots and spills can be prevented by careful work habits. As mentioned above, a tray is extremely helpful in catching spills. Unpleasant accidents, such as dropping a pie or placing one tray of unbaked cookies on top of another, can usually be prevented by care and thought. For example: Remove spills from the floor at once before someone slips. Check the oven shelf to be sure it is clear. Replace lids tightly onto the proper jars. Put utensils and appliances back into their proper places, and always turn off appliances rather than merely unplugging them. Plan ahead in all respects rather than proceeding haphazardly. (All of these precautions apply to the sighted as well; however the blind person learning new techniques may need to be reminded.)

Often the need for cleaning or washing can be felt tactually. It is important, however, to anticipate dirt which may not be so readily noticed, and to do routine general cleaning such as wiping off the entire counter after mixing on it. In cleaning a surface such as the counter or floor, a planned approach is very important: clean in strips rather than random strokes here and there.

Dishwashing usually presents no particular problems.

Cleanliness and neatness should be considered at every stage of the food preparation procedure. Organize equipment and supplies beforehand; keep your hands thoroughly clean; plan carefully; clean up spills when they occur; wash all utensils and wipe off the entire cooking area afterwards. Double check after the cleanup is completed, to be sure nothing was missed.

Conclusion

A positive attitude is essential to success.

If you really believe that the blind cook necessarily takes many safety risks, needs a great deal of special equipment, has only a limited repertoire, and produces questionable products–then you will do a poor job. If you really believe that the blind cook may choose among many good methods to work with all kinds of food and produce high-quality products–then you will find a way to succeed.

If you have questions which have not been resolved by the suggestions in this booklet, we cordially invite you to write to the National Federation of the Blind for further information on cooking techniques or any other subject pertaining to blindness.

APPENDIX D

SEWING

By Ramona R. Walhof and Doris M. Willoughby

THE BLIND CAN SEW: SOME HOW-TO IDEAS

By
Ramona Walhof

[The following is reprinted from the article by the same title, originally appearing in *The Braille Monitor,* June, 1973.]

In sewing, a blind person uses most of the same methods a sighted person uses, but here are a few suggestions and gadgets that are often helpful.

Many people use needle threaders to thread needles. There are a variety of types available. The simplest of these is available in sewing departments in most cities. It consists of a small piece of metal with a wire loop attached. This delicate wire loop is passed through the needle; the thread is passed through the loop; and the threader is removed, pulling the thread with it. With a little practice the process can be done quickly and easily. Many people also like to use self-threading needles. For hand sewing, these needles are also widely available, but self-threading needles of machines are more difficult to find. Either means of threading needles is workable.

Most sewing machines come equipped with a seam guide to be screwed onto the machine table to the right of the presser foot. Such a guide is most useful to sew a half-inch or five-eighths-inch seam or hem. These guides can generally be purchased separately if desired, and other types of guides are also available. Some blind people like to put tape on their machines as guides. Some people find they can guide the material by keeping one finger on the edge of the material and another finger on the presser foot. For top-stitching or very narrow seams – such as are often recommended for sewing knitted fabrics – the presser foot is the best guide for most people. Regardless of the kind of sewing guide used, the procedure is the same. Just determine where the edge of the fabric should be in relation to the needle and the guide; then keep it there as the needle moves under the presser foot.

To make a good-looking garment, one must be a good ripper. To rip, one needs to feel the threads of the seam to be ripped and get the point of a standard ripper under the stitches. If the fabric is lightweight or knitted, this can be delicate work. Again, practice will prove that ripping need not be a problem to a blind person.

Then what should be said for patterns and cutting? Picking patterns and fabric depends on getting someone to serve as a reader and getting her to give you the information wanted in shopping. When the pattern has been purchased, a blind person needs to have a sighted person cut off the extra tissue paper around the edges of pieces, trimming on the regular cutting line. Then the blind person merely needs to cut at the edge of the pattern. Some sewing teachers recommend that blind students have their patterns cut out of brown paper in order to feel it better, but I have never found this necessary, nor have my students.

An experienced seamstress can identify the different pieces of the pattern by their various shapes. The beginner needs to learn to do this. Then it is possible to pin on the pattern, cut it out, and put it together with no more sighted help than is given at the time of trimming the pattern. Darts and other markings, if needed, can be marked with pins, tape, or by cutting out a pattern for the dart itself from another piece of paper.

In guiding the scissors when cutting out the garment, most of my students have found that one can be more exact in her work by curving the left hand (assuming you are a right-handed cutter) over the top blade of the scissors, thumb and fingers coming together at the edge of the tissue pattern between the blades of the scissors when the scissors are open. It is really a simple means of following the edge of the pattern as you cut. [See Figure D-1. Note that in this illustration, two separate pieces of the paper pattern were previously cut apart and then pinned onto the cloth, close together. The blind seamstress is now cutting out the piece on the right.] Generally, this method enables the blind person to do a neater job of cutting than she does with the left hand guiding the scissors from beyond the tip.

Sometimes labeling thread for color can be a problem. One unique solution to this problem is to obtain pill bottles with large tops from your local pharmacy and stick Braille labels on them. Braille labels glued to the spool of thread itself will be pushed off by the spindle if the spool is put on the machine.

These are the things that seem to bother blind people who want to sew, and these are the solutions that my students and I have found. With confidence and a bit of imagination blind people can sew whatever they wish with very little assistance. There may be other ways of doing some of the things also. Good luck as you proceed with your sewing.

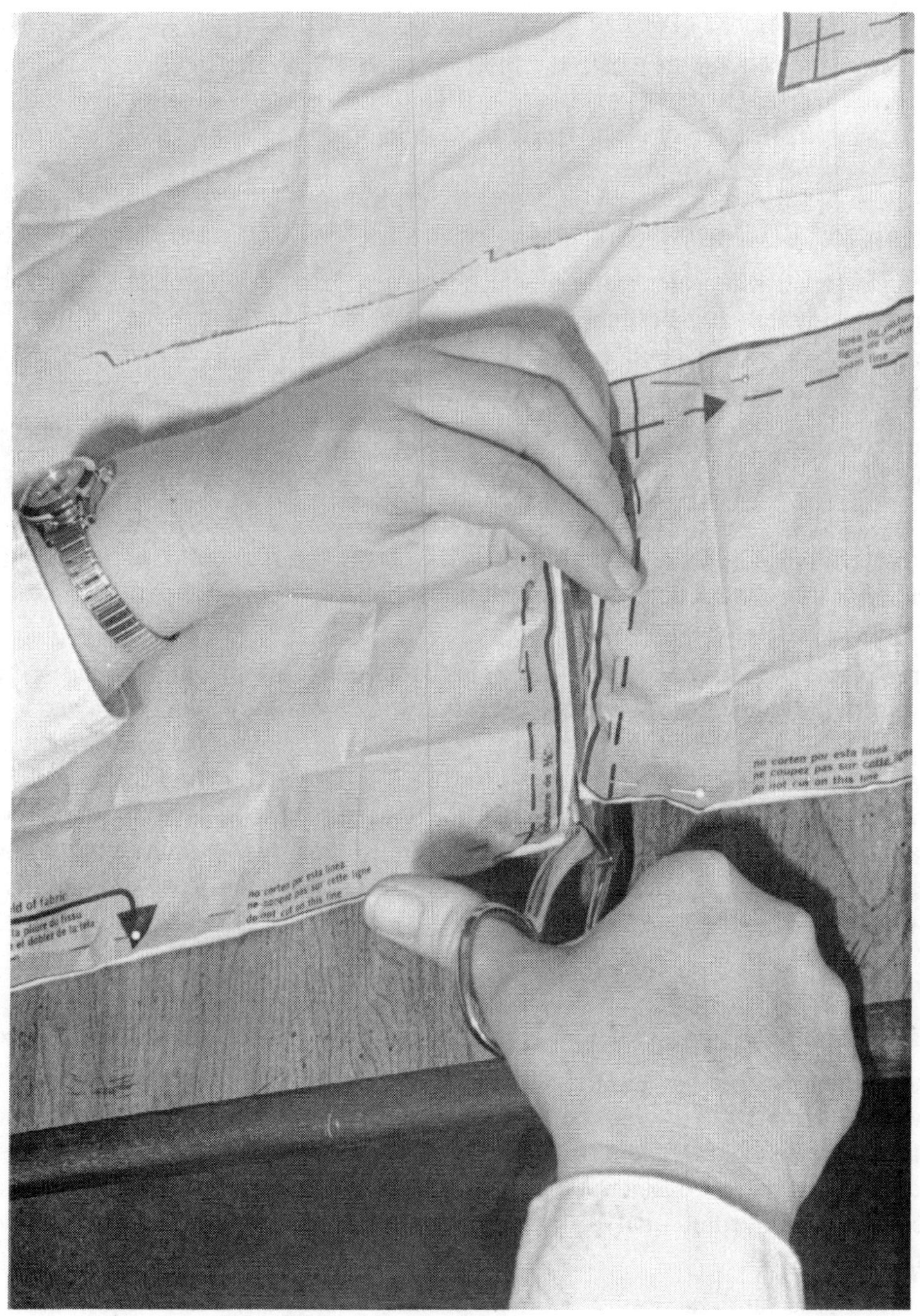

Figure D-1
Cutting

SEWING:
NOTES FOR HELPING YOUNGER STUDENTS
By
Doris M. Willoughby

Preparation for Sewing

A young beginner will prefer material which is easy to handle, which is not flimsy, and on which stitching can be easily felt. It is best not to have a print which requires matching at the seams.

If the material has a "right side," this should be learned at the time of purchase. The student can then keep track of this by memory, touch, and/or a labeling system.

The advanced student should be able to work with any material. Alternative techniques include placing a pin at the edge of each major print figure in key areas, for matching and for overall appearance.

Each pattern piece may be labeled in Braille to show the name of the piece, the grain of the material, etc. For long instructions, it is best to transcribe them onto a separate piece of paper, or to use a reader and take Braille notes.

In some places tape may be preferred to pins as a method of tactual marking. Notches may be cut outward from the edge of the pattern piece, rather than inward.

The Sewing Machine

Although Braille diagrams are helpful in many educational situations, learning the parts of the sewing machine is generally not one of them. The real machine is always available. Both instruction and tests should be given by allowing the student to examine the part in question and its relationship to the rest of the machine.

THREADING

Threading may seem impossible for an "all thumbs" beginner, but it can be achieved.

If your student has not learned to use a needle threader, or if hand sewing is the task at hand, you may want to begin by threading hand needles. Stick the needle upright in a stable pincushion. Have plenty of wire needle threaders (found in any sewing store) available; they are easily destroyed in the hands of a beginner. Consider teaching your student to thread hand needles in the same direction as most machine needles–that is, inserting the wire loop from back to front, and pulling the thread from front to back.

The entire procedure can easily be accomplished without any use of sight. For the partially-sighted person, using a threader is far easier than attempting to see the delicate thread and tiny hole. (As always, the use of sleepshades greatly facilitates learning.)

Grasp the needle with the free hand and locate the end containing the eye. With the other hand, bring the point of the wire loop to touch the needle in the vicinity of the eye. Use the point of the threader as a probe to locate the hole; push the wire through. See Figure D-2.

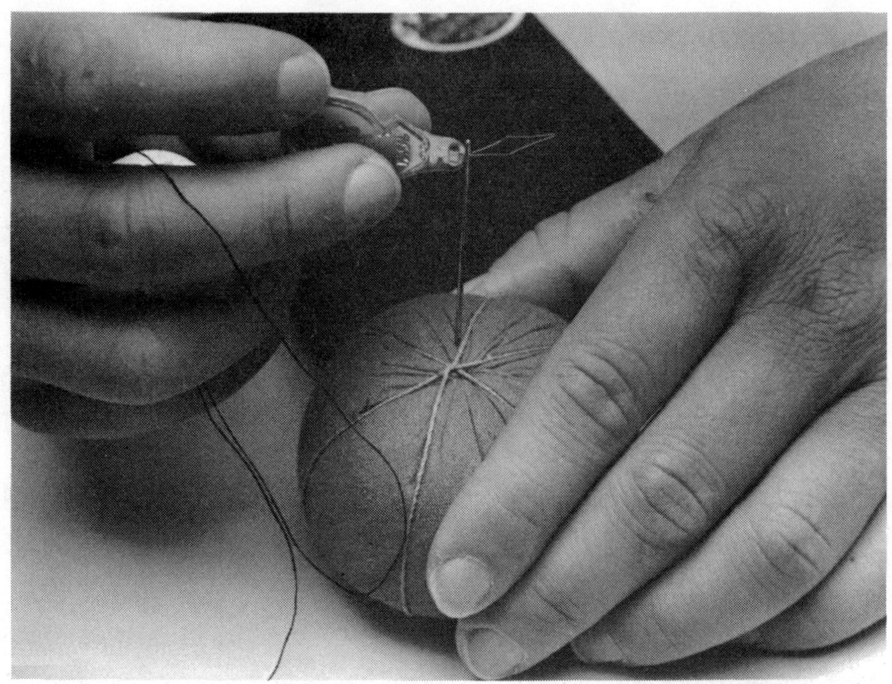

Figure D-2
Wire Threader Inserted

With the wire loop remaining in the eye of the needle, the thread is now drawn through the wire loop. (Figure D-3) The young beginner will find it easier to practice with a heavy thread and a large-eyed needle. It also may be helpful to roll up the end of the thread, tape it, or wrap it around a pin, in order to get it through the loop. The experienced student will use thin, delicate thread without difficulty.

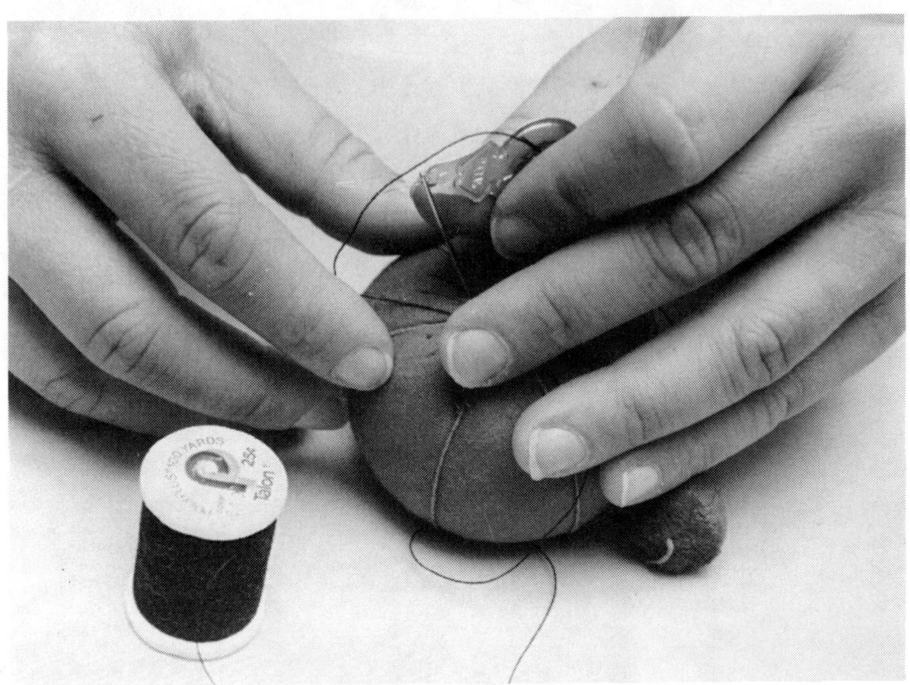

Figure D-3
Thread Through Wire Loop

At least two inches of thread should be drawn through the wire loop. Then the threader is pulled out of the eye of the needle – thus pulling the thread through the eye (Figure D-4). When the shorter end of the thread comes through the eye, the threader is removed. The needle is now threaded and ready for use.

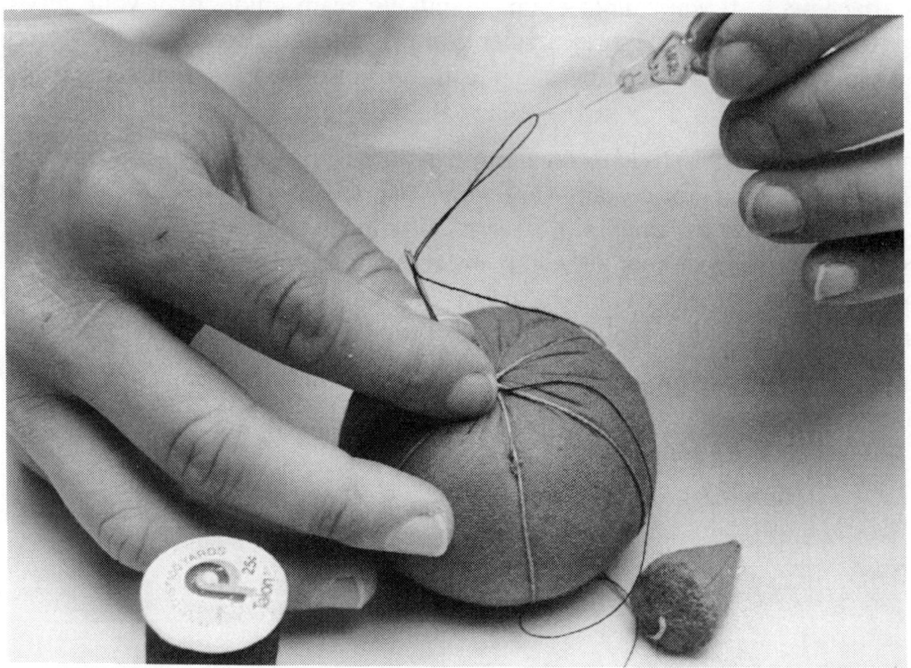

Figure D-4
Drawing Thread Through the Eye

A wire needle threader can be used with a machine needle. Note that the wire must be inserted the opposite direction from the way the thread will go through – i.e., if the thread is to be pulled from front to back, the wire loop must be inserted from back to front.

For threading parts of the machine other than the needle, various ideas can be used: e.g., rolling up the end of the thread, taping it, or wrapping it around a pin. In late-model machines, often the thread is intended to slip through a slot rather than being actually threaded. Also note that a needle threader can be used on parts other than the actual needle, although it rarely is necessary.

Show your student self-threading needles and mechanical needle threaders also. Different individuals have different preferences. However, it is especially important that the student know how to use the simple wire threader, since it is so readily available.

SAFETY

The student with low vision will do neater and more reliable work if sleepshades are used to cover the eyes and alternative techniques are learned. On the sewing machine it is not only a question of preventing inaccuracy and strain, but also a matter of real physical danger. Attempting to watch the moving needle and material with inadequate eyesight is a gamble. Using a tactual guide is not a gamble.

STARTING TO SEW

Screw the seam guide down firmly. (Note: I have seen one machine which would not run at all when the seam guide was screwed down tightly. We used a felt washer under the head of the screw, thus raising the bottom tip of the screw to keep it from interfering with machine operation.) The beginner will probably benefit from a relatively large and long seam guide, which may be available as an additional attachment. If you cannot obtain a suitable seam guide, or if your very inexperienced student seems to need something more, a ruler can be fastened down to make a very long tactual guide. Heavy tape can also be used as a guide in the absence of a seam guide attachment. Be creative!

An advanced and careful student, on the other hand, may prefer to use the right edge of the presser foot as a tactual guide for certain work with a narrow margin. In sewing a zipper, many blind persons find that a very narrow double presser foot (with the finger kept against the right edge) is preferable to the single "zipper foot." Sewing an applique onto the center of a piece is a situation where a seam guide attachment cannot be used: a solution is to run the right-hand edge of the presser foot along the edge of the applique.

Everyone, sighted or blind, must frequently check that the seam really is being sewn correctly–no broken thread, loose thread, etc.

APPENDIX E

ALTERNATIVE TECHNIQUES WITH POWER TOOLS

By John Cheadle and Doris M. Willoughby

This appendix consists of technical descriptions of the use of certain power tools, measuring instruments, and other devices. It is assumed that the reader already has a background in industrial arts.

Note that the chapter, "Industrial Arts and Related Skills," contains descriptions for the hand-held power saw and the drill press, as well as general basic information.

Measuring Devices

THE ROTOMATIC

The Rotomatic (available from the National Federation of the Blind) permits accuracy greater than 1/64"–much more precise than a Braille ruler, an adapted tape measure, or a click-rule. The basic device is a threaded rod slightly over 6-1/2" long. (See Figure E-1.) With the extensions usually supplied, it can measure up to 42 inches with great accuracy. Additional extensions can easily enable measurements up to eight or ten feet.

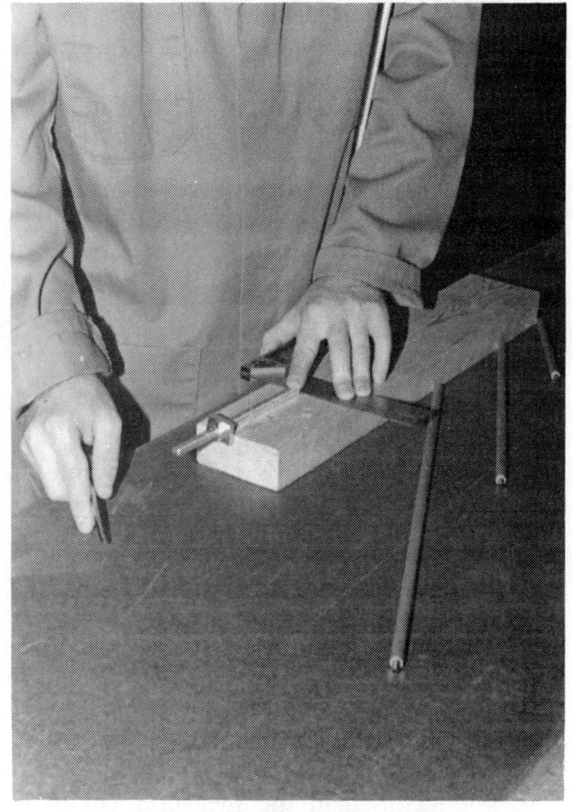

Figure E-1
Rotomatic Measuring Device

There are 16 threads per inch, and at every half-inch there is a tactual mark on one side. A large rectangular nut is used for measuring; each complete revolution changes the measurement by 1/16", and each quarter-turn changes it by 1/64". One side and one end of the nut are grooved for identification. The tapped end of the rod (i.e., the end to which an extension may be attached) and one face of the rectangular nut are the surfaces between which measurements are taken. (The nut itself is 1/4" thick; its thickness is included when making an "inside" measurement, and not included when making an "outside" measurement.) When the measurement is exactly a multiple of 1/16", the marked side of the nut is on the marked side of the rod. When the measurement is exactly on a multiple of 1/2", the leading edge of the nut is at a half-inch mark on the rod.

A smaller nut is used as a locknut.

Following is an example of use in measuring a board which is 4-3/32" wide:

(1) Unlock the locking nut (if necessary).

(2) Place the large nut against one edge of the board, with the locking nut away from the board.

(3) Turn the large nut and/or the rod, until the tapped end of the Rotomatic is flush with the other edge of the board (thus, the device is now spanning the interval to be measured).

(4) Remove the Rotomatic and observe the orientation of the large nut with respect to the marked side of the rod. Also note that the large nut is beyond the 4" mark. Turn the large nut back toward the tapped end of the rod until it exactly reaches the 4" mark (the leading edge of the nut is on the 4" mark, and the marked side of the nut is on the marked side of the rod), meanwhile carefully counting the number of turns.

(5) Note that the thickness of the nut itself is not included in the measurement in this case.

(6) If it is 1-1/2 turns back to the 4" mark, that would be 3/32". One must add 4" to 3/32", and thus the total measurement would be 4-3/32".

(7) Note that in this instance the locknut was not used. For still greater precision, or for the purpose of cutting another board to exactly this length, the locknut could be used to lock the measurement. Then the Rotomatic could be taken elsewhere to mark an identical interval.

BRAILLE MICROMETER

(Note: Micrometers are chiefly used in metal work, which is beyond the scope of this book. A description is included here, however, since this is an important measuring device readily available to the blind.) Braille micrometers are basically the same as print micrometers, and are accurate to .001". Markings can be read tactually, and are arranged somewhat differently than those on a print micrometer.

On a print micrometer, the graduations are spread in a single line on the sleeve. But on the Braille micrometer, the graduations are in three separate lines on the sleeve. The top row of grooves show .025, .075, etc. The grooves in the center are for tenths of an inch. The bottom row of marks are .050, .150, .250, etc.

On the thimble, the thousandths markings are grooved, with a group of five raised dots indicating zero or twenty-five thousandths. Single dots indicate five thousandths.

The micrometer is a sophisticated instrument, used for very fine accuracy. By using the proper model, one can measure either outside or inside dimensions, or the depth of a hole. Braille micrometers are available from the National Federation of the Blind.

Power Tools

Note: Names given here are those most familiar to the authors. Names may vary with local usage – i.e., the same tool may be given various names in different parts of the country.

BAND SAW

The band saw can cut a curved line, which should be scribed (grooved) into the piece of wood.

Attach a guide which has a notch in the bottom directly in front of the blade (see Figure E-2). This notch can be felt with the thumbnail, as can the scribed line in the piece of wood.

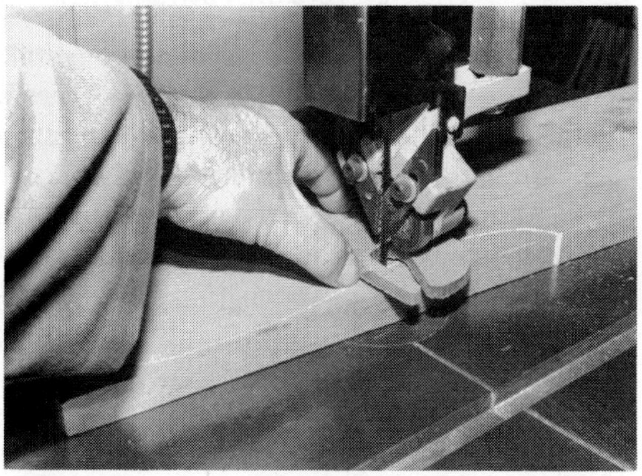

Figure E-2
Band Saw

With the guard about 1/8" above the wood, the thumbnail can feel both the notch (above) and the scribed line (below) at the same time. Power is then turned on, and the other hand feeds the piece on through, while the thumbnail of the first hand continues to keep track of proper positioning. Cut on the scrap side of the line, to allow for sanding.

To cut a straight piece, set the fence so that the desired width of the piece is the same as the distance between the fence and the blade. Lock the fence into place and proceed.

A template may be helpful when making several pieces exactly the same.

SCROLL SAW

Usually there is a small bar in front of the blade. If a notch is filed directly in front of the blade, the thumbnail can be used with a scribed line or template, in the same manner as for the band saw.

RADIAL ARM SAW

Suggested procedure:

(1) Using the Rotomatic, measure the desired distance between the right end of the board and the right side of the blade. Use the locknut to hold the interval.

(2) Place the board against the fence.

(3) To measure the length of the cut, place one end of the preset Rotomatic against the right end of the board, and the other end against the right side of the blade. (Figure E-3)

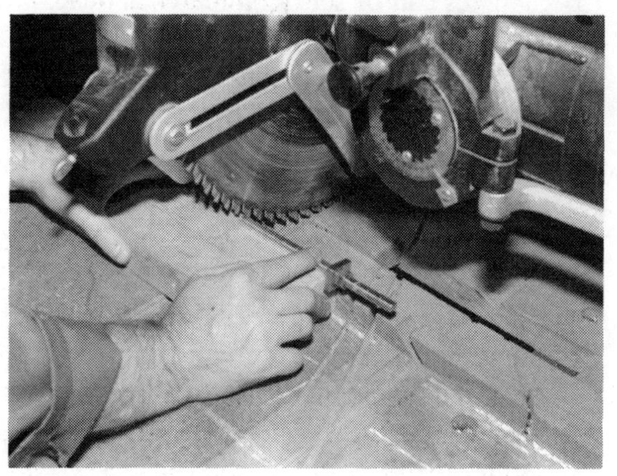

Figure E-3
Measuring Length of Cut

(4) Hold the board against the fence with the left hand. Check to make sure there is at least a hand's width between your left hand and the path of the blade. (Figure E-4)

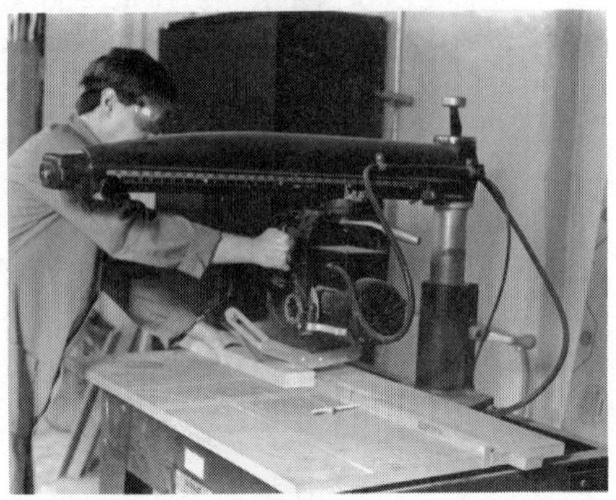

Figure E-4
Checking Safe Distance

(5) Angles can be set up in the usual way. The stops for the common angles can be felt. For less common angles, a sliding "T" bevel square may be used. Also, the American Printing House for the Blind offers a protractor for the hand-held power saw. Protractors which are not especially manufactured for the blind often have marks which can be felt; otherwise tactual marks can be added.

(6) Cut the board in the usual manner.

(7) Make sure the blade has stopped turning before removing any pieces. If the shop is so noisy you cannot hear the blade stop turning, check the motor shaft at the right end of the saw.

ROUTER

Clamp a scrap board on as a guide, in a manner similar to that described for the Skill Saw. If the path is to stop before reaching the end of the wood, place another guide board crossways.

For curves or figures, prepare a jig or template. Ready-made templates are often available for letters or other standard patterns.

In starting the router, pull it back a little at first to be sure it is turning freely.

POWER SANDER (DISK-BELT SANDER)

This is a common machine, generally regarded as easy to use, but requiring careful safety precautions as any power tool. It is the same for the blind student–he/she should use the sense of touch to greatest advantage, but be careful to keep fingers away from the belts.

Other Devices

PUSH STICK

Sometimes it seems that a person would need to reach very close to the blade, despite the suggestions above. A "push stick" is useful for manipulating small or narrow items. Typically this resembles a very large key (see Figure E-5), with a slight lip to extend over the top edge of the item to be pushed. Something like this should be used if the fingers would otherwise come within about 4" of the saw blade. These are available commercially, or may be made individually.

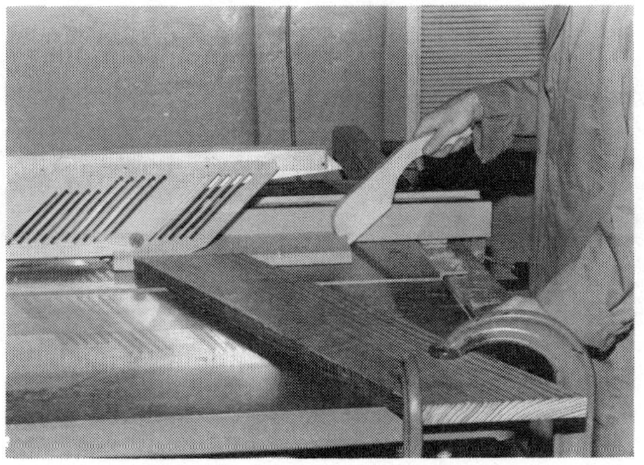

Figure E-5
Push Stick

FEATHER BOARD

As the piece moves toward the blade, use of a feather board can prevent unwanted lateral motion. This device is available commercially, but may be homemade:

A piece of wood approximately 1" x 4" x 10" is a convenient size. Cut slots, approximately 6" long and 1/8" apart, with the grain. Then cut off one end of the board, making the cut at an angle of about 30 degrees.

Clamp the feather board beside the piece of wood being cut, on the side away from the fence. The slots should be facing the piece of wood being cut. When the feather board is used in this way, the "comb" against the wood permits motion to proceed forward only.

APPENDIX F

EASY GUIDE TO THE NEMETH CODE

By
Sharon L. M. Duffy

Over the years, a number of people have asked me to write them a list of the basic math symbols. Rather than continue to give these out piecemeal, here is a list. This is not intended as a comprehensive guide to the Nemeth Code, but as a reference for the most commonly used applications, and as a means to begin learning the Nemeth Code.

EDITOR'S NOTES: For the print version of this paper, certain conventions will be used so that Braille can be represented. Some Braille symbols have no counterpart in inkprint. Therefore, certain inkprint signs (e.g., ⊂) will be used in arbitrary ways other than their mathematical meaning, to represent certain Braille symbols.[1]

In this paper, the beginning fraction indicator will be represented by ⊂ and the ending fraction indicator by ⊃. Dots 4-5-6 will be represented by the | (vertical bar).[2]

Parentheses ( ) will be shown in their usual way. However, as explained below, in actual Nemeth Code Braille they are not the same as in literary Braille. To illustrate Braille usage, brackets and braces will not be shown in their usual inkprint form. Instead, brackets [ ] will each be represented by a "grave accent" mark ` and the appropriate parenthesis:

`( and `) respectively

Braces {} will each be represented by a colon and the appropriate parenthesis:

:(and :) respectively

Books on the Nemeth Code refer to parentheses, brackets, and braces as "signs and symbols of grouping."

---

[1]When ⊂ appears with its conventional mathematical meaning in a math textbook, and the textbook is transcribed into Braille, there is a Braille counterpart for the regular usage of ⊂.

[2]Like ⊂, the vertical bar is used in an arbitrary way in this paper, to illustrate Braille usage. When the vertical bar | appears with its conventional mathematical meaning on a page being transcribed into Braille, there is a counterpart for the conventional usage of |.

The "dot 4" alone will be represented by the ` (grave accent).[3]

The numeric indicator (dots 3-4-5-6, comparable to the number sign in literary Braille and identical in its appearance) is indicated by the inkprint number sign wherever it would appear. Note that the numerals themselves are, as described below, always in the lower part of the cell in Nemeth Code.

Precise description of symbols will be given by dot numbers. As in literary Braille, each cell is composed of six dots. The three dots on the left side of a cell, from top to bottom, are dots 1-2-3. On the right side, from top to bottom, are dots 4-5-6. The description will consist of the word "dots" followed by the dot numbers connected by hyphens. If a symbol occupies two or more cells, a comma will follow the dot numbers for each individual cell.

Occasionally it will be difficult to make it clear whether a number is meant to represent an actual numeral or a dot number. To avoid this confusion, sometimes the name of a numeral (never a dot number) will be spelled out.

Some of the Nemeth Code symbols have the same appearance as certain symbols in literary Braille. For example, the "divided into" symbol (dots 1-3-5) has a shape identical to the letter *o*. The beginning fraction indicator (dots 1-4-5-6) has a shape identical to the *th* symbol. In this paper, this comparison will sometimes be used to simplify explanation; the literary expression will be in italics. However, the reader needs to understand (and children must be taught) that the meaning is not the same. This matter is comparable to the fact that in inkprint a "zero" is not the same thing as a letter "O" even if the appearance is exactly the same.

General Rules

Books on the Nemeth Code give detailed rules for when each symbol must be used. For example, the Nemeth comma (dot 6) is used only with actual mathematical expressions; the literary comma (dot 2) is used with words which are not in math expressions – even on the same page. This paper does *not* explain all provisions and all exceptions for the rules discussed here.

First, it is important to note that numbers in the context of Nemeth Code are dropped within the Braille cell. That is, they utilize the bottom four dots of the Braille cell (dots 2-3-5-6) instead of the top four as in literary Braille (dots 1-2-4-5). This is done for easy distinction between numbers and letters. Also, before each string of numbers, the numeric indicator must be used. However, the numeric indicator need not be repeated so long as there is no space between characters. If a string of numbers is preceded by an initial fraction indicator or another "numeric" symbol containing dot 1 and/or dot 4, the numeric indicator is unnecessary.

In materials which are not "mathematics or science" overall, the Nemeth Code is not used at all. Suppose, for example, that a *reading* textbook has the following sentence in inkprint:

Patty won't add 2+2=4.

The Braille version would appear as:

Patty won't add #2 plus #2 equals #4.

The words "plus" and "equals" would be spelled out. The numerals would be in the upper part of the cell. Punctuation indicators, etc., would not be used. Literary Braille rules would apply, not Nemeth Code.[4]

Some Common Symbols

Since punctuation marks also utilize the bottom four dots of the cell, a punctuation indicator (dots 4-5-6 in actual Braille, and represented in this paper by the vertical bar |) must precede punctuation marks which

[3]As with ⊂, the grave accent and the colon are used here in an arbitrary way to illustrate Braille usage.

[4]In a math or science book, Nemeth numerals (in the lower part of the cell) are used everywhere except for page numbers and the title page. Literary Braille numerals (in the upper part of the cell) are used for page numbers and the title page. "Literary Braille" is also called "English Braille."

immediately follow numbers or other numeric symbols.

Following is a list of some basic symbols, and examples of their use:

Plus +
Dots 3-4-6

Minus -
Dots 3-6

Times x
[Cross]
Dots 4, 1-6

Times ·
[Dot]
Dots 1-6

Division ÷
["Divided by"]
Dots 4-6, 3-4

Divide into
$\overline{)}$
Dots 1-3-5
(Same shape as the letter "o")[5]

Fraction line
/ (Dots 3-4)
or
| / (Dots 4-5-6, 3-4)

Equals =
Dots 4-6, 1-3

Decimal point .
Dots 4-6

Comma ,
[Mathematical comma][6]
Dot 6

Examples of Usage

Here are some simple problems using these symbols. Note that a "symbol of comparison" such as "equals" requires a space before and after. "Symbols of operation" (+ - x ÷) do not have spaces.

3 plus 4 equals 7
#3+4 = #7

10 minus 3 equals 7
#10-3 = #7

2 times 5 equals 10
#2x5 = #10

18 divided by 3 equals 6
#18÷3 = #6

3 goes into 26
#3o26

Fractions and Mixed Numbers

Fractions and mixed numbers are written differently in Nemeth Code than they are in literary Braille.

In literary Braille, the number "three and one-half" is written:

#3-1/2

However, this must be modified in the Nemeth Code, since numerals are in the lower part of the cell and the hyphen is the minus symbol. Also, it is often necessary to indicate exactly where a fraction begins and ends in an algebraic expression.

The opening fraction indicator is the *th* (dots 1-4-5-6) and the closing fraction indicator is the *ble* symbol (dots 3-4-5-6).

---

[5]Usually this symbol is indicated by Dots 1-3-5, the same shape as the letter "o." The complete format is: divisor; dots 1-3-5; dividend. However, if the problem is shown in a spatial arrangement, so that the quotient and/or subtractions can be written in, then additional symbols (not explained in this paper) are used.

[6]The "mathematical comma" (dot 6) is used with all mathematical expressions. The regular literary comma (dot 2) is used with words which do not appear in a mathematical expression as explained in reference books on the Nemeth Code. Thus both kinds of commas may be used on the same page.

In the case of mixed numbers, each of these fraction indicators is preceded by dots 4-5-6.

Here are examples of each.

NOTE: Refer to the note in boldface type at the beginning of this paper, for explanation of conventions used to represent Braille in this paper.

Often a fraction is written in inkprint with the numerator and the denominator directly above each other and separated by a horizontal line:

$$\frac{1}{3}$$

In Braille this requires the fraction indicators:

⊂1/3⊃

If, however, the fraction is written horizontally in inkprint:

1/3

fraction indicators are not used in Braille, and dots 4-5-6 must appear before the fraction line:

#1|/3

The distinction between these two ways of writing a fraction is not usually considered significant in inkprint, but it affects the Braille transcription.

Below are examples of Nemeth Code usage for mixed numbers.

NOTE: It should be assumed that in inkprint the fractions below are shown vertically–that is, with the numerator physically above the denominator and separated by a horizontal line. The numerals and other symbols below illustrate the Nemeth Code Braille usage for fractions and mixed numbers, not the inkprint appearance.

Three and one-half
#3|⊂1/2|⊃

Six-eighths equals three-fourths.
⊂6/8⊃ = ⊂3/4⊃

Two and one-fourth equals nine-fourths.
#2|⊂1/4|⊃ = ⊂9/4⊃

Signs and Symbols of Grouping

Parentheses, brackets, and braces are a necessary part of mathematical experience. The regular parentheses cannot be used because they would be confused with the 7. Therefore, the opening mathematical parenthesis is the *of* symbol (dots 1-2-3-5-6), and the closing mathematical parenthesis is the *with* symbol (dots 2-3-4-5-6). To make brackets, the opening parenthesis is preceded by dot 4, and the closing parenthesis is also preceded by dot 4. Following is the precise description of parentheses, brackets, and braces:

Opening mathematical parenthesis (
Dots 1-2-3-5-6

Closing mathematical parenthesis)
Dots 2-3-4-5-6

Opening mathematical bracket [
Dot 4, 1-2-3-5-6

Closing mathematical bracket]
Dot 4, 2-3-4-5-6

Opening mathematical braces {
(Also called "curly brackets")
Dots 4-6, 1-2-3-5-6

Closing mathematical braces }
("Curly brackets")
Dots 4-6, 2-3-4-5-6

Following are examples of usage.

Refer to the note in boldface type at the beginning of this paper, for explanation of conventions used to represent Braille in this paper.

2 times opening parenthesis 6 minus 3 equals 6.
#2(6-3) = #6

3 times opening brackets 16 over opening parenthesis 10 minus 6 closing parenthesis closing bracket equals 12.
#3`(16|/(10-6)`) = #12

2 times opening brace 3 plus opening bracket 8 minus opening parenthesis 2x minus 2 closing parenthesis closing bracket closing brace equals 18.
#2:(3+`(8-(2x-2)`):) = #18

Remember that all symbols of grouping (parentheses, brackets, etc.) must be mathematical and not the literary Braille symbols.

Representing Shapes

Geometric shapes are represented by an *ed* symbol (dots 1-2-4-6) immediately followed by a code letter or number. The code letter or number may in turn be followed by a space and then the coordinate points or letter identifying the shape. Here are a few common shapes.

Refer to the note in boldface type at the beginning of this paper, for explanation of conventions used to represent Braille in this paper.

Note that in this paper, italics are used for letters representing the literary Braille symbol which looks the same. Note also that there is no space after the *ed* in these expressions.

Angle
edow
[The "ed" symbol
and the "ow" symbol]

Intersecting lines
*ed*i

Perpendicular lines
*ed*p

Parallel lines
*ed*l
[Use the letter l, not the number 1]

Triangle [equilateral]
*ed*t

Circle
*ed*c

Square
*ed*4
[Following the *ed*, use dots 2-5-6 without a numeric indicator]

Rectangle
*ed*r

There is no space between parts of the symbol of shape itself (e.g., there is no space between the *ed* and the "t" in the symbol for "triangle"). However, when a symbol of shape is followed by its identification, there must be a space between the shape symbol and its identification. For example,

Square y
□ y
is Brailled as
*ed*4 y

"Levels" (Including Superscripts and Subscripts)

Superscripts and subscripts are also a part of Nemeth Code:

Superscript (exponent) indicator
Dots 4-5

Subscript indicator
Dots 5-6

For example:

Three to the fourth power
3^4
Numeric indicator, three, dots 4-5, four

Three subscript four
3_4
Numeric indicator, three, dots 5-6, four

When a letter has a numeric subscript (e.g., x_1), the subscript indicator is not used.

The "multipurpose indicator" is dot 5. Among other things, it is used to terminate superscripts and subscripts–that is, to show that the rest of the expression is on the baseline or normal line. The multipurpose indicator is not used if a space follows the superscript or subscript, as it usually does.

The multipurpose indicator (dot 5) is also used in a division problem when a remainder is written. For example, suppose that the remainder is 4, and it is to be written as r4. A dot 5 must appear between the "r" and the "4" to indicate that the "4" is not a subscript.

Sometimes a math expression is not so simple as an ordinary superscript (exponent) which is raised and to the right, or an ordinary subscript which is lowered and to the right. Symbols may be directly above others, directly below, superimposed, etc. Nemeth symbols used to arrange this are called "Modifiers."

Radicals

Square roots and other roots are defined by a set of symbols equivalent to the radical sign $\sqrt{\ }$. To write "the square root of three," an *ar* symbol (dots 3-4-5) should precede the three, and the *er* symbol (dots 1-2-4-5-6) should follow the three.

For cube roots and above, the "index of the radical" must be given (three for a cube root, four for a fourth root, etc.) A *gh* symbol (dots 1-2-6) should precede the index. The rest of the expression then follows (without a space) in the same way as for square root.

Here are some examples. Note that there are no spaces within the expression, until the space that comes before the "equals."

Refer to the note in boldface type at the beginning of this paper, for explanation of conventions used to represent Braille in this paper.

The square root of sixteen equals four.

$\sqrt{16} = 4$

*ar*16*er* = #4

The cube root of twenty-seven equals three.

$\sqrt[3]{27} = 3$

*gh*3*ar*27*er* = #3

Money

The dollar sign and the cent sign are represented differently than in literary Braille. In Nemeth Code they are:

Dollar sign $
Dot 4, s

Cent sign ¢
Dot 4, c

The comma in the above examples represents the end of a cell, and does not appear in Braille. These symbols are written in the same place as in print – that is, the symbol for "dollars" before its number, and the symbol for "cents" after its number.

The decimal point (dots 4-6) is the same as in literary Braille. It is not the same as the period.

Here are some samples of Nemeth Code usage:

Three dollars and fifty cents
Inkprint: $3.50
Braille: `s3.50
[No numeric indicator is required because the dollar symbol is a mathematical symbol.]

Eighty-five cents
Inkprint: 85¢
Braille: #85`c

Working a Problem

Math problems can be set up in the same way as inkprint problems written vertically. This is easiest to do with a Braillewriter. A problem can be worked similarly to the way it would be done in print. However, many Braillewriters tend to flatten the dots and have irregular line spacing if the paper is rolled up and down. Therefore it is helpful for the student to learn to remember carried/borrowed numbers mentally, and write down only the answer.

Writing a vertical problem for addition, subtraction, or multiplication, or setting up a problem for long division, is done with essentially the same arrangement as in inkprint. A book on the Nemeth Code will call these "spatial arrangements." Rules for spacing will be given, including rules for the length of the "separation line" (the horizontal line, made up of dots 3-5, separating the answer from the problem).

Here is an example of a problem involving fractions. The fraction lines / must be lined up above one another.

NOTE: It should be assumed that the fractions below were shown vertically in inkprint–that is, with the numerator physically above the denominator and separated by a horizontal line. The numerals and other symbols below illustrate the Nemeth Code Braille usage for fractions and mixed numbers, not the inkprint appearance.

Five-sixths minus one-fourth equals seven-twelfths.

⊂5/6 ⊃
- ⊂1/4 ⊃
―――――
⊂7/12⊃

The chapter on "Mathematics" and the Appendix on "The Paper-Compatible Abacus" in this *Handbook* offer detailed suggestions on methods for working problems.

Other Common Symbols

Here are a few miscellaneous symbols which may be useful.

Refer to the note in boldface type at the beginning of this paper for explanation of conventions used to represent Braille in this paper. Commas are used here to show the end of a Braille cell, and do not appear in Braille.

Omission symbol
[To show where a missing element must be filled in]
Dots 1-2-3-4-5-6
[Full cell]

Is less than
<
Dots 5, 1-3

Is greater than
>
Dots 4-6, 2

Degrees
°
[Both angle and temperature]
Dots 4-5, 4-6, 1-6

Percent
%
Dots 4, 3-5-6

The degree symbol and the percent symbol immediately follow the number, without a space, just as they appear in print.

Pi π is written:
Dots 4-6, p

Pi r squared is written:
Dots 4-6, p, r, dots 4-5, two
[no spaces]

Conclusion

A Braille edition of this "Easy Guide to the Nemeth Code" is available from:

Braille Action Laboratory
Perceptual Alternatives Laboratory
Life Sciences Building
University of Louisville
Louisville, KY 40292

To promote maximum clarity for each group of readers, the Braille edition is not identical to this inkprint edition.

This "Easy Guide to the Nemeth Code" is *not* a complete guide to the Nemeth Code. For more detailed information, consult *The Nemeth Braille Code for Mathematics and Science Notation*, from the American Printing House for the Blind.

APPENDIX G

THE PAPER-COMPATIBLE ABACUS

By Doris M. Willoughby

In Consultation With

Dr. T. V. (Tim) Cranmer

"The abacus is so *different* from working out a problem with pencil and paper or on the Braillewriter. Why do we have to have two completely different systems?" Many blind students and their teachers have echoed this lament.

Indeed, we do *not* need to have two completely different systems. This paper presents a new approach to the abacus, conforming to the traditional patterns of addition, subtraction, multiplication, and division in this country. At the same time, it incorporates many of the elements of the traditional Oriental method which has proven so helpful to so many blind students.

The Cranmer Abacus – A Valuable Tool

Before the 1960's, blind children worked math problems in Braille (or large print), by mental arithmetic, and with various devices such as the Taylor Slate and the Cubarithm Slate. A tremendous tool for speed and efficiency was added in the early 1960's, when Dr. T. V. Cranmer adapted the Japanese abacus for use by the blind, and Fred Gissoni developed a system of instruction. With the Cranmer Abacus, which is designed so that beads stay in position while being examined by touch, blind students could work problems with great speed. Fred Gissoni's instruction book made the Japanese method of calculating widely accessible. An instruction book by Mae Davidow followed in 1966. The book by Nancy Jacquat Foster provided particularly clear explanations and a great many well-chosen practice problems. (See "References" for complete bibliographical information on each instruction book above.)

Nevertheless, this method, derived from the Japanese with few adaptations, had several serious disadvantages when used by American schoolchildren.

Disadvantages of Traditional Japanese Method

As the social climate in America has changed to bring most blind children into regular "mainstream" classes, several serious disadvantages have become apparent with the Oriental method on the abacus:

(1) Work proceeds from left to right, instead of from right to left.

(2) Conventional "borrowing" and "carrying" are not used; instead a differing system of "secrets" (as they are called in instruction books) must be learned – e.g., to add 9, you might "set 4, clear 5, and set one left."

These "secrets" actually are a form of borrowing and carrying, but are very different from the conventional Western method.

(3) In the Japanese system, the number facts are not organized in the "families" well-known to U.S. schoolchildren (e.g., 4+3, 3+4, 7-4, 7-3). Instead, combinations are organized as "secrets" for a given addend (e.g., 1+3, 2+3, 3+3, 4+3, 5+3, 6+3, 7+3, 8+3, and 9+3 are grouped together). The "commutative property of addition" (e.g., 4+3=3+4) is not easy to demonstrate with such a system. Furthermore, there are more total "number facts" to be learned.

(4) Children below third grade find it very difficult to grasp these "secrets" as being logical. This is unfortunate, because modern education stresses that children should understand mathematical processes. Moreover, the Oriental method discourages a logical approach as being slower than memorized "secrets."

(5) If a child is to become skilled in traditional on-paper computation, it is difficult to devote the time to developing skill on the abacus. If, on the other hand, much time and attention is devoted to learning abacus skills, the child may not understand on-paper computation.

(6) If a child does manage to understand both the abacus and on-paper computation, he/she finds that one skill actually interferes with the other. They proceed in opposite directions and use different combinations.

(7) Because of all these difficulties, blind students often are not taught to use the abacus until the upper grades. Valuable time is lost, and high proficiency and speed are rarely attained.

The Oriental method of calculation on the abacus is extremely fast. It is also efficient, and time-tested – in fact, tested over a time span that may boggle the mind of the typical Western teacher. (Whereas Western on-paper methods only became common in very recent history, the abacus has been in use in the Orient in virtually the same way since ancient times.) Nevertheless, in the setting of general education in the United States today, the Oriental method does have the disadvantages stated above.

Why Not Calculators?

"Why not just use calculators?" is a question often asked today. Many adults (blind and sighted) do just that. However, schoolchildren are still taught to work problems on paper, and blind children should learn along with others. The abacus is not a "calculator," since the actual computation must be done by the operator; hence it is appropriate for situations in which others are required to use pencil and paper. When sighted children are permitted to use calculators, as they are in some situations, then the blind child should be permitted to use a calculator (with speech or Braille output) also.

Advantages of the New Method

In contrast, the new method is compatible with computation on paper (print or Braille), and very similar to it:

(1) Addition and subtraction proceed from right to left, just as on paper.

(2) The Oriental "secrets" are not used. Instead, the ordinary number facts (e.g., 5+6=11) are used directly.

(3) Borrowing and carrying are done in essentially the same way as on paper.

(4) Real understanding of the computation is facilitated, in accordance with modern educational philosophy. If the child already understands borrowing, carrying, and other aspects of on-paper calculation, he uses the same principles to which he/she is already accustomed. If he/she has not yet learned these things, work on the abacus helps with this understanding instead of interfering with it.

(5) If a first-grader has learned only some of the number facts (for example, those totaling less than ten), he/she can easily be taught to add or subtract with these on the abacus. As the student learns more

combinations, he/she can include them.

(6) In multiplication, the partial products are positioned in the same way as on paper.

(7) The subtractions which are part of traditional long division are seen on the abacus almost exactly as on paper.

(8) Learning can proceed in the same sequence and at the same pace as for sighted students. Regular arithmetic textbooks are entirely suitable. (Note: For this reason, no lists of practice exercises are included in this paper. If a particular student needs supplementary exercises, the teacher should obtain another regular textbook, possibly from a lower grade level.)

(9) Many elements of this new method are the same as the method derived from the Japanese and described by Foster (Jacquat), Gissoni, and Davidow. Thus the changes which a teacher must make in converting to this new method are minimized.

Disadvantages of the new method, together with some disadvantages of the abacus *per se,* are discussed below.

How the New Method Came to Be

Delores Hornocker, an experienced teacher of blind children, was frustrated by her young students' difficulty with the Japanese "secrets." She said, "Why not just add and subtract with conventional borrowing and carrying?" and proceeded to do just that.

I (Doris Willoughby), teaching in a neighboring district, had given up on teaching the abacus below third grade. I observed Mrs. Hornocker's method, and was excited to note that it could easily be taught to very young children. Inspired by her idea, I added some aspects to make it even more compatible with on-paper computation (especially the matter of proceeding from right to left). My husband, Curtis, a blind electrical engineer, helped us to make optimum adaptations in multiplication and division.

"This is too good to be true," I kept thinking. "Why haven't other people, especially Dr. Cranmer himself, used this approach already if it is so good? There must be something wrong with it." So I called Dr. Cranmer and described the idea.

"I like it!" he exclaimed, to my great relief. "I agree that compatibility with the written problem is highly desirable. I think it will work, and I'd like to help you publicize it. Send me a written description (in Braille, of course), and let's look it over together. We've always used the other approach because that's how the Japanese do it. Nobody has really tried anything that's compatible with American computation on paper."

Since that conversation, I have learned that a number of other people are indeed using this method, to one degree or another. Newly blinded older students (including adults) often adapt the abacus to parallel the inkprint computation they formerly used.

Disadvantages and How to Handle Them

Nothing is perfect, and this new method is not perfect, especially in the context of the widespread current use of the Japanese method. Following is an acknowledgement of the major disadvantages and how they can be handled.

DISADVANTAGES OF THE PRINT-COMPATIBLE METHOD

(1) *"Students already skilled on the abacus should not be forced to change."* -They need not change. If a student really is skilled and comfortable in the Oriental method, he/she should be encouraged to continue. If, however, he/she is having difficulty with that method, the advantages of a changeover should be considered. If the student already knows how to work problems on paper, there is relatively little new learning involved.

(2) *"A teacher will need to teach two different ways, because so many students already use the Oriental method."* -In some situations this is true, and a substantial disadvantage. We believe that this is outweighed,

however, by the great advantages of the new method. An itinerant teacher can simply begin teaching the new method to younger students. In a special school with many blind students, it is possible that some groups may need to be subdivided for certain activities.

(3) *"If a child moves, the new school may not use this new system."* –This is no greater obstacle than many others encountered in changing schools. Provide the parents with information about this method so that they may tell others about it.

DISADVANTAGES OF THE ABACUS AS SUCH

(1) *"A partially-worked problem (e.g., the display after two of three partial products have been figured) is not the same as the written problem."* –This need not be a major barrier. If the teacher wishes to check the student's work at that point, he/she need simply work out the addition (in appropriate position) of the partial products which have already been set. Overall, this new method is much more easily reconciled with the written problem than is the Oriental method.

(2) *"In division, the procedure for correcting an error in the quotient is not the same as an equivalent erasure in print."* –Again, this is a minor difference which can easily be analyzed. The method for division, as a whole, is quite similar to long division on paper.

(3) *"Teachers want to see how a problem was worked. Afterwards you cannot see that."* –When a student is first learning, or if he is having difficulty, certain problems should be worked while a teacher is watching. (It may be helpful–for many reasons–for the child to explain aloud what he is doing, as he proceeds to work the problem.) Otherwise it usually is not essential that the teacher see a record of how the problem was worked.

(4) *"The child has to learn that some beads are worth 5 and are moved down, while others are worth 1 and are moved up."* –Learning the values and motions of the beads should require very little time and effort.

Any disadvantages of the abacus are very minor compared to the immense advantages to the student in terms of speed and convenience.

Many Procedures Unchanged

In many respects, this paper does not substantially change the way the use of the Cranmer Abacus was taught by books previously published in this country. However, all procedures –even those unchanged–will be described in some detail for the convenience of the reader.

Even where there are major differences between this method and the Oriental method, many aspects in common will be noted.

Reading the Cranmer Abacus

Figure G-1 shows the number 5270 on the Cranmer Abacus (both on a real abacus and on a diagram).

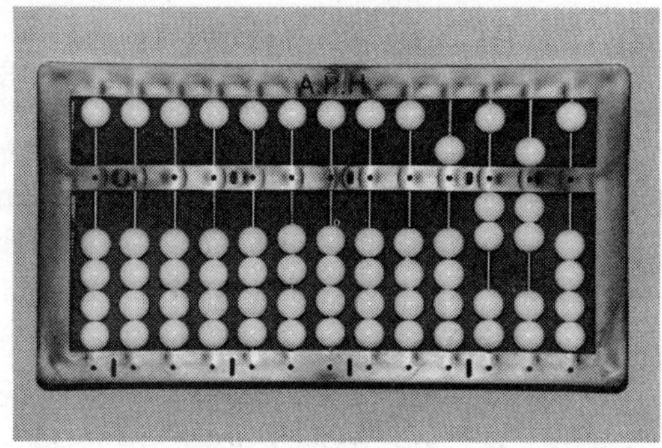

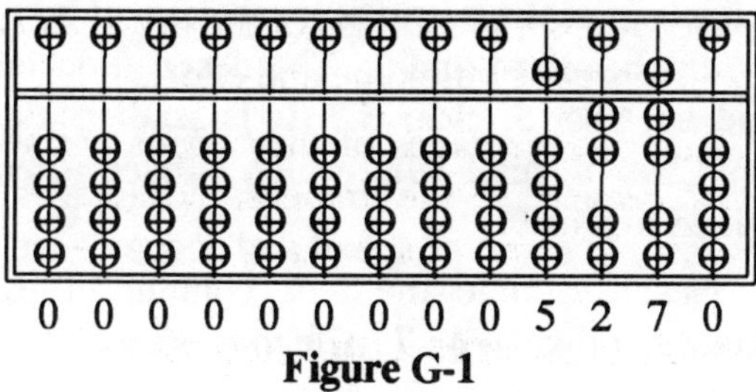

Figure G-1

To set a number on the abacus, beads are brought *to the horizontal bar* -that is, upper beads are brought down and lower beads are moved up. Each bead above the bar is worth 5 in its respective column, and each bead below the bar is worth 1 in its column. Column positioning is the same as on paper-units at the extreme right, tens in the next column to the left, etc. Thus Figure G-1 shows 5270.

On the horizontal bar itself, and also at the bottom of the abacus, a small raised dot appears at each column. Also, as one moves from right to left, one finds a small raised vertical mark dividing off each group of three columns. These coincide with comma placement in Braille or inkprint. (They also can be used for other purposes, as described for fractions and decimals.)

In this conventional position, the number is read as 5270 (rather than 527) because it ends at the extreme right edge of the abacus. For many kinds of computation this placement remains the same. In other procedures, other rules are used for determining where a number begins and ends.

Use a Real Abacus

The descriptions of computation, below, are detailed and contain many illustrations. Nevertheless, we strongly recommend that the reader have an actual abacus in hand and work out each step as described. Despite our efforts at clear explanation, it is difficult to follow the descriptions without moving the beads of an actual abacus.

Fingering

Efficient, consistent hand and finger movements are very important. Detailed suggestions are given at the end of this *Appendix*, in the Suggestions for Teaching.

In the descriptions of computation, finger motions as such will generally not be discussed.

Addition

TWO ADDENDS (NO CARRYING)

Example: **243 + 532 = 775**

$$\begin{array}{r} 243 \\ +532 \\ \hline 775 \end{array}$$

Place 243 at extreme right on the abacus. Place 532 at extreme left. (Figure G-2)

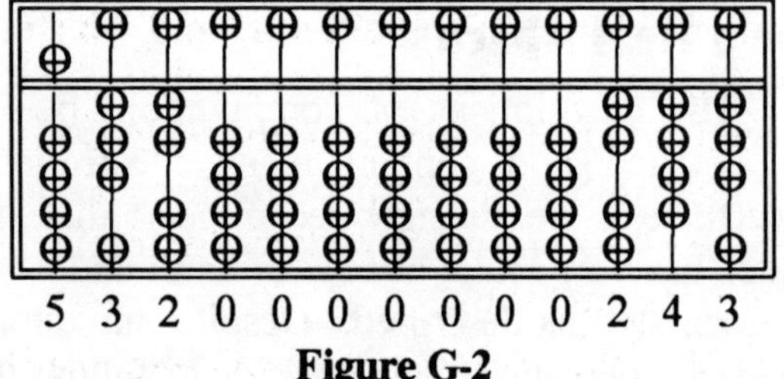

Figure G-2

[*For the convenience of the instructor, numerals have been written at the bottom of each column in abacus diagrams.*]

Examine the units column in both addends. Think 3+2=5. In the units column of the first addend (which is in the location where the sum will appear), "erase" (i.e., clear off) the 3, and replace it with a 5 (that is, a bead from above the bar). Thus the sum is now beginning to appear. See Figure G-3.

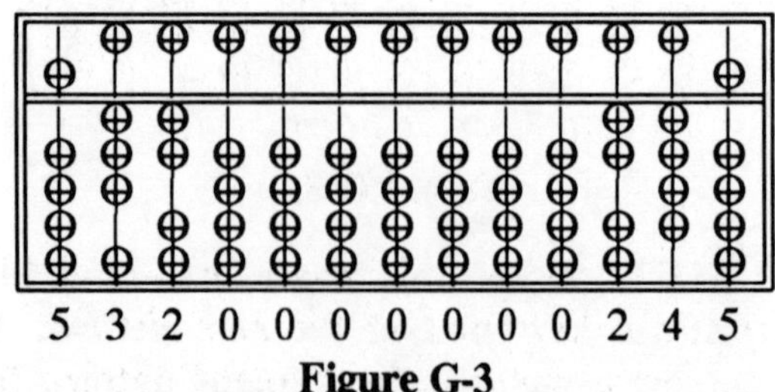

Figure G-3

Clear the 2 in the units column of the second addend (on the left side of the abacus). (Note: The student may find it more efficient to clear the digit of the left-hand addend just before he does the computation on the right side of the abacus; or he may do both acts simultaneously. For simplicity in description, however, this paper will assume that the digit in the left-hand addend is cleared after it has been added in.)

NOTE: This way of handling 3+2 illustrates a key point of the new method. As in traditional on-paper computation in the U.S., 3+2 is studied as part of the grouping of facts which equal 5: 0+5, 1+4, 2+3, 3+2, 4+1, 5+0. The emphasis is on the sum. The student simply changes the 3 to a 5; it is rather like erasing a chalk number and replacing it with another.

In the Oriental method, in contrast, the emphasis is entirely on the mechanics of how to move the beads to add 2. The description here would be, "Set 5, clear 3." It is studied along with "Clear 8, set 1 left," which is used when 2 is added to 8 or 9.

Next, examine the tens column in each addend. Think 4+3=7. Clear ("erase") the 4 and replace it with a 7. Also clear the 3 of the second addend (at the left).

In the hundreds column of the right-hand area, think 2+5=7. The idea here is the same. However, note that in a mechanical sense it is even simpler: to change the 2 to a 7 does not require replacing any beads, but merely bringing the "5" (upper) bead to the bar. The 5 in the second addend (at the left) is then cleared.

The sum, 775, appears in the right-hand position. (Figure G-4)

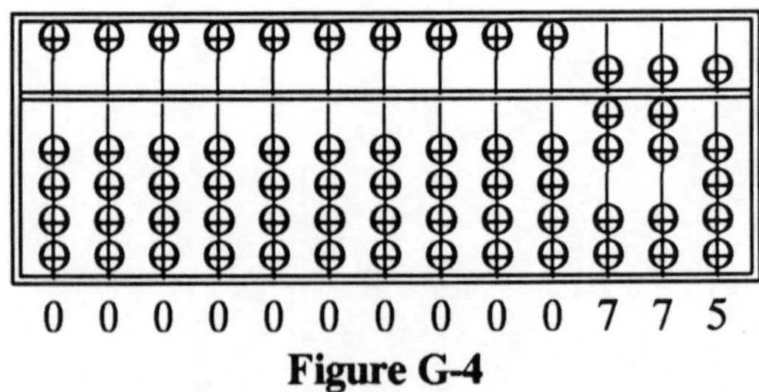

Figure G-4

ALTERNATIVE OPTIONS

Some teachers have young beginners always use the *four* columns at the extreme left for the second addend. That is, while a second addend of 2524 would be placed at the extreme left, a second addend of 24 would be placed in the third and fourth columns from the left (as though it were 0024). With young children just learning about place value, this helps reinforce the idea of "thousands, hundreds, tens, and ones." With this option, there is even a small vertical mark in the location for the comma.

The above alternative idea will not work for addition problems using long numbers. The older student should learn to set the addend at the extreme left regardless of its length. The illustrations in this paper show the second addend at the extreme left.

As a different alternative, placing the second addend at the left is regarded by some teachers as unnecessary. The student may prefer to keep the second addend in his head, or to refer to the written problem. However, we recommend that the student be taught to place the second addend onto the abacus as explained, and then clear off each digit as it is added in.

TWO ADDENDS (*WITH CARRYING*)

```
  11
 476
+ 56
----
 532
```

Place 476 at extreme right on the abacus. Place 56 at the extreme left, and clear those digits as they are added in.

(Note: The student needs to remember that this addend is 56 and not 560. For the beginner, it may be helpful always to use *four* columns at the left, as described above under Alternative Options, and set 56 as 0056. The advanced student, who should remember whether or not there are zeros, and who may need the space on the abacus elsewhere, should place the second addend at the extreme left. The illustrations in this paper will continue to show the second addend at the extreme left, without leading zeros.)

The following description will be somewhat abbreviated, since the idea has been explained in the previous example.

Think 6+6=12. Change the units column (at the right) to a 2. Carry 1 to the tens, changing the 7 to an 8. Also clear the 6 from the second addend, at the left. Abacus now reads 482. (Figure G-5)

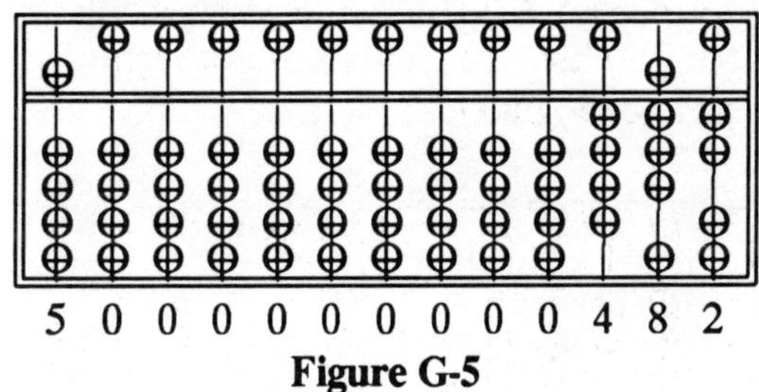

Figure G-5

NOTE: Again, this way of handling 6+6 illustrates a key point of the new method. In the Japanese method, the thought pattern for adding 6 would be, "Set 1 and clear 5 [in the units column]; then set 1 left [in the tens column]." In the new method, the thought pat-

tern is the familiar, "6+6=12: note down the 2 and carry 1."

Think 8+5=13. Change the tens column to 3. Carry 1: In the hundreds column, think 4+1=5, and simply change the 4 to a 5. Also, clear the 5 in the second addend, at the left. Abacus now reads 532.

Note that in the hundreds column there is nothing more to add, since the second addend has nothing in the hundreds column. Therefore the problem is finished, and 532 is the final sum.

COLUMN ADDITION (MORE THAN TWO ADDENDS)

$$\begin{array}{r} \mathit{22} \\ \mathbf{487} \\ \mathbf{359} \\ \mathbf{24} \\ \mathbf{+198} \\ \hline \mathbf{1068} \end{array}$$

Add 487+359 as you would for a two-addend problem, above. This sum, 846, now becomes the first addend for the problem 846+24=870. Then in turn add 870+198 to achieve the final sum, 1068.

Although this is not exactly the same as the traditional paper method for manual addition of several numbers [see note at the end of this description], it has many important advantages:

(1) This method is not dependent on having the problem written on paper in columnar format. This advantage is especially important when a problem is dictated orally, or when it is presented as a story problem ("Mr. Brown is taking inventory at his grocery store. He has 487 cans of chicken soup, 359 cans of vegetable soup, 24 cans of mushroom soup...")

(2) When adding numbers written in columnar format, it is easy to make mistakes in reading down each separate column (7+9+4+8, etc.) This is especially true when, as in this example, the addends have differing numbers of digits.

(3) This method is the same as the procedure on a calculator.

(4) This is the same as the two-addend method on the abacus.

Note: If the problem is set up in columnar format in Braille (or large print), it is possible to proceed all the way down each column in turn. However, Tim Cranmer, Sharon Duffy, and other blind adults strongly recommend the regular method as described above (that is, the abacus method identical to that for two addends). The advantages to the regular method are major ones. The only clear advantage to the alternative (described below in this footnote) is its greater similarity to the traditional manual method for column addition.

Here is the alternative method for column addition:

Do not set the addends onto the abacus. Instead, refer to the written problem.

Read down the column on paper, and add the units mentally: 7+9+4+8=28. Set the 8 in the units column, and set the 2 (carry) in the tens column.

Again refer to the written problem to add the tens column: 2(carry)+8+5+2+9=26. Change the tens column to a 6, and set the 2 (carry) in the hundreds column.

Read the next column to the left (hundreds) and think 2(carry)+4+3+nothing+1=10. Change the hundreds column to zero, and set the 1 (carry) in thousands. The complete sum is 1068.

Subtraction

SUBTRACTION WITHOUT BORROWING

$$\begin{array}{r} 945 \\ -203 \\ \hline 742 \end{array}$$

Subtraction is set up in a manner comparable to addition. In this example, 945 is set at the extreme right, and 203 at the extreme left. Again, the digits of the number which is set at the left of the abacus are cleared as they are processed. (As with addition, some teachers prefer to have beginners always use the *four* columns at the left for the number to be subtracted. However, illustrations in this paper will show the second addend at the extreme left without leading zeros.)

In the units column, think 5-3=2. Replace the 5 with a 2, thus beginning to record the answer (difference). Clear the 3 of the second addend. Figure G-6 shows the work at this stage.

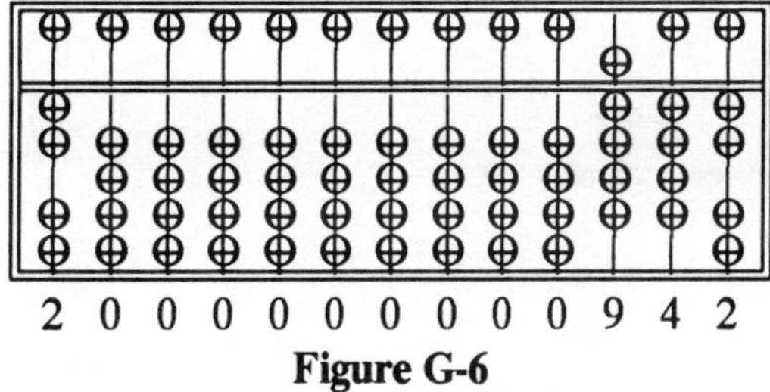

Figure G-6

In the tens column, think 4-0=4. (It is important to notice that there is a zero, and avoid slipping over to the hundreds column by mistake). In the tens column, no movement of beads is needed. The 4 is already there, and we must merely consider this numeral to be part of the answer which is being formed. In the second addend, at the left, there is a zero, and the student must only understand that the column has now been processed.

In the hundreds column, think 9-2=7. Change the 9 to a 7; in this case, it is just a matter of removing two beads. Clear the 2 from the second addend, at the left. We have the answer: 742.

SUBTRACTION WITH BORROWING

51
~~6~~~~2~~4
-398
226

Set 624 at extreme right. Set 398 at the left, and clear those digits as they are processed.

It is not possible to subtract eight from four [in elementary arithmetic]. Therefore, borrow 1: that is, change 2 to 1 in the tens column on the abacus. Mentally consider the 4 to be a 14 instead. Then think 14-8=6, and change the units column to 6. Clear the 8 from 398. Abacus now reads 616. (Figure G-7)

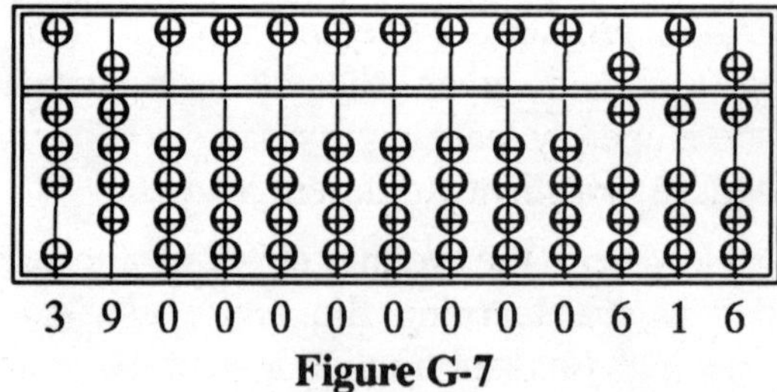

Figure G-7

NOTE: Once more, this illustrates a key point. In the Japanese method, the directions for subtracting 8 would be, "Clear one left [in the tens column]; then [in the units column] set 5 and clear 3." With the new method, in contrast, the thought pattern is the familiar "Borrow 1 from the tens column, then think 14-8=6: put down a 6 in the units column." The student simply changes the 4 to a 6, rather like erasing one chalk number and replacing it with another.

In the tens column, it is not possible to subtract nine from one. Borrow one from the hundreds – that is, change the 6 to a 5. In the tens, mentally consider the 1 to be an 11 instead. Then think 11-9=2, and change that column to a 2. Clear the 9 of 398. Abacus now reads 526.

In hundreds, think 5-3=2, and change that column to a 2. Clear the 3 of 398. The abacus now reads 226, which is the final answer.

Borrowing Across Zeros

Example: **6003 - 358 = 5645**

599
~~600~~3
- 358

5645

When borrowing is necessary and a zero appears in the column immediately to the left–and especially when there is another zero to the left of that–the beginner may need additional explanation. The procedure is basically the same as in the previous example, but some added understanding is necessary.

An older student accustomed to borrowing in written problems (whether in inkprint or in Braille) should grasp the idea immediately; he/she is merely learning to carry out a familiar procedure in a slightly different medium.

However, the young child in the early grades is still learning the entire concept of "borrowing" (and subtraction in general) as well as the specifics of how to do this on the abacus. Regular elementary arithmetic texts generally avoid examples with zeros during the first few lessons on borrowing, and give added explanation when borrowing across zeros is introduced. This is a good policy with a young learner.

To solve the above example, set 6003 at the right and 358 at the left (Figure G-8).

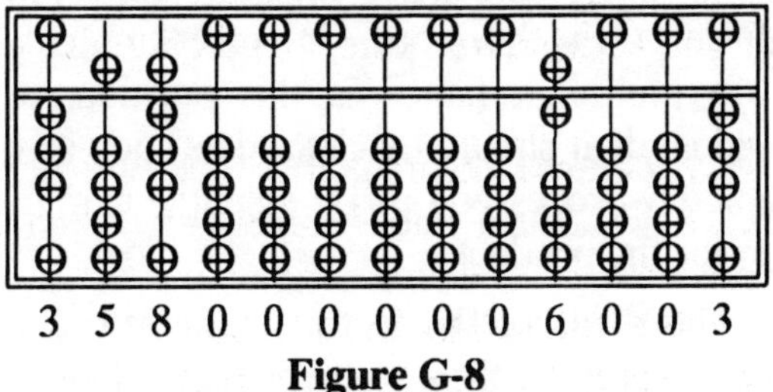

Figure G-8

It is not possible to subtract 8 from 3, and therefore we must borrow. But as we examine the tens column in 6003, we find that we are "borrowing from a zero." We must look as far to the left as necessary to find a digit other than zero; borrow from that non-zero digit; and then change the intervening zeros to nines.

Specifically in this example, change the 6 to a 5 and change the zeros to nines. Then mentally consider the 3 to be a 13. Think 13-8=5, and change the units column to 5. At the left end of the abacus, clear the 8 from 358. The abacus now reads 5995 (Figure G-9).

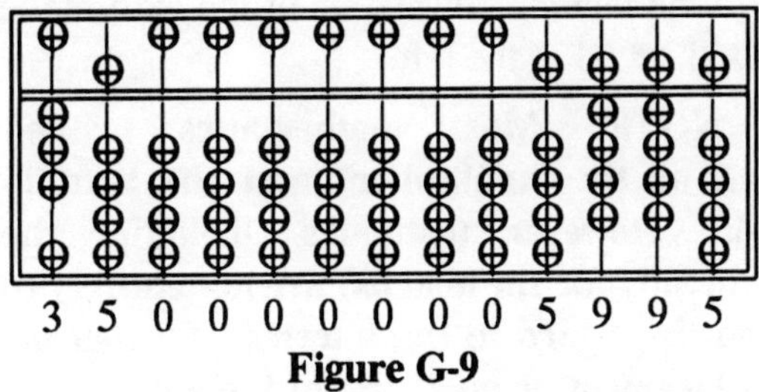

Figure G-9

In the tens column, think 9-5=4, and change the 9 to a 4. Clear the 5 of the 358.

In the hundreds column, think 9-3=6. Change the 9 to a 6, and clear the 3 of 358.

The number which was at the left (358) has now been entirely subtracted and cleared. Therefore the 5 in the thousands column stands. The abacus reads 5645, which is the final answer (difference).

Multiplication

MULTIPLYING BY ONE DIGIT

First Example: **3x94=282**

```
  94
 x 3
 ---
 282
```

One factor is always set at the extreme left. We will set 94 at the left.

NOTE: Most mathematics textbooks speak of the "multiplier" and the "multiplicand." However, textbooks (including those specifically for the abacus) are not entirely consistent in regard to these terms. Furthermore, the placement of numbers on the abacus is not perfectly analogous to placement on paper–especially in regard to a problem written both vertically and horizontally. Therefore this paper will refer to the multiplier and the multiplicand simply as "factors" (an inclusive term), to avoid confusion. Since multiplication is commutative (i.e., 3x94=94x3), it does not matter which factor is placed on which side of the abacus. If the student finds it easier to place the smaller number in a particular position, he/she may choose to "reverse" a problem when one factor has more digits than the other.

The position of the other factor (3) on the abacus is determined by the total number of digits in the entire problem (excluding the answer)–in this case, three digits. This number of digits, plus one, shows where to start placing the other factor (i.e., where the most significant, or leftmost, digit of the other factor is placed). In this example, the 3 should be placed four columns from the right: two digits in "94" plus one digit in "3" plus one extra equals four. See Figure G-10.

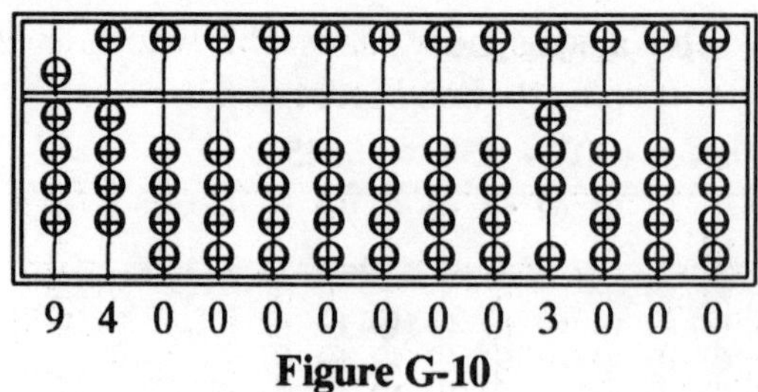

Figure G-10

When the product is found, it will end at the extreme right.

Think 3x4=12; set 2 in the units column (extreme right) and 1 in the tens column.

The two rightmost columns constitute the location for the product of the first multiplication fact (12 in this case). The product of the next multiplication fact will *overlap* and be allotted the second and third columns from the right. The next (if there were one) would have the third and fourth columns from the right; etc. This thought pattern is not precisely the same as that for on-paper computation, but it is compatible with it.

Now think 3x9=27. The allotted position for 27 is the second and third columns from the right. We note that the 7 (of 27) falls on the same column as the 1 (of 12) which is already there; thus we must mentally add 1+7 and change the 1 to 8. The 2 falls into the third column from the right, which had been vacant.

NOTE: All addition should be done as explained for "Addition," above. However, the precise movement of the beads will not be described here.

Clear the 3. It is important to clear this factor so that the answer may be read without confusion. Furthermore, in problems which have a multidigit factor in this position, each individual digit should be cleared as soon as it is completely processed–this is essential in making room for the product.

The digits of the factor at the left should *not* be cleared as they are processed. Doing so may cause confusion in multidigit problems where the same digit will be multiplied more than once.

The abacus now reads 282, which is the answer (product). See Figure G-11.

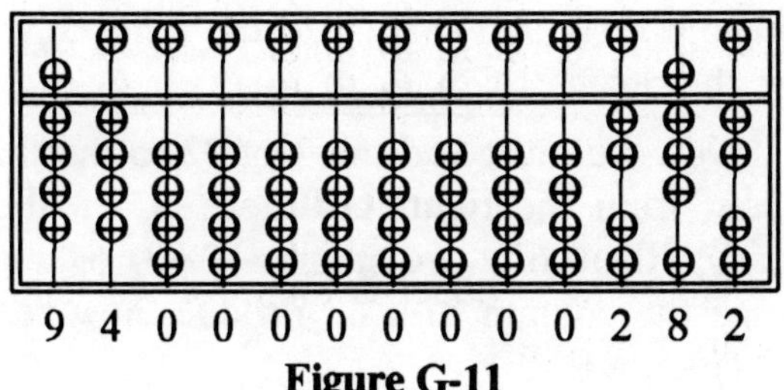

Figure G-11

Second Example: **6x981=5886**

$$\begin{array}{r} 981 \\ \times\ 6 \\ \hline 5886 \end{array}$$

Set one factor (981) at the extreme left.

In this example there are four total digits. By adding one extra column, we determine that the first digit of the other factor (in this case, the only digit) should be placed on the fifth column from the right.

Think 6x1=6, and place 6 at the extreme right. (It is often helpful to think of the one-digit answer as "06," as is done when filling in a computerized space which requires two digits. This helps to maintain the concept of overlapping two-digit locations for the products of individual multiplication facts.)

Think 6x8=48, and place the 48 in the second and third columns from the right. (At this point, some students may become confused about left-to-right *vs.* right-to-left progression, and try to place the 4 to the right of the 8. Explanation is comparable to what would be done for a similar error made on paper.) (See Figure G-12)

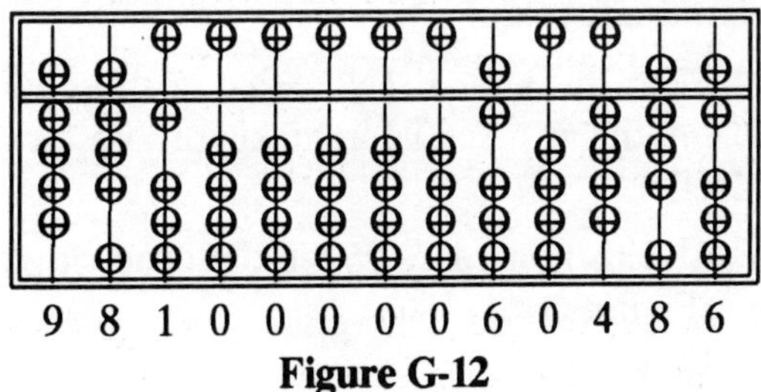

Figure G-12

Think 6x9=54, and prepare to place the answer on the third and fourth columns from the right. There is already another 4 in the column where this 4 should be placed, so it is necessary to think 4+4=8 and change that column to 8. Then a 5 is placed in the fourth column from the right.

Clear the factor, 6.

The complete product, 5886, is now displayed at the extreme right on the abacus.

MULTIPLYING BY TWO OR MORE DIGITS

Example: **83 x 94 = 7802**

```
  94
 x83
 ---
 282
752
----
7802
```

Set one factor (94) at extreme left. By noting the total number of digits in the problem, plus one extra, we determine that the other factor (83) should start in the fifth column from the right. (Figure G-13)

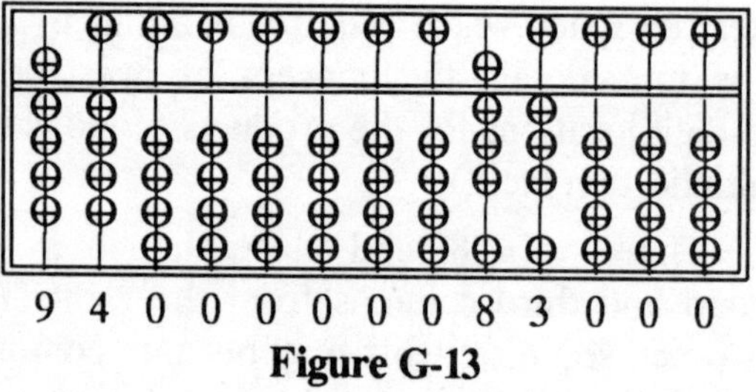

Figure G-13

Determining the first partial product is just like working the problems above with a one-digit factor. 3x4 = 12; therefore, set 2 in the units column and 1 in the tens. 3x9 = 27; change the tens column to 8 (because 1+7=8), and set 2 in the hundreds column.

Clear the 3 of 83. (Note that in a multidigit problem, this is essential in making room for the product.)

Abacus now reads 282 in the product position. (Figure G-14)

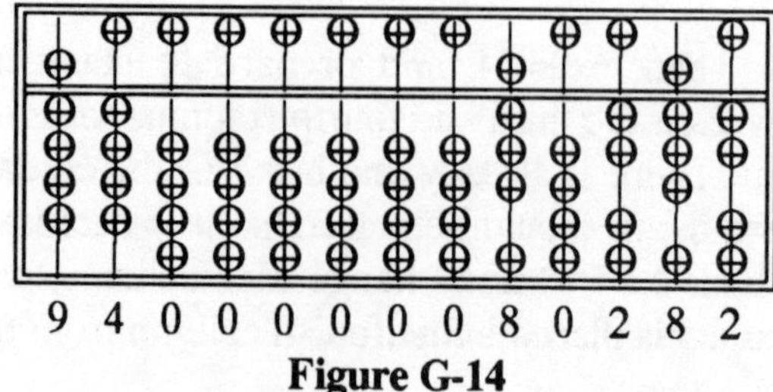

Figure G-14

Now prepare to set the next partial product, which will be offset just as in the written problem. Think 8x4 = 32. We want to place the 2 in the the second column from the right; but there is an 8 there already. Therefore, we think "8+2=10," change the second column from the right to a zero, and carry 1 to the third column from the right.

Now we must add the 3 of 32 to the third column from the right, but there is a 3 there already; therefore we think "3+3=6," and change the column to a 6. Product now reads 602. (Figure G-15)

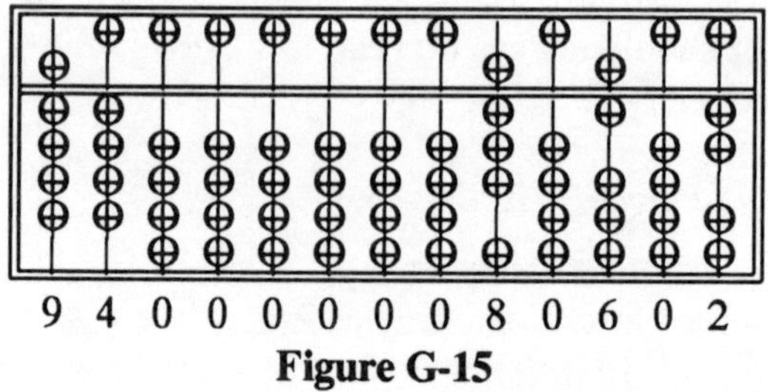

Figure G-15

For the next position in this second partial product, think 8x9 = 72. (Remember the concept of two-column overlapping positions.) Add the 2 onto the third column from the right: 6+2=8. The 7 of 72 is then set on the fourth column from the right. Clear the 8 of 83.

The final product is 7802 (Figure G-16).

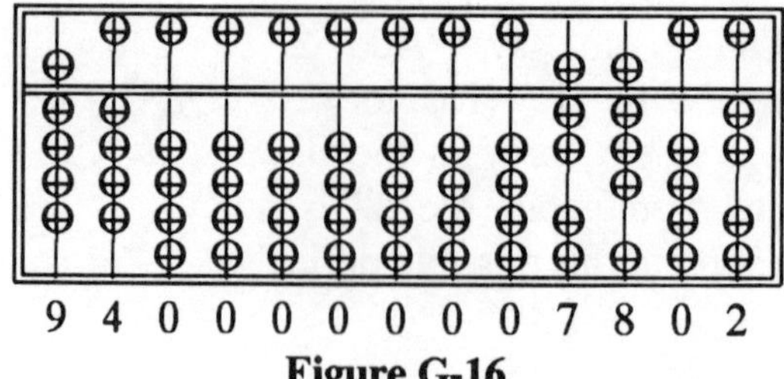

Figure G-16

REMARKS

Factors

As explained above, this discussion will refer to both the multiplier and the multiplicand simply as "factors." Placement on the abacus is explained in connection with examples.[1]

Care must be taken not to forget a final zero in a factor (example: 350x780). (In the *product* there is no difficulty, since it always ends at the extreme right. A vacant column at the right should always be read as a zero in the final product.)

Don't Forget Digits

Another matter of "easy forgetting" deserves attention. In the example 83x94, consider the first number fact in multiplying by 8 (when 94 has already been multiplied by 3). The student thinks "8x4=32;" mentally adds the 2 (of 32) to the 8 which is there already; changes the second column from the right to zero; and carries 1 to the third column from the right. Having done this much (including having some contact with the third column from the right), the student may forget all about the *3* of 32.

To prevent this difficulty, the student might be taught to say, "Add 2, carry one, and *remember the 3.*" (Do not say "carry the 3," as this is not a carry in the usual sense. But to recite "remember the 3" is helpful in calling attention to this possible difficulty.)

[1] It is possible to place the products as described without actually placing the factors on the abacus at all. Instead, the student could simply refer to the written problem if it is available. It is recommended, however, that the entire problem be placed on the abacus.

Division

ONE-DIGIT DIVISOR

First Example: **658 ÷ 3**

```
   219 R1
3)658
  6
  05
  03
   28
   27
    1
```

This procedure on the abacus closely parallels the way long division is done on paper.

The divisor (3) is always set at the extreme left. The dividend (658) is always set at the extreme right.

First, consider whether or not the one-digit divisor will go into the first digit of the dividend. Since it will, the first digit of the quotient must be placed two columns to the left of the beginning of the dividend, as in Figure G-17. (This makes it possible always to have a two-column position for the product when the divisor is multiplied by a digit of the quotient. Further explanation of overlapping positions appears below under Generalizations.) This analysis of position is only necessary for the first digit of the quotient; each succeeding digit is simply placed immediately to the right of the preceding one.

The rule is a simple one, but may seem hard to remember. An amusing mnemonic device may help: "When the divisor *will* go in, it makes the quotient so happy that it skips!"

Just as would be done with on-paper computation, mentally determine that the first digit of the quotient should be 2. The 2 is placed two columns to the left of the dividend, leaving one column blank. (See Figure G-17.)

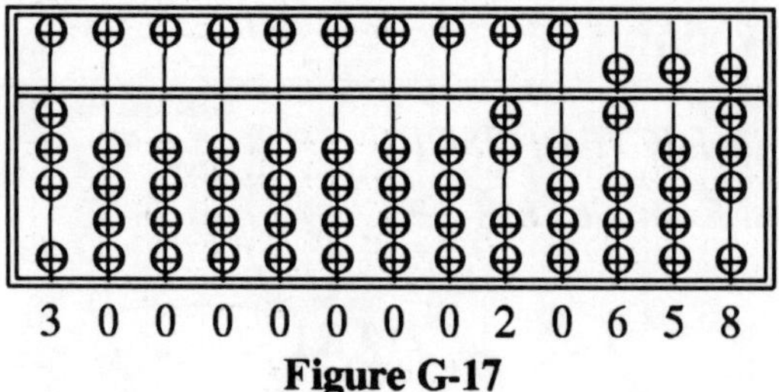

Figure G-17

As we multiply with the 2 of the quotient, we will be working only with the 6 of the dividend (with the vacant column on its left, it constitutes a two-column position for consideration). Think 2x3 = 6, and subtract 6, leaving another column vacant. (Note: To facilitate thinking of overlapping two-column positions, you may wish to look at the problem as 0658÷3. Writing this out in long division, as below, illustrates that the first subtraction [as well as the subsequent ones] actually involves a two-column position. This is clearly seen on the abacus but is not apparent in the traditional on-paper form.)

```
    219 R1
  ________
3)0658
  06
  --
   05
   03
   --
    28
    27
    --
     1
```

Now consider the 5, which technically may be considered to be 05, occupying the next (overlapping) two-column position. Determine (mentally) that the next digit in the quotient should be 1, and place a 1 to the right of the 2 in the quotient. Think "1x3 = 3" and subtract the 3, leaving 2. (Figure G-18)

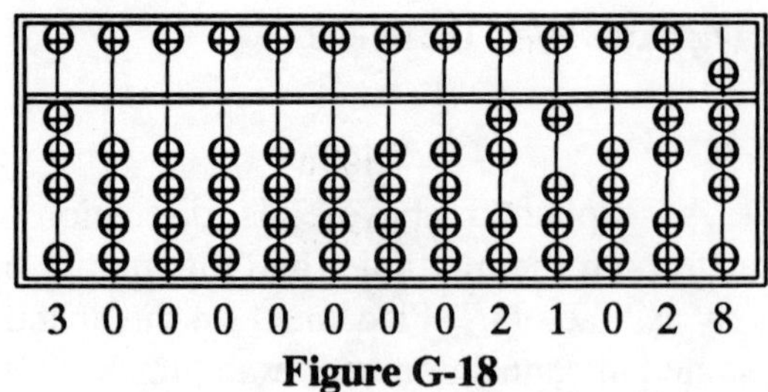

Figure G-18

NOTE: All subtractions should be done as explained for "Subtraction," above. However, the precise movement of the beads will not be described here.

Now consider the next (overlapping) two-column position, which reads 28. The nearest appropriate division fact is 9x3 = 27. Place a 9 in the quotient position, to the right of the 1. Think 9x3 = 27, and subtract: 28-27 = 01.

We have now reached the end of the quotient, since we have reached the last two-column position in the dividend. [This assumes the dividend to be a whole number.] Another way of checking is to compare the method that would be used to set up the multiplication problem 219x3: The total number of digits in 219 and 3 together, plus one extra, equals the number of columns from the right where the first digit (2) of 219 appears.

The 1 at the extreme right is not part of the quotient, but is a remainder. (Figure G-18)

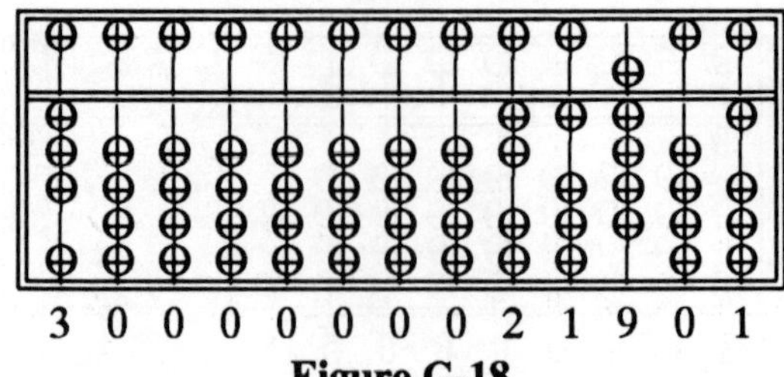

Figure G-18

Second Example: **16218 ÷ 3**

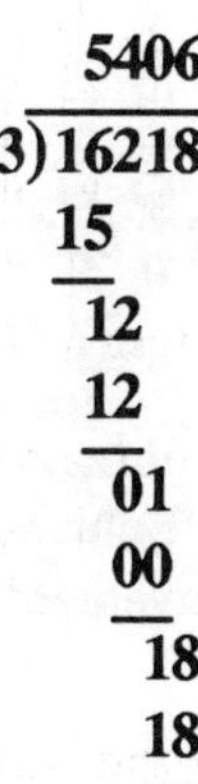

The divisor (3) is set at the extreme left. The dividend (16218) is set at the extreme right.

First, consider whether or not the one-digit divisor will go into the first digit of the dividend. Since it will *not* go in (1 cannot be divided by 3), the first digit of the quotient will be placed *immediately* to the left of the dividend. Remember that this analysis of position is only necessary for the first digit of the quotient; each succeeding digit is simply placed immediately after the preceding digit.

Determine (mentally) that the first digit of the quotient should be 5. Place the 5 immediately to the left of the dividend. (Figure G-19)

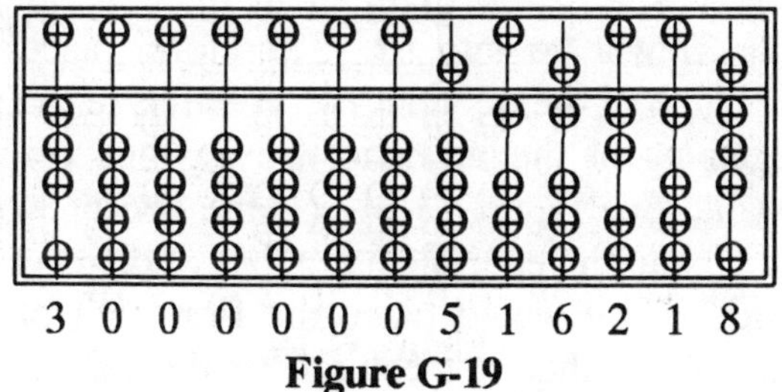

3 0 0 0 0 0 0 5 1 6 2 1 8

Figure G-19

As we multiply with the 5 of the quotient, we will be working only with the first two digits of the dividend (16) just as in a written problem. Think 5x3 = 15, and subtract the 15: change the 6 to a 1, then clear the 1 to the left. (Figure G-20)

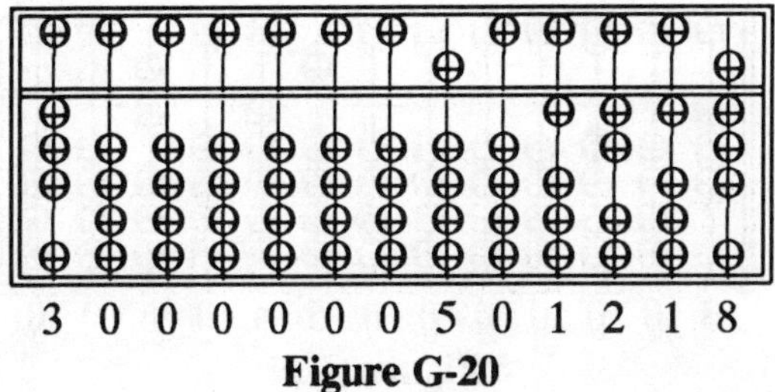

3 0 0 0 0 0 0 5 0 1 2 1 8

Figure G-20

Note that the 1 which remains (in the fourth column from the right) corresponds to the 1 which is found by subtraction during long division on paper.

Now consider the 12 in the next overlapping two-column position. Determine (mentally) that the next digit in the quotient should be 4, and place a 4 to the right of the 1 in the quotient. Think 4x3 = 12; subtract the 12, leaving zero (actually 00).

It is helpful to think of the next position in the dividend as 01, to aid in keeping the pattern of two-digit overlapping positions. Since 3 will not go into 01, the next digit of the quotient is 0, and a column is left vacant (Figure G-21).

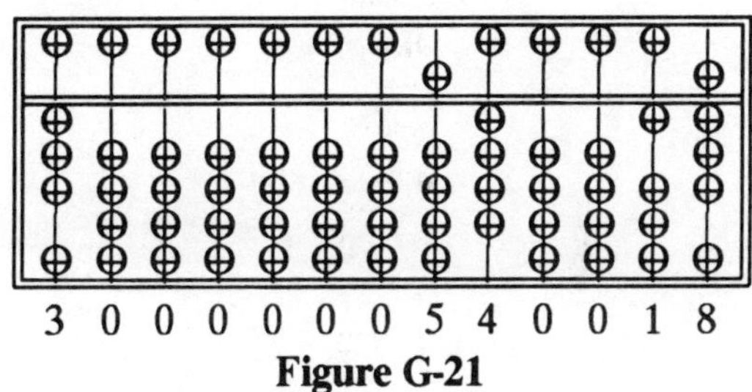

3 0 0 0 0 0 0 5 4 0 0 1 8

Figure G-21

Finally, consider the last two digits of the dividend (18). Since 18 ÷ 3 = 6, place a 6 after the 0 in the quotient (i.e., place a 6 in the third column from the right on the abacus). Subtract 18-18 = 0, thus clearing the dividend position and leaving no remainder. (See Figure G-22)

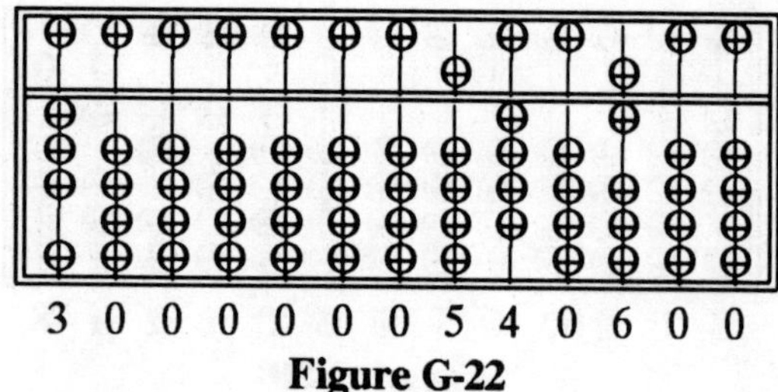

3 0 0 0 0 0 0 5 4 0 6 0 0

Figure G-22

Verify that the quotient is 5406 (not 54060 or 540600): The total number of digits in 3 and 5406 together, plus one extra, equals the number of columns from the right where the first digit of 5406 is placed.

DIVISOR HAVING TWO OR MORE DIGITS

Example: **626 ÷ 27 = 23 R5**

```
    23 R5
27)626
   54
    86
    81
     5
```

Set the divisor (27) at extreme left. Set the dividend (626) at extreme right. (Figure G-23)

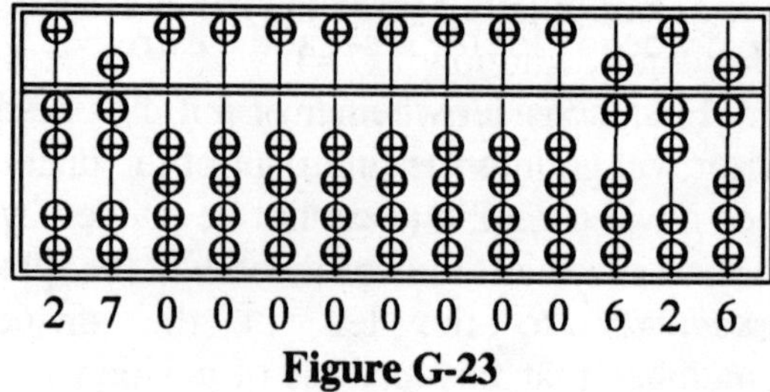

2 7 0 0 0 0 0 0 0 0 6 2 6

Figure G-23

In the first example for division, in deciding where to place the first digit of the quotient for a *one*-digit divisor, we asked whether or not that one digit would go into the first digit of the dividend. With a two-digit divisor, we consider whether or not those *two* digits will go into the first *two* digits of the dividend.

27 will go into 62. Therefore, place the first digit of the quotient two columns left of the beginning of the dividend, leaving one column vacant. See Figure G-24. (If the divisor would *not* go into the equivalent number of digits of the dividend, we would place the first digit of the quotient in the first column to the left of the dividend, leaving no columns vacant.)

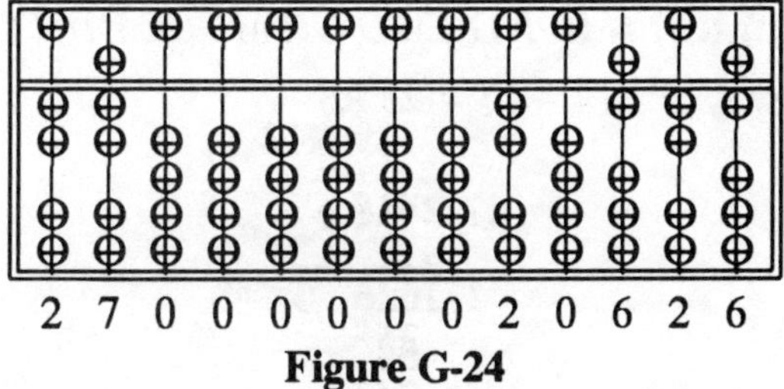

Figure G-24

Just as in doing long division on paper, we must mentally estimate each digit of the quotient. Estimate "2." Place a 2, two columns to the left of the beginning of the dividend. (Refer again to Figure G-24.)

Note that as we multiply with the 2 of the quotient, we will be subtracting from the first two digits of the dividend (62), just as in a written problem. First observe the 2 in the dividend, and mentally multiply 2x7=14. Four cannot be subtracted from 2, so we must borrow 1 from the next column to the left, making that a 5. Think 12-4=8, and change the 2 to an 8. Now we must subtract the 1 of the 14 (5-1=4). See Figure G-25.

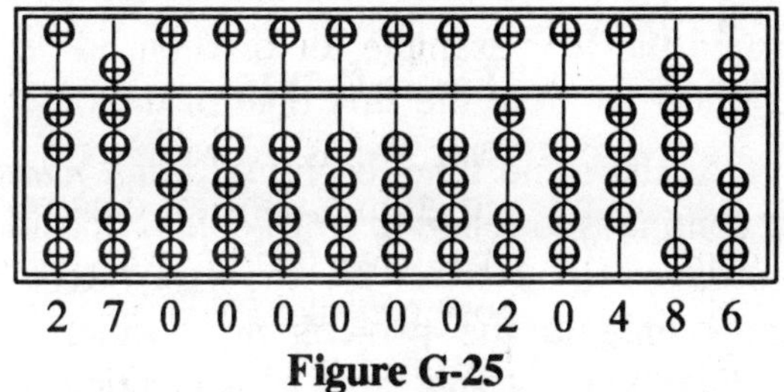

Figure G-25

Multiply the 2 in the quotient with the 2 of the divisor (2x2=4). Subtract the 4 in the dividend (4-4=0).

The abacus now reads 86 in the dividend position. In the quotient we still have just the 2 so far.

Now estimate 3 as the next digit in the quotient, placing it just to the right of the original 2. We now deal with the next (overlapping) two-column position: 86. Think 3x7=21. Subtract 1 from the column farthest right, leaving 5 in that column. Subtract 2 from the tens column, leaving 6. See Figure G-26.

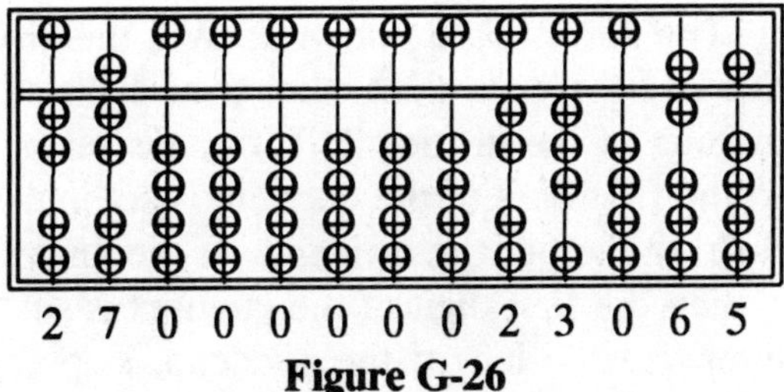

Figure G-26

Then think 3x2=6. Subtract 6 from the tens, leaving the tens column vacant.

Only 5 remains in the dividend position on the abacus. Since 27 cannot go into 5, this is a remainder of 5, and we do no further computation.

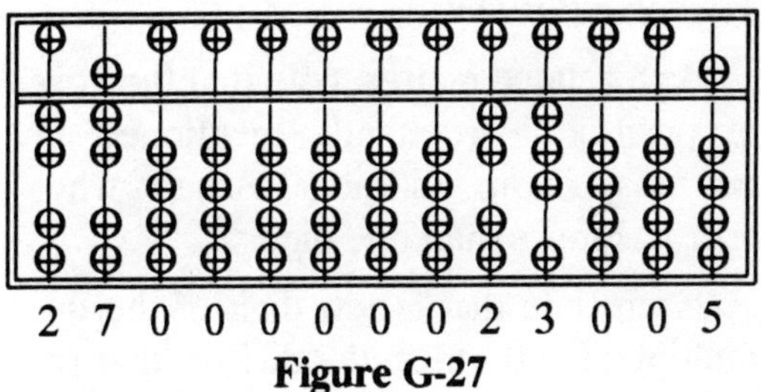

Figure G-27

The final answer is a quotient of 23 with a remainder of 5. (Figure G-27)

As an alternative confirmation, we know that the quotient is 23 (and not 230 or 2300, etc.) because on its right are the appropriate three columns: two corresponding to the two digits of the divisor, plus one extra. This is like the arrangement for setting up a multiplication problem.

GENERALIZATIONS ABOUT DIVISION

Don't Make This Mistake

When students (and teachers as well) first learn to skip a column to the left of the dividend when starting the quotient (if the divisor will go into the beginning of the dividend), they sometimes make an incorrect generalization. They may wrongly assume that the quotient should move over one column in the case of a one-digit divisor, two columns for a two-digit divisor, three columns for a three-digit divisor, etc. This is not correct.

The governing question is: Will the divisor divide into the equivalent number of digits at the beginning of the dividend? If the answer is no, then the first digit of the quotient is set immediately to the left of the dividend. If the answer is yes, then the first digit of the quotient is set two columns to the left of the dividend, skipping a column. *Always one column skipped!* If a one-digit divisor will go into the first digit, then skip *one* column. If a two-digit divisor will go into the first two digits, then skip *one* column. If a three-digit divisor will go into the first three digits, then skip *one* column – and so on, *ad infinitum.*

Overlapping Positions

As a related matter, note that the "overlapping positions" frequently mentioned in this paper acquire an additional aspect when the divisor has more than one digit.

Each time that a new digit of the quotient is multiplied with the *entire* divisor, that product is subtracted from a field which is one digit longer than the number of digits in the divisor. (Always *only one* digit *longer,* regardless of the number of digits in the divisor.) These fields overlap, moving one column to the right each time. All of this is analogous to the subtractions in long division on paper. For example, consider 626 ÷ 27, above. When 27 is multiplied by the 2 of the quotient, the result (54) is subtracted from the field *062.* Then 81 is subtracted from *086.* The fields in this example happen to have leading zeros. However, in many problems there is indeed a three-digit number to be subtracted from, when the next number of the dividend is considered (or "brought down," as it is often called when working on paper). Here is an example:

2415 ÷ 27 = 89 R12

```
     89 R12
27)2415
   216
    255
    243
     12
```

Note that in this example, a column would *not* be skipped between the first quotient digit and the dividend. The first field is 241, not 0241. Figure G-28 shows 2415 ÷ 27, with the first digit of the quotient in place, but with no subtraction having been done.

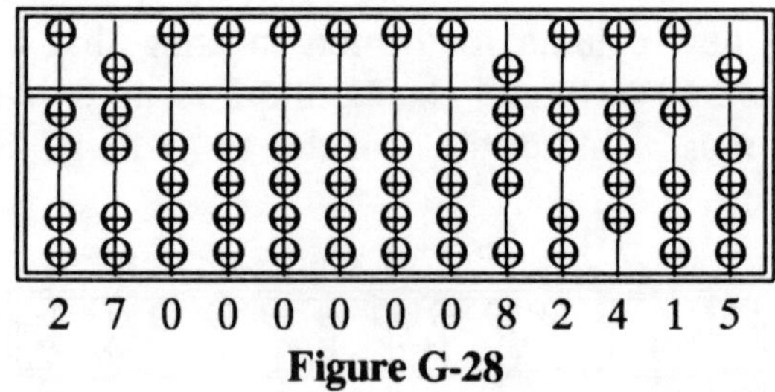

Figure G-28

At the same time, each *individual number fact* continues to relate to a *two-column* position, regardless. In 2415 ÷ 27, the fact "8x7=56" relates only to the two-column position now occupied by the 4 and the 1 (this position overlaps the two-column position which is now occupied by the 2 and the 4, and which is related to the fact "8x2=16"). However, the complete multiplication "8x27" relates to the entire three-digit field now occupied by 241.

Which Direction to Move

In this paper, computation usually is directed from left to right, or right to left, to agree with the traditional procedure on paper. In division, for example, the dividend is processed from left to right. However, when a subtraction is done during the division process, the right-hand column is subtracted before the left. (For example, the first subtraction for 626 ÷ 27 is 62-54. The 4 is subtracted before the 5 is subtracted.) In this paper, deviations from the directionality of traditional procedures are made only when essential. It is, however, possible in most cases to proceed in the reverse direction.

ADJUSTMENT FOR INCORRECT TRIAL QUOTIENT

When working long division on paper, sometimes we misjudge a digit of the quotient and need to erase a segment of computation. On the abacus we can make a similar correction without needing to work the entire problem over. The method described here is essentially the same as that in other instruction books; however the subtraction or addition itself is done in the manner of this new method.

Trial Quotient Too Low

```
    22 ?
27)626
   54
    86
    54
    32 ?
```

Suppose, in the example, that we expect the second digit of the quotient to be 2 instead of 3. The following steps describe correct calculation for the first digit, a too-low second digit, and correction of the error:

(a) Place the first 2 of the quotient and subtract 54 from the first two digits of the dividend, as described above. 86 remains in the dividend.

(b) Place another 2 to the right of the first 2 in the quotient.

(c) Subtract 54 from the 86 which had remained in the dividend position. (See Figure G-29)

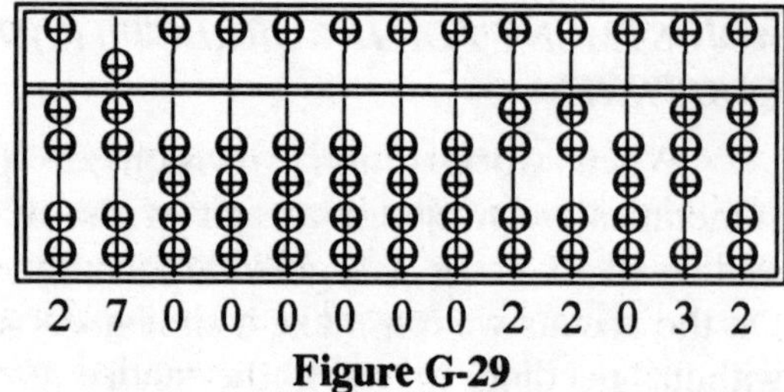

2 7 0 0 0 0 0 0 0 2 2 0 3 2

Figure G-29

(d) Note that we have an apparent remainder of 32. This is not appropriate, since the divisor of 27 is smaller than the remainder.

(e) Note that we do not need to re-compute with the first 2 in the quotient, as there was no difficulty with that.

(f) To make the correction, change the second (right-hand) 2 in the quotient to a 3.

(g) Multiply 1x27 (mentally), and subtract 27 from 32.

(h) We now have a remainder of 5, which is appropriate. The abacus is now as it should be for the completed problem. (Refer back to Figure G-27.)

Trial Quotient Too High

```
     24 ?
27)626
    54
    --
     86
     ??
     --
```

Suppose that we misjudge in the opposite manner and expect the second digit of the quotient to be a 4. The following steps describe correct calculation for the first digit, a too-high second digit, and correction of the error:

(a) Place the first 2 of the quotient and subtract 54. 86 remains in the dividend.

(b) Place a 4 to the right of the 2 in the quotient.

(c) Think 4x7=28. Subtract 28 from 86, leaving 58 on the abacus.

(d) Think 4x2 for subtraction from the tens column. However, 8 cannot be subtracted from 5, and we recognize the mis-estimation. (Figure G-30)

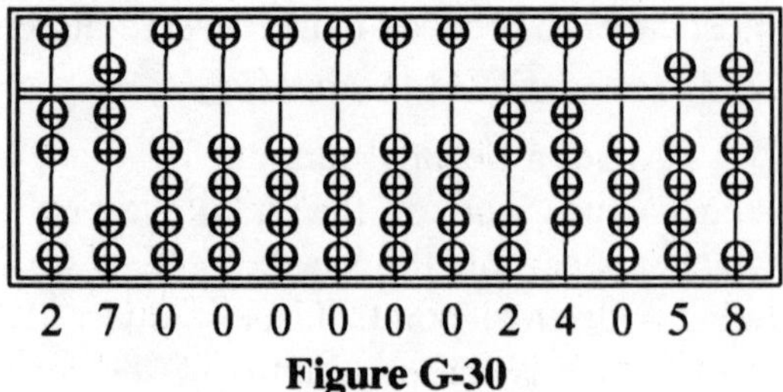

2 7 0 0 0 0 0 0 0 2 4 0 5 8

Figure G-30

(e) To make the correction, change the second digit of the quotient from 4 to 3.

(f) Recall that the second digit of the quotient had only been multiplied with the 7 of the divisor, and not with the 2 of the divisor. Therefore we need not make any correction in regard to the 2 of the divisor.

(g) Think 1x7=7 (because of the 1 which has now been removed from the second digit of the quotient), and add 7 back onto the dividend: 58+7=65. (Figure G-31)

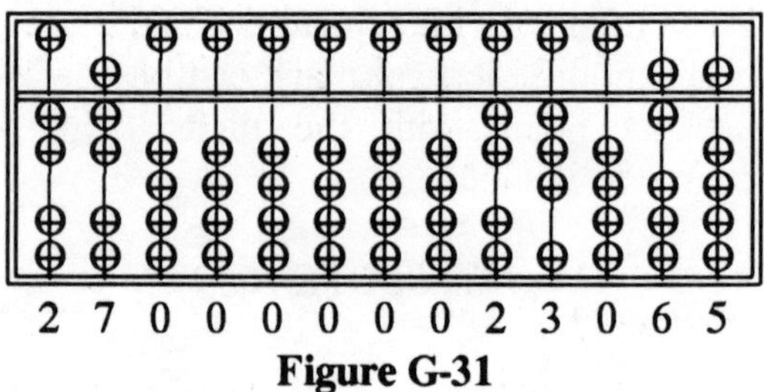

2 7 0 0 0 0 0 0 0 2 3 0 6 5

Figure G-31

(h) Now multiply the 3 of the quotient with the other digit of the divisor: 3x2=6. The 6 is subtracted from the tens column.

(i) Note the remainder of 5. (Refer back to Figure G-27.)

Decimals

Note that any problems involving percentages are actually decimal problems.

SETTING DECIMAL NUMBERS

To set a decimal number on the Cranmer Abacus, use one of the small vertical marks which appear on the plastic, and regard it as being a decimal point. Usually this will be the mark which is three columns to the left of the right-hand edge. Figure G-32 shows **47.39** [or 47.390] on the abacus. Note that between the 7 and the 3, there is a vertical mark on the plastic bar.

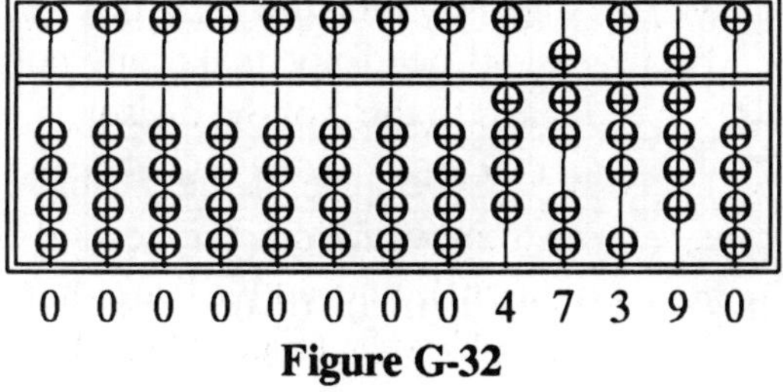

Figure G-32

For a number with several decimal places, however, another vertical mark can be used for the decimal point, with the digits being placed farther to the left.

ADDITION AND SUBTRACTION OF DECIMALS

For addition and subtraction, decimal numbers are set up in the way just described. That is, instead of having the units column at the extreme right, the units appear to the left of the chosen vertical mark (decimal point). Columns to the right of the chosen mark are tenths, hundredths, etc. Addition or subtraction then proceeds as described previously, except that all numbers are read in relation to the chosen decimal-point mark.

Temporary Adaptation for Beginners

First- and second-grade books often include addition and subtraction problems which use the dollar sign and have two decimal places. If the young child is just learning the regular position for whole numbers, he may be badly confused if asked to use the decimal position described above.

A child at this level may simply work the problem as though there were no decimal points. He can be told, "When you are older, you will learn a special way of working with decimals. Then you will have decimal points in lots of different places, and you will use the abacus in a different way. Right now, just be sure to remember whether a problem shows dollars and cents. If it does, then when you write down your answer on paper, put in a decimal point so that there are two numbers to the right of it. And remember to write the dollar sign at the beginning of the answer."

MULTIPLICATION OF DECIMALS

In multiplication, the decimal point is irrelevant during the actual computation. On paper, the decimal point is not shown in a partial product. On the abacus, also, simply ignore the decimal point(s) until the final product is found. Then, place the decimal point in the same manner as on paper – move it to the left according to the total number of decimal places in the two factors together. (Note: Especially if a problem is given orally, the student must take care to remember the number of decimal places until he is ready to mark them off.)

DIVISION OF DECIMALS

With No Decimal Places in Divisor

Example: **Solve the following, rounding off the quotient to two decimal places.**

$$7\overline{)62.5}$$

In previous examples of division, it was stated that "the dividend is set at the extreme right on the abacus." This assumed the dividend to be a whole number. The "end" of the dividend coincided with the decimal point and the end of the abacus.

When the dividend has one or more places to the right of the decimal point, a second abacus should be attached at the right (using a coupler from the American Printing House for the Blind), so that work may proceed farther to the right. Figure G-33 shows the above problem ready to be worked:

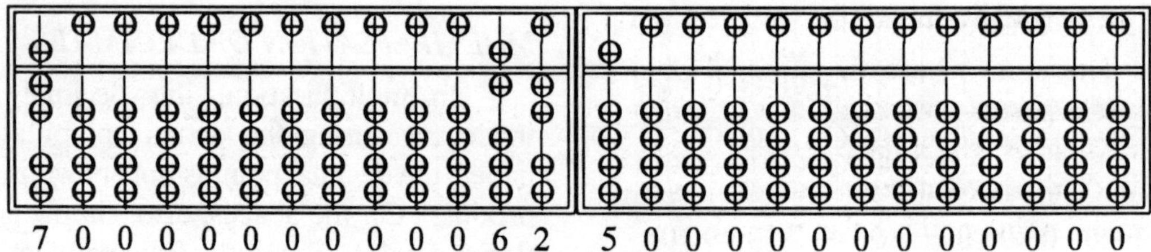

Figure G-33

```
     8.928
  7)62.500
    56
     65
     63
      20
      14
       60
       56
        4
```

Since 7 will not go into 6, the first digit of the quotient (8) is set immediately to the left of the dividend. Computation proceeds as with whole numbers, but continues across the boundary between the two abacuses. Figure G-34 shows the abacuses when 7 has been divided into the first three digits of the dividend (i.e., the 8 and the 9 of the quotient have been set).

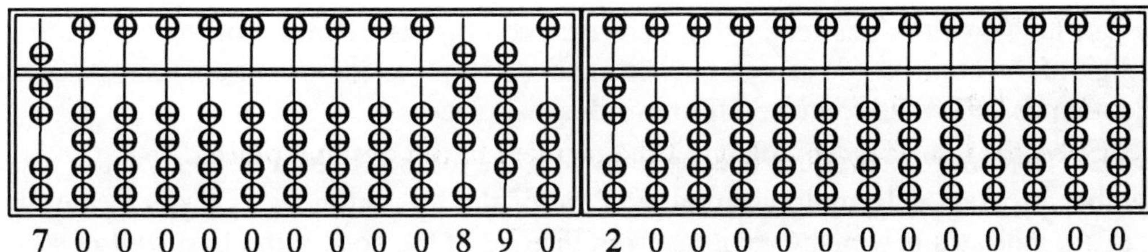

Figure G-34

To solve the problem we must determine not only what digits have been set to form the quotient, but where the decimal point belongs within them. Three elements, together, provide this information:

(a) In the quotient, note the last digit which has been *set.* (A zero may be "set" when the divisor will not go into a particular digit of the dividend.) The last digit of the quotient that has been set thus far is 9.

(b) In the dividend, note the last digit which has been processed thus far (that is, used in actual computation) – the digit 5 currently. (It is possible for one or more digits to be zeros to the right of the originally-stated dividend, just as on paper.)

(c) To determine where the decimal point should appear in the *quotient,* count the number of decimal places processed in the *dividend* thus far – that is, the number of columns on the right-hand abacus which have been processed. Thus far we have proceeded one column beyond the boundary between the abacuses. Therefore the quotient has just one place to the right of the decimal point, and is 8.9 currently.

As is done on paper, to carry out this problem to more decimal places merely requires extending the dividend with zeros at the right. (The decimal point in the quotient will remain in the same place.)

In Figure G-35 the work has been carried out farther by processing two zeros on the right-hand edge of the dividend:

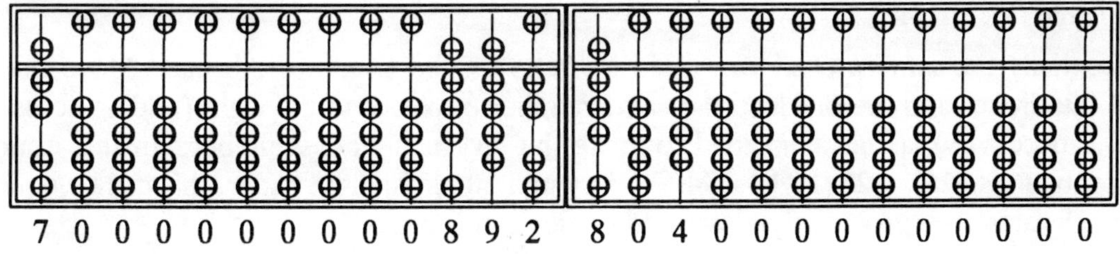

Figure G-35

At this point, consider again the three elements in understanding the quotient:

(a) In the quotient, the digits set thus far are 8, 9, 2, and 8. The last digit set is 8.

(b) In relation to the dividend as it originally appeared, the last digit processed is now the second zero after the 5 (i.e., the third column on the right-hand abacus).

(c) If we wish to check where the decimal point belongs in the quotient, we consider that the dividend now has been processed *three* columns/digits to the right of the boundary between the abacuses. This means that the quotient has *three* digits to the right of the decimal point, and is read as 8.928 currently.

Note that the 4 which appears still farther to the right is *not* part of the quotient, but instead is a remainder. It would not be correct to read the quotient as 8.92804. It is 8.928 with a remainder of .004 (though it is not customary to give the answer in these terms).

We can now give the answer in the form desired–that is, rounded off to two decimal places. The last digit of the quotient (8) causes the second decimal place to be rounded off to a 3 instead of a 2. The quotient is 8.93 when rounded off to two decimal places.

NOTE: This entire procedure is consistent with the methods given earlier for the placement of whole-number problems. In multiplication, a count of the total number of digits in the two factors, plus one extra, indicates how many columns from the end of the abacus the first (leftmost) column of the second factor should be. The quotient in division is equivalent to the second factor in multiplication.

In a decimal division problem, this same principle applies if *only whole numbers* are considered (that is, if digits after the decimal point are disregarded). In the above example, the two total digits in the whole-number factors 7 and 8, plus one extra, equal *three.* The quotient begins in the *third* column from the right-hand side of the [first] abacus.

With Decimal Places in Divisor

On paper it is traditional, if the divisor has digits after the decimal point, to place carets in the divisor and dividend. A decimal point is also placed in the quotient position, above the caret in the dividend.

Suppose that the example described above under whole-number Division (626 ÷ 27) had been, instead, 626 ÷ 2.7. Long division on paper would place carets, thus:

2.7‸)626.0‸

Despite modern educational efforts at explanation, most sighted students use the caret method by rote without really understanding why it works. It works because the divisor and dividend are multiplied by the same "power of ten," to derive numbers which have the same relationship *to each other* as the original two numbers.

Essentially the same procedure should be done on the Cranmer Abacus. Move the decimal point on the divisor and the dividend the same number of places to the right (adding zeros onto the dividend if necessary), as far as needed to make the divisor a whole number. In this example, the revised problem is 6260 ÷ 27 (Figure G-36). As with long division on paper, this can be done by rote learning. Division then proceeds as described earlier in this paper.

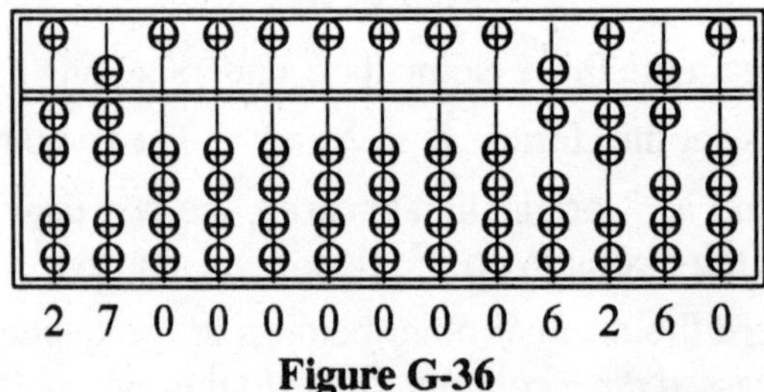

Figure G-36

The example above has been converted into a problem which has whole numbers in the divisor and dividend positions. If it were desired to find only a whole-number answer (quotient), the abacus would appear as in Figure G-37 when the problem was finished. The quotient would be 231 R23.

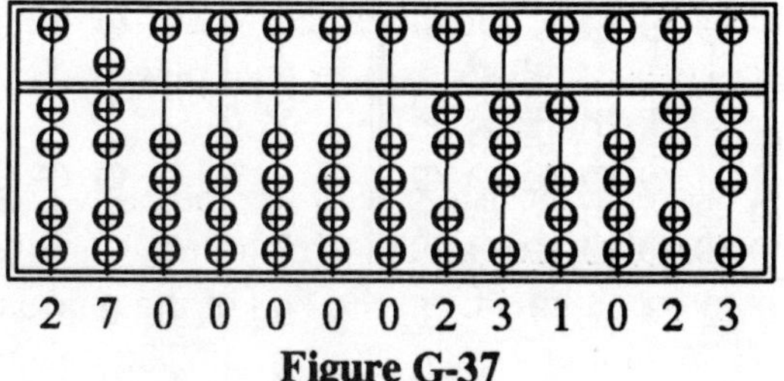

Figure G-37

The 23 is a remainder and *not* an additional decimal place of .023. Division has not been continued past the decimal point. If this remainder of 23 were used to "round off" the answer, it would be noted that 23 is more than half of the divisor (27), and therefore the answer would round off to 232 instead of 231.

However, with problems involving decimals it is not usual to seek a whole-number answer with a remainder. Instead it is customary to carry out the quotient to a given number of decimal places:

```
          23 1.851
      ____________
2.7^)626.0^000
      54
      --
       86
       81
       --
        5 0
        2 7
        ---
        2 3 0
        2 1 6
        -----
          1 40
          1 35
          ----
             50
             27
             --
             23
```

As explained previously, another abacus should be attached at the right. Figure G-38 shows this same problem carried out to three decimal places. The decimal point of the quotient (231.851) in Figure G-38 is between the 1 and the 8. Since there are three columns to its right [on the left-hand abacus], the decimal point is in the correct place for the "end" of the whole-number quotient.

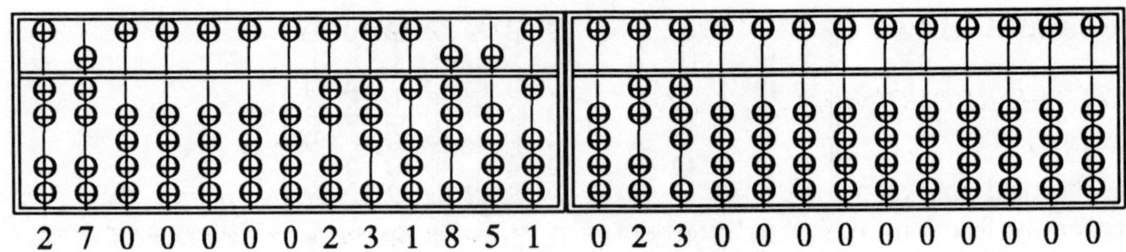

Figure G-38

When the problem has been carried out to three decimal places, it may be rounded off to two decimal places in the conventional way: because the third decimal place is a numeral less than 5, the quotient rounds off to 231.85 rather than 231.86.

Again, the 23 remaining to the right of the quotient (on the second abacus) is a remainder and not a decimal figure. The quotient must *not* be read as 231.851023. It is 231.851 with a remainder of 23 (actually .023). The remainder is usually not reported, since instead an additional decimal place is generally used for rounding off. When a problem is carried out beyond the decimal point, the end of the quotient ceases to coincide with the decimal point. Anything beyond the end of the quotient is still a remainder.

This entire procedure is easily correlated with long division on paper.

Note, incidentally, that this particular problem is a "repeating decimal," in which the same numerals appear over and over if the quotient is carried out to more places. The student must recognize this possibility and not become confused.

An Alternative

With many problems, it is possible to set the dividend farther to the left, if desired, and fit everything onto one abacus. The above problem, for example, could have been set up with the dividend (and therefore the quotient) three columns farther to the left, with the decimal point between the sixth and seventh columns from the right. It would then have fit onto one abacus. (If this idea is used, the student should consider beforehand how far he wishes to carry out the problem beyond the decimal point.)

For the beginner, however, the regular procedure described above is recommended. When the decimal point is in the same place as for whole-number division, it is much easier to grasp the idea of going beyond the decimal point.

A Hint for the Teacher

While helping a student, you should have an abacus also. You are much better able to analyze each example, and to help the student with possible difficulties, when you actually work it out on an abacus yourself. Sit *beside* the student, rather than facing her, to avoid reversal confusion.

In following a complicated problem, it may also be helpful to write it out in long division for your own benefit. Keep the numbers precisely aligned vertically. Consider drawing vertical guidelines or writing the numbers in the squares of graph paper, with vertical lines separating the numerals. This is especially helpful when there are confusing repetitive numerals. Also note that, although carets and decimal points seem to take up space in a handwritten problem, they do not actually occupy a position like a numeral, and they do not take up space on the abacus. If vertical guidelines are used, carets and decimal points should be *on* the vertical lines rather than between them.

Fractions and Mixed Numbers

SETTING AND REDUCING A FRACTION (or mixed number)

The vertical marks on the abacus frame are also used for fractions and mixed numbers.

Consider the nine columns at the right, and regard these as three groups of three (marked off by the vertical marks on the plastic). The three columns farthest to the right constitute the location for the denominator; the next three (as we move to the left) are for the numerator; and the next three (as we move to the left) are for the whole number, if any. See Figure G-39, which shows 14 6/8. Note that each number is placed as far to the right in its respective location as possible. In the descriptions below, this placement will be called the "regular position."

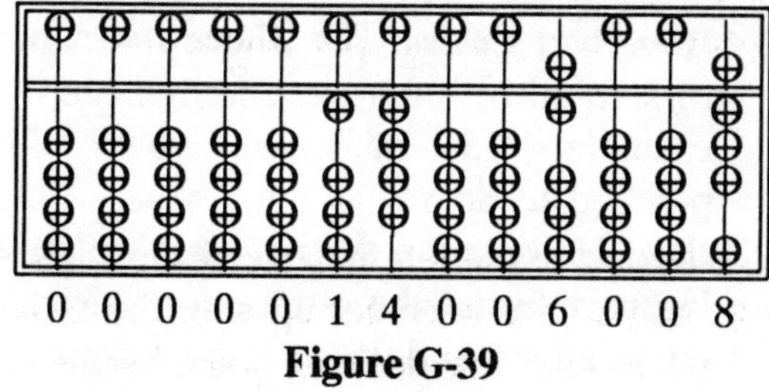

Figure G-39

Reducing to lowest terms is done just as on paper. Think of a number which can be divided into both the numerator and denominator. Simply divide (mentally) this number into both the numerator and the denominator. In this example, one realizes that 2 can go into both 6 and 8. Change the 6 to a 3, and change the 8 to a 4.

Suppose that the example is 14 17/8. Then one must realize that there is an improper fraction, and again proceed essentially as on paper. 8 will go into 17 twice. Therefore we have two "wholes," and must add 2 to the whole-number position. 1 was left over, however, so there is still 1 in the numerator. The answer is 16 1/8.

ADDITION OF FRACTIONS AND MIXED NUMBERS

Example: **14 1/3 + 2 3/4**

NOTE: All adding within this procedure is done in the manner described for "Addition" in this paper. Exact motion of beads will not always be described here.

To add two or more fractions or mixed numbers, set the first addend in the regular position.

(a) Set 14 1/3 in the regular position.

(b) Do not set the entire second addend, but proceed as in the steps below.

(c) Adding the whole numbers is done easily and directly. In the units column of the whole-number position (that is, the farthest column to the right in the whole-number position), think 4+2=6, and change the 4 to a 6. The whole number in the regular position is now 16.

(d) We must find a common denominator before proceeding to add the fractions. Set the second fraction in a different position to facilitate this process: place the numerator (3) at the extreme left of the abacus, then skip one column and place the denominator (4). See Figure G-40.

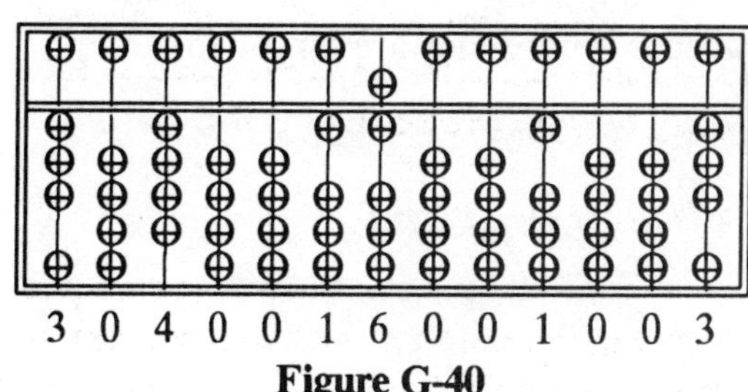

Figure G-40

(e) Now think of a common denominator: 12.

(f) Look at the first fraction (1/3) in the regular position. Use the same mental process that is used in figuring on paper: "3 must be multiplied by 4 to become 12. Therefore multiply each part of the fraction by 4, and we have 4/12." Change the fraction of the first addend (in the regular position) to read 4/12. We now have 16 4/12 in the regular position, where the final answer will eventually appear.

(g) Examine the 3/4 at the left. To convert to twelfths, each part must be multiplied by 3; thus we must change it to 9/12.

(h) Add 9 to the 4 which is now in the regular numerator position, making the answer read 16 13/12.

(i) Reduce to lowest terms, and we have the final answer of 17 1/12.

The above procedure assumes that the young student does not find this example easy. An experienced student will prefer to do easy problems in his/her head, partially or completely. In this example, a more experienced student probably would not actually place the 3/4 onto the abacus at all. Instead the student would convert the 3/4 into 9/12 in his/her head, and then add the numerator 4 onto the regular position. An even more advanced student might do this entire problem mentally, and not use the abacus at all for such an easy example.

Caution students, however, against carelessly attempting to work problems in their heads without thinking them through. One must convert the fractions into common terms before adding the numerators.

Also note that if a problem is given orally, it is important to set the fractions onto the abacus before they are forgotten.

SUBTRACTION OF FRACTIONS AND MIXED NUMBERS

Example: **14 1/3 - 2 3/4**

NOTE: All subtraction within this procedure is done in the manner described for "Subtraction" above. Exact motion of beads will not always be described here.

What if our previous example had been subtraction instead of addition?

Steps a-f are done in almost exactly the same way. The only difference is that the whole numbers are subtracted instead of added. Therefore, at the end of step f, the regular position reads 12 4/12.

Complete the procedure as follows.

(g) Exactly as for addition, change the fraction in the left-hand position to 9/12.

(h) If we had an example where the numerators could be subtracted immediately (for example, 4/5 - 3/5), we would simply proceed to do so, as the reverse of addition. However, in this problem we are trying to subtract the numerator 9 from the numerator 4, and this cannot be done.

(i) We must "borrow" from the whole-number position. Subtract 1 from the whole-number position, leaving 11 there. The 1 (whole) which was subtracted is now converted into 12/12; thus we add 12 to the regular numerator position, making it 16. The regular position overall now reads 11 16/12. (Figure G-41)

(j) Now it is possible to subtract the numerators. Think 16-9=7, and change the numerator in the regular position to 7. We then have 11 7/12. This cannot be reduced, so it is the final answer.

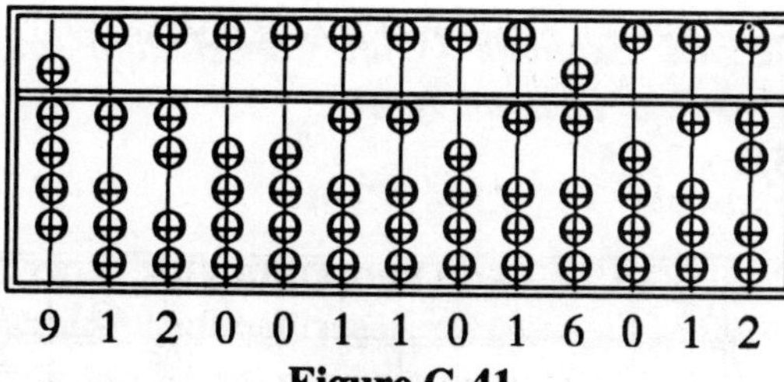

Figure G-41

MULTIPLICATION OF FRACTIONS AND MIXED NUMBERS

Multiplication of Fractions

First Example: **2/3 x 4/7**

For multiplication, fractions are set differently than for addition or subtraction. The regular position is not used at first. Instead, both numerators are set toward the left of the abacus, and both denominators are set toward the right of the abacus. With the example above:

(a) For the first fraction (2/3), set the 2 at the extreme left and the 3 at the extreme right.

(b) To set the numerator of the 4/7, skip one column at the left (thus moving inward toward the center of the abacus) and set the 4.

(c) For the denominator of the fraction 4/7, move to the left from the 3 (again moving inward) – skip one column and set a 7. See Figure G-42.

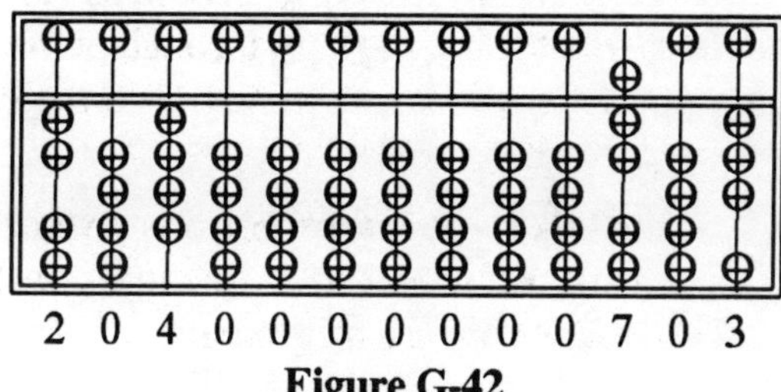

Figure G-42

(d) Examine the denominators, and mentally multiply them together. Clear them off and place that product (21) at the extreme right on the abacus.

(e) Examine the numerators, and mentally multiply them together. Clear them off and place the product (8) so that it ends at the vertical mark which is three columns from the right. Note that the answer to the example is now appearing in the regular position. (Figure G-43)

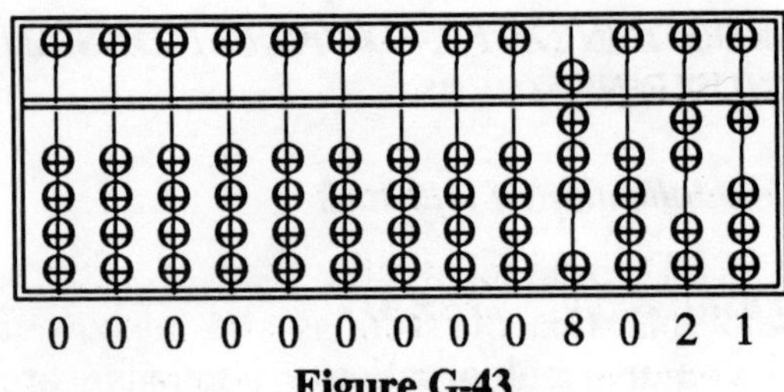

Figure G-43

(f) We now have 8/21. If the answer were not already in lowest terms, we would reduce it as described above for "reduction of fractions." Since the regular position is now being used, the normal location for the whole number is available.

Second Example (With Cancellation and with Two-Digit Denominator):
5/9 x 3/25

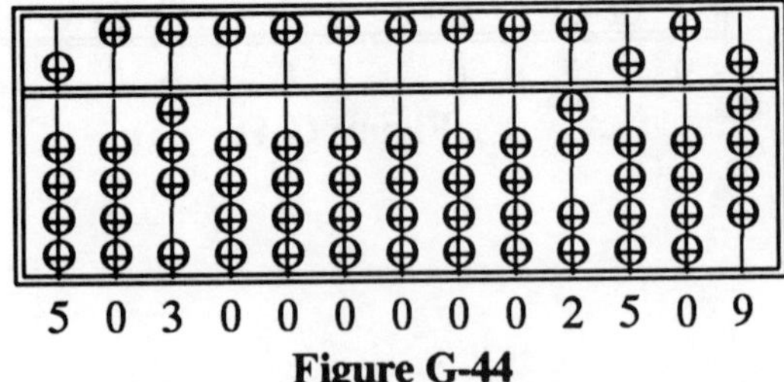

Figure G-44

(a) As in the example above, place the numerator and denominator of the first fraction at the extreme left and extreme right, respectively.

(b) Skip one column at each side; set the 3 and the 25 inward from the respective edges. (Figure G-44)

(c) Consider whether any number may be evenly divided into both the first numerator (5) and one of the denominators. Think 25÷5=5, and change the 25 to a 5. Think 5÷5=1, and change the 5 to a 1. Since the first numerator is now a 1, no further cancellation is possible with this combination.

Consider whether any number can be evenly divided into both the second numerator and one of the denominators. Change the 9 to a 3, and the 3 to a 1.

Mentally multiply the denominators together (3x5=15). Clear them off and replace them with a 15 at the extreme right.

(d) Mentally multiply the numerators together (1x1=1). Clear them off and place a 1 in the regular numerator position (fourth column from the right).

(e) The answer, 1/15, is now shown in the regular position.

Multiplication of Mixed Numbers

Mixed numbers must be converted into improper fractions before computation. Work then proceeds as above.

DIVISION OF FRACTIONS AND MIXED NUMBERS

Example: **2/3 ÷ 4/7**

Division follows the same procedure as for multiplication of fractions and mixed numbers, except that it is necessary to reverse the numerator and denominator of one fraction.

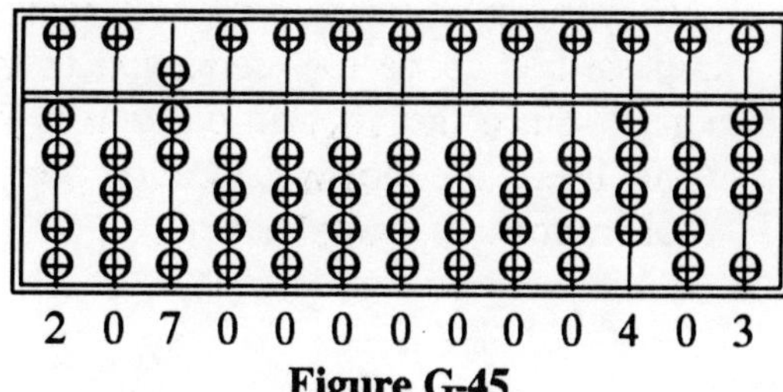

Figure G-45

(a) Place 2/3 onto the abacus just as in the multiplication problem above.

(b) Place 4/7 onto the abacus in reverse position. (Figure G-45)

(c) Perform cancellation with the 2 and the 4, replacing them with 1 and 2, respectively.

(d) Mentally multiply 2x3. Clear the 2 and the 3, and place 6 at the extreme right (in the regular position for the denominator).

(e) Mentally multiply 1x7. Clear off the 1 and the 7, and place 7 in the regular numerator position (just to the left of the vertical mark which is three columns from the extreme right).

(f) Observe the current answer (7/6) now in the regular position, and note that this is an improper fraction. Reduce to lowest terms.

(g) The answer, 1 1/6, is now shown in the regular position. See Figure G-46.

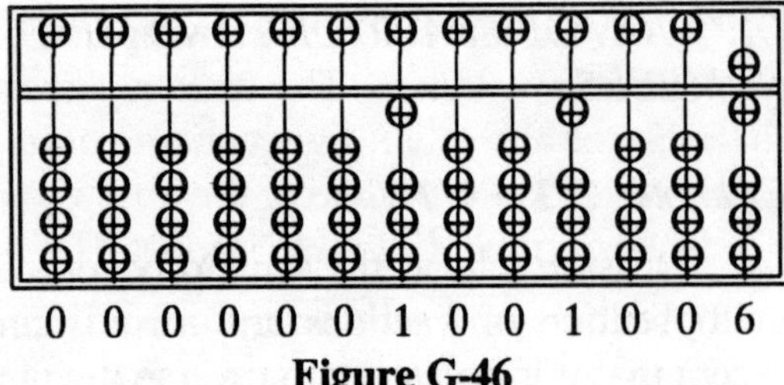

Figure G-46

Suggestions for Teaching

PLANNING APPROPRIATE LESSONS

This description of the use of the abacus does not include many suggestions for actual lesson planning. If you are accustomed to teaching adults or high school students, or even somewhat younger students who have already learned to work problems on paper, give extra thought to methods for teaching younger children. Remember that younger children are still learning to understand *arithmetic,* as well as the mechanics of the abacus. Do not assume that a student in the primary grades is already skilled in carrying and borrowing, for example.

In beginning to teach any new process, select relatively easy tasks at first (e.g., teach division with a one-digit divisor before attempting problems with two-digit divisors.) A regular mathematics textbook will generally do this anyway for all students, and this new abacus method is much more easily correlated with a regular American textbook than is the Oriental method.

Look ahead and anticipate new procedures (e.g., division with a two-digit divisor). The headings and subheadings in this Appendix may be used as a guide, although parts of the sequence will vary with the curriculum. It may be advisable to show the student (and the classroom teacher) the mechanics before the class arrives at that point.

If a supplementary textbook is needed for a student needing extra practice, another regular text may be used–possibly one from a lower grade level.

Additional suggestions on lesson planning appear in the chapter on "Mathematics" in this *Handbook.*

EFFICIENT USE OF THE FINGERS

Emphasize the efficient use of the fingers.

When one finger is busy–for example, keeping track of the position for starting each partial product in multiplication–that hand is limited as to what else it can do. However, usually it can do more than one thing.

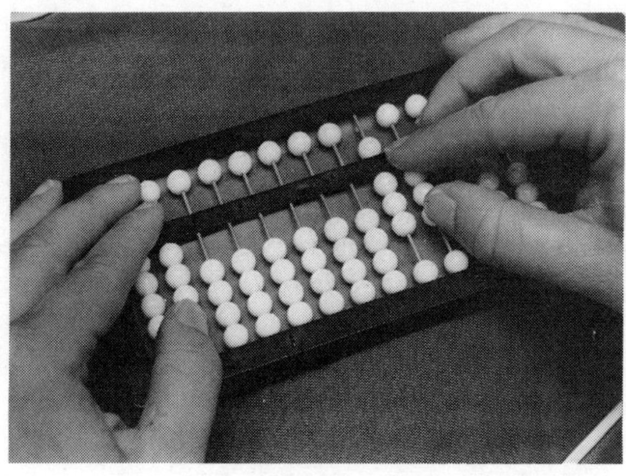

Figure G-47

Efficient and consistent hand and finger motion is very important. Even if the teacher is sighted, the teacher should learn to work the abacus efficiently by touch (without using the eyes), in order to advise the student correctly.

In multiplication, for example, this approach is effective: The left hand stays on the factor at the far left (moving from one digit to another as the work is done). The forefinger of the right hand is placed on the factor in the middle of the abacus (also moving from one digit to another). The remaining fingers of the right hand (including the thumb) manipulate the product.

The hand position for multiplication will work also for division. The divisor corresponds to the factor at the left; the quotient corresponds to the factor in the middle of the abacus; and the dividend corresponds to the product.[2]

Addition and subtraction are less complex in regard to fingering patterns, since they are more compact. However, it is important that the student make use of both hands and more than one finger.

The thumb is advantageous in moving the lower beads.

An individual may also devise her own method for movement of the fingers. Whatever is done, it is very important that both hands and various fingers be used in an efficient pattern.

GENERAL EFFICIENCY

Encourage mental arithmetic, partial or complete. For example, an older student should not need to use the abacus for problems such as 304+9001, or 200 ÷ 25. Many students learn to use mental arithmetic reliably for problems much harder than these. Mental arithmetic is also discussed elsewhere in this paper.

Consider the creative use of two abacuses. For an advanced student, use the coupler available from the American Printing House for the Blind to provide twice as many columns. For a beginner, consider occasionally trying a procedure on a separate abacus while keeping a partially-worked problem on the first abacus (e.g., experiment with different estimates of the quotient in division).

---

[2]The regular fingering method for multiplication and division, described in the text above, works well for most students. However, if a given student seems to have difficulty with that approach, particularly if the student is left-handed, a possible alternative is as follows: Keep the little finger of the left hand on the factor at the left, and keep the forefinger of the left hand on the factor in the middle of the abacus. The entire right hand then manipulates the product. This plan also may help the student remember which are the factors and which is the product.

Conclusion

All this explanation may seem complicated at first. To a person who figures on paper automatically and quickly, the abacus may at first seem difficult or cumbersome. However, it is experience that makes the difference. If a person spends 12 years learning a given system of computation, and then uses it throughout her life, it will be fast and automatic. This is no less true of the abacus than of the traditional written method. Moreover, with the Paper-Compatible system, there are actually very few differences.

For procedures not covered specifically here, compatible methods can easily be devised.

REFERENCES

General Bibliography

American Association of Workers for the Blind, et al. *Code of Braille Textbook Formats and Techniques, 1977.* Louisville, KY: American Printing House for the Blind, 1977.

American Association of Workers for the Blind, et al. *English Braille, American Edition, 1959.* Louisville, KY: American Printing House for the Blind, 1986.

American Association of Workers for the Blind, et al. *The Nemeth Braille Code for Mathematics and Science Notation* (1972 Revision). Louisville, KY: American Printing House for the Blind, 1973.

American Foundation for the Blind. *AFB Directory of Services for Blind and Visually Impaired Persons in the United States.* New York, NY: American Foundation for the Blind, 1988.

American Printing House for the Blind. *The Central Catalog: Volunteer and Commercially Produced Materials for Visually Handicapped Children.* Louisville, KY: American Printing House for the Blind. (Published annually.)

Anderson, Mary Ellen (Ed.). *Competing on Terms of Equality: The Goal and the Reality.* Baltimore, MD: National Federation of the Blind, 1982.

Barth, John L. *Tactile Graphics Guidebook.* Louisville, KY: American Printing House for the Blind, 1983.

Benson, Stephen O. *So What About Independent Travel.* Baltimore, MD: National Federation of the Blind.

Betker, Janiece. *Lifeskills: A Can-Do Program for Living With Blindness.* Published by Janiece Betker (1886 29th Ave. NW, New Brighton, MN 55112), 1989.
(*Helpful suggestions on daily living skills.*)

Betker, Janiece. *Parent Tips: The Challenge Years.* Published by Janiece Betker (address above).
(*Information for blind parents of school-age children.*)

Betker, Janiece. *Parent Tips: A Guide for Blind and Visually-Impaired Parents.* Published by Janiece Betker (address above), 1988.
(*Information on baby and child care.*)

Blind Childrens Center. *Talk To Me: A Language Guide for Parents of Blind Children* and *Talk To Me II: Common Concerns* (two booklets). Los Angeles, CA: Blind Childrens Center.

Braille Authority of North America. *Code for Computer Braille Notation.* Louisville, KY: American Printing House for the Blind, 1987.

Brown, Adelle. *So What About Sewing.* Chicago, IL: The Guild for the Blind.

Brown, Donnise, Vickie Simmons, and Judy Methuin. *The Oregon Project for Visually Impaired and Blind Preschool Children.* Medford, OR: Jackson County Education Service District, 1979.

Butler, Debbie, and Sharon L. M. Duffy. "Materials for Teaching Braille." National Association to Promote the Use of Braille *Newsletter,* Fall 1986, pp. 10-14.

Cheadle, John. "For Fathers (And Others): Some Tips on Alternative Techniques." *Future Reflections,* March-April 1983, pp. 11-15.

Cheadle, John. "On Driving Nails and Hitting the Mark With 'Attitudes.'" *Future Reflections,* March-April 1983, pp. 6-8.

Coalition in Oregon for Parent Education. *Parents Rights Card.* Salem, OR.

Coudron, Jill M. *Alphabet Puppets: Songs, Stories, and Cooking Activities for Letter Recognition and Sounds.* Belmont, CA: Fearon Teacher Aids (a division of David S. Lake Publishers), 1983.
(*Not written specifically for teaching the Braille alphabet, but extremely suitable for this purpose.*)

Davidow, Mae E., Ed. D. *The Abacus Made Easy.* Philadelphia, PA: Overbrook School for the Blind, 1966.

DeGarmo, Mary Turner. *Introduction to Braille Music Transcription.* Washington, DC: Division for the Blind and Physically Handicapped, Library of Congress, 1970 with 1983 Addendum.

Dodd, Tami. "Looming Lettered Monsters: Helpful Hints for Standardized Testing." *The Student Slate* (Publication of the National Federation of the Blind Student Division), Spring, 1987, pages 5-6.

Dorf, Maxine B., in collaboration with Barbara H. Tate. *Instruction Manual for Braille Transcribing.* Washington, DC: Library of Congress, 1984.

Drouillard, Richard, and Sherry Raynor. *Move It!!! (A Guide for Helping Visually Handicapped Children Grow).* Mason, MI: Ingham Intermediate School District, 1977.

Duffy, Sharon L. M. "Braille For Sale." National Association to Promote the Use of Braille *Newsletter,* Spring 1988, pp. 24-31.

Duffy, Sharon L. M. "A Braillewriter In My Pocket." *Future Reflections,* September-November 1984, pp. 6-8.
(*This article is reprinted in this Handbook as part of the chapter by the same title.*)

Duffy, Sharon L. M. "Grade Three Braille Compared to Other Abbreviated Forms of Braille." National Association to Promote the Use of Braille *Newsletter,* April 1987, pp. 17-19.

Edmister, Patricia, and Richard K. Ekstrand. "Lessening the Trauma of Due Process." *Teaching Exceptional Children,* Spring 1987, pp. 6-10.

Fernandes, Joanne. "About Dating, Blindness, and the 'Little Things' of Life." *Future Reflections,* January-February, 1984, pp. 1-5.

Ferrell, Kay Alicyn. *Parenting Preschoolers: Suggestions for Raising Young Blind and Visually Impaired Children.* New York, NY: American Foundation for the Blind, 1984.

Foster, Nancy Jacquat. *Detailed Instruction on the Use of the Cranmer Abacus.* Published by Poudre R-1 School District, Mountain View School, 2540 LaPorte Ave., Ft. Collins, CO 80521. (Previously published with author's name as Nancy Jacquat.)

Gilkerson, Linda, *et al.* "Point of View: Commenting on P.L. 99-457." *Zero to Three* (Bulletin of the National Center for Clinical Infant Programs, 733 15th Street NW, Suite 912, Washington, DC 20005). February 1987, pp. 13-17.

Ginott, Haim G. *Teacher and Child; A Book for Parents and Teachers.* New York, NY: Avon, 1975.

Gissoni, Fred L. *Using the Cranmer Abacus for the Blind.* Louisville, KY: American Printing House for the Blind, 1964.

Grannis, Florence. *Beginning a Transcribing Group.* Baltimore, MD: National Federation of the Blind.

Halverson, Mary Ellen. "I Remember." *National Federation of the Blind Newsletter for Parents of Blind Children* (This publication is now called *Future Reflections*). January 1982, pp. 5-7.
(*A blind adult recalls her experiences while growing up.*)

Hauge, David. *Techniques for the Blind Student in Industrial Arts.* Des Moines, IA: Iowa Commission for the Blind, 1985.

Hayden, Ruth R. *The Braille Code: A Guide to Grade Three.* Louisville, KY: American Printing House for the Blind, 1985.

Jernigan, Kenneth. *Blindness: A Left-Handed Dissertation.* Baltimore, MD: National Federation of the Blind.

Jernigan, Kenneth. *Blindness: Concepts and Misconceptions.* Baltimore, MD: National Federation of the Blind.

Jernigan, Kenneth. *Blindness: Discrimination, Hostility, and Progress.* Baltimore, MD: National Federation of the Blind.

Jernigan, Kenneth. *Blindness: Handicap or Characteristic.* Baltimore, MD: National Federation of the Blind.

Jernigan, Kenneth. *Blindness: Is Literature Against Us?* Baltimore, MD: National Federation of the Blind.

Jernigan, Kenneth. *Blindness: The Myth and the Image.* Baltimore, MD: National Federation of the Blind.

Jernigan, Kenneth. *Blindness: The New Generation.* Baltimore, MD: National Federation of the Blind.

Jernigan, Kenneth. *Blindness: New Insights on Old Outlooks.* Baltimore, MD: National Federation of the Blind.

Jernigan, Kenneth. *Blindness: Of Visions and Vultures.* Baltimore, MD: National Federation of the Blind.

Jernigan, Kenneth. *Blindness: That's How It Is at the Top of the Stairs.* Baltimore, MD: National Federation of the Blind.

Jernigan, Kenneth. *Competing on Terms of Equality.* Baltimore, MD: National Federation of the Blind.

Jernigan, Kenneth. *A Definition of Blindness.* Baltimore, MD: National Federation of the Blind.
(*Note: This paper is reprinted as an Appendix in this Handbook.*)

Jernigan, Kenneth. "Fighting a Straw Man." *The Braille Monitor,* August-September 1986, pp. 363-370.

Jernigan, Kenneth. *Jargon and Research – Twin Idols in Work with the Blind.* Baltimore, MD: National Federation of the Blind.

Jernigan, Kenneth. *To Man the Barricades.* Baltimore, MD: National Federation of the Blind.

Job Opportunities for the Blind (JOB). *Have You Considered...?* Baltimore, MD: Job Opportunities for the Blind.
(*Descriptions of blind employees in many different regular, competitive jobs*)

Mangold, Sally S., Ed. *A Teachers' Guide to the Special Educational Needs of Blind and Visually Handicapped Children.* New York, NY: American Foundation for the Blind, 1982.

Moor, Pauline M. *Toilet Habits – Suggestions for Training a Child Who is Blind.* New York, NY: American Foundation for the Blind.

National Association to Promote the Use of Braille. *Newsletter.* Louisville, KY: National Association to Promote the Use of Braille.

National Braille Association, Inc. *Manual on Foreign Languages to Aid Braille Transcribers.* Midland Park, NJ: National Braille Association, 1970.

National Federation of the Blind in collaboration with Daniel Finkelstein, M.D. (Associate Professor of Ophthalmology, The Wilmer Eye Institute, Johns Hopkins

University). *Blindness and Disorders of the Eye.* Baltimore, MD: National Federation of the Blind, 1989.

National Federation of the Blind. "Annual Braille Reading Contest for Blind Children." *Future Reflections,* special insert.

National Federation of the Blind. *The Blind Child In the Regular Preschool Program.* Baltimore, MD: National Federation of the Blind.

National Federation of the Blind. *The Braille Monitor.* Baltimore, MD.
(*A monthly magazine on topics related to blindness.*)

National Federation of the Blind. *Braille: What Is It? What Does It Mean to the Blind?* Baltimore, MD: National Federation of the Blind.
(*Note: This paper is reprinted in this Handbook as part of the chapter, "Braille – What Is It?"*)

National Federation of the Blind. "Cane Travel." *Future Reflections,* March-May 1984, pp. 10-17.

National Federation of the Blind. *Comments on Dog Guides.* (Pamphlet)

National Federation of the Blind. "Distinguished Teacher of Blind Children Award." *The Braille Monitor,* September-October 1988, pp. 410-11.

National Federation of the Blind. *Future Reflections.* Baltimore, MD: National Federation of the Blind.
(*Magazine for parents and educators of blind children. Four or more issues per year. Published in inkprint and on cassette.*)

National Federation of the Blind. "Life After High School: College and Your Blind Son Or Daughter." *Future Reflections,* July 1982, pp. 7-10.

National Federation of the Blind. *Model White Cane Law.* Baltimore, MD: National Federation of the Blind.

National Federation of the Blind. *Postsecondary Education and Career Development – A Resource Guide for the Blind, Visually Impaired, and Physically Handicapped.* Baltimore, MD: National Federation of the Blind.

National Federation of the Blind. "They Put On Blindfolds and Play at Being Blind." *The Braille Monitor,* July 1985, pp. 348-50.

National Library Service for the Blind and Physically Handicapped, Library of Congress. *Volunteers Who Produce Books: Braille, Large Type, Tape.* Washington, D.C.: Library of Congress, 1973.

Olson, Carl. *The Encounter.* Baltimore, MD: National Federation of the Blind, 1980.
(*In humorous cartoon format, public misconceptions about blindness are analyzed and dispelled in this booklet.*)

Raynor, Sherry, and Richard Drouillard. *Get a Wiggle On (A Guide for Helping Visually Handicapped Children Grow).* Mason, MI: Ingham Intermediate School District, 1975.
(*This book is primarily about infants.*)

Roberts, Helen, *et al. An Introduction to Braille Mathematics.* Washington, DC: National Library Service for the Blind and Physically Handicapped, 1978.

Rottman, Robert. *When Your Best Efforts Fail: Open Letter to Eye Specialists.* Baltimore, MD: National Federation of the Blind.
(*This publication helps eye doctors to advise patients whose sight cannot be improved medically, but who can benefit from education and rehabilitation.*)

Scholl, Geraldine T., and Kay Alicyn Ferrell, Editors. *Foundations of Education for Blind and Visually Handicapped Children and Youth: Theory and Practice.* New York, NY: American Foundation for the Blind, 1986.

Schroeder, Ruth, and Doris Willoughby. *Suggestions for the Blind Cook.* Baltimore, MD: National Federation of the Blind.

Spock, Benjamin, and Michael Rothenberg. *Dr. Spock's Baby and Child Care.* New York, NY: E. P. Dutton, 1985.

U.S. Congress. *Education for All Handicapped Children Act.* Public Law 142, 94th Congress, 1975, U.S. Government Printing Office.

U.S. Congress. *Education of the Handicapped Act Amendments of 1986.* Public Law 457, 99th Congress, 1986, U.S. Government Printing Office.

U.S. Congress. *Family Educational Rights and Privacy Act,* Public Law 380, 93rd Congress, 1974, U.S. Government Printing Office.

U.S. Congress, *Rehabilitation Act of 1973,* Public Law 112, (Title V, Section 504), 93rd Congress, 1973, U.S. Government Printing Office.

Vermeij, Geerat J. "To Sea With a Blind Scientist." *Future Reflections,* Spring-Summer, 1989, pp. 2-7.

Walhof, Ramona. "The Blind Can Sew-Some How-To Ideas." *The Braille Monitor,* June, 1973, pp. 306-7.

Walhof, Ramona. "I Am a Blind Mother Fighting to Keep My Children From Corruption," *The Braille Monitor,* April, 1978, pp. 96-101.

Weiss, Johnette, and Jeff Weiss. "Teaching Handwriting to the Congenitally Blind." *Journal of Visual Impairment and Blindness,* September 1978.

Willoughby, Doris M. "Dating and Marriage." *National Federation of the Blind Newsletter for Parents of Blind Children* (This publication is now called *Future Reflections*). January 1982, pp. 10-12.

Willoughby, Doris M. "Part-Time and Summer Jobs." *Future Reflections,* April 1982, pp. 3-6.

Willoughby, Doris M. *A Resource Guide for Parents and Educators of Blind Children.* Baltimore, MD: National Federation of the Blind.

Willoughby, Doris M. *Your School Includes a Blind Student.* Baltimore, MD: National Federation of the Blind Teachers Division.

Zambone, Alana M., PhD., Barbara McCarry, and Alan Dinsmore. "Your Response Is Needed: Early Childhood, P.L. 99-457." *DVH Quarterly* (Division for the Visually Handicapped, Council for Exceptional Children). June 1987, pp. 5-11.

Inkprint Books for Children and Young People

Aiello, Barbara, and Jeffrey Shulman. *Business Is Looking Up* (*The Kids on the Block* book series). Frederick, MD: Twenty-First Century Books, 1988.
(*An enjoyable story based on the blind puppet character, Renaldo Rodriguez.*)

Bawden, Nina. *The Witch's Daughter.* Philadelphia, PA: J. B. Lippincott, 1966.

Eyerly, Jeannette. *The Seeing Summer.* New York: J. B. Lippincott, 1981.

Kent, Deborah. *Belonging.* New York: Dial Press, 1978.
(*This autobiographical book tells about a blind teenager's successful struggle to "belong" in a regular public school.*)

Litchfield, Ada B. *A Cane In Her Hand.* Chicago, IL: Albert Whitman & Co., 1977.

McIntyre, David J. *Movin' On Out* (*Starting Out on Your Own*). New York: G. P. Putnam's Sons, 1984.
(*This is a general trade book for young adults, with advice about finding an apartment, managing money, meeting people, etc.*)

Petersen, Palle. *Sally Can't See.* New York: John Day Co., 1974.

Walhof, Ramona. *Questions Kids Ask About Blindness.* Baltimore, MD: American Brotherhood for the Blind, 1979.

Yolen, Jane H. *The Seeing Stick.* New York, NY: Crowell Junior Books, 1977.
(*A Chinese folk tale: The princess is sad because she is blind, until she learns to "see with her fingers."*)

Braille Instruction Materials

(INCLUDING RECREATIONAL READING FOR YOUNG CHILDREN)

American Brotherhood for the Blind. Twin Vision Books.
(*Lending library of books featuring print and Braille together; materials for the deaf-blind.*)

American Printing House for the Blind. *Modern Methods of Teaching Braille.* Louisville, KY: American Printing House for the Blind.
(*Volume I develops tactile readiness; Volume II teaches the alphabet and Grade II Braille.*)

American Printing House for the Blind. *Touch and Tell.* Louisville, KY: American Printing House for the Blind, 1969.
(*Braille reading readiness.*)

Braille Institute of America. *Expectations.*
(*Annual Braille anthology of children's literature, available free of charge to blind children in grades 3-6.*)

Caton, Hilda, Eleanor Pester, and Eddy Jo Bradley. *Patterns: The Primary Braille Reading Program.* Louisville, KY: American Printing House for the Blind, 1980-83.
(*This is a basal reading series teaching general reading skills, comprehension, phonics, and Grade II Braille. It begins at the "Readiness" level, which includes letters and words, and continues through the third reader. Worksheets and tests are included. Also, correlated library books for recreational reading are available for most reading levels.*)

Curran, Eileen P. *Just Enough to Know Better: A Braille Primer."* Boston, MA: National Braille Press, Inc., 1988.
(*Intended for parents of blind children to help them learn Braille along with their children, this primer is written in an easy-to-use style.*)

Duffy, Sharon L. M. *The McDuffy Reader: A Braille Primer for Adults.* Baltimore, MD: National Federation of the Blind, 1989. (*Suitable for adults and high school students. Student's cassette available, with lesson-by-lesson guide. Teacher's Guide is available in inkprint and in Braille, and includes lesson-by-lesson guide; suggestions for teaching the Braille slate; brief descriptions of the Nemeth Code, Braille music, and Grade III Braille; comments on overall philosophy, methods, and problem-solving.*)

Jones, Pauline A., *et al. Braille for Beginners: A Phonetic Approach to Reading and Writing Braille.* Dept. of Education, Michigan School for the Blind: 1973. (*For young children.*)

Krebs, Bernard M. *ABC's of Braille.* New York, NY: Jewish Guild for the Blind, 1973. (*Grade II Braille is presented in rather quick succession, with reading matter geared to ages 9-12.*)

Krebs, Bernard M. *Braille in Brief.* New York, NY: Jewish Guild for the Blind, 1968. (*Grade II Braille is presented quickly.*)

Krolick, Bettye. *How to Read Braille Music.* Champaign, IL: Stipes Publishing Co., 1975. Braille transcription by Bettye Krolick, University of Illinois Braille Service, Champaign, IL.

Kurzhals, Ina, Hilda Caton, and Eleanor Pester. *Patterns Prebraille Program.* Louisville, KY: American Printing House for the Blind.

Kurzhals, Ina W., and Hilda Caton. *A Tactual Road to Reading (A Developmental Program for Young Children).* Louisville, KY: American Printing House for the Blind, 1974. (*Braille Reading Readiness.*)

Mangold, Sally. *The Mangold Developmental Program of Tactile Perception and Braille Letter Recognition.* Castro Valley, CA: Exceptional Teaching Aids, 1977. (*Teaches prereading skills and the alphabet.*)

Nading, Mabel, and Ramona Walhof. *Beginning Braille for Adults.* Baltimore, MD: National Federation of the Blind, 1980.

National Braille Press. *Children's Braille Book-of-the-Month Club.* Boston, MA: National Braille Press. (*Braille books for young children, available for purchase at reasonable prices.*)

Porter, Marie. *Children's Series* books. Chicago, IL: The Guild for the Blind. (*Several sets of books for beginning Braille readers are available. Raised pictures are used creatively.*)

Seedlings Braille Books for Children. (*Braille books for young children, available for purchase at reasonable prices.*)

Weiss, Johnette, and Jeff Weiss. *Braille: A Different Approach.* Louisville, KY: American Printing House for the Blind.

Videotapes and Films

Iowa Commission for the Blind and Heartland Area Education Agency #11. *Industrial Arts: Methods for Blind Students.* Videotape, 25 minutes. Des Moines, IA.

KOLN/KGIN Television, Lincoln, NE. *It's Not So Different: A Talk With Blind Parents.* Videotape, 10 minutes. (*Available from POBC Videos.*)

Nebraska Services for the Visually Impaired. *Kids With Canes.* Videotape, 35 minutes. (*Available from POBC Videos.*)

Dramas and Puppet Shows

Eyerly, Jeannette, and Beth Couch. *The Seeing Summer* playlet. (*This playlet is included as an appendix in this Handbook. It is also available separately from the National Federation of the Blind. The playlet consists of selections from the book of the same title, above.*)

The Kids on the Block. (1712 Eye Street NW, Washington, DC 10006.) (*A puppet show about disabilities.*)

Addresses – General

Aids Unlimited, Inc.
1101 N. Calvert St.
Baltimore, MD 21202

American Brotherhood for the Blind, Inc.
National Center for the Blind
1800 Johnson Street
Baltimore, Maryland 21230
(*General information about blindness; materials for the deaf-blind; lending library of "Twin Vision" books, featuring print and Braille together. Alternate address for Twin Vision Books: 18440 Oxnard Street, Tarzana, CA 91356.*)

American Council of the Blind
1010 Vermont Avenue NW
Suite 1100
Washington, DC 20005

American Federation of Teachers (AFT)
11 Dupont Circle NW
Washington, DC 20036

American Foundation for the Blind (AFB)
15 W. 16th Street
New York, N.Y. 10011
(*Source of aids and appliances, games, etc. Also offers a variety of publications.*)

American Printing House for the Blind (APH)
1839 Frankfort Avenue
Louisville, KY 40206
(*Source of books and maps in Braille and large print, and many other teaching aids. Most materials may be obtained with Quota funds.*)

American Thermoform Co.
2311 Travers Avenue
City of Commerce, PA 90040

Association for Education and Rehabilitation of the Blind and Visually Impaired
206 N. Washington St.
Suite 320
Alexandria, VA 22314

Blind Childrens Center
4120 Marathon Street
P.O. Box 29159
Los Angeles, CA 90029-0159
(*Services for blind and partially-sighted children aged birth through seven years, and their families.*)

Blind Children's Fund
230 Central Street
Auburndale, MA 02166-2399
(*Services for young children. Also known as International Institute for Visually Impaired 0-7, Inc.*)

Braille Institute of America
741 North Vermont Avenue
Los Angeles, CA 90029

Canadian National Institute for the Blind (CNIB)
1929 Bayview Avenue
Toronto, Ontario M4G 4C8 Canada

Christian Record Braille Foundation, Inc.
4444 So. 52nd Street
Lincoln, NE 68506
(*Specializes in Christian religious materials.*)

Closer Look
National Information Center for the Handicapped
P.O. Box 1492
Washington, DC 20013
(*This agency may be able to suggest sources of help for a multiply handicapped child.*)

Council for Exceptional Children (CEC)
1920 Association Drive
Reston, VA 22091
(*This organization may be able to suggest sources of help for a multiply handicapped child.*)

ERIC Clearinghouse on Handicapped and Gifted
Council for Exceptional Children
1920 Association Drive
Reston, VA 22091

Exceptional Teaching Aids
20102 Woodbine Avenue
Castro Valley, CA 94546

The Guild for the Blind
180 N. Michigan
Chicago, IL 60601

The Hadley School for the Blind
700 Elm Street
Winnetka, IL 60093
(Note: This is a correspondence school, generally tuition-free for blind students. It also offers courses for parents of blind children.)

Howe Press of Perkins School for the Blind
175 North Beacon Street
Watertown, MA 02172

Independent Living Aids, Inc.
27 E. Mall
Plainview, NY 11803

Jewish Braille Institute of America, Inc.
110 E. 30th Street
New York, NY 10016
(Specializes in materials about Judaism or written by Jewish authors.)

Job Opportunities for the Blind (JOB)
National Center for the Blind
1800 Johnson Street
Baltimore, MD 21230

Learning Pillows
Box 631
New Town Branch
Boston, MA 02258
(Source of teaching aids for Braille readiness.)

National Association to Promote the Use of Braille (NAPUB)
National Center for the Blind
1800 Johnson Street
Baltimore, MD 21230

National Braille Association (NBA)
1290 University Avenue
Rochester, NY 14607

NBA Braille Book Bank
1290 University Avenue
Rochester, NY 14607

National Braille Press, Inc.
88 Saint Stephen Street
Boston, MA 02115

National Education Association (NEA)
1201 16th Street NW
Washington, DC 20036

National Federation of the Blind (NFB)
National Center for the Blind
1800 Johnson Street
Baltimore, MD 21230

National Library Service for the Blind and Physically Handicapped (NLS)
Library of Congress
1291 Taylor Street NW
Washington, DC 20542

National Society to Prevent Blindness
70 Madison Avenue
New York, NY 10016

Oakmont Visual Aids Workshop
6637 Oakmont Drive
Santa Rosa, CA 95405
(Braille readiness and concept-development books and other materials.)

Parents of Blind Children (POBC)
National Federation of the Blind
1800 Johnson Street
Baltimore, MD 21230

POBC Videos
National Federation of the Blind
1800 Johnson Street
Baltimore, MD 21230

Rainshine Canes
158 Jackson Street
Madison, WI 53704

Recording for the Blind, Inc.
20 Roszel Road
Princeton, NJ 08540
(*Source of recorded textbooks.*)

Royal National Institute for the Blind (RNIB)
224-6-8 Great Portland Street
London, WIN 6AA England

Science Products
Box A
Southeastern, PA 19399

Seedlings
Braille Books for Children
8447 Marygrove Drive
Detroit, MI 48221

The Smith-Kettlewell Eye Research Foundation
2232 Webster Street
San Francisco, CA 94115
(*Offers advice on technical matters, including methods for use by blind technicians and engineers.*)

Texture-Touch
Rural Route 2
Albion, NE 68620

Traylor Enterprises, Inc.
830 NE Loop 410
Suite 505
San Antonio, TX 78209

U.S. Office of Special Education and Rehabilitative Services
330 C Street SW
Washington, DC 20202

Vis-Aids
102-09 Jamaica Avenue
Box 26
Richmond Hill, NY 11418

Xavier Society for the Blind
154 E. 23rd Street
New York, NY 10010
(*Specializes in Roman Catholic books and materials, including a free Braille calendar.*)

Addresses – Computers and Computer-Related Technology

Apollo Electronic Visual Aids
6357 Arizona Circle
Los Angeles, CA 90045

ARTS Computer Products
145 Tremont Street, Suite 407
Boston, MA 02111

Artic Technologies
55 Park Street
Suite 2
Troy, MI 48083

Automated Functions, Inc.
6424 N. 28th Street
Arlington, VA 22207

Computer Aids, Inc.
124 West Washington Boulevard
Suite 220
Ft. Wayne, IN 46802

Computer Conversations
6297 Worthington Road SW
Alexandria, OH 43001

Enabling Technologies
3102 Southeast Jay Street
Stuart, FL 33497

Henter-Joyce, Inc.
7901 Fourth Street N
Suite 211
St. Petersburg, FL 33702

HumanWare
Horseshoe Bar Plaza
Unit P
6140 Horseshoe Bar Road
Loomis, CA 95650

Interface Systems International
11306 NE Thompson
Portland, OR 97220

Kansys, Inc.
1016 Ohio
Lawrence, KS 66044

National Braille Press
88 Saint Stephen Street
Boston, Massachusetts 02115

National Federation of the Blind
in Computer Science (NFBCS)
National Center for the Blind
1800 Johnson Street
Baltimore, MD 21230

Omnichron
1438 Oxford Street
Berkeley, CA 94709

Raised-Dot Computing
408 South Baldwin Street
Madison, WI 55703

Sense-Sations
919 Walnut Street
Philadelphia, PA 19107

Street Electronics
1140 Mark Avenue
Carpenteria, CA 93013

Telesensory Systems, Inc. (TSI)
455 N. Bernardo Avenue
Mountain View, CA 94043

VTEK
1625 Olympic Boulevard
Santa Monica, CA 90404

Willoughby Enterprises
2711 54th Street
Des Moines, IA 50310